ACUTE CARE NURSING IN THE HOME

A Holistic Approach

ACUTE CARE NURSING IN THE HOME

A Holistic Approach

Edited by

Catherine Malloy, RN, DrPH

ASSOCIATE PROFESSOR, GRADUATE PROGRAM
COLLEGE OF NURSING
MEDICAL UNIVERSITY OF SOUTH CAROLINA
CHARLESTON, SOUTH CAROLINA

Jeanette Hartshorn, RN, PhD, FAAN

ASSOCIATE PROFESSOR, GRADUATE PROGRAM
COLLEGE OF NURSING
MEDICAL UNIVERSITY OF SOUTH CAROLINA
JOINT APPOINTMENT, MEDICAL UNIVERSITY HOSPITAL
CHARLESTON, SOUTH CAROLINA

with 23 contributors

J.B. Lippincott Company   Philadelphia
London   Mexico City   New York
St. Louis   São Paulo   Sydney

Acquisitions/Sponsoring Editor: Patti Cleary
Manuscript Editor: Lorraine D. Smith
Indexer: Ellen Murray
Senior Design Coordinator: Anita Curry
Cover Design: Anne O'Donnell
Production Coordinator: Pamela Milcos
Compositor: Digitype Inc.
Printer/Binder: R.R. Donnelley & Sons Company

135642

Library of Congress Cataloging-in-Publication Data

Acute care nursing in the home.
   Includes bibliographies and index.
   1. Intensive care nursing.   2. Home nursing.
3. Holistic medicine.   I. Malloy, Catherine.
II. Hartshorn, Jeanette.   [DNLM: 1. Acute Disease—
Nursing.   2. Critical Care—nurses' instruction.
3. Home Care Services—United Services—nurses'
instruction. WY 154 A189]
RT120.I5A28   1989   649'.8   88-26607
ISBN 0-397-54661-0

Any procedure or practice described in this book should
be applied by the health-care practitioner under appropriate supervision in accordance with professional standards of care used with regard to the unique circumstances that apply in each practice situation. Care has
been taken to confirm the accuracy of information presented and to describe generally accepted practices.
However, the authors, editors, and publisher cannot accept any responsibility for errors or omissions or for
consequences from application of the information in this
book and make no warranty, express or implied, with
respect to the contents of the book.

Every effort has been made to ensure drug selections and
dosages are in accordance with current recommendations and practice. Because of ongoing research, changes
in government regulations, and the constant flow of information on drug therapy, reactions, and interactions,
the reader is cautioned to check the package insert for
each drug for indications, dosages, warnings, and precautions, particularly if the drug is new or infrequently
used.

This book is dedicated to the people in my life who, through their love, have given me the gifts of courage and faith: to Laura, my daughter, for her continuous encouragement

to Tim, my son, for believing in me

to Brian Duffy, my husband, for urging me to reach beyond myself

Catherine Malloy

This book is dedicated to my husband, Ed Hartshorn, for his unconditional support and love.

Jeanette Hartshorn

CONTRIBUTORS

Nancy L. Bohnet, RN, MN
Adjunct Instructor, Medical–Surgical Nursing
School of Nursing
University of Pittsburgh
Pittsburgh, Pennsylvania

Corine Bonnet, RN, PhD
Associate Professor, Coordinator, BSN
    Program
Midwestern State University
Wichita Falls, Texas

Angela P. Clark, RN, PhD
Lecturer, Graduate Program
University of Texas
Austin, Texas

Charmaine Cummings, RN, MSN
Clinical Nurse Educator—Neuroscience
Clinical Center Nursing Department
National Institutes of Health
Bethesda, Maryland

Carol Jean DeMoss, RN, MSN, CS
Oncology Nurse Clinician
Visiting Nurse Association of Allegheny
    County
Pittsburgh, Pennsylvania

Barbara J. Edlund, RN, MS, MNP
Associate Professor
College of Nursing
Medical University of South Carolina
Charleston, South Carolina

Karen S. Edmonson, RN, MN
Instructor in Nursing
Neonatal Clinical Specialist
Medical University of South Carolina
Charleston, South Carolina

Vicki Embiscuso, RN, MSN, CNM
Bethlehem, Pennsylvania

Karen Evans, RN, MSN
Galveston, Texas

Linda E. Evans, RN, MS
Nutrition Clinician
Visiting Nurse Association of Allegheny
    County
Pittsburgh, Pennsylvania

Patricia D. Fedorka, RN, MPH
Faculty Member
School of Nursing
Duquesne University
Pittsburgh, Pennsylvania

Cheryl Gardner, RN, CRNI
Director, IV Team
Spartanburg Regional Medical Center
Spartanburg, South Carolina

Mary Gokey, RN, MSN, CCRN, CNRN
Fargo, North Dakota

Barbara Kavanagh Haight, DrPH, RNC
Associate Professor
College of Nursing
Medical University of South Carolina
Charleston, South Carolina

Jeanette Hartshorn, RN, PhD, FAAN
Associate Professor, Graduate Program
College of Nursing
Medical University of South Carolina
Joint Appointment, Medical University
    Hospital
Charleston, South Carolina

Barbara Hastings, RN, MN
Director, Clinical Services
Visiting Nurse Association of Allegheny
    County
Pittsburgh, Pennsylvania

Catherine Malloy, RN, DrPH
Associate Professor, Graduate Program
College of Nursing
Medical University of South Carolina
Charleston, South Carolina

M. Carroll Miller, RN, MSN, MA
Associate Professor of Nursing
School of Nursing
Duquesne University
Pittsburgh, Pennsylvania

Sue Reitz Perdew, RN, PhD
Associate Professor of Nursing
Marywood College
Scranton, Pennsylvania

Barbara Kovalcin Piskor, RN, MPH
Director, Long-Term Care Assessment and
    Management Program
Allegheny County Department of Aging
Pittsburgh, Pennsylvania

Nancy Pratt, RN, MSN, CCRN
Charleston, South Carolina

Martha M. Skoner, RN, PhD
Assistant Professor
School of Nursing
University of Southern Maine
Portland, Maine

Cansas Deitz Smith, RN, MSN
South Carolina Department of Health and
    Environmental Control
Clinical Nurse Specialist
Trident Home Health Services
Mt. Pleasant, South Carolina

Bonnie Wesorick, RN
Clinical Nurse Specialist
Butterworth Hospital
Grand Rapids, Michigan

JoAnn B. Wise, RN
Program Nurse Specialist
Medical University of South Carolina
Charleston, South Carolina

PREFACE

Sweeping changes occurring in the health care field have drastically altered the delivery of health care. Competition, cost-containment, and corporatization have created an environment in which the turnover of patients from the hospital to home care occurs at a dizzying rate. Not only are hospital days shorter, but patients are still sick when they are sent home. The acuity of illness often requires technology-intensive remedies. The home serves as the care setting for persons who customarily would have been assigned to the intensive care unit.

High-tech care has created new levels of knowledge and skill for the practicing home-care nurse. Formerly, nurses did not provide services to clients with Hickman catheters, with IV feeding requirements, or with ventilators. What the present situation requires is a combination of traditional home care and complex high-tech care. Nurses must have the technical skills required of practitioners in intensive care units as well as community nursing skills. Truly, a marriage of community health and acute care nursing is needed. Additionally, nurses in the home need to know how to relate technical information and skills to the clients and families they serve,

since the latter will be responsible for most of the client care. This makes the nurse's role more critical than ever to the health and well-being of the family. Given the fact that critical care nurses in increasing numbers are being recruited to home care, a conceptual framework for integrating traditional community health nursing with critical care nursing is essential.

The purpose of this text is to provide nurses with an organizing framework to use in considering care for acutely ill clients in their homes. Practical, relevant information is presented within the context of the nursing process through discussion of specific nursing diagnoses approved by the North American Nursing Diagnosis Association (NANDA).

"Acute Care Nursing in the Home" is comprised of 17 chapters covering the holistic needs of acutely ill clients and their families in the home. The first eight chapters deal with the broader psychosocial–spiritual–cultural aspects of home health care. An overview of the home-care environment is followed by a chapter on the coordination of care, with particular emphasis on discharge planning principles. A chapter on liability is particularly instructive, alerting nurses to potential malpractice problems that might occur in the home setting. With the technology-intensive procedures now performed in the home, nurses need to be more aware and better informed about their risks and responsibilities. Patient teaching is thoroughly addressed to assist nurses in anticipating the types of learning needs that may be found with acutely ill clients at home. A chapter on the family presents information the nurse can use in establishing a supportive and effective relationship with both the client and his family. In essence, these first eight chapters establish a holistic overview of home care.

The remaining nine chapters present the major clinical problems a home care nurse will face in today's practice arena. The chapters are written within the framework of nursing diagnoses and discuss alterations in respiration, circulation, nutrition, elimination, sensory perception, locomotion, endocrine control, reproduction, and body integrity. Each of these nine chapters identifies a specific medical condition found with the nursing diagnosis and discusses pathophysiology and nursing interventions. Sample care plans are provided to illustrate the main points of care, and to clarify pertinent interventions and desired outcomes. Specific attention is paid to assessing the home environment, adapting the home for various technologies, and identifying troubleshooting points that may be encountered.

Certain features of the book are intended to assist the nurse in learning about specific home care needs of acutely ill clients. Each chapter specifies NANDA-approved nursing diagnoses relevant to the content presented. This framework is designed to guide the nurse in applying theory to practice.

We have tried to present this material in an understandable, practical manner. While avoiding a "cookbook" approach to the care plans, we have tried to give the practicing nurse relevant, appropriate information on managing the care of the acutely ill client—incorporating a holistic orientation.

Objectives of the book are sixfold:

1. To provide a conceptual framework for acute care nursing in the home by using the nursing process with nursing diagnoses as the unifying theme.
2. To synthesize the disciplines of critical care nursing and community health nursing, and thus to define the changing role of home care nursing.
3. To provide home care nurses with a practical guide to use in their practice of high-tech care.
4. To contribute to the educational process of undergraduate students and graduate students by assisting faculty to focus on the practical demands of home care.
5. To provide nurse case managers in hospitals with a practical reference guide to use in planning for home care coordination.
6. To provide a resource that continuing education program directors may use in presenting practical approaches to the most common acute care problems in the home.

We hope this text will serve as a useful reference to the nurses actively involved in the care of acutely ill clients in their homes.

Catherine Malloy, RN, DrPH
Jeanette Hartshorn, RN, PhD, FAAN

ACKNOWLEDGMENTS

We wish to express our appreciation to our families, friends, and colleagues who encouraged and supported us throughout the process of conceptualizing and actualizing this book. Special thanks go to the administration and faculty of the Medical University of South Carolina College of Nursing for their interest and support.

This book would not exist without the contributors whose expertise in the domains of critical care and community health nursing provided rich information of practical significance. The mix of contributors reflects a blend of acute care and home care nurses representing service, education, and administration in a variety of nursing organizations from different parts of the country. They responded to the challenge of creating a combined critical care–community health approach to areas known to be problems in home care. Their cooperation in meeting deadlines and their patience with the production process is greatly appreciated.

We are especially indebted to Cansas Smith and Marge Wheeler, who reviewed the entire manuscript for accuracy and relevance to home care nursing, and to Laurie Watson, who reviewed the Reference listings. Also, we thank Pat Fedorka for assuming the difficult task of reviewing, in each chapter, those sections on assessment of the home environment. She diligently ensured that information would be timely and appropriate for nurses to incorporate into their practice.

Mention is also due to those individuals, agencies, and authors who gave us permission to reproduce their materials for this book.

We wish to extend special appreciation to the J.B. Lippincott Company and especially to Patti Cleary, Diana Merritt, and Lorraine Smith for their support, interest, advice, and friendliness in assisting us through delays, revisions, and deadlines in fine-tuning the manuscript. Their patience, sense of humor, and general goodwill made our work much easier.

CONTENTS

ACUTE CARE NURSING IN THE HOME

A Holistic Approach

Overview of Acute Care Nursing in the Home

Catherine Malloy

The decade of the 1980s has witnessed dramatic changes in the health-care system. Cost-containment pressures, shortened hospital stays, and increasing client acuity levels have contributed to the unprecedented expansion of home-care services. As the primary professionals delivering care in the home, nurses are faced with new demands on their practice.

The purpose of this chapter is to present a holistic framework that nurses can use when providing acute care nursing in the home. Major trends influencing the demand for home care will be reviewed, and use of a systems approach to understanding home care will be presented. The chapter will conclude with a discussion of the nursing process and nursing diagnoses as an organizing theme for this text.

MAJOR TRENDS INFLUENCING HOME CARE

Words used to describe the change in the health-care system and the demand for home care include "revolution," "dramatic escala-

tion," "skyrocketing growth," and "burgeoning field." The forces that have contributed to the increased growth and the demand for home health care as described by Louden (1984) include

1. Cost-containment pressures
2. An increasing elderly population
3. Reduction in the number of care-givers (primarily women)
4. Consumer health awareness
5. Advances in medical technology

The influence of each of these forces on home care will be discussed separately to provide a background for understanding the environment in which the nurse practices.

COST-CONTAINMENT PRESSURES

Runner-Heidt (1984, 1985) discussed statistics related to home-care expenditures. In 1982, home-care expenditures amounted to $2 billion, only 2% of the Medicare bill. But this figure was expected to reach $7 billion to $9 billion in the late 1980s. Louden (1983) noted that forecasters varied in their projections concerning market expansion. However, most agreed that the expected growth would be about 13% to 20% annually through 1990. Of all the forces influencing the growth of the home-care market, the cost-containment pressures brought about by the prospective payment system are probably the most important (Louden 1984; Coleman and Smith 1984). The Medicare prospective payment system bases reimbursement on fixed rates, not on actual hospital costs. This policy provided hospitals with an incentive to reduce the client's length of stay, that is, to get the client in and out of the hospital as quickly as possible. One way to accomplish this was to move clients into the home setting, which was perceived to be a less expensive way of providing health care.

Halamandaris (1984) has summarized the cost figures obtained from several studies of delivering care in the home. The average annual cost of hospital care for ventilator-dependent patients was $270,000 compared to $21,000 for such care at home. Moreover, a study of children who were ventilator-dependent showed that hospital costs were $400,000 per year as compared to $75,000 for home care. Rogatz (1985) warned health professionals to scrutinize the meaning of these cost statistics. He asserted that significant methodologic problems have resulted in inconclusive evidence when comparing hospital and home-care costs. He further suggested that home care may be more costly than had been expected. Home-care agencies are also concerned about cost-containment pressures. Decreasing Medicare reimbursement, confusing reimbursement mechanisms, increasing rates of denials for claims, and the complexity of required care have placed burdensome demands on the providers of home care.

AN INCREASING ELDERLY POPULATION

Among current demographic trends with the greatest impact is an increasing older population, most of whom are women. In fact, the fastest growing minority in the country is the elderly population. With the prolongation of the life span also comes an increase in the numbers of chronic health conditions. Older persons live longer because of advances in medical technology, but they suffer more physical disability and functional impairment than the general population and are frequent consumers of the health care system. Elderly persons account for 29% of health care in the United States, 25% of prescription drug costs, 15% of physician visits, 34% of days in short-stay hospitals, and 87% of nursing home occupants (Louden 1983).

Andreoli and Musser (1985) see the graying of America as the most influential trend affecting health-care delivery and the roles of health practitioners. They noted, "Because most health care for the elderly is given at home, the home health-care industry will explode." These authors also cited the growth of biomedical technology as having a revolutionary effect on the practice of nursing. They predicted that "the future will belong to those nurses who develop skills and behaviors to meet health-care trends."

The U.S. Bureau of Census statistics on the age distribution of the population indicated that by the year 2030, 20% of the total U.S. population will be 65 years of age and older, and by 2040, those 75 years of age and older will represent the majority of the elderly population.

REDUCTION IN NUMBER OF CARE-GIVERS

Runner-Heidt (1984) identified fewer family care-givers as an influence on the demand and market for home care. At a time when more clients are being moved to the home for care, this society has fewer extended family supports, due to social and economic pressures influencing today's family. The number of women in the work force has reached an all time high, as has the number of two wage-earner families. This means there is no one at home to serve as care-giver. Much of the burden falls on adult children and their families. The literature reports that many working women leave their jobs to take care of elderly relatives.

The implications of an increased demand for home care and a decreased supply of family care-givers are serious. Reduced numbers of care-givers at home place more stress on the family trying to cope with someone who is acutely ill. In effect, this creates another "at risk population," the family care-givers, who are dealing with added responsibility and the demands of 24-hour care over an indefinite period of time, sometimes even years.

CONSUMER HEALTH AWARENESS

The public has become disenchanted with the traditional form of health-care delivery. Many persons believe they would prefer to be treated in their homes. Comprehensive insurance coverage, increasing sophistication of the lay public in regard to self-care, and the ability to deliver technical care in the home have contributed to the consumer's growing acceptance of home care. Clients enjoy a more normal life-style at home with family and friends. They can set their own schedules, free of the regimentation of the hospital setting. By remaining in their homes, clients can sleep in their own beds, spend time in their favorite room, enjoy their pets, talk on the phone, dress in their own clothes; in short, control their own lives.

MEDICAL TECHNOLOGY

More acute care *is* taking place in the client's home. Gelinas (1985) noted that restrictions on length of stay due to Diagnostic Related Group (DRG) regulations meant that clients were leaving hospitals "quicker and sicker" than ever before and this phenomenon was placing an even greater demand on the home-care delivery system.

Technology allows clients to return to their homes for care. Some of the treatments being performed in the home today were not even commonplace in many hospitals 10 years ago. The needs of clients at home are actually similar to the needs of hospitalized clients in critical care units. Some clients are being discharged to home directly from intensive care units. The situation also places new demands on the role of nursing.

DIFFERENCES IN CARING FOR THE ACUTELY ILL AT HOME

In 1984 Elsie Griffith, director of the New York Visiting Nurse Service and chair of the National Association of Home Care (NAHC), explained the effect of changes in health care on the practice of nursing in an interview for the *American Journal of Nursing*. She indicated that the complex client care seen today demands greater expertise in decision making. She also emphasized the autonomous nature of home-care nursing, in which nurses must assess not only the client but the client's total environment. According to Griffith, greater synthesis of knowledge is required for nurses to make sound judgments.

Home care differs from the system of care delivered in the hospital. By its nature the hospital system gives health professionals control of the situation on *their* terms, meeting *their* schedules. The home-care system differs because the nurse's role is to facilitate clients and families in assuming responsibility for the client's own care. The nurse teaches the client and family to manage their health care with the goal of independence. The level of care and expertise requires nurses who are knowledgeable and highly skilled in dealing with families, in teaching, and in coordinating care. Home-care nurses function in an independent manner, without the security of the institution. The work of home care is diverse and nurses must be able to deal with a variety of clients and home environments.

NEW PROVIDERS

The movement of medical high tech into the home has brought about a change in the identity of providers on the home-care scene. Community health was once the domain of the Visiting Nurse Association, the Public Health Department, and some private community health agencies. Now, the situation shows a tremendous increase in the number and types of providers. One of the newest providers in home care is the distributor of durable medical equipment. Most notable are medical companies such as Abbott Laboratories, American Hospital Supply Corporation, Travenol Laboratories, and Johnson and Johnson. They employ highly specialized nurses who visit clients and care-givers in the hospital prior to discharge to plan for home care. They also assist hospital and home-care nurses to learn the complex care required in many situations. Zucker and Barisonek (1984) discussed the impact that the competitive home-care environment has had on the nurse's role. ". . . The professional nurse, long the mainstay of home health care, must now decide if she should discuss care with the physician, the family, the vendor of equipment, or all of them." In many agencies, clinical nurse specialists are being hired for home care. This practice has been a cause of some concern for community health nurses. The concern deals with a philosophy of nursing.

While critical care nurse specialists are comfortable with the range of technical equipment used, there is a concern that they might not have the personal attributes or the desire to work in the home environment. The

critical care environment of the hospital is dramatically different from that of the home. There is a very definite lack of control in the home environment and there are no team members next door with whom to consult. The ability to work with families and their peculiarities on their own turf can be distressing to those who are accustomed to the structure of a hospital setting. What is really required is a marriage of community health nursing principles, including public health science, and acute care nursing.

FRAME OF REFERENCE — ATTITUDE

Caring for a client in the home calls for a change in basic attitudes about the "receiver and giver" of care. The client must be seen as part of a family and a community in a different way than before. The focus is on dealing with the client/family system — the family unit. The center for planning care has to be from the home *outward*, rather than from the traditional health agency *inward* to the home. In the traditional setting, the nurse is in command of the schedule, but in the home the mode of operation has to be developed from the family's point of view. If the nurse does not incorporate this frame of reference into her value systems, she will experience great difficulty in working with the family when dealing with high-tech procedures.

There are three major areas of difference that need to be understood by nurses: turf, control, and decision making.

Turf

The territory is the client–family's environment. It is defined and controlled by the family unit. The nurse is the stranger, the outsider, the guest, not unlike the client when he enters the hospital system. As such, the nurse is dealing with an unstructured environment and each client/family's environment will be unique. The nurse must be tolerant of the differences, habits, and life-styles of family members. This has particular significance when working with families in managing high-tech care. The environment may be less than desirable. There may be inadequate space, poor order in the home, lack of refrigeration, or inadequate attention to cleaning equipment. This calls for careful assessment by the nurse and restraint of judgmental conclusions. The nurse must deduce the client's perceptions about the reality of his environment. The primary responsibility is to assist the family to function at its optimum in managing acute care in the home. The nurse needs to gain the family's trust and support in order to help the family function effectively.

Control

Nurses who deal with high-tech home care find that they are not in control of the situation to the same degree that they are in a more structured setting. Nurses must be aware of the total environment and its influence on the family unit. They need to understand the inner workings of the family. Who is in charge of the family unit? Who seems to be in control? Who makes the decisions? Is it a small group, that is, mother and the eldest daughter, or is it one person? How is the family unit managing? What is its style? Who is the action-taker?

Interpersonal skills are very important. By making the family feel comfortable in the care situation, the nurse builds confidence and trust. Feedback is necessary, and the nurse conveys to the client and family that they are managing the care effectively. Nurses are often the stumbling blocks to clients' success by not "letting go." For nurses who have functioned in an environment where they were "in charge," it can be difficult to relinquish knowledge and skill to

untrained nonprofessionals. One nurse expressed her dismay by saying skills that had taken her years to develop were being performed by family members in the home. Nurses often find it uncomfortable to permit the family to be responsible for acute care.

Decision Making

The nurse who deals with the acutely ill client and his family is an autonomous, adaptable practitioner who strives to prevent family dependency. The goal is to enable the family to function without extensive nursing support. Families are assisted in identifying their problems and working through the problem-solving process. Often families' solutions may be at odds with the nurse's approach, but their choices must be respected. The *whole family* must be involved in planning to ensure that the client can be cared for appropriately. Everyone who is involved needs to be included. The nurse carefully tailors the nursing process to the client/family and environment. This total environmental perspective is fundamental to all nursing care provided by the home-care nurse.

Kratz (1985) wrote that "the care of patients or clients in their own homes is potentially the most advanced form of nursing." She further commented, ". . . anybody who works outside the institutional setting must be prepared to deal with a whole individual, with his needs and problems, his idiosyncracies, and his downright unacceptable habits as a whole."

Statistics show that more and more persons will be cared for in the home. The logical conclusion is that there are more opportunities for nurses from a variety of clinical disciplines to be involved in home care. In order to expand the nurse's conception of home-care practice, it is useful to look at home care from a systems perspective.

SYSTEMS THEORY AND HOME CARE

A system is an entity made up of separate parts or elements. The parts or elements are interrelated, interact, have a common purpose, and form a whole (Hall and Weaver 1985; Braden 1984). A system is purposeful in nature and uses a process to reach its goal (Clemen and associates 1981). A home-health agency can be viewed as a system composed of people (nurses, administrators, social workers, physical therapists, occupational therapists, home-health aides, speech therapists, accountants, data processors), equipment, the office, and the policies and procedures or rules of operation. Each part of the agency is necessary for its operation. These parts are sometimes referred to as *subsystems*. Also each of the parts (the people, the policies, the equipment) interact with other components within the system as well as with other systems in the external environment, such as the Health Care Financing Administration and third-party payers. When the home-care agency functions properly, sufficient services are provided, and sufficient revenue is generated to maintain the system.

A system has a process of information exchange that assures its viability: input, throughput, output, and feedback. *Input* is the information or materials introduced into the system. In a home-care agency, input includes the clients requiring care, the personnel qualified to deliver care, and adequate materials to conduct the business of the agency. *Throughput* refers to the processes required to transform the input for use. The assessment, diagnosis, planning, implementation, and evaluation of the clients receiving care refer to the throughput or processes of the home-care agency. *Output* is the outcome or end result of a system. In a home-care agency, output consists of the services provided and the revenue generated.

Each system maintains a *feedback* mechanism that enables a system to regulate itself. Through the feedback process, the output of the system is returned as input. The circular nature of the feedback system enables the system to regulate the flow of inputs and outputs, and to achieve a dynamic balance between what is coming in and what is being released to the environment. In the system example of the home-care agency, revenues are returned to the system, enabling the ongoing operation of the home-care agency (Fig. 1-1).

The nurse caring for an acutely ill client at home is quite aware of the informational processes that contribute to the regulation of the system of care. The nurse obtains input and receives feedback from many components of the home health-care system. Planning for high-tech care in the home requires coordination with the health agency and pertinent community resources as well as consultation with medical equipment suppliers, the local electric company, and the nearest emergency medical services back-up, not to mention working with the family care-giver. All of the individual elements contribute to the self-regulation of the system.

Factors influencing the environment also have an effect on the system. In the home-care agency system, if a change in the environment occurs, such as an unusually high number of cases requiring complex technologies, the product (nursing services) of the agency will be affected. The demand for volume of services requiring a high level of technical skill and sufficient time to perform them places a strain on the agency's ability to deliver care to all clients in the system.

The final consideration is that a system continually responds to changes affecting its input, output, and feedback. As new information enters the system, the system builds up or breaks down. Using the home-care agency example, the services are provided with little build-up in growth until an influx of very ill

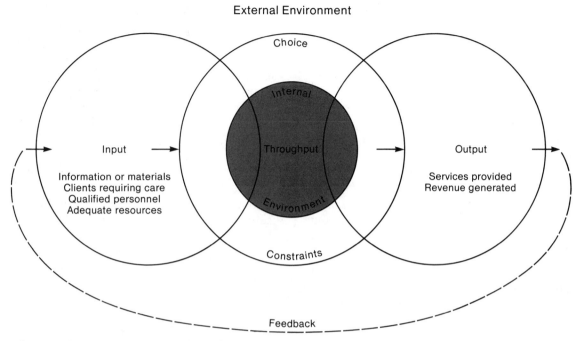

Figure 1-1. System function: home-care agency.

clients requiring sophisticated treatment enters the home-care system. As the agency responds and gears up for the new service demands, more services are provided, and the output of the system is increased. After a period of time, the system regains balance and is able to deliver the increased volume of services more comfortably.

Systems theory is a useful framework for dealing with complex home-care problems and changing relationships (Helvie 1981). The systems approach can be used to determine if the appropriate services are being provided in a cost-effective manner. When systems thinking is applied to a home-care agency, each component of the agency, such as the input and output, is scrutinized. Agency outcomes are measured in relation to the overall goal of the system, which is to provide services, generate an adequate income, and maintain the business.

NURSING PROCESS AND HOME CARE

The nursing process is consistent with a systems approach to care in the home. As the method or activity of professional nursing practice, the nursing process is directed to achieving specific outcomes in the client's (and family's) health situation. Each step of the nursing process is interrelated and interdependent with all other steps. Each step influences and is influenced by the other steps. Information generally flows in a circular manner from assessment to diagnosis, to planning, to implementation, and then to evaluation. Feedback can occur at any step.

The components of the nursing process — assessment, diagnosis, planning, implementation, and evaluation — have at their centers the nurse and client/family relationship, which also influences and is influenced by each subsystem (Fig. 1-2). To discuss the components of the nursing process in more detail, its steps will be reviewed.

ASSESSMENT

Assessment is an ongoing process of data collection and analysis. Potential as well as actual health problems are assessed. This permits the nurse to take action to prevent the occurrence of problems. The input to the assessment subsystem includes both subjective and objective information about the acutely ill client, the family, its strengths and limitations, available resources, and agency constraints and resources.

Subjective information provides important data because it is obtained directly from the acutely ill client and the family. They provide first-hand information about the health problem and their perceptions of their situation.

Objective information can be obtained via the nurse's skill in observation. By using the skills of watching and listening, the nurse can assess the adequacy of the home environment for care, the attitude of family members toward the client and each other, the atmosphere of concern and support, and the absence or presence of conflict.

Members of the health-care team, involved agencies, neighbors, associates, published reports in the literature, and the client's medical record may be used to obtain additional data.

Communication, as a powerful tool to elicit information, cannot be understated. Verbal and nonverbal behaviors can give the astute nurse important information about the

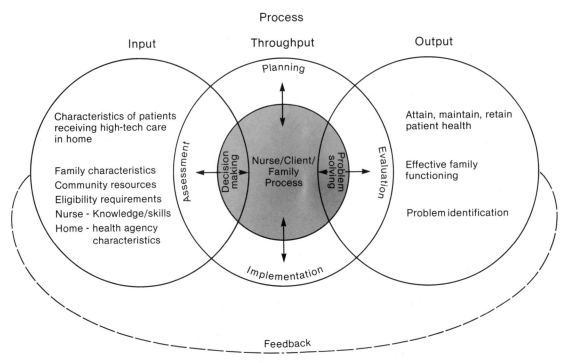

Figure 1-2. Nursing process with home-care client.

client–family interaction and about actual or potential troublespots. It is important to assist the client and care-givers to express both their thoughts and their feelings. Often clients and family members experience stress because of their negative feelings. At times unexpressed anger and resentment about the situation lead to feelings of guilt, anxiety, and depression. Helping those involved to express these feelings often ameliorates this guilt and stress.

Talking with the client and family using quasi-interview techniques can assist the nurse in obtaining complete information. Alternatives to what the client and family say, and the nonverbal behaviors that accompany their words can provide many useful clues. Often families express the desire to become involved in the care of their loved ones at home but other behaviors appear that seem to indicate they might not be equipped to carry out such a commitment.

NURSING DIAGNOSES

The analysis of the assessment data and the arrangement of information into patterns along with their scientific bases concludes in the selection of nursing diagnoses. The latter are client-centered statements describing health situations in which the nurse can intervene. Nursing diagnoses are statements of actual or potential health problems derived from the interpretation of the collected information. Each nursing diagnosis is the outcome of the inferences drawn from the nursing assessment and history.

The diagnosis needs to be validated with the client and the family. Once there is agreement on the diagnosis, the planning step can be undertaken. Validation is necessary to ensure that the nurse has interpreted the data correctly.

Nurses from all areas of the profession have been working on a taxonomy of nursing diagnoses since 1973. Seven national conferences have been held since that time to continue the work. It was during the fifth national conference in 1982 that a new title was given to the group—The North American Nursing Diagnosis Association (NANDA). NANDA has identified 82 diagnostic categories that have been recognized and are being tested by nurses. The taxonomy of nursing diagnosis is seen as a scientific basis for nursing practice (Griffith-Kenny and Christensen 1986; Carpenito 1983).

The taxonomy provides a definition of the diagnostic category, etiological and contributing factors, and definitive characteristics of the problem. A specific nursing diagnosis reflects the health problem of the individual, and provides direction for nursing activities. For the purpose of this text, the nursing diagnostic categories accepted by NANDA will be used to illustrate the content in each chapter.

PLANNING

The planning phase of the nursing process follows assessment, begins with the validated nursing diagnosis, and concludes with the formulation of mutual goals and objectives and the selection of priorities and nursing orders. Planning is a decision-making and problem-solving process that is conducted *with* the client and family. The multidisciplinary aspect of planning care is especially important for ill clients at home. Many different members of the team work together to coordinate care. It is particularly critical to have mutual agreement between the nurse and the acutely ill client and his family in planning for complex treatments in the home. It is essential to learn what motivates the client and family to assure that the care will be carried out appropriately.

Priority Setting

The process of priority setting begins with rank–ordering the nursing diagnoses. Usually the client's health concern can be categorized by short-term, intermediate, or long-term needs. Then, each of these is ranked in order of importance. The concerns that are life threatening obviously would be ranked first. An immediate concern must sometimes be addressed before proceeding to a more important long-term concern. Moreover, a specific condition may warrant a higher place on the list of priorities because of the degree of importance assigned to it by the client and family. Nursing standards, agency policies and procedures, health rules and regulations must all be considered in assigning priorities.

Goals and Objectives

Goals, in this instance, may be defined as broad statements that describe expected outcomes. Objectives are the observable, measurable steps taken to meet the goals. Goals and objectives must be realistic and achievable. They are written in terms of the client and family and reflect the nursing diagnoses for which they were formulated. As the nurse develops the action plan for the acutely ill client at home, it is important to consider alternative approaches and options in meeting the goals. By considering all available options, the home-care nurse can decide on appropriate strategies consistent with the client's and family's needs, resources, constraints, and abilities. Since the bottom line of any intervention strategy is the achievement of the goals in terms of improved outcomes and function, individualized goals valued by the client and family are essential.

The action plan may be expressed through written nursing orders. Nursing orders reflect the precise activities used to meet the objectives and are specific, sequential, and current. They include designated actions by the client, family, and the nurse, and must be revised and modified according to the changing needs of the client and family. Nursing orders reflect the home-care nurse's concern for health promotion, health maintenance, anticipatory guidance, and restorative care. In addition, the collaboration inherent in the multidisciplinary home-care team is shown in the nursing orders. Nursing orders are somewhat like a prescription for the who, what, and when of specific intervention strategies. In formulating the action plan with the client and family, the nurse uses specific principles as the basis for planning, as well as judgment and technical skill. The plan guides and directs the nursing actions and can be used to measure the progress in meeting the designated goals and objectives.

IMPLEMENTATION

Implementation includes the decisions and activities performed in carrying out the written plan of action. It is based on the nursing orders and includes activities performed by the client and family as well as the nurse and the multidisciplinary health team. Implementation of nursing orders ensures that all dimensions of nursing care are performed efficiently and competently, including the technical, interpersonal, and the judging elements of care. Yura and Walsh (1983) identified three skills as necessary for implementation of the nursing plan of action. These are *intellectual, interpersonal,* and *technical* skills. They are not seen as distinct and mutually exclusive but rather as integrated skills of the professional nurse.

It is important to document the care provided in the home accurately and appropriately. Documentation provides a comprehensive record of care and ensures continuity for all members of the health team involved with the care of the acutely ill individual. It provides evidence as to the progress the client and family are making in meeting their goals and objectives. It assists the agency in quality assurance and utilization review. Documentation is also critical to the financial health of the home-care agency (Jacob 1985). The home-care nurse must know and follow the requirements and regulations stipulated by the federal government and third-party payers to ensure reimbursement for services rendered by agency personnel (Holloway 1984; Connaway 1985).

EVALUATION

Evaluation judges the effectiveness, efficiency, and adequacy of the nursing care plan. Outcomes of client and family functioning and health are measured in relation to the progress or lack of progress in meeting goals. The effectiveness of the nursing intervention relates to actual client and family outcomes as compared with the planned goals and objectives. Positive outcomes are expected changes in client and family health consistent with the stated goals and objectives. Evaluation of efficiency examines whether or not the goals and objectives were realistic for the given time frame. Adequacy refers to the degree to which the client and family needs were met by the nursing intervention. Depending on the client's response, the nursing order may be eliminated, modified, or continued.

Evaluation is an ongoing systematic process and includes formative as well as summative evaluation. Formative evaluation is continuous and occurs with the implementation and appraisal of each nursing order. The client's and family's responses to the intervention provide feedback to the assessment, planning, and implementation subsystems. Summative evaluation refers to the determination of overall results in meeting goals. Based on this information, the plan is revised and updated to reflect changes occurring in the acute care situation in the home.

References

Andreoli KG, Musser LA: Trends that may affect nursing's future. Nurs Health Care 6 (1): 47–51, 1985

Braden CJ: (1984) The Focus and Limits of Community Health Nursing. East Norwalk, CT, Appleton-Century-Crofts, 1984

Carpenito LJ: Nursing Diagnosis: Application to Clinical Practice. Philadelphia; JB Lippincott, 1983

Clemen SA, Eigsti DG, McGuire SL: Comprehensive Family and Community Health Nursing. New York, McGraw Hill, 1981

Coleman JR, Smith DS: DRGs and the growth of home health care. Nurs Econ 2 (6): 391–395, 1984

Connaway N: Documenting patient care in the home—legal issues for home health nurses. Home Healthcare Nurse 3 (5): 6–8, 1985

Gelinas L: Interview. Nurs Life May/June: 18–21, 1985

Griffith E: Interview. Am J Nurs 84 (3): 342, 1984

Griffith-Kenny JW, Christensen PJ: Nursing Process: Application of Theories, Frameworks, and Models. St. Louis, CV Mosby, 1986

Halamandaris VJ: President's Page. Caring 3 (7): 112, 1984

Hall JE, Weaver BR: Distributive Nursing Practice: A Systems Approach to Community Health, 2nd ed. Philadelphia, JB Lippincott, 1985

Helvie CO: Community Health Nursing. Philadelphia, Harper & Row, 1981

Holloway VMc: Documentation: One of the ultimate challenges in home health care. Home Healthcare Nurse 2 (1): 19–22, 1984

Jacob SR: The impact of documentation on home health care. Home Healthcare Nurse 3 (5): 16–20, 1985

Kratz C: Advances in non-institutional care. Nurs Mirror 160 (18): 48–49, 1985

Louden TL: Opportunities—and competition in home healthcare are on the rise. Mod Healthcare, 13 (Dec): 109–112, 1983

Louden TL: Opportunities on the rise in home health care. Caring 3 (7): 12–14, 1984

Rogatz P: Home health care: Some social and economic consideration. Home Healthcare Nurse 3 (1): 38–43, 1985

Runner-Heidt C: Where does the hospital discharge planner go from here? Home Healthcare Nurse 3, (4): 30–35, 1984

Runner-Heidt C: Initiating hospital-based home care. Home Healthcare Nurse 3 (4): 33–36, 1985

Yura H, Walsh MB: The Nursing Process: Assessing Planning, Implementing, Evaluating. New York, Appleton-Century-Crofts, 1983

Zucker E, Barisonek L: Shaping our destiny in the age of competition. Home Healthcare Nurse 3 (4): 1–2, 1984

DISCHARGE PLANNING

Cansas Deitz Smith

During 1985 in the United States, 35.1 million persons were discharged from hospitals (National Center for Health Statistics 1986). Many of these individuals required further care in the home. While exact statistics of hospital discharges to home care are not compiled on a national level, the significant increase in home-care clients signifies that their numbers are substantial. To facilitate the client's transition from the acute care setting to the home, discharge planning is required.

Discharge planning focuses upon the identification of the client's needed services, equipment, medical supplies, planning, client education, and the client's follow-up. This chapter will examine the discharge planning process, and the potential problems involved in the transition from the hospital to the home.

DISCHARGE PLANNING DEFINED

Discharge planning has been defined by various professional groups. The American Nurses' Association (1975) defined discharge planning as

that part of the continuity of care process which is designed to prepare the patient or client for the next phase of care and to assist in making any necessary arrangements for that phase of care, care by family members, or care by an organized health-care provider.

Every client admitted to an acute care facility should be assessed for present and future physiological and psychosocial needs. When needs are identified, plans for client education to provide self-care should be implemented. If the client or family cannot provide care, referrals to community health-care services should be made (American Nurses' Association 1975).

The American Hospital Association (1984) defined discharge planning as "an interdisciplinary hospital wide process that should be available to aid patients and their families in developing a feasible post-hospital plan of care." In 1972 the American Hospital Association stated in the "Patient's Bill of Rights" that a patient has a right to be informed of his anticipated health-care needs after discharge from the hospital.

The Joint Commission for the Accreditation of Hospitals (JCAH) has developed standards relative to the client's right to transfer and continuity of care. The commission maintains that discharge planning is a vital part of the client's plan of care. On a site visit to the facility, the JCAH surveyor seeks validation that discharge planning has occurred and the effectiveness has been evaluated (Accreditation Manual for Hospitals, 1983). The reader is referred to the JCAH standards for nursing services, social work services, and utilization review relative to discharge planning.

To participate in the Medicare and Medicaid programs, hospitals must meet the requirements established by the Health Care Financing Administration (HCFA) known as the "Conditions of Participation." The Hospital Conditions of Participation as they appeared in the June 17, 1986, Federal Register, reflect a change in how "patient health and safety" will be protected. The government surveyors focus has been changed to "comprehensive" needs of clients rather than "procedural" requirements. The surveyors will be evaluating client outcomes and the effectiveness of interventions. Documentation of discharge planning and follow-up will be expected.

The manual of the Professional Review Organization (1974) states that discharge planning should begin at admission. This is necessary to prepare the client for discharge to the next level of care with appropriate referrals and arrangements included. A history of health-care needs prior to admission may be helpful in assessing present and future needs after discharge. Identification of the expected length of stay provides a time frame in which teaching, identification of resources, and arrangements for referrals will have to be made.

Fagan (1984) identified three stages when discharge planning information may be collected. The stages are (1) prior to admission;

(2) during admission; and (3) during hospitalization. A system to collect information and assessment criteria must be developed for each stage.

REGULATION AND DISCHARGE PLANNING

Many private insurance companies have required preadmission review prior to authorization of coverage for services. Dumbaugh and Neuhauser (1975) studied the effect of preadmission testing on the length of stay and found that length of stay was reduced. The effects were lower costs to third-party payers, fewer days away from work for patients, and improved bed utilization for hospitals.

Medicare began using a prospective payment system called *Diagnosis Related Groups* (DRGs) when the payment system became law in October 1983 (Federal Register, 1983). There are 467 DRGs within the 23 *Major Diagnostic Categories* (MDCs) that are based on anatomical organ systems. Each DRG has an assigned mean *Length of Stay* (LOS), which is the number of days Medicare will pay for services. The *Outlier Cutoff* is the maximum number of days per DRG for which the hospital may charge Medicare. The hospital must negotiate payment for the days between the mean length of stay and the outlier cutoff and the request must be justified by the severity of the client's condition.

Hospitals are assigned *Relative Weights* (RW) for each DRG length of stay based on cost data and category. The three categories are *acute or chronic, teaching or nonteaching,* and *urban or rural.* Each DRG has a cost outlier that is the maximum Medicare will pay for services. Resource consumption is the total cost of services per hospitalization.

PREADMISSION DISCHARGE PLANNING

For Medicare clients, DRGs provide the discharge planner with the time frames and cost limits within which to assess clients, arrange interventions, and ensure follow-up care. The discharge planner could consult the admissions department and identify clients who have been scheduled as elective admissions. The expected needs of clients could be identified early and planning could begin. Client teaching could be implemented prior to or at admission. Rice and Johnson (1984) found that teaching of physical exercises prior to admission reduced the hospital length of stay.

Preadmission discharge planning should provide assessment and identification of high risk clients who may need instruction and post-hospital care (Fagan 1984). The client's age, home environment, support systems, financial status, and diagnoses should be assessed to identify potential problems (Smeltzer and Flores 1986).

DISCHARGE PLANNING IN HOSPITAL

On admission to the hospital, assessment of every client for discharge should be completed. Basic information should include the client's age, past and potential health-care needs, expected level of function at discharge, anticipated instruction needed, and where post-hospital care will be provided. Coordinated efforts by all members of the health-care team in the assessment, potential or actual problem identification, and intervention will enhance the client's effective discharge.

High-risk clients must be identified and assessed for discharge planning needs as soon as possible. Clients who are over the age of 65 years and live alone should be considered in the high-risk category. Potential care-givers should be identified. If the client will need assistance and no care-giver is available, other arrangements must be made before discharge.

Clients who have had radical or mutilating surgery should be assessed for discharge planning needs. The neonate, the young mother, and pediatric clients should be included in the high-risk categories. Any client who is expected to have a decrease in his level of function should receive careful discharge planning.

During hospitalization, discharge planning includes the assessment and identification of needs that the client must have met before being discharged from the hospital (Fagan 1984). If follow-up care and referrals are indicated, they must be arranged in conjunction with the client and family. Community resources must be identified and referrals made.

There are varying degrees of client discharge planning assessment and intervention. Some hospitals have developed comprehensive assessments that include every possible need. A comprehensive assessment focuses on the client's physical, psychosocial, financial, and environmental needs. Basic superficial assessments may focus only on the client's age or medical diagnoses.

The evaluation of the discharge planning process should include follow-up with clients and community support service providers through telephone calls or a written questionnaire. Whether or not health-care needs were met and services were provided should be addressed, as should the outcome of the planned interventions.

The Client Assessment and Plan of Care for Discharge tool (shown on pages 16 and 17) may be used as a guide to gather important information. Potential problems are easily identified. The form provides space to docu-

CLIENT ASSESSMENT AND PLAN OF CARE FOR DISCHARGE

NAME _____

ADDRESS _____

PHONE NUMBER _____ DATE OF BIRTH _____

DIAGNOSIS:

Primary diagnosis for this admission _____
_____

PHYSICIAN _____ PHONE NUMBER _____

POTENTIAL CARE-GIVERS

Name	Address	Phone Number	Relationship
_____	_____	_____	_____
_____	_____	_____	_____
_____	_____	_____	_____

Support Systems _____

LIVING ARRANGEMENTS PRIOR TO ADMISSION

_____ Lived alone
_____ Prior outside support — list _____
_____ Lived with relative — list _____
_____ Boarding home
_____ Nursing home
_____ Other _____

Will previous arrangements be adequate? _____

SUPPORT SERVICES PRIOR TO ADMISSION AND PROVIDERS _____
_____

FINANCIAL*

_____ Medicare # _____
_____ Medicaid # _____
_____ Champus
_____ Veterans Administration
_____ Private Insurance _____
_____ Indigent

* (Monthly income – to determine eligibility for services)

TREATMENTS

Has client/care-giver been instructed and correctly returned demonstration? _____
_____

CLIENT ASSESSMENT AND PLAN OF CARE FOR DISCHARGE (continued)

MEDICATIONS

Will client be capable of administering? _____

If no, who will administer? _____

MEDICAL SUPPLIES NEEDED _____

  Supplier: _____

ACTIVITIES OF DAILY LIVING

  _____ Requires no assistance

  _____ Requires assistance with   _____ eating   _____ transfers

                                      _____ bathing   _____ treatments

  _____ Requires total assistance with _____ eating   _____ transfers

                                        _____ bathing   _____ treatments

---

IN-HOSPITAL SERVICES

  _____ PT   _____ OT   _____ ST   _____ Nutritionist

Response to treatment _____

SERVICES NEEDED IN THE HOME

  _____ Private-duty   _____ Nursing   _____ Sitters

Hours per day _____   Provider _____

_____ Home Health/Visiting Nurses

  _____ Nursing   Frequency _____

  _____ Home-Health Aides   Frequency _____

  _____ Physical Therapy   Frequency _____

  _____ Speech Therapy   Frequency _____

  _____ Occupational Therapy   Frequency _____

  _____ Medical Social Worker   Frequency _____

  _____ Nutritionist   Frequency _____

_____ Oxygen Therapy   Provider _____

_____ IV Therapy   Provider _____

Other Services:

  _____ Transportation

  _____ Meal Preparation/Home Delivered Meals-Provider _____

---

ment needs and the names of providers after referrals are made. The client will not be ready for discharge until all referrals and arrangements for home care have been made. A copy of this tool could serve as a client referral form from the hospital to a home-health agency to avoid duplication of effort by the discharge planner.

NURSING DIAGNOSES RELATED TO DISCHARGE PLANNING

The discharge planner assesses the client, family, and home environment in preparing for the client's transition to the home setting.

After acquiring the data base, the discharge planner establishes nursing diagnoses. A nursing diagnosis is a diagnostic statement dealing with actual or potential problems that might affect the client's health needs in the home.

As a framework for analyzing the typical nursing diagnoses that might be relevant, the following will be discussed:

- Lack of knowledge related to self-care needs
- Potential/actual inadequate support system
- Potential/actual inadequate home environment
- Lack of knowledge regarding financial resources
- Lack of knowledge regarding community resources
- Lack of financial resources

LACK OF KNOWLEDGE RELATED TO SELF-CARE NEEDS

The client must be assessed to determine if he will be capable of meeting his needs *independently* after discharge. Assessment should include the client's knowledge regarding his diagnosis, health status, treatments, medications, level of activity, and follow-up care. A review of anatomical organ systems may assist the nurse in her assessment.

Clients who lack knowledge related to self-care needs may be provided instruction that will allow them to function independently. Development of a teaching plan by the health-care team and prompt intervention

will assist the client to meet the goal of competent self-care. The theories of learning and client teaching are covered extensively in another chapter of this text.

POTENTIAL/ACTUAL INADEQUATE SUPPORT SYSTEM

The client and family support system must be explored by the discharge planner. Clients must be assessed to determine whether there are relatives in the community to assist with care. The discharge planner may wish to interview the client's visitors as part of the assessment process. This will assist in the identification of potential care-givers and relief for the immediate family in a crisis.

Identification of a competent and willing care-giver is critical when it is determined that a client is dependent in any activity. The discharge planner should meet with the family members or significant others. They should be asked directly if they are willing to care for the client when he goes home. If their response is yes, then their availability and other responsibilities must be discussed. If the care-giver works outside the home, other arrangements for provision of care must be made prior to discharge.

Unfortunately, many care-givers are unable to perform tasks correctly or are simply unable to manage the client's needs. The ineffective care-giver is often poorly instructed or unable to learn the necessary care. This person may be physically or psychologically unable to cope with the client's demands. Alternate placement outside the home should be considered if the care-giver cannot provide adequate care.

Once the client is home, the care should be evaluated to determine if it is appropriate for the client's needs. For example, an elderly woman brought her son home after he had suffered a severe head injury. The son had abandoned the family 20 years previously. The mother punished the son by deliberately neglecting to feed him. If a home-health nurse had not been involved, the man would have died of malnutrition. Another case involved an elderly woman who was confined to bed. Her sister, the care-giver, placed newspapers under her because she was incontinent. She also restricted her fluids to decrease her urinary output. A home-health nurse intervened and made the appropriate protective services referrals. Another very willing care-giver was giving her husband water and orange juice only through his feeding tube. She had misunderstood the instructions given in the hospital.

There are hundreds of such examples of neglect and improper care. Most could be prevented with appropriate referrals to community agencies or proper client placement. Only through assessment can the need for referrals be identified and made.

When a client has had multiple recent hospital admissions, this is usually due to medical complications. The health-care team must assess whether the complications could have been prevented. Follow-up by a home-health agency might have provided the assessment and supervision necessary to prevent readmission. If the home environment or care-givers are inadequate or absent, alternate placement should be considered.

If the client is over 65 years of age, a thorough assessment is indicated. The ability of the individual to provide self-care must be assessed. The older client may have few friends or family members. His income may be limited. He may not recall when medications are to be taken. He may not be able to arrange for the help he needs and become frustrated. Older clients are often discharged to the home and soon reenter the hospital with more complications. To determine the effectiveness of discharge planning in a hospital, examine the readmission rate.

POTENTIAL/ACTUAL INADEQUATE HOME ENVIRONMENT

From the hospital setting, it is difficult to assess the adequacy of the home environment. Many clients are discharged to the home when no assessment of its adequacy has been made. The basic modern conveniences, such as heat or indoor plumbing, are not always available. Before the hospital admission, the client may have been capable of preparing meals and performing his own activities of daily living. Who will now provide the basic necessities of food, water, and meet the hygienic needs of the client? Assessment of the home environment in relation to specific conditions is explored in each of the physiological chapters in this book.

Maslow's (1954) hierarchy of needs could be used by the nurse to guide in the assessment of the home environment. Assessment of the heating and cooling systems is necessary to determine the temperature range of the home. If the home has no cooling system and the temperature may rise above 90° F in the summer, a client with severe respiratory disease could not tolerate this environment safely. The nurse should determine whether the client is capable of adjusting the controls or maintaining adequate temperature and humidity in the home.

If the nurse determines that the home temperature is not adequate due to a lack of funds, she may assist by contacting community agencies who provide heating and cooling assistance. Social service organizations often provide such assistance to lower income individuals. With the client's permission, the nurse may contact the local fire department or utility company in order to provide a home evaluation to determine if the systems are safe or pose a possible fire hazard.

The availability of hot and cold running water and indoor plumbing should be assessed. In older homes the plumbing may be broken or not work properly. The nurse may intervene by assisting the client in finding a repairman. Baptiste and Feck (1980) found that the elderly and infants were the most often burned by hot tap water. Intervention should assure that the hot water heater setting be adjusted to 120° F to decrease the probability of burns.

Assessment of the living space for adequate lighting, fire detectors, and uncluttered walkways is important. As individuals become older, vision and hearing are impaired. Improved lighting of clear walkways free of hazards may prevent accidents. In the event of a fire, a fire detector will provide warning to the elderly person. Intervention might include changing the light bulbs to a higher wattage to provide improved lighting, clearing of walkways, and installation of fire detectors.

If modifications of the home must be made to accommodate the client, the discharge coordinator may need to direct these efforts. It is easy to tell the family they may need a ramp, but few individuals are aware of community agencies who will provide this service. The discharge planner should make every effort to assist the family in making arrangements for needed modifications in the home. A local home-health agency and durable medical equipment provider will gladly assess the home and make recommendations. Many times a predischarge home visit from the nurse, physical therapist, or occupational therapist is helpful. Equipment needs and home adaptation needs can be identified more clearly. This helps to ease transition from hospital to home.

Minor adaptations such as elevated toilet seats, a hand-held shower adaptor, oversized handles, and faucet adapters can make activities of daily living easier. The addition of safety bars in the bathroom may prevent falls. The discharge planner might recommend items such as transfer boards, bath benches, and lifts to assist the client and care-giver. Figure 2-1 illustrates some of these devices.

LACK OF KNOWLEDGE REGARDING FINANCIAL RESOURCES

Most clients or families will be capable of determining whether they have Medicare, Medicaid, or other types of insurance benefits. Few individuals will be aware of exactly which services are covered by their policies. Financial assessment is necessary since most services, equipment, and supplies must be purchased.

The hospital discharge planner must first assess the client's financial resources before services can be planned. Identification is necessary of any third-party payers and of the benefits provided by insurance policies. The discharge planner may have to determine what services will be covered, such as private-duty nurses, therapy services, pharmaceutical needs, and equipment. Most payers have specific criteria that must be met.

The client or family will usually have to pay some portion of costs that the third-party payer will not cover. The deductibles are usually 20% or more. The discharge planners will have to inquire about available funds to meet these costs.

Intervention by the discharge planner will include client and family education regarding the financial resources available to the client. Specifically to be clarified are the portion the third-party payer will cover and the portion for which the client will be responsible. If the client is financially unable to purchase the services required, the discharge planner must investigate other possible resources.

Major potential payment sources to be explored are Medicare, Medicaid, Veteran's Administration, Champus, or private insurance. Each has specific eligibility requirements.

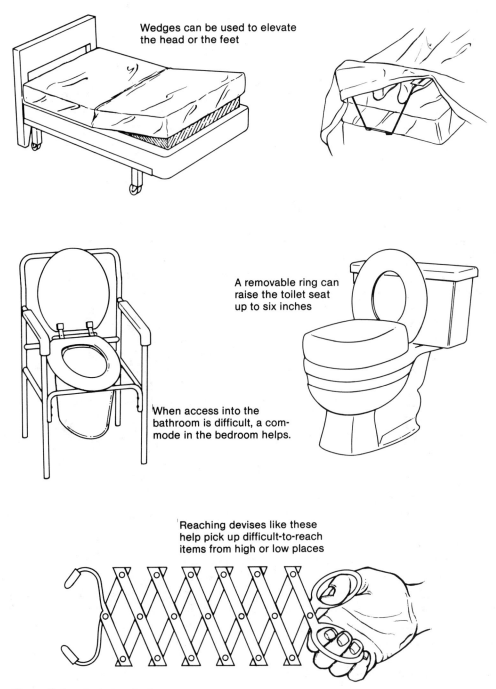

Wedges can be used to elevate the head or the feet

A removable ring can raise the toilet seat up to six inches

When access into the bathroom is difficult, a commode in the bedroom helps.

Reaching devises like these help pick up difficult-to-reach items from high or low places

Figure 2-1. Assistive devices.

Payment Source

Medicare

Title XVIII of the Social Security Act created Medicare in 1965. Medicare will pay for home-health care and "necessary" durable medical equipment in the home. In order to qualify, a beneficiary must meet the eligibility criteria (Medicare Home Health Agency Manual).

The beneficiary must be over 65 years of age and have paid into the Social Security or Railroad Retirement systems. An individual who is under 65 years of age, but who has been disabled for 2 years, may become eligible. End-stage renal disease also qualifies an individual for Medicare benefits. Spouses of beneficiaries, who are over 65 years of age, may also be eligible for Medicare benefits.

Medicare has two parts. Hospital insurance (*Part A*) provides benefits to beneficiaries who have paid into the Social Security or Railroad Retirement systems. Supplemental Medical Insurance (*Part B*) is an optional insurance that a beneficiary can purchase by paying a monthly premium.

Medicare will pay only for those home-health services that are skilled, intermittent, and medically necessary. The beneficiary must be "homebound." The "homebound" client leaves the home only for medical care and is not able to perform housework or walk more than 20 feet without difficulty. *Skilled* care can only be performed by a nurse or therapist. The services provided must correlate with the client's medical diagnosis, the problems identified, and the actual condition. The services must be reasonable and necessary, with precise documentation that progress is being made as a result of services.

Intermittent means that the need must be medically predictable and not indefinite. Daily visits should not exceed 21 days or this is deemed continuous care that should be provided in a hospital or nursing home. To ensure payment, prior authorization for daily visits must be obtained from the fiscal intermediary *before* services are rendered. A fiscal intermediary is a financial middleman. Private insurance companies serve as the fiscal intermediary between the client and the provider. Services of a preventive or maintenance level, such as homemakers, sitters, or private-duty nurses are not covered by Medicare.

The client must require at least one of these three "primary" services: skilled nursing, physical therapy, or speech therapy. As long as a primary service is provided, a medical social worker, home health aide, occupational therapist, or nutritionist may also provide services if ordered by the physician. A laboratory result must be normal on two occasions before services are no longer covered. The exception to this is blood coagulation studies for clients on sodium warfarin (Coumadin). These are covered at least monthly and indefinitely. Medicare services are reviewed retrospectively and may be denied—and therefore unpaid—after services are rendered. In such a case, the provider (not the client) is liable. If a primary service had been provided and then was terminated, the occupational therapist may continue to provide services.

The physician must order all services, the frequency and duration of services, supplies, equipment, and also must certify that the client is homebound on a home treatment plan provided by the Health Care Financing Administration. At least every 60 days, the physician must recertify the client's services on a home-treatment plan.

Documentation is the key to reimbursement. Clear, descriptive explanations of clinical problems related to services provided should be documented, particularly with regard to skilled care. Skilled nursing for observation and assessment of an unstable client is usually covered if frequent physician contact resulting in changes in treatment orders is documented. If the physician does not change treatment orders, services will not be covered.

Services to clients with chronic diagnoses are usually not covered unless there has been a recent hospital admission due to an acute exacerbation of the condition. Infrequent procedures or treatments that require the skills of a nurse are generally covered. When procedures and treatments are ordered which are to be performed frequently, the nurse should so instruct the client or care-giver since Medicare will cover the nurse for a short time only. When laboratory studies are ordered and the results are normal, services may not be covered. It should be noted that the services of a nutritionist are not reimbursable, but are often provided as a "service" and considered an administrative cost by some agencies. If the physician does not order changes in medications or treatment when findings are abnormal, services are not covered.

Medicaid

Title XIX of the Social Security Act created the Medicaid program in 1965. Each state individually administers the Medicaid program. The federal government matches 50% of every dollar the state provides. Every state has an income requirement for client eligibility (Federal Register, 1976).

In most states Medicaid will reimburse Medicaid-certified home-health agencies for skilled nursing services that are certified medically necessary and ordered by a physician. Therapy services, and home-health-aide services are reimbursed on a much more limited basis than skilled nursing services. Most states limit the number of health-aide visits to the client that will be reimbursed in one year. Medical social worker and occupational therapy services are not covered by Medicaid.

Most medical services require prior authorization.

Private Insurance

Clients may have private insurance policies that will cover home-health services, supplies and equipment. Coverage varies greatly from 75% to 90% of the cost, depending on the individual policy. There is generally a deductible the client must meet every year. Typically, the services, equipment, and supplies must be medically necessary and ordered by a physician. Many states have now enacted legislation requiring home health coverage to be an option offered by insurance companies. Many private insurance companies require pre-authorization and some initiate their own utilization review—mandated to the physician that the client be discharged from the hospital and home health be used. In addition, even if a client's insurance coverage does not include home-health benefits, insurance companies are frequently willing to negotiate or make an exception if it will allow discharge from the hospital (and thus a substantial cost-savings for the insurance company).

Veterans Administration

Home-health services may be reimbursed by the federally funded Veterans Administration. Eligibility is determined by the local Veterans Administration facility and is limited to skilled care to veterans with disabilities related to military service or follow-up care after discharge from a facility. Only medically necessary services that are related to the client's diagnosis and ordered by a Veterans Administration facility physician will be covered. When follow-up appointments at the facility are scheduled, a client must comply or home-health services will not be reimbursed. Necessary supplies and equipment are provided by the Veterans Administration.

Champus

Civilian Health and Medical Programs of the Uniformed Services (CHAMPUS) provides reimbursement for medically necessary hospitalization, outpatient, and home-health service care for spouses and children of active duty members of the uniformed services, retired servicemen and spouses, and children of retired and deceased members of the uniformed services. Each beneficiary must meet a deductible every year, with a maximum per family. The CHAMPUS fiscal year begins October 1 and ends September 30. Active duty members must also pay 20% of the approved charges after the deductible has been met. Retirees and their dependents and dependents of a deceased retiree must pay a cost share of 25%. It is important to note that CHAMPUS would pay before Medicaid if the individual has both benefits. Frequent use of CHAMPUS requires that the client pay the agency first, then CHAMPUS may (or may not) reimburse the client, and that is a major drawback.

LACK OF KNOWLEDGE REGARDING COMMUNITY RESOURCES

Most communities have many services available to their residents. The discharge planner must stay abreast of every service in the community and maintain a close working relationship with the providers of such services. When the needed services, equipment, and supplies are identified, the discharge planner can assist the client and family by providing information concerning their availability in the community and by making the appropriate referrals.

Many home-health agencies provide a wide range of services, including intermittent visits, private duty nursing, home-health-aide/homemaker care, medical equipment, and pharmaceuticals. The trend seems to be toward "one stop shopping." However, in some locales there is still a need to coordinate services through a variety of arrangements with separate organizations.

Private-Duty Nursing Services

Most communities have individuals or agencies who will provide private-duty nursing or sitter services to clients in the home setting. The hospital nursing office often keeps such a list. The discharge planner may need to provide the client or family with this information. The discharge planner and other members of the health-care team can help the client or family determine the hours needed per day for such services. Many private insurance policies cover a portion of the cost for private-duty nursing services if they are medically necessary and ordered by a physician. Most policies will cover only the services rendered by a registered nurse, licensed practical nurse (LPN), or a licensed vocational nurse (LVN), In fact many insurance companies prefer the services of an LVN, as the cost is generally several dollars less per hour. Individual coverage will need to be verified with the company by the discharge planner, client, or a family member.

Visiting Nurses and Home-Health Agencies

Visiting Nurses Association (VNA) and home-health agencies provide a full range of intermittent services to clients in their homes. Services may include nursing, physical therapy, speech therapy, occupational therapy, medical social work, home-health aide, and nutritional counseling. The discharge planner must identify the agencies that can provide the ordered services and allow the client, family, and physician to choose which agency will be utilized. The referral can then be initiated. It is important to assess whether the agency is available to provide services 24 hours a day, 7 days a week. The replacement of feeding tubes or catheters, the administration of drugs, and dressing changes may be needed after normal business hours, on holidays, or weekends.

Community Groups

Local Red Cross units, senior citizens groups, and the Long-Term Care Project may provide homemaker or chore services. Churches and other volunteer groups sometimes offer more limited homemaker services to the elderly, together with Meals on Wheels.

Typical support services include private-duty nursing and home-health agency services. Both services are usually available and accessible in communities. However, it may be difficult to gain access to free or low-cost homemaker services, transportation, and home-delivered meals, if available, due to long waiting lists. Transportation services may not be available at all.

Durable Medical Equipment and Supplies

Durable medical equipment involves much more than hospital beds, wheelchairs, and bedside commodes. Respiratory care in the home includes liquid, gaseous, and oxygen therapy. Aerosol and ventilator therapy, infant apnea monitoring and phototherapy, and parenteral and enteral nutrition therapy can all be provided more cost effectively in the home. All the necessary supplies are provided. Durable medical equipment companies also provide specialized wheelchairs, splints, and electrical modalities. The physician must certify and provide documentation of the medical necessity for such equipment and supplies.

There are two types of equipment and supplies (Buyers Guide 1986). Durable medical equipment can be used repeatedly. Examples of durable medical equipment include hospital beds, monitors, and wheelchairs. Supplies are either disposable or replaceable. Disposable supplies include clean gloves, sterile dressings, disposable pads, and any sterile item. Replaceable supplies include thermometers and nonsterile irrigation equipment.

Vendors are the suppliers of durable medical equipment and supplies. The discharge planner should assist the client in the selection of a vendor who will provide all the required equipment and supplies. Some vendors deal only with oxygen equipment and may not provide other equipment such as hospital beds or wheelchairs. Many vendors do not provide supplies. Maintenance of equipment and prompt delivery of all equipment and supplies should be guaranteed.

Clients may elect to rent or purchase durable equipment. Items such as hospital beds and ventilators are usually rented, while walkers, canes, and commode seats are usually purchased. Lease-purchase agreements are available for all items and should be considered if the length of time the equipment will be used is uncertain. The charges of leasing the equipment will be applied toward the purchase of the equipment. At the point the lease charges reach the purchase charges, the client will own the equipment. Medicare now has rental-purchase regulations requiring purchase of the equipment if the monthly rental times the length of rental exceeds the purchase cost.

The client and family may improvise household items instead of purchasing expensive equipment and supplies. For example, a client's physician ordered a hospital bed and air mattress for the client. The client and family could not afford the equipment. A nurse determined that the family already owned a waterbed. The client was placed on the waterbed and pillows were utilized to elevate the client to a 90° angle when necessary. Before equipment and supplies are ordered, an assessment of what is available should be completed. Family, friends, neighbors, community organizations, and churches may loan the client the needed equipment, avoiding unnecessary expenses.

A vendor of durable medical equipment and supplies can provide a comprehensive listing of all available items on the market. A review of the list (categorized into respiratory, mobility, elimination, adaptive, nutritional, and safety equipment and supplies) will assist the discharge planner in the planning phase. Intervention will be the ordering of all needed equipment and supplies.

In order for Medicare to cover the cost of any type of hospital bed for the home, the client must spend at least 50% of the time in bed. Similar restrictions may also apply to other medical equipment items before Medicare will provide coverage. Medicare rarely covers the cost of an electric bed for the home. If coverage is to be considered, the client must be able to operate the controls and an immediate need for position change due to respiratory distress must be documented. Alternating air mattresses and kinetic or continuous motion beds are available for clients with an alteration in skin integrity, but they are not paid for by Medicare.

The availability of home oxygen therapy allows many clients to be maintained at home. Gaseous oxygen is available in the conventional tank. The tanks may be large and prevent easy mobility, necessitating a small, portable tank. Liquid oxygen is available in a reservoir that is stationary. An oxygen concentrator is smaller and can easily be moved about the home. Consumption must be carefully calculated to avoid running out of oxygen unexpectedly. When selecting a provider for oxygen therapy, the discharge planner should ask if services are available 24 hours a day in the event of equipment malfunction or other problems. Abnormal arterial blood gas studies and physician certification of medical necessity will be required for reimbursement.

LACK OF FINANCIAL RESOURCES

Many clients will need services, equipment, or supplies, but have no means of paying for them. The discharge planner's knowledge of available community resources may make the difference between whether or not the client's needs are met. Most durable equipment providers have a "loan closet" with equipment they will loan to clients. Public health home-health agencies may provide care to indigent clients, and in many communities, private home-health agencies provide a limited amount of care to such clients. Some agencies have a sliding-scale fee structure. Needed supplies may be donated by private individuals, companies, or community organizations. Community organizations may provide free homemaker services, transportation, and meals.

In some instances the needed services, equipment, supplies, or alternate placement cannot be secured. Discharge planners and home-health staff frequently face this frustrating dilemma. The physician and hospital administration staff must be informed of the problems. Often home care will be tried as a last resort, even when the outcome is likely to be poor.

References

Accreditation Manual for Hospitals. Chicago, Joint Commission on Accreditation of Hospitals, 1983

Baptiste M, Feck G: Preventing tap water burns. Am Public Health 70(7): 727–759, 1980

Continuity of Care and Discharge Planning Program. New York, American Nurse's Association, 1975

Dumbaugh K, Neuhauser D: The effect of pre-admission testing on length of stay. In Shortell SM, Brown M (Eds): Organizational Research in Hospitals. Chicago, Blue Cross–Blue Shield, 1975

Fagan JL: Developing an information system for

discharge planning under prospective pricing. Dishcarge Planning Update, Spring, 5–9, 1984

Federal Register: 41(166): 35847, August 25, 1976

Federal Register: 42(405J), June 17, 1986

Guidelines: Discharge Planning. Chicago, American Hospital Association, 1984

Health Care Financing Administration (HCFA). Department of Health and Human Services Medicare Program: Prospective payments for medicare inpatient hospital services. Federal Register 39752-39890, September 1, 1983

Health Care Financing Administration (HCFA). U.S. Department of Health and Human Services: Medicare Home Health Agency Manual (Pub No 11. 1-10-32. 2)

Health Care Financing Administration (HCFA). U.S. Department of Health and Human Services: Medicare Provider Reimbursement Manual (Pub No 11. 15-1, 21-2. 5-26-12. 1)

Hospital Discharge Survey. Hyattsville, MD, National Center for Health Statistics, September 25, 1986

Maslow A: Motivation and Personality. New York, Harper & Row, 1954

U.S. Department of Health, Education, and Welfare: Professional Standards Review Organization Manual. Washington, DC, U.S. Government Printing Office, 1974

Rice V, Johnson J: Pre-admission self instruction booklets, post admission exercise performance, and teaching time. Nurs Res 33(3): 147–151, 1984

℞ home care. Buyer's Guide, 50–53, 1986

Smeltzer C, Flores S: Preadmission discharge planning. JONA 16(5), 1986

Statement on a Patient's Bill of Rights Chicago, American Hospital Association, 1972

LIABILITY ISSUES*

3

Sue Reitz Perdew

Today's practicing home health-care professionals worry about risk related to malpractice litigation. A general unease and discomfort finds its way into formal and casual discussions of professional issues that touch on the relationship of home-care nurses to the law.

Are home-care nurses and organizations *really* going to be sued more frequently? What causes people to sue? How can nurses protect themselves, individually and organizationally? Is there any theoretical framework likely to provide nurses with a useful structure for considering the complex issues involved in these questions? Can the nursing process be useful in analyzing risk in the area of malpractice? Should nurses be conducting research to find answers to these questions? If so, who should conduct the research, and what are the questions?

This chapter is speculative, in the sense that home-care providers have not yet seen

the anticipated sharp rise in numbers of malpractice suits. Those who believe that the profession may be in for "hard times" could be viewed as negative, alarmist, overly pessimistic.

Nevertheless, the signs of trouble are already here, and it would be worse than foolish to ignore the possibility that the health-care industry is heading for a new, albeit unwanted, phase in its history. This discussion of present and future situations is offered in the spirit of positive assessment. If this assessment is incorrect, the home health-care industry will be relieved; if it is correct, the speculation will have served the purpose of preparing nurses to meet a new, and very dangerous, challenge to the health-care industry and to the nursing profession.

PREDICTING THE DIRECTION OF CHANGE IN LITIGATION

Nationwide, home health-care nurses confront the necessity of predicting change that will affect their practice. Prediction can be

*The information in this chapter is intended to be general in nature, and is not to be understood as legal advice. Those nurses who have specific questions should seek advice from legal counsel.

accomplished by comparing what *was* before with what *is* today and by identifying major forces likely to influence the legal situation for nurses. Issues of major importance to a discussion of malpractice in home-care nursing include reimbursement of nurses, scope of practice, and expectations of the public concerning nursing care.

The reimbursement of nurses is a complex issue with legal implications. Will nurses be employees of agencies or will they be independent contractors? Who will pay for the various professional nursing services?

Since the practice of nursing is linked to remuneration, it becomes necessary for nurses as individuals and as a professional body to influence decisions about reimbursement. A great many home-care nurses are paid with tax money, and legislators make decisions about the use of tax dollars. How will nurses influence these legislators in the future?

What clients will nurses care for? For how long? What can nurses do for their clients. How often will they see them? And for what services, accomplished with what level of expertise, will nurses be held accountable by the public? Nurses must know what the public expects, not only in order to provide acceptable care, but also to avoid legal action.

Litigation against nurses is a subject that seems to be emphasized in advertisements by insurance companies interested in selling malpractice insurance, or in justifying the fact that rates for such insurance are increasing. This is not to suggest that these "scare techniques" are not useful. Nurses who become aware of risks, by whatever means, may be motivated to protect themselves. The advertisements of the insurance companies seem to serve such a purpose.

For years, several major professional journals have consistently provided readers with vital legal information in monthly articles written by highly qualified attorneys and nurse-attorneys. *The Hospital Law Newsletter* and *The Regan Report on Nursing Law* have been staples for those nurses who are interested in current legal issues. More frequently articles dealing with malpractice written by and for practicing nurses are appearing in professional journals and newsletters.

Although it seems likely to this author that litigation efforts against home health-care nurses and agencies will increase dramatically in the next few years (Perdew 1986), it should be noted that not all authors agree with this perspective. Some have suggested that home health nurses may be sued less frequently (Creighton 1985). This argument places emphasis on the system used to pay lawyers, the typical elderly clinical population, and potential changes in state laws to limit types of litigation and amounts of rewards.

GENERAL TYPES OF ACTIONS TO BE TAKEN IN RESPONSE TO CHANGE

Nurses dealing with change can be categorized into two quite different types. One type responds to knowledge of change by gearing up for self-protection. The premise on which this nurse acts is that by familiarizing herself with this new knowledge, she can protect against unwanted changes. "Forewarned is forearmed" is this person's motto.

The other type of nurse seeks knowledge of change for an entirely different reason. This person is looking for information about change in order to use it to influence the *direction* of the change for the benefit of herself, her colleagues, the nursing profession, and its clients. Although the nursing profession has been ably led by nurses in the second group, implementation of change within the profession has been and will continue to be influenced by the size of the first group.

At this point, there are certain actions likely to increase our chances of dealing effectively with the changes we encounter. These actions will be taken by nurses as professional persons and by nurses in their positions as employees in an agency. Nurse managers in home-care agencies can also take action—in support of the work of nursing (client care), in support of nursing research, and in assuring that appropriate policies are developed and applied. If nurses must risk making a mistake—and they must—then they are safer to come down on the side of action!

STRENGTHS OF HOME-CARE NURSES

Fortunately, there are several factors that home health nurses can use to help them deal with the new and potentially litigious climate in home care. These factors include the evolving standards of practice; the fact that home health nurses have some knowledge of the law; recent increased experience of nurses with documentation of care provided; and increased individual malpractice insurance coverage. Each of these factors is considered below.

STANDARDS OF PRACTICE

Accepted standards of practice of the profession are used in court to establish the specific duty of a health-care practitioner to the client (Southwick 1978). The trend in nursing has been to upgrade standards to improve quality care.

Knowing that nurses have these various standards could improve public confidence, so that clients are less likely to sue. The caveat here is that these standards, once articulated, must be met and documented in order to protect the nurse from successful malpractice litigation (Fiesta 1983).

KNOWLEDGE OF THE LAW

As a result of involving themselves in the political and legal problems of client care and reimbursement, nurses practicing in the community have traditionally been quite aware of the law. These nurses should be in an excellent position to accept the new legal situation and to work, professionally and legislatively, to solve the problems that changes present.

INCREASED USE OF DOCUMENTATION SKILLS

Nurses employed in home-care agencies are complying with recent management directives to document care more accurately and thoroughly. While this documentation has been primarily geared toward obtaining reimbursement, improved skill in documentation will be important in efforts to stay out of court.

INCREASED INSURANCE COVERAGE

Many home-care nurses do carry their own personal malpractice insurance. Nurses, agencies, and insurers need to examine the extent and limits of coverage to determine if the coverage for specific types of practice settings is appropriate and adequate.

FACTORS SUGGESTING A POTENTIAL FOR INCREASE IN LITIGATION

The factors that increase a nurse's chance for involvement in litigation are categorized, for the purposes of this discussion, as *forces*. Two major forces, technology and economics, appear to be driving social, political, professional, and educational efforts.

TECHNOLOGICAL FORCES

At the beginning of this decade, families placed their loved ones in a nursing home when they were unable to care for them at home. Now families care for clients at home when the highly skilled care needed is not available in nursing homes, and when acute care hospitals are no longer willing or financially able, under new systems of reimbursement, to provide care for the chronically ill client.

Some technological changes to be considered are the increased use of machines in the home, the malfunction of these machines, and the increase in specialization necessary to deliver modern home care.

Increased Use of Machines in the Home

There has been and will continue to be an increased use of complex machines at home (Weinstein 1984). This situation arises from continuing advancement in technology and relates to early discharge from hospitals. No matter how many complex machines a client is using in the hospital, if his condition is "stable," he may be a candidate for home care. With the increase in use of machines in the home there is an increased risk of suit.

Machine Malfunction

In the hospital there are back-up machines, maintenance services, engineers, and other health-team members who can share the responsibility for identifying a problem involving a machine. In the home it is the nurse who will be teaching the operation of these increasingly complex machines so that clients and families can identify problems. In many home-care situations, days or weeks would be needed to assure that a family truly understands a sophisticated machine. As nurses provide a wider variety of higher in-

tensity care strategies to more and sicker clients, more mistakes will occur. Thus, the likelihood increases that suits will arise when a machine malfunctions and a client is hurt.

Specialization in the Delivery of Care

There is no doubt that, with increasing technological advancement, it will be even more important to provide client care through nurses and others who have expertise in specialized areas. Home-care agencies will employ nurse specialists in the delivery of chemotherapeutic agents, in rehabilitation, in cardiovascular-pulmonary care, in home renal dialysis, or in care of the skin.

However, it would be simplistic to believe that our sicker clients will be sicker only in one physiological system; they usually have serious problems in more than one area. Increasingly, they will need the services of more than one nurse specialist.

When applied to client care, specialization often promotes a fragmented view of persons. It is precisely this perspective that home-care agencies need to guard against if they wish to prevent lawsuits.

ECONOMIC FORCES

A short time ago, prospective reimbursement began to force changes in amounts and types of care given to individual clients. This payment system will influence changes in litigation patterns against health-care providers (Creighton 1985).

It is widely accepted that the perception of the client and family about the care received influences the decision to sue (Bernzweig 1981; Southwick 1978). Clients observe, and generally support, changes in technology. But, while they live in a society in which complex economic decisions are made, they often do not understand these decisions and feel a loss of control over their lives.

The economic situation provides premises on which clients base their perceptions. In greater numbers and with more serious conditions, clients are being discharged into home care. Less time in the hospital enabling nurses in acute care to complete the necessary teaching plan for a client and family has resulted in clients coming to the home-care nurse with less information and more anxiety (Creighton 1985). It remains a nursing responsibility to teach these clients, a responsibility for which nurses will be held legally accountable (Cushing, Key Court Cases, 1984).

When considering economic forces that may cause trouble and litigation, some factors are increased depersonalization of care; loss of the coordination role of the nurse; a perception by clients that the health-care system has failed them; inability of a family to handle increased stress; the present system used to pay lawyers. Additional factors include the perception that the home-care agency is "rich;" that a poor client does not receive care as good as a more affluent client; that one agency is inferior to another; finally, increased public knowledge that nurses carry malpractice insurance (Perdew 1986).

Increased Depersonalization of Care

Community nurses today pay shorter visits to clients. Reasons for these shorter visits relate to lower reimbursement, increased costs, and agency administrators mandating a specific number of visits per day (usually five to six visits). Also, nurses are being paid "per visit." Without the time that clients once had to tell nurses all about their health patterns and coping responses, the element of a personal relationship with good communication between client and nurse is likely to be lost (Creighton 1985). Clients expect personal care, and they may sue if they perceive that they do not receive it (Southwick 1978).

Loss of Coordination Role of the Nurse

Other professional and nonprofessional health-care providers now share the client relationship. Even the generally accepted role of the nurse as coordinator of care is being eroded through practice and legislation as other professional groups push for autonomy in the home setting. As it becomes less clear which professional should be allocating responsibility when several professionals are actively involved with client care, litigation may be necessary to clarify legal accountability.

Perception That Health-Care System Has Failed

Home-care agencies are accepting very sick clients in an increasingly competitive environment. Clients who feel they were discharged from hospitals too quickly are likely to transfer their anger to the present care provider. Once home health agencies accept these clients, the agency is telling the client that it can meet his needs. When an agency finds it cannot, the agency may be sued. Northrup seems to support this point of view, as she states ". . . lawsuits against home-care nurses and agencies for failure to detect situations requiring care beyond or different from the skills of the nurse and agency will probably increase . . ." (Northrup 1986).

Inability of Family to Handle Stress

Even with careful preparation, families face overwhelming physical and emotional demands when caring for a seriously ill person at home. One predictable reaction is to be angry at the system. The family may feel guilty about its inability to deal with the situation; it then may transfer blame to the representative of the system who is not helping them as much as they want to be helped. Even when the nurse is doing all that is possible, the family may expect something more; anger and frustration may find outlet in litigation.

The System Used to Pay Attorneys

A major influence on litigation against health-care providers is the system of payment for legal services in this country. Paid on a contingency basis, attorneys receive a given percent of the dollar amount of an award for a successful malpractice suit. Contingency fees are generally higher when the award is to a young client, because the court considers the loss of "productive years of life."

There has been speculation that elderly persons may have difficulty securing quality legal services because their attorneys may choose those cases of younger clients that are likely to be more lucrative for them (Creighton 1985). Home-care agencies today are accepting younger and sicker clients, thereby increasing the pool of clients for potential litigation.

Perception That the Home-Care Agency Is Rich

In all of the history of home-care nursing, the public has never viewed the home-care agency as rich. These agencies have given service to the indigent without question.

However, as the home-care business proliferates, both not-for-profit and proprietary agencies have gradually come under suspicion in the public mind. Home-care agencies may now be seen as part of a rich and incomprehensible system. Clients who seek revenge for perceived wrongs are much more likely to sue in such a situation.

Perception That an Agency Provides Inferior Care

In one metropolitan area known to this author, there are 32 home-care agencies competing for clients. Competition is heavy, and the effort to convince physicians and clients that one agency is better than another is regarded as a sound marketing strategy. A clear implication of this strategy is that if one is better, others are worse. It is not hard to see why a client may judge care given by nurses in one agency as being "bad." Poor service, from the point of view of the client, is substandard care; lawsuits follow.

Increased Public Awareness That Nurses Carry Malpractice Insurance

Many home-care nurses, recognizing their legal accountability, have protected themselves against litigation by carrying ever more malpractice insurance. At the same time, the public has become aware of the fact that nurses carry this protection, and today it has become much more lucrative for a client to sue a nurse.

WHERE IS MAJOR RISK LIKELY TO APPEAR?

Home-care agencies have historically addressed the traditional risk-management activities of safety programs, insurance coverage, and asset management—tasks that have frequently been the responsibility of the financial manager. However, the responsibility for managing litigation risk, long believed to be minimal in home care, has not traditionally been assigned to any one person within the organization.

A rational approach for home care today, however, demands an aggressive and comprehensive program of litigation risk management (Gould et al 1986). The major goals of such a program will be to reduce exposure of the agency to litigation and to minimize the severity of financial loss should successful litigation occur. Areas of increasing vulnerability involve, in the main, personnel management and individual clinical practice in the provision of client care.

PERSONNEL MANAGEMENT AS A RISK AREA

Managers of direct client care must assure the public that competent staff has been hired, that staff members continue to maintain their competence in a rapidly changing work environment, and that the quality of the care provided is meeting "industry standards." Another area of increasing concern to personnel managers is that of potential legal action against the employer by employees.

Hiring Competent Persons

It seems obvious to the public that an agency should hire competent persons to provide client care. While a lack of understanding of the complexity of professional nursing has contributed to a simplistic view of what that work involves, it is true that a competent nursing staff member will not only have the necessary credentials but will also possess the skills and judgment necessary to provide quality client care.

Assuring Proper Credentials

One finds both dramatic and subtle changes in the qualifications considered to be "basic" in an applicant for a position in home-care nursing. In recent years directors of nursing in home-care agencies have said they would not hire a recent graduate of any nursing program. While advertising for nurses with "at least a year of medical–surgical experience," these directors often accepted experience in a nursing home as meeting this requirement.

In today's growing home-care industry, an increased need for nurses is coupled with an understanding of the "new client" as a person who requires complex, specialized care. This situation leads the home-care agency administrator to seek professional nurses with experience, not just in "medical–surgical" nursing, but also in critical care nursing. A nurse with nursing home experience only is no longer acceptable to most home-care agencies.

Although many agency directors say that they do not hire recent graduates, in actuality, many do so. While one director explained this by saying that new graduates were "special" in some way, the changing job market was more likely to be the real reason. Home-care agencies are expanding, and hospital medical–surgical positions for new graduates in that area are scarce. It is legally risky for a home-care agency to accept new nursing graduates unless a structured, sophisticated, in-service program is in place.

Identification and Evaluation of Relevant Skills

One major problem in home-care agencies is that of determining, at the time of hire, that a new employee's abilities meet agency standards. This is true, of course, even when an experienced nurse is hired. In order to assure that a potential employee has the requisite competence, it is necessary to identify and provide accurate measures of those skills and judgments that define competent practice.

The primary problem with satisfactory demonstration of relevant abilities seems to be that agencies have not identified precisely what these abilities are and how best to measure them. Nursing is not alone in facing this problem; other professions are also struggling with the same issue.

The professional competencies needed by home-care nurses are changing, not only in the direction of increasingly complex technical skills but in the direction of increasingly complex interpersonal and cognitive skills. It has become even more important that nurses who practice in the home be able to use these sophisticated professional abilities in the implementation of the nursing process and in the integration of research knowledge into client care.

The legal risk to a home-care agency is that an employee will perform a procedure resulting in client harm. An accurate evaluation of the employee's relevant abilities at time of hire can only be accomplished through an analysis of the nursing work to be done and the development of a description of expectations of staff based on that work. Policy decisions about hiring can then be made nationally and tests of knowledge and competence instituted.

One of the results of the increasing emphasis placed on medication management (initiated several years ago in home-care agencies) has been the administration to potential employees of "medication tests" to provide evidence of minimum knowledge regarding basic calculation skills and drug information. This practice is now common. It is reasonable to assume that as such additional knowledge becomes increasingly important, concerned agencies will administer tests to applicants related to subjects such as physiology, disease process, educational measurement, nursing process, or the operation of certain machines.

Assuring Continued Competence

In the present expanding market for home-care services, agencies will not be able to hire only persons with expertise in every area. Therefore, the agency must undertake orientation and in-service programs that are much more intense than has been considered necessary in the past.

Orientation Program

The orientation programs in home-care agencies are likely to change dramatically in the near future. Although the majority of small home-care agencies will not be able to afford an in-service educator, the middle-sized units will follow the lead of the large, long established home-care systems in developing a sophisticated system of meeting the agency's educational objectives. Small agencies are likely to seek the services of businesses that will provide packages of education materials.

Continuing Education

Agencies that have provided continuing education for employees know that it is very costly to present "updates" on drugs, machines, treatments, and laws. In the past, nurses often resisted these efforts by agencies on their behalf, sometimes stating that the continuing education was a waste of time or that the program took time away from the "real work" of client care.

If there are still nurses practicing in home-care today who do not understand that the changing nature of the profession demands constant personal learning, they will not remain in the business very long. So, while it is true that with increasing acute care demands, the needs for continuing education will increase, it is also true that nurses will be likely to view the opportunities to learn in a more positive light.

Assuring That Professionals Meet "Industry Standards"

If a nurse does find herself in court, what "standards" will be applied to her as a home-care nurse? After first consulting the state nurse practice act and rules and regulations, an attorney for the plaintiff will look at the general professional standards of practice, code of ethics, and definitions of nursing accepted by the professional association. From there the attorney will move to those standards that are more specific to the home-care specialty area, the Standards of Community Health Nursing and the Standards of Practice for Home-Care Nurses. Practicing home-care nurses will be held accountable in court for meeting these standards, and nurses who do not take the opportunity to read and respond to developing standards are placing themselves at increased legal risk.

After the applicable standards are considered, what can agencies do to assure that employees meet these standards? Responses of agencies are likely to include the use of contracting for the provision of specialized services involving complex skills, the institution of improved documentation systems, and the development of increasingly sophisticated educational programs for both staff and clients.

Use of Contractors

There is a risk that the small agency, involved in intense competition, may try to meet client care needs beyond its scope. To avoid this risk, some home-care agencies consider the use of independent contractors to provide complex, specialized services beyond the competence of its employees. Home-care agencies also contract out particular shifts they are unable to fill. Contracts should be in place between agencies.

Documentation System

The organization must provide effective documentation of its efforts to hire competent employees, keep them competent, and release them if they do not measure up to standards. The recurrent organizational problem of how to do this efficiently will not be eased by the increasing types and amounts of information to be documented. The only practical relief in sight is the use of computer technology available to organize, process, and store information.

Client Education System

While client education is the direct responsibility of the nurse, the health-care organization is responsible for setting up a system of documentation of the client education program. Allocation of responsibility for educational efforts, documentation of how well the client has learned, and planning for future efforts will be among the primary decisions to be made by managers in home-care agencies.

It will become increasingly common to use the computer as a tool in managing the complex information systems. For small operations, managers may feel that computers are too expensive, but this expense must be reviewed in the light of potentially successful litigation against the agency or its personnel.

Preventing Suits by Personnel

The subject of prevention of litigation by personnel against the agency presents complexities beyond the scope of this text. It is mentioned here only briefly because of the increasing importance to home-care agencies of potential litigation by employees.

Agencies have a responsibility to provide personnel with safe working conditions. A suit by an employee is likely to come about because the employee believes this responsibility has not been met. The assignment of employees to duty in an area of the community which the employee believes to be dangerous has led some agencies to send teams of two into the "high-risk zones."

The assignment to "dangerous cases" becomes another potentially serious problem when more agencies accept clients with serious communicable diseases. In some agencies, home-care employees assigned to care for clients with Acquired Immune Deficiency Syndrome (AIDS) or AIDS-Related Complex (ARC) have responded negatively.

It is very risky for an agency to ignore or make light of the fear or anger of its employees. Employees also sue because of real or perceived discrimination, firing practices, and alleged injuries (Workman's Compensation). Rational education programs are available, or can be developed, to meet the needs of employees for information, reassurance, and support.

INDIVIDUAL CLINICAL PRACTICE AS A RISK AREA

Probably the most important risk area for litigation in home-care nursing today is related to the individual practice of the direct-care provider. Clinical practice has had some risk in the past, even though home-care nurses were not sued frequently. This section will discuss where risks develop, what these risks have been up to the present, and where the risks are likely to develop in the future.

How Do Legal Risks Develop?

Suits against the professional home-care nurse can come from civil or criminal action. Risk of litigation results if someone (the state or an individual) believes that a nurse has committed either a crime or a civil wrong.

Civil Action

The most common civil action against a professional nurse today is the charge of malpractice. While nurses do commit crimes, and they can be sued for acts not covered under professional negligence, the focus of this discussion is on the increasing risk of malpractice litigation in a new clinical environment.

Malpractice A tort is a wrong committed against a person or property rendering the person who commits it liable for damages in a civil action. Redress in a civil action is by financial award — sometimes quite large.

Negligence is a tort; malpractice is a special kind of negligence — professional negligence.

In order to prove that malpractice has occurred, a client must show that his case meets all of the following four conditions: that the professional owed a duty to the client; that this duty was breached; that harm occurred; and that the breach of duty was responsible for the harm that occurred (direct cause).

Duties Owed. After a client has been officially accepted by the home-care agency, the home-care nurse owes a duty to that client. This fact alone makes it very important to both nurse and agency that quality decisions be made as to which individuals will be accepted as clients. For every agency the possibility exists that the needs of certain clients cannot reasonably be met. Risk increases dramatically if an agency adds these clients to case rolls.

Duties Breached. Breach of duty is the condition that attorneys on both sides will emphasize. Often the duty of the nurse in a particular case is unclear. As has been noted, the standards that a professional nurse must meet come from many sources and are changing rapidly.

Expert testimony by nurses other than those involved in the case will likely play a larger part in future malpractice cases. Meeting standards will be the best defense for a nurse defendant in a malpractice action.

Damages (Harm). Attorneys for clients do not usually proceed with a case unless it is reasonable to assume that some damage, or harm, did occur. Ordinarily the defendant home-care nurse is not involved in trying to prove, in her own defense, that damage to a client did not occur.

Direct Cause. On the other hand, a nurse will frequently be involved in attempting to sever the alleged link between the professional action in question and whatever harm may have occurred to the client. Severing this link is accomplished effectively when there is sufficient evidence that the care provided by the nurse was reasonable evidence that is provided by clear documentation of care.

The nurse and her attorney will also be involved in attempting to identify causes, or contributing causes, of the damage to the client other than the actions of the defendant nurse. Precise documentation of actions and time sequence of events leading up to and following the incident will be important.

Criminal Action

A crime is a wrong punishable by the state. Redress for a crime is by fine or imprisonment. Criminal law provides another avenue of attack by a plaintiff's attorney against a home-care nurse, since there are some actions of nurses that may be prosecuted as crimes. That is, the state has declared that these actions are specifically prohibited and, if committed, it is the public that is harmed. Of course, murder is a crime; so are assault (threatening a client), battery (touching a client without his consent), and false imprisonment (inappropriately restraining a client). Nurses have been charged with all of these crimes.

Civil action, however, is much more likely than criminal action, when the client has a choice. Punishment of a defendant in a successful civil suit involves the payment of money to the injured person; punishment in criminal cases, as noted above, is by set fine or by imprisonment. Both lawyers and injured clients will generally prefer the financial reimbursement for wrongs done.

ASSESSMENT OF RISK: PAST AND PRESENT

Home-care nurses today are likely to be sued for the same mistakes, and under the same legal doctrines, as are their colleagues in acute care settings. For whatever reasons, nurses sometimes fail to prevent clients from falling, or they administer medication incorrectly, or let obvious defects in machines go unnoticed, or provide inadequate supervision for other health-care workers, or carry out procedures poorly, or neglect to document that actions have met appropriate standards of care.

These are the mistakes that have resulted in legal actions against hospital-based nurses. It is likely that, at least in the near future, these are the mistakes for which home-care nurses will be sued. As the volume of clients seen by home-care agencies increases, as new machines go into homes, as sicker clients are sent home from the hospital sooner, risk increases for the home-care nurse.

Falls

Falls in the home can be the responsibility of the nurse if she neglects to obtain appropriate assessment information about the client. She is also responsible when, having obtained the correct information, she does not make proper decisions or does not communicate the information in a timely manner to some other appropriate decision-maker. Her chance of a legal problem increases as the quantity of information needed increases and as the speed with which it must be communicated increases.

Medication Administration

Nurses do not generally administer oral medication to clients in the home. Nevertheless, nurses are responsible for maintaining a current evaluation of the client's total medication picture, including a description of the client's need for information. In addition, a system must be devised to assure that the client or family has actually learned about the medication effects and side-effects. The nurse is also responsible for reviewing all medications a client is taking and for determining if inappropriate combinations are present.

The nurse is responsible for recording, during each visit, any changes that clients or physicians have made in medication, and for assessing the client's potential for side-effects. She is responsible for notifying the physician immediately, often by telephone from the client's home, of any present or potential problem. Added to this responsibility, nurses administer intramuscular, subcutaneous, and intravenous medications in the home and assess intended effects and potential or actual unwanted effects.

The management of medication administration poses the greater possible risk for increasing numbers of malpractice actions against community health nurses today. Yet systems for managing information about medication remain inadequate in many home-care agencies. A major reason for this problem lies in the difficulty of providing care through at least semi-traditional methods in a home setting where clients have autonomy.

Supervision of Machines

The increased use of sophisticated machines in the home involves nurses in issues concerning placement of responsibility when something goes wrong with the machine (Borovetz 1984). In this age of new technology, agency policies will include, for example, directives to nurses about how to seal a defective machine part in a package, whom to notify, and what to document.

There is risk, too, in inadequate education of clients and families concerning their responsibility in caring for, or detecting problems in, a machine. Written instructions for the client about correct machine operation,

and who to call if a problem occurs, are essential.

Supervision of Other Direct Care Providers

At the present time, by law and by tradition, the professional nurse coordinates care for clients served by the home-care agency. Implications of liability for breach of duty in the coordination function of the nurse have not been adequately explored. When another professional, a physical therapist for example, is accused by a client of malpractice, what responsibility will the nurse have as coordinator of care? The nurse could be liable if poor coordination contributed to the injury.

The responsibility for supervising nursing assistants is one which the profession has taken quite seriously. Policies among agencies differ, however, as to the tasks assigned to the nursing assistant. Some agencies, for instance, require assistants to obtain vital signs, including blood pressure; others do not allow assistants to obtain this information.

Differences in policy generally reflect different philosophies concerning just how the information is used. For instance, is the blood pressure reading a "piece of data" to be relayed, according to some set protocol, to a decision-maker? Or is this information only a small part of a comprehensive cardiovascular assessment? The risk is that an inadequate analysis of the appropriate use of the information will lead to a missed nursing diagnosis, resulting in harm to the client.

Procedures

Almost any nursing procedure, when done poorly, can prompt a lawsuit. An epileptic client suffers mouth injuries from biting on a glass thermometer; a client suffers colonic burns from an enema given with scalding water. As the procedures nurses perform become more complicated, as the numbers of procedures needed by each client increase, as the client comes home in poorer physical condition so that his tolerance for complex and time-consuming procedures is decreased, the legal risk for the nurse increases.

Documentation

Nursing literature has frequently addressed the need for improved documentation: to provide better care, to avoid court appearances, to provide data for research. There have been numerous articles concerning improved methods of documentation.

Nevertheless, home-care agencies frequently make decisions without viewing the choice of a documentation system as a rational need when coordinating the distribution of information. In this new age, overall policy must address what information is needed, by whom, for what purpose, how it is to be shared, and how it is to be stored.

FUTURE RISKS

It is obvious that our future risks are likely to increase as numbers of seriously ill clients come to us. To treat them, we will need to use new medicines, some of which may be experimental in nature.

For example, among these very sick clients there will be large numbers of newborns, infants, and children—age groups that have not generally been managed by home-care nurses in the recent past. The treatments they will need will involve the use of complex machines; many of these machines are so new that they have not yet been proved reliable. Other, sicker clients will include those with malignancies who are being treated at home with nutritional therapy and chemotherapy, and clients with bacterial disease requiring intensive intravenous antibiotic therapy.

It is reasonable to assume that more experimental drugs will be used in home therapy, and that numbers of clients with depressed immune systems will increase. These clients will require intensive physical and emotional care from home care nurses.

Based on this analysis of our past and present risks for litigation, and on knowledge of the dramatic changes in the business of home care, we can predict where the future may take us in our efforts to prevent legal action against nurses.

A more difficult issue remains, however. How do we deal with possible legal action? We need to find answers that will not only improve client care and decrease our risk of litigation, but will also preserve the integrity of the profession.

USING THE NURSING PROCESS TO ANALYZE RISK

When a nurse becomes aware that she may be at legal risk for a malpractice suit, anxiety can be diminished through a rational analysis of risk, using a problem-solving process. Since the process of problem solving with which the nurse is most familiar is the nursing process, the following hypothetical case will be analyzed through assessment, planning, intervention, and evaluation of the situation.

Case Study

Mrs. G is 78 years old and has a 15-year history of hypertension. She returned to her daughter's home one week ago after having been hospitalized with a "mild cerebrovascular accident."

Mr. T, a professional nurse, is visiting Mrs. G for the medically prescribed purpose, among others, of "monitoring medication." He takes and records Mrs. G's vital signs as she sits in her chair. He asks her if she is walking "better," to which she responds, "Yes, much better." He asks if she is taking her antihypertensive medication as prescribed and again she answers, "Yes."

The following day Mrs. G takes her blood pressure pill and diuretic at breakfast. On arising from the breakfast table, she becomes very dizzy and falls, breaking her hip. On her admission to the hospital emergency room, the nurse on duty discovers that Mrs. G is under the care of the home-care nurse, and telephones Mr. T to let him know what has happened. The emergency room nurse tells Mr. T that, on arrival in the emergency room, Mrs. G's blood pressure, taken when she was supine, was slightly low but within normal limits. The physician, however, suspecting that the medication may have contributed to the client's dizziness, has changed the medication order by discontinuing all antihypertensives until further evaluation has been made.

Given this information, Mr. T is able to begin to assess his situation for risk in a malpractice suit against him.

Assessment

Mr. T decides that, although the client and family were friendly toward him, there had not been time to develop a significant trust relationship with them. If the family believes that the client has been harmed by any act of the nurse, they may well initiate legal action. He also concludes that there is no reason to believe there would be any suggestion of criminal liability in this case.

In assessing whether or not a malpractice case could be successful, Mr. T reviews the four "D's" of malpractice.

Duty Did he owe a duty to this client? Clearly he did, because the client had been accepted by the agency, and he was employed to provide nursing care for the agency.

Breach of Duty Did he breach this duty? On consideration, Mr. T realizes that he did not fully assess Mrs. G. He did not take her blood pressure while she was standing and compare it to her sitting or lying pressure. He did not observe her while she stood, but took her word that she was "walking better." Although he was quite aware of the untoward effects of her medication, he did not advise her to stand slowly, nor did he caution her about the possibility of dizziness.

Would an expert nurse witness state that these actions were below the standard for a reasonably prudent nurse? Mr. T believes this would be the case. His conclusion is that he did not act as a reasonably prudent nurse should act in similar circumstances.

Damages Were there damages to the client? Obviously, the injuries to the client are unquestionable.

Direct Cause Direct cause will be the key issue in this case. The possibility is present that if Mr. T had taken Mrs. G's blood pressure in a standing position, it would have been essentially normal. If recorded as such there would have been less question of breach of duty in this case.

The physician's immediate change in the client's medication as soon as Mrs. G arrived in the emergency room would indicate that the physician may have believed a decrease in blood pressure from medication was a likely cause (or a contributing factor) to the fall. This would support a client contention of causal relationship, in that the nurse's omission of a standing blood pressure (information) on which to base a communication with the physician was the cause of the client's fall.

Plan

After assessing his legal situation, and concluding that he is at legal risk for a malpractice action, Mr. T will make a plan for protecting himself as much as possible.

Goals of the Plan

The goals of this plan will be to:

1. *Obtain legal advice.*
   Legal counsel should be sought. Depending on his malpractice insurance, he may discuss the situation with the attorney for his own carrier, or the attorney for his employer, or both.
2. *Obtain the assistance of his supervisor.*
   Mr. T should notify his supervisor immediately of the problem, and request legal counsel. Waiting until a formal charge is filed would, in this instance, be foolish.
3. *Assure that all relevant information about his actions and the client and family situation is written as soon as possible in his own personal record.*
   At this time, everything he can remember about the client, about his relationship with the client and the family, and about his actions and the reasons for his actions should be described, dated, and retained in Mr. T's own personal record for possible later use.
4. *Review the written record (client chart) for accuracy and potential implications for his defense.*
   Mr. T. will search for information that could be useful to him in his defense or could be used against him by the client. What he is seeking is any information that could break the presumption of the chain of events—information that would cast doubt on the assumption that his breach of duty caused Mrs. G's fall.

If, for instance, Mrs. G were alcoholic, with a recent history of alcohol abuse, this fact could conceivably be useful in his defense. On the other hand, such knowledge should have been incorporated into Mr. T's care plan, and would indicate an even greater responsibility to record accurate and complete blood pressure measurements.

If a neighbor of Mrs. G, also a client, says on his next visit, "It sure was too bad about Mrs. G's fall. I talked to her daughter right after it happened, and she told me that Mrs. G had spilled some milk at breakfast, and they had forgotten to wipe it up before she stood up," this should be recorded, in writing, in the nurse's personal record. The information should also be given to the supervisor and legal counsel.

Implementation

Mr. T will not, of course, discuss the potential problem with anyone except his supervisor and legal counsel at this point.

Evaluation

In this case, Mr. T will be involved in evaluating and changing his own practice behaviors. This example has not included an evaluation of agency policy. In all likelihood, the agency would also be named in a suit against Mr. T. For instance, if the agency had no written policy to the effect that all clients on antihypertensive medications should have their blood pressure taken sitting and standing, then the agency could also be held liable. And if Mr. T had a written history of reprimands for inadequate performance, the supervisor and the agency may both be held liable. □.

ACTIONS TO TAKE TO PROTECT AGAINST LITIGATION

While home-care agencies bear major responsibility in devising effective policies to protect the agency and its employees from a malpractice suit, some effective actions can be taken by the nurse.

ACTIONS BY THE INDIVIDUAL NURSE

As a professional nurse, the four major actions to be taken to assure preventive management of personal malpractice risk are choosing the right insurance; maintaining a quality practice; documenting professional actions; and participating in major policy decisions of the employing agency.

Choosing the Right Malpractice Insurance

Aspects of malpractice litigation of greatest concern to nurses will be state laws relating to malpractice and issues related to insurance coverage.

Relevant State Laws

Every nurse should be familiar with present and proposed legislation concerning malpractice. In addition to the nurse's state legislators, valuable information may be obtained from the professional association, home health-care associations, and from major insurance carriers in the area. Of particular importance to the home-care nurse should be information about proposed legislation that would limit the dollar amount of recovery by the plaintiff; change the statute of limitations for malpractice actions; establish screening panels for malpractice cases.

Issues Related to Coverage

Issues related to coverage include choosing a type of insurance and choosing an insurance that provides good value.

Types of Insurance. The two basic types of insurance coverage are "claims-made" and "occurrence." For "claims-made" insurance, the policy must be in effect when the suit is filed, even if several years have elapsed since the event occurred. Although this makes it necessary for nurses with this type of insurance to carry the policy even after retirement, continuation policies on claims-made malpractice insurance may be available at lower rates. Malpractice insurance of the "occurrence" type will provide coverage if premiums were paid at the time of the alleged occurrence of the incident, even if the nurse is no longer paying premiums on the policy.

Cushing points out that some policies require that the nurse notify the insurance carrier of an "incident," even if no suit has been filed (Cushing, Malpractice: Are you covered?, 1984). If this is not done, the company may later refuse to cover any costs of the litigation process or awards.

Value in Insurance. Rates of malpractice insurance are rising, as are the dollar amounts of coverage. In comparing insurance policies, it is important to note how much coverage is allowed, the conditions of the coverage, and the specific risks covered by the policy. It is interesting to note that, generally, malpractice insurance is available at lower rates through professional nursing associations.

MAINTAINING A QUALITY PRACTICE

Maintaining a quality practice involves practicing according to current nursing standards.

Knowledge

Since primary responsibility for quality client care rests with the nurse, it is important to know current regulations and standards, current and proposed legislation affecting practice, current and precedent-setting malpractice cases, current medications and treatments, and current agency policies related to client care.

Regulations and Standards

In addition to the nursing documents previously discussed, practicing nurses need access to Medicare and Medicaid regulations. Nurses should insist that copies of the documents important to their practice be available in the office. If they are not available, nurses can obtain their own personal copies of necessary documents. Many practicing nurses today do not even have a copy of their own nurse practice act available to them; no one but the nurse is to blame for this inattention to professional responsibility.

Legislation

Information on current and proposed legislation affecting home-care nurses is available. Membership in the national nursing organizations will provide nurses with essential information about legislation. (Most states also have state associations for home care, usually affiliated with the National Association for Home Care.)

Monitoring this mountain of information, however, is far too much for any one nurse. For help, nurses will need to depend on nursing association lobbyists at the national level. State nurses' associations, too, frequently employ lobbyists who can assist the nurse with this task. Many times nurses have worked with their legislators long enough so that the legislator and staff are aware of the special interests of nurses. Invaluable information is often obtained in this way.

Court Cases

Although information on current or recent malpractice cases would be very useful, such information is difficult to obtain. This is particularly true for cases settled out of court. Even when cases go to court, trial court opinions may not be published (Fiesta 1983). Organizations such as the National Association for Home Care may be able to assist nurses in keeping informed about current cases.

Medications and Treatments

Agencies are sometimes willing to "sell" inservice programs to home-care organizations not affiliated with the agency. Depending on the status of competition in the home-care business within the area, several agencies may join in efforts to develop continuing education programs. Hospitals often allow home-care agency personnel access to their inservice, particularly if they are members of the Hospital Satellite Network (HSN). Nurses can also obtain assistance from libraries and instructors in local nursing schools. Moreover, it is likely that nurses will spend more money and time on their own continuing education.

Documentation

While the organization as a whole must treat documentation as a system of information exchange and storage, each nurse must document her own actions in such a way as to leave no doubt that the client care provided met current standards. Provision of care and incident reports must be documented.

Care

Documentation of the care given, based on current standards, is the best defense in a legal action. Many systems in current use in home-care agencies do not provide sufficient "clues" or direction for documentation. Insufficient space for nurses to write on specific documents has also been a recurrent problem.

The documentation systems used by some home-care agencies are not only inadequate, but are legal disasters. For example, the system used in some agencies of applying "post-it notes" to chart pages is indefensible; notes fall off and are reapplied in the wrong place, or lost entirely.

The policy of the agency will offer no protection in court if a nurse's note is lost, so nurses must insist that the system used maintains a permanent record. Since the emphasis in home care has previously been on documentation to gain reimbursement, not prevention of litigation, this issue has not been sufficiently emphasized in many agencies.

A nurse can request a review of a sample of her own documentation by someone in the agency whose judgment she trusts. She can also try to obtain permission to have her notes reviewed by an outside person—an experienced nurse in an acute care setting, for example.

If the agency is not ready to address the documentation issue in a comprehensive way, the nurse may feel a need to manage information personally. In this case, the purchase of a personal computer system could be considered.

Incidents

As has been previously noted, the nurse or designated agency representative may be required to report to the insurance carrier any incident which could precipitate a legal action. This depends on the type of malpractice insurance carried and on state law. The nurse is also bound by agency policy in the reporting of an incident.

Within an agency, incident reports have one major function: to alert managers that an action has occurred that is unusual or has the potential for client harm. Obviously, this information should be kept confidential. A potential suit could become an actuality if a client becomes aware that a nurse believes a legal action could be initiated because of a nursing action.

Incident reports must be complete in every detail. While the incident itself is clearly documented in the client's clinical agency record, no reference to the fact that an incident report has been filed should be placed in the client's current "chart."

Only one original copy of the report should be made; this copy will usually be filed either in the office of the agency person designated as responsible for risk management, or in the office of the legal counsel for the agency. Insurance carriers may also receive a copy. In some cases, the courts may find that these incident reports are "discoverable," or available to a prosecuting attorney.

Participation in Policy Decisions

Policies of the agency control the daily practice of the nurse. Policies at state and national levels affect the nurse less directly, but yet significantly.

Nurses must influence these policies. Such influence will demand a commitment, over time, to being active in the political system. The payoff is in seeing the emergence of legislation and regulations that support quality client care and the ongoing development of the nursing profession.

In addition to requesting membership on agency policy committees, nurses can pool their information by creating or participating in a forum for community home-care nurses. This group, while recognizing the problems of competition within an area, can share information of benefit to all.

ACTIONS TO BE TAKEN BY MANAGEMENT

The possibility exists that the actual care provided by nurses and other direct care personnel in an agency is inadequate. Professional personnel may not hold the appropriate credentials or may not know essential information about new treatment for a disease or operation of a new machine.

There are also unique client factors to be addressed by managers in home care. These arise from the fact that health-care providers are guests in the home and cannot ultimately control the compliance of a client and family. Nor can a provider assure that quality care is consistently provided by unsupervised family care-givers. In addition, environmental factors related to housing, cleanliness, and availability of utilities influence client outcomes.

COMPREHENSIVE RISK MANAGEMENT PROGRAM

An effective risk management program should be viewed as essential in today's home health care business environment. With careful analysis of risks, an agency should be able to develop an economical yet comprehensive system that will improve the quality of client care and keep litigation at a minimum.

Definition of Risk Management in Home Care

Risk management may be viewed as a set of activities designed to address all risks to which an organization is exposed, with the aim of protecting the organization's income and assets (Gould et al 1986). Identifying, preventing, and controlling all risks of economic loss due to litigation are the primary activities of a litigation risk management (LRM) program.

Risk Management and Quality Assurance

The aspects of a quality assurance program designed to discover and resolve problems must be an inherent part of any LRM program. However, quality assurance has the broad goal of promoting optimal care while the LRM concerns prevention of loss due to legally unacceptable care. Integrating those

quality assurance and LRM activities in a systematic approach to identifying and resolving problems should enable the agency to change policies and procedures and to initiate in-service education.

Costs and Benefits of an LRM Program

A decision to institute a litigation risk management program in an agency will have serious implications regarding costs and benefits. The development, implementation, and evaluation of any such program, no matter how basic its design, will be costly. Costs will arise from involvement of significant amounts of time for administration and staff. Costs of the educational component will include time lost from income-generating activities.

Benefits of programs aimed at prevention are always difficult to assess in financial terms. Some benefit to an agency will inevitably occur through the process of carrying out an activity that provides information needed to make quality decisions. Beginning a program of risk management is likely to provide a sense of direction for all of the employees within an organization. An increase in the good will of the community and of clients as a result of such a program can also be anticipated.

What Are Its Objectives?

The goal of an LRM program is to minimize the potential for economic loss arising from litigation. This goal can be accomplished by meeting the following five program objectives (Gould et al 1986):

1. Reduce the probability of all types of compensable events.
2. Reduce the severity of loss from an incident.
3. Avoid risks where feasible.

4. Retain risk when severity of loss is insignificant.
5. Transfer risk where possible.

Who Is Responsible?

Responsibility for a successful LRM program must rest with one person who will coordinate litigation risk management activities, including the education component of the system. In a small agency, the risk manager is probably the chief executive officer (CEO) or owner; in a large agency, the risk manager may be on the CEO's staff.

What Are Significant Issues Related to Cost and Management?

Coordination of activities and responsibilities may best occur through an interdisciplinary committee that will include top level managers from administrative, personnel, financial, and clinical departments. This committee will be responsible for policy development and overview of LRM activities. Legal counsel may be included on a regular or on an intermittent basis.

Development of LRM Program

Medicare-certified home-health agencies will find that they already have certain crucial pieces of a risk management program in place. A comprehensive program can then be built incrementally by adding to existing activities. Budget allocation for design, implementation, and management of the LRM program will reflect the seriousness of the agency's commitment to litigation loss control. The Joint Commission on Accreditation of Hospitals (JCAH) home-health agency standards contain some standards relating to risk management and clearly outline the minimum risk management program (3rd revision, to be in effect in 1988).

Process Model for Use in Development of the LRM

A process model for an agency to use in identification of risk and in implementation of an LRM plan has been suggested by Gould and associates (Gould et al 1986). The five-step approach suggested is outlined here.

1. Analyze area of exposure for its risk potential.
2. Suggest a set of preventive strategies likely to decrease risk to acceptable levels.
3. Establish a plan for identifying and responding to unanticipated problems that have escaped preventive efforts.
4. Design protocols for addressing legal questions once an actual suit has arisen.
5. Activate a comprehensive evaluation plan permeating the entire LRM program, which effectively utilizes timely, accurate information for decision-making.

SPECIFIC MANAGEMENT POLICIES UNDER CONSIDERATION

DOCUMENTATION POLICIES

Policies related to documentation will be among the first to be addressed in a new LRM program. Developing a documentation system that is easy to use and sufficiently thorough to demonstrate adherence to all relevant procedures and standards will prove an invaluable asset for both the individual and the agency.

Documentation of Educational Efforts

Among the first areas to be addressed by agencies is the documentation of all educational efforts on behalf of staff and clients.

The agency must provide client education materials that are clear and comprehensive, thus enabling all professionals and technicians involved in education to instruct clients in a consistent manner. Clients or family members may check the written materials for guidance between visits of the professionals.

Policies Related to Client Care Responsibility

Direct client care has been discussed earlier as having serious litigation risk potential. Having a clearly identified clinical care manager who coordinates the client's care can reduce the possibility of legal action.

Policies Related to Reporting of Incidents

In the event that all prevention and problem-resolution efforts have failed, the client's official clinical agency record should be sent immediately to the risk manager for safekeeping; the risk manager will notify the chief executive officer, legal counsel, and the insurance company.

Clinical staff should be informed of a lawsuit in the event they might encounter the client in a clinical or nonclinical setting. Staff may inadvertently provide opinions and information that could be used as evidence against the agency. To prevent this, all communications are directed to the identified risk manager.

POLICIES ADDRESSING CONSISTENCY IN TECHNIQUE

Promoting consistency among staff in following basic technical procedures (obtaining vital signs, handwashing, dressing changes, bag technique) will provide baseline protection to the agency if an issue of quality care is raised. Policy manuals developed to assure consistency must reflect current standards of client care.

There is a legal risk when using photographs or detailed diagrams of equipment in policy manuals. If the equipment actually used in the agency is different from the equipment pictured, a case could be made that a nurse did not follow agency policy. Since today's technological environment changes too quickly to allow for development of new policy manuals for each new piece of equipment, only general diagrams of equipment should be included in policy manuals.

The practice, common in smaller agencies, of using a published procedure book with pictures is obviously risky. The written manual needs to be specific enough to provide direction to the nurse, but general enough to allow for safe variations in procedures and equipment.

Another type of policy important in today's home-care agency is related to communicable disease control. For example, the Centers for Disease Control (CDC) guidelines for disposal of used parenteral needles recommend that no needle ever be recapped (Centers for Disease Control 1985).

The policy in many home-care agencies today not only permits, but encourages or actually mandates, the recapping of needles. Agencies have not adhered to the CDC guideline (standard) because, in part at least, systems of simple, economical, and safe disposal of used needles have not been available. However, if a staff member should sue the agency for harm incurred (hepatitis B, for instance) from following an agency policy contrary to CDC guidelines, the suit would have a good chance of success.

In nursing there are many ways to accomplish the same task, all of which may be satisfactory. However, we have reached that point in our history of litigation where we must value consistency among nurses more than independence if we are to protect nursing against the suspicion of the public and against legal action.

POLICIES REGARDING EQUIPMENT

The agency must provide sufficient equipment to do the job. For example, agencies that allow nurses to take only one urinary catheter into a home are putting the agency and the nurse at unnecessary legal risk.

SUGGESTIONS FOR FUTURE STUDY

Nursing research in the area of malpractice litigation could be of benefit to nursing and health care in the USA. However, since research is costly, and answers are needed quickly, precious resources must not be wasted on poorly designed or poorly conceptualized research. The right questions must be asked and must be answered in an efficient manner. Some important questions to be addressed immediately are these:

Who Is Being Sued?

All legal actions concerning nurses must be considered, whether or not these actions are settled out of court. Information must be obtained and disseminated while preserving the anonymity of the principles in the cases.

Present Risk of Suit?

Have more suits been brought against nurses involved in home chemotherapy than against those who are pulmonary specialists, for instance? Or, is the risk of suit unrelated to specific specialties?

Factors Contributing to Suits Against Home-Care Nurses?

A descriptive study of families and clients might yield important information about *who* sues, and *when,* and *how* the decision was made to sue. It will be important in such research to gain the cooperation of plaintiffs, even if the case is settled out of court.

Knowledge of Home-Care Nurses Re: State Malpractice Laws, Case Law, Precedent, Regulations?

Information concerning nursing knowledge would be relatively easy to obtain. Nurses would want to participate in such a study because they would want to know the results.

Curriculum Efforts To Better Prepare Nurses for Legal Risks of Home Care?

The practice of nursing is moving into the community, but we are not presently educating nurses to face the legal realities of changing practice. Nursing programs in which legal accountability is an identifiable thread in the curriculum would provide a service to the profession by sharing and publicizing objectives and learning activities.

Present Status of LRM Program Development in Home-Care Agencies?

What pieces of a comprehensive program are presently in place in home-care agencies around the country? Is there a correlation between the litigation risk management program and size of the agency, type of organization, funding sources, or length of time the agency has been in business? What constraints are experienced by agencies related to the development of comprehensive risk management programs? Research of national scope could be supported by government, insurance companies, and national home-care groups, as well as other interested organizations.

Certain Nursing Diagnoses To Pose Special Legal Risks?

Is there a specific nursing diagnosis or complex of diagnoses that would provide an early warning system, identifying clients who may need special attention or intervention to prevent legal actions? It may be that the use of nursing diagnosis in the home-care setting is not sufficiently sophisticated at present to provide adequate information, but the possibility of such research could definitely be considered for the future.

SUMMARY

As home-care nurses throughout the country begin to view in a new way their risk of being sued for malpractice, that risk will become manageable. The key to successful management of any risk is full awareness of the potential harm and the ability to take action and protect against the risk. Working as individuals and as members of a professional group, home-care nurses can make and influence decisions to protect against malpractice litigation in a changing world.

For many years home-care nurses have known that their practice was "special." They are invited guests in the homes of their clients. Nevertheless, these clients expect the nurse to be competent in the care she provides. That is, the nurse must have the knowledge, skills, and judgment to help the client. While advice must be given, and is expected, the nurse often does not know if information is used or advice followed. Evidence shows that a client who perceives the nurse as kind and caring is less likely to sue. Taking time with clients, listening, and showing respect are proactive responses.

Nurses are most certainly accountable for the quality of the advice, information, and physical care provided. Yet nurses are now facing a period of increased accountability for assuring, where possible, that the *results* of taking the advice are results the client desires.

In the face of difficulties encountered in a fast-paced, highly technological home-care environment, the most effective defense for the nurse is likely to be recognition of the value of a therapeutic nurse–client relationship. Could it be that the "new age" is forcing nurses to put their faith in the older values of caring and trust?

If this is true, then home-care nurses can go forward confidently, knowing that no matter what else changes, it is the relationship that is primary. Our history, our future, is in the maintenance of that relationship.

References

Bernzweig E: The Nurse's Liability for Malpractice: A Programmed Course, 3rd ed. New York, McGraw-Hill, 1981

Borovetz S: Biomedical equipment problems: Strategy for the hospital and physician. Hosp Law Newsletter 1(11): 1, 1984

Creighton H: Legal implications of the DRG's. Nurs Manage 16(7): 17–19, 1985

Cushing M: Key court cases: Where are they now? Am J Nurs 84(12): 1469–1470, 1984

Cushing M: Malpractice: Are you covered? Am J Nurs 84(8): 985–986, 1984

Department of Health and Human Services/Public Health Service, Centers for Disease Control: Recommendations for preventing transmission of infection with human T-lymphotropic type III/lymphadenopathy associated virus in the workplace. MMWR 34: 681–686, 691–694, 1985

Fiesta J: The Law and Liability: A Guide for Nurses. New York, John Wiley & Sons, 1983

Gould F, Ginsberg A, Perdew S: Litigation risk management: Today's home care challenge. Caring V(9): 74–83, 1986

Northrup C: Home health care: Changing legal perspectives. Nurs Outlook 34(5): 256, 1986

Perdew S: Litigation in home care: What the future holds. CARING V(9): 84–88, 1986

Southwick A: The Law of Hospital and Health Care Administration. Ann Arbor, University of Michigan Health Administration Press, 1978

Weinstein S: Specialty teams in home care. Am J Nurs 84(3): 342–345, 1984

PATIENT TEACHING

4

Barbara Kovalcin Piskor

The need for client education and health teaching requires little justification. Indeed most health professionals have a favorite story about a client's misunderstanding of a particular illness, treatment, or health fact. The basis for most of these stories is that teaching, real teaching, and learning, real learning, never occurred. The knowledge deficit remained and the targeted health behavior was never achieved.

Case Study

Mrs. A had a Hickman catheter inserted for the purpose of administering chemotherapy and drawing blood for laboratory tests. On a home visit, the nurse discovered an infection at the exit site. The area was edematous and the patient had a low-grade fever. Mrs. A had noticed the swelling but had not called the nurse. Why not? The nurse had told her to call at "the first sign of an infection" but had not taught Mrs. A what these signs were. What had occurred? Mrs. A thought redness and drainage always accompanied infection and the nurse

assumed that a college-educated mother of three knew the signs of infection! □

While this anecdote emphasizes that

- Telling is not teaching, and
- Never assume

it also stresses that the client/family requiring home health care usually has many knowledge needs. These must be identified with learning methods recognized and teaching strategies implemented before they are able to carry out many aspects of care. Unless round-the-clock, private-duty nursing is desired and available, the client, family, or a friend is the primary care-giver. The home health nurse must teach the care-giver about all aspects of the care.

Health education is any planned combination of teaching methods designed to facilitate voluntary adaptations of behavior conducive to health. Patient education is a subset of health education. It orients itself to secondary and tertiary prevention such as early case finding, disease treatment, and rehabilitation. (Green 1980)

51

The profession of nursing has gradually evolved to include health/client teaching as an integral part of its function. As early as 1918, statements from the National League for Nursing showed concern for the teaching function of nursing and a 1937 curriculum guide stated, "The nurse is essentially a teacher and an agent of health in whatever field she may be working" (Redman 1984).

In practice, however, many nurses have not seen themselves as teachers. In her classic early 1960s study of the teaching activities of the nurse practitioner, Margaret L. Pohl found that 37.2% (107 nurses) of her study population did not complete her questionnaire, indicating, on follow-up, that they gave direct nursing care and did not teach (Pohl 1968).

Teaching has always been central to community health nursing. The primary role of the visiting nurse is teaching. This was recognized by English leaders in nursing by the mid-1800s when they stressed teaching families about sanitation, cleanliness, and sick care. When the first visiting nurse associations were established in Buffalo, Boston, and New York during the late 1800s, teaching was viewed as a necessary way of extending their services (Redman 1984).

This long tradition, combined with today's universal expectation of teaching within nursing, brings both professional and legal responsibilities to the activity. Health-care agencies and individual professionals have been held liable for failing to instruct clients (Cushing 1984). Despite these strong motivators, some nurses continue to avoid teaching opportunities or respond only to the most pressing learning needs. The following information details some of the reasons contributing to the problem.

WHY SOME NURSES DON'T TEACH

1. *Do not view themselves as teachers.* The activity and role expectation must be stressed not only in schools of nursing but also in job expectations and new staff orientation.

2. *Have low self-esteem and do not believe they have important information to share.* Unfortunately, this problem plagues female-dominated professions. It needs to be addressed in both pre-service and in-service education.

3. *Do not know what to teach.* This is, perhaps, the most easily addressed problem since basic information of the cognitive variety requires pure transmission of knowledge without attitude or motivational interference.

4. *Do not know how to teach.* Many nurses believe that telling a client is the same as teaching. These nurses need to learn *how* to teach.

5. *Presume the client knows the information.* This is a particular problem with clients from an above-average socioeconomic status or who have a college or beyond education. Obviously, a mechanical engineer, even if he has become the company chief executive officer, does not necessarily understand diabetes.

6. *Presume the client is not motivated or interested in learning.* Sometimes nonverbal communication and/or socioeconomic status make professionals assume incorrect levels of interest.

7. *Think teaching is too much trouble or takes too much time.* This is unacceptable practice and must be altered through employer intervention, peer pressure, or reassignment.

8. *Do not receive the system support necessary to be an effective teacher.* For teaching to be carried out uniformly it must be

an activity that is rewarded and one that is easily carried out on a day-to-day basis.

THE HOME AS A SETTING FOR TEACHING AND LEARNING

The fact that the nurse is a guest in the client's home has an overriding influence not only on the total care plan but also on the teaching/learning climate. The nurse who does not involve the client and primary care-giver in the development of the teaching plan may find disparate outcomes or even a closed door on her next visit. The client is, indeed, in the driver's seat! The following information outlines advantages and disadvantages of teaching in the home setting.

Advantages of the Home Setting

* *The reality of the situation.* No "mock" setup is required. The actual chair the client must learn to transfer to is in the room. The cooking baster that will be used to irrigate the wound is available for demonstration.
* *A less anxious client and family.* It is recognized that learning progresses more quickly in familiar, reality-based surroundings. Sometimes even the anxiety and questions from the primary care-giver about whether or not the care can be managed at home can contribute to learning motivation. Too much anxiety, of course, works against learning. If this occurs, the nurse should carry out the care while helping to decrease the anxiety and delaying teaching until the next visit, if possible.
* *Opportunities for health promotion and illness care teaching.* After the immediate crisis abates, the nurse can respond to general health teaching concerns of the client and family while continuing to visit for the primary skilled care activity.
* *Being on the client's turf.* This contributes

to the learning climate. The nurse who is able to demonstrate acceptance of the client and his environment through verbal and nonverbal communication enhances learning.

Disadvantages of the Home Setting

* *The time-limited nature of the visit.* An injection required "as circumstances dictate" (*prn*) challenges the nurse's timing since a demonstration followed by a return demonstration is mandatory. Bladder training and Foley catheter removal are also difficult since re-visits, even on the same day, must be considered in terms of geography and timing.
* *The effect of the burden of care.* The physical care, emotional drain, and time commitments required of a care-giver when there is a seriously ill person at home are great. The home health nurse must teach an often overburdened and sometimes reluctant care-giver. The nurse can help relieve this stress by recognizing it, involving several family members/friends in the care, and anticipating respite needs. However, a primary home care-giver should be identified to lessen confusion and communication difficulties.
* *Limited equipment and resources.* The nurse who learns to modify dressing changes creatively and to adapt a third floor walk-up to the needs of an intravenous therapy patient can turn this liability into an asset. The basic teaching/learning process is, of course, the same in any health-care setting. However, the variety of client needs and home situations plus the fact that, in most instances, the nurse is the lone professional visiting the client brings an additional challenge. Most home health nurses function as generalists and may visit various types of clients on any given day. The nurse may teach exercises to the 80-year-old

woman who fractured her hip, pain management to the wife of a 45-year-old cancer client, intravenous antibiotic methods to the 30-year-old client with osteomyelitis, ventilator care to a family member of a syringomyelia client, a sodium-restricted diet to the 60-year-old cardiac client, and insulin injections plus total diabetic care to the juvenile diabetic. Combining all of this with teaching plan accommodations for clients from a cross section of socioeconomic settings, educational levels, and ethnic backgrounds requires maximum flexibility and skill.

EDUCATIONAL DIAGNOSIS

Client education, though historically a recognized component of health care, has been highlighted in recent years as knowledge from the field of education and has combined with health-belief theory and scientific study. Together this has given validity to the process of educational diagnosis and client teaching. The process of health education helps clients bridge the gap between knowledge and action since the acquisition of knowledge alone does not necessarily lead to action (Figure 4-1).

In order to select the appropriate intervention, the nurse must make an educational diagnosis. Making such a diagnosis parallels the nursing process. A systematic assessment, diagnosis, goal establishment, intervention, and evaluation occur. Green, a leading health educator, defines an educational diagnosis as *the delineation of factors that predispose, enable, and reinforce a specific health behavior* (Green 1980). The educational diagnosis, in effect, becomes an important as nursing and medical diagnoses. All contribute to the total palliative, curative, or health-promotive picture of the client.

Making an educational diagnosis means assessing client and care priorities, influenc-

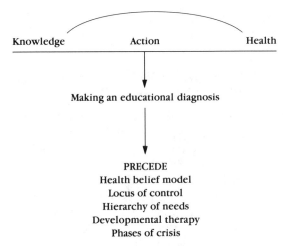

Figure 4-1. Health education bridges gap.

ing factors, health beliefs, psychological controls, needs, and crisis orientation. These considerations determine the patient's readiness to learn, psychologically, physiologically, and experientially.

Case Study

On her first home visit to Mr. B, the nurse determined, after talking with him and his daughter, that pain control was the priority care issue. A medication order permitted morphine injections *prn*. His daughter was initially willing to learn, but she said he didn't want her to give him injections. She then became hesitant about learning and said "I thought only nurses gave injections."

Possible nurse responses:

1. "I can teach your daugher to give you injections safely. You don't need to worry about it."
2. "The doctor wants you to receive these injections and I can't always visit you when you need them. There's no other way."
3. "Have you had experience with morphine injections? Tell me about it."

Using Approach #3, the nurse found that he received many morphine injections in the hospital. They left him drowsy; he disliked this because he wanted to be more in control and to be able to talk with his grandchildren. After discussion with him, his daughter, and his physician, Brompton's mixture and relaxation therapy using visual imagery was utilized.

The educational diagnosis was not the daughter's unwillingness to learn, but the patient's desire to stay in control. Likewise, while the primary nursing diagnosis was "Alteration in Comfort: Pain," a secondary diagnosis might have been "Ineffective Coping: Individual and Family." ☐

HEALTH BEHAVIOR: RELEVANT THEORIES

A sound health-teaching plan must consider not only the physical care priorities of the acutely ill client at home, but also relevant education, health belief, and behavioral science theories. Theories such as the health-belief model, locus of control, hierarchy of needs, development stages, and phases of crises provide health professionals with an understanding of—and an assessment base for—a client's readiness or motivation to learn. Health-related actions seem dependent on motivational levels, since many studies in health education demonstrate that knowledge alone seldom leads to action (Suchman 1967).

HEALTH-EDUCATION PLANNING MODEL

PRECEDE

PRECEDE is a health-education planning model developed by Green and colleagues. It utilizes a sequential process based on the consideration of multiple factors.

PRECEDE is an acronym for *predisposing, reinforcing,* and *enabling causes* in *educational diagnosis* and *evaluation.* This planning model starts with the desired goal or outcome and works back to original causes. This is a seven-phase process with applicability to individuals and groups (Green 1980, Redman 1984). Phase 4 and its various factors are especially relevant since these might be the etiology of the primary or secondary nursing diagnosis.

Phase 1: Consider the quality of life for the group or individual involved.

Phase 2: Identify specific health problems that appear to be contributing to the problems noted in Phase 1 and select the most pressing or resolvable problem.

Phase 3: Identify the specific health-related behaviors that appear to be linked to the health problem chosen.

Phase 4: Categorize the factors that seem to have direct impact on the behavior selected in Phase 2 into

Predisposing factors: any characteristics of the patient or community that motivate behavior related to health. For example, attitudes, beliefs, values, and perceptions that facilitate or hinder motivation for change.

Enabling factors: any characteristics of the environment that facilitate or block health behavior. These are usually created by societal forces or systems.

Reinforcing factors: any reward or punishment following or anticipated as a consequence of a health behavior. These are related to the feedback the learner receives from others resulting in the encouragement or discouragement of behavioral change.

Phase 5: Decide exactly which of these factors is to be the focus of the intervention.
Phase 6: Select interventions and assess problems and resources.
Phase 7: Evaluate.

HEALTH-BELIEF MODEL

The Health-Belief Model (HBM) is a paradigm used to predict and explain health behavior based on a value-expectancy theory. It provides a framework for understanding why individuals do or do not engage in preventive and sick-role behavior. Studies demonstrate its helpfulness in predicting the acceptance of health and medical care recommendations.

The HBM (Figure 4-2) was developed in the early 1950s by a group of social psychologists at the U.S. Public Health Service in order to understand the failure of persons to seek screening tests for the early identification of health problems or to practice disease-prevention activities. Later HBM was applied to clients' response to symptoms and compliance with medical regimens. (Becker 1974, 1977).

HBM considers the individual's perceptions, modifying factors, and the likelihood of action. This allows for both readiness and motivation to play a role in health action. The following example, involving a diabetic client who needs to balance insulin, diet, and foot care with the likelihood of gangrene complications and amputations, illustrates the perceptual factors emphasized in the Health Belief Model.

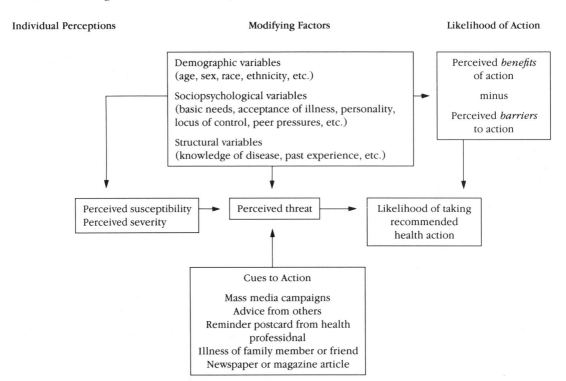

Figure 4-2. Health belief model. (Adapted from Becker MH et al: Selected psychosocial models and correlates of individual health-related behaviors. Med Care 15:27–46, 1977)

Perceived susceptibility. Does he believe that an amputation "could never happen?"

Perceived severity. Does he believe that losing a leg is significant? Would it influence his preferred life-style? Are there secondary gains that would be achieved?

Perceived benefits. Does he believe that the insulin, diet, and foot care reduce complications? Or does he believe there is no relationship?

Perceived barriers. Does a balanced diabetic regimen fit into his activities of daily living? Does the risk of losing "drinking buddies" mean more than the possible, future loss of a leg?

In addition, modifying factors such as demographic, sociopsychological and knowledge variables and cues to action such as peer advice, mass media campaigns, family illness, and provider reminder cards play a role.

Recent studies "provide substantial empirical support for the HBM with findings from prospective studies at least as favorable as those obtained from retrospective research. 'Perceived barriers' proved to be the most powerful of the HBM dimensions across the various study designs and behaviors. While both were important overall, 'perceived susceptibility' was a stronger contributor to understanding preventive health behaviors than sick-role behaviors, while the reverse was true for 'perceived benefits.' 'Perceived severity' produced the lowest overall significance ratios; however, while only weakly associated with preventive health behaviors, this dimension was strongly related to sick-role behaviors" (Janz and Becker 1984).

LOCUS OF CONTROL

A social learning theory developed by Rotter forms the base for locus of control and its influence on health-related behaviors. Many health educators believe, and some studies support, the theory that individuals can do a great deal to promote, maintain, or regain their health. Rotter's theory states that "the potential for a behavior to occur in any specific psychological situation is a function of the expectancy that the behavior will lead to a particular reinforcement in that situation and the value of that reinforcement" (Rotter 1975).

The application of this theory leads to the belief that reinforcement is either under the control of the individual (termed *internal*) such as a positive life outlook and control of destiny or under the control of outside forces such as fate, luck, chance, or powerful others (termed *external*). This is referred to as the internal or external locus of control (Wallston and Wallston 1978).

Research efforts are still in an early stage in applying and evaluating this theory, but it serves as the foundation of many health-education techniques. Relaxation therapy and imagery are two examples. The theory has application to health-related behaviors to promote, maintain, or regain health.

In considering this theory, one needs to assess whether the previously discussed diabetic client believes it is his fate to have a leg amputated or whether his actions can possibly avoid this consequence. Mr. B, who was having difficulty with pain control, desired control over his situation and believed he could influence it. His strong internal locus of control made relaxation therapy a viable alternative.

HIERARCHY OF NEEDS

Most nursing students have studied Maslow's theory related to human needs (Maslow 1962). He organized these needs in a pyramid with physiological or basic survival needs at the bottom of the hierarchy. Safety needs are next, followed by the need to love and to feel loved and to belong. The next higher need is for self-esteem. All of these lead to the need for self-actualization (Figure 4-3).

The client with limited income and no third-party reimbursement for sterile suction catheters is likely to reuse equipment rather than go without daily food. Sometimes medication is bypassed or taken only every other day, even if prescribed daily, when there is insufficient money to support other basic needs. Compliance is not the issue; rather, insufficient funds are the culprit.

DEVELOPMENTAL THEORY

Erik Erikson's theory of development is a psychosocial model that presents eight stages of development, with each stage presenting certain crises or conflicts to which the individual must adjust (Table 4-1). The degree of adjustment influences the way the person handles crises and conflicts at the next and subsequent stages (Craig 1980).

If the diabetic client is not able to achieve a view of himself as a contributing person during his years of middle age, he may "give up" and feel that it does not matter if he has both legs or not—or if he lives or dies.

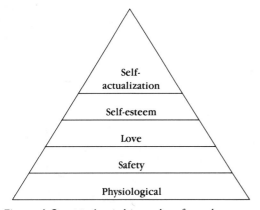

Figure 4-3. Maslow's hierarchy of needs.

TABLE 4.1 Erickson's Theory of Development

Life Stage	Life Stage Tasks
Infant	Sense of trust *vs.* mistrust
Toddler	Sense of autonomy *vs.* shame and doubt
Preschool	Sense of initiative *vs.* guilt
School age	Sense of industry *vs.* inferiority
Adolescent	Sense of identity *vs.* role confusion
Young adult	Sense of intimacy *vs.* isolation
Middle-aged adult	Sense of generativity *vs.* stagnation
Older adult	Sense of integrity *vs.* despair

PHASES OF CRISES

Since many of the clients and families visited by the home health nurse are grappling with a catastrophic illness, theories related to the phases of crisis and the stages of dying are important to consider. A theoretical model (Table 4-2) useful with clients who have incurred a physical disability or a diagnosis requiring major life-style adjustment is one that looks at the psychologic phases of crises (Fink 1967).

Much has been written about Dr. Elizabeth Kubler-Ross' five stages of dying (Kubler-Ross 1969). She identified the following: (1) denial—"No, not me . . ."; (2) Anger—"Why me?"; (3) Bargaining—"Yes, me but . . ."; (4) Depression—"Yes, me . . ."; and (5) Acceptance. Clients and families are likely to pass through, and sometimes repeat, these stages. They need to be considered as teaching needs surface.

Facts or activities taught prior to the last stage in both Fink's and Kubler-Ross' theories simply are not learned. However, the reality

TABLE 4.2 Phases of Crises

Phase	Reality Perceptions	Emotional Experience
Shock (stress)	Perceived as overwhelming	Panic; anxiety: helplessness
Defensive threat	Avoidance of reality; wishful thinking; denial	Indifference or euphoria (except repression when challenged, in which case, anger, low anxiety)
Acknowledgement (renewed stress)	Facing reality; facts impose themselves	Depression with apathy or agitation; bitterness; mourning; high anxiety; possibility of suicide
Adaptation and change	New reality testing	Gradual increase in satisfying experience; gradual lowering of anxiety

of care for the acutely ill at home sometimes demands that teaching be initiated before the final stage. The teaching effect from both of these theories is that repetition is necessary, not only to reinforce information but also, sometimes, for it to be heard for the first time.

The family care-giver who insists on maintaining maximum pressure in the client's cuffed tracheostomy tube may believe that erosion will not be a problem since "the tube won't be necessary when he gets well." This defensive retreat interferes with putting knowledge into action. The nurse who acknowledges how the family member might be feeling reinforces the teaching, and discusses a possible referral for counseling and/or care-giver supports, thus using this theoretical information in a very pragmatic way. On the surface, the primary nursing diagnosis may have appeared to be a "Knowledge Deficit" or "Noncompliance;" however, it might really have been "Fear" or "Ineffective Coping."

THE PROCESS OF TEACHING AND LEARNING

Teaching is the activity of helping another person learn while learning is usually defined as the acquisition of knowledge or skills.

Teaching and learning are interactive processes with each dependent on the other and each requiring active involvement of the other so that behavioral outcomes can be achieved. Teaching and learning do not stand alone but rather are dependent on learning methods tailored to the knowledge needs of clients and families.

LEARNING METHODS

There are two methods by which persons learn. One is through information-processing and the other is by experience. Both methods are influenced by the previously described internal and external factors such as health beliefs, education, age, readiness, peers, and others.

Information Processing

In order for persons to change behavior utilizing the interactive teaching/learning approach, they must process information in a sequential format. The learner must be "exposed" to the new information, listen/hear the message and comprehend it, accept and retain the information. Only then can the knowledge be translated into action. See Table 4-3 for information processing and related teaching considerations.

Experiential Learning

This method is popularly termed the "trial and error" method or "learning by experience." This is a time-consuming, slow method of learning that requires a great deal of self-motivation. However, it is learning that is not likely to be forgotten. One of the advantages of working with adults is that the teacher can and must build the information-processing method onto an already existing experience base.

TABLE 4.3 Information Processing and Related Teaching Considerations

	Learner	Teaching Considerations
Step 1.	Be EXPOSED to new information.	Barriers to availability and accessibility of new information must be removed.
Step 2.	ATTEND to the message.	Message is denied or rejected due to an emotional reaction to the health problem. Client is not ready to learn.
Step 3.	COMPREHEND the meaning of the communication.	Sometimes too little time is spent, or technical information is used, or no opportunity for questions is allowed.
Step 4.	ACCEPT the intent of the message.	Interference with learning can be attitudes to health or of health personnel, health problem, or prescribed behaviors don't work into preferred life-style. Suggestions relate new behavior to an old, favorable attitude. Attitude change is helped by: small group discussions with peers; health worker seen as peer or viewed as highly creditable or empathetic, increasing the perceived severity and susceptibility to the problem/disease and involvement of family members.
Step 5.	RETAIN given information.	The first third of education is most remembered; one half is usually forgotten. Reinforcement and follow-up are essential through printed materials, revisits, and family involvement.

Adapted by Health Education Center, Pittsburgh, PA, from McGuire GH: Attitude change: The information processing paradigm. Physician's Patient Educ Newsletter 1: 7–8, 1979.

Bloom's Taxonomy

Psychologists and educators classify the types of learning outcome behaviors into three areas: (1) cognitive, dealing with knowledge and intellectual abilities; (2) affective, including attitudes, values, and feelings; and (3) psychomotor, dealing with motor skills. This taxonomy was first described in the literature by Bloom (1956). Further work has related it to behaviorally stated educational objectives.

The cognitive and psychomotor areas generally move from simple to complex while the affective areas increase in intensity of internalization or commitment to a feeling (Redman 1984). For example, the cognitive domain usually progresses in this fashion: basic knowledge or identification ability . . . comprehension . . . application . . . analysis . . . synthesis . . . evaluation. Simple tasks and procedures should be taught first, with a gradual progression to the complex. Handwashing techniques and clean *vs.* dirty should be taught before teaching a suction procedure.

After the procedure is taught, using demonstration and return demonstration, the next step is to present a problem situation to allow for analysis, synthesis and evaluation. Examples for testing synthesizing skills and evaluating cognitive learning could include the following:

Case Studies

In working with a recently bedfast client related to physical reconditioning, the nurse would first present the facts about immobility, then relate these to movement and exercise. To evaluate, she could ask the question, "If you stay in bed for several more weeks, what can you expect to happen to your body?"

After teaching the use of a manual resuscitation bag and related problem solving to the primary home care-giver of a ventilator-dependent client, the nurse could ask "What would you do if the ventilator stopped functioning?" □

The affective domain moves from receiving the information to responding then valuing, organizing, and utilizing. The client who begins to ask questions related to the dangers of immobility and then gradually changes behavior to some regular activity demonstrates progress in the affective area.

The psychomotor or skill domain moves from a basic perception or recognition to a set or ability to demonstrate, then to guided response with increasing skill to adaptation. Ultimate activity in this area would move to origination or the development of a new, related skill. The nurse begins by demonstrating a conditioning exercise then has the client or primary care-giver return the demonstration. Correctly carrying out the exercises at times other than the professional's home visit shows client progress in this area (as well as in the affective area).

LEARNING PRINCIPLES

The culmination of education, social, and developmental theories combined with information processing methods and the types of learning form the basis of learning principles. Consideration of these principles is crucial to effective client teaching. (Format courtesy of Visiting Nurse Association of Allegheny County, PA, 1986, based on general information from Redman, Bloom, and Knowles.)

Principle 1. **Interest and motivation are increased when one understands and perceives the relevance of the learning.**

This principle relates to one's readiness to learn. The relevant human behavior theories include Health Belief Model and the various stages of crisis. One can think of readiness in terms of physical (*e.g.,* does client have strength to transfer?), emotional (*e.g.,* is client still in denial?), and experiential (*e.g.,* does the client know how to calculate dosages?). It is, however, sometimes imperative that teaching begin before true readiness, especially emotional, occurs. Sometimes the combination of the actual teaching and the teaching approach can assist with the affective learning, which can lead to cognitive and skill learning. Just as the hospital nurse sometimes must begin teaching during the crisis of the brief hospital stay, the home health nurse must, at least, set the stage for teaching on the first visit.

Principle 2. **Learning is increased if the content moves from simple to the complex or the concrete to the abstract.**

Teaching one step at a time lays a better groundwork and tends to avoid overwhelming the client and family. The learner needs to be carefully assessed, however, since simple and complex are relative terms. While the concept of the immune system and the susceptibility of the chemotherapy client is simple to the biochemist, it may be complex for the chief executive officer of a department store.

The building technique is easily obtainable since the nurse can develop a plan with the client. "Today I will teach you how to suction the opening of the trachea. First I'll do it and explain the steps. Then I'll want you to practice. Tomorrow we can review cleaning and changing the inner tube (cannula)." Using the word "teach" approaches the effort in an organized, serious, and important manner. This leads to credibility and the perceived value of the learning.

Principle 3. **Anxiety affects learning, attention span, and retention of information.**

A certain degree of anxiety is necessary to motivate persons to learn; however too much anxiety interferes with learning, usually causing poor retention of information. The client or primary care-giver who moves in and out of the room, whose eyes dart in many directions, or whose hands are in constant motion is probably too anxious. Asking the question "How can I be of most help to you?" or "What are you most concerned about? can sometimes alleviate the pressure. It allows the person to state his priority.

Principle 4. **Active learning is more meaningful than passive learning.**

The learner who participates either through discussion, actual practice, or problem-solving generally learns more quickly and retains the information. A good rule of thumb is to involve two senses, at least, in the learning process. Skill-learning is enhanced by listening to instructions and by viewing a demonstration followed by practice. Consider how poor the learning would be if one only described how to tie shoelaces and never demonstrated it. Most treatment procedures are more complicated, yet many professionals fall back on giving verbal instructions only, which limits the client's perception to the sense of hearing.

Studies on how information is processed in the brain have shown that "brain-sidedness" or hemisphericity is important (Torrance et al 1977). It is believed that the information is processed in a different manner on each side of the brain. In general, it is thought that the left hemisphere responds to verbal instructions and depends on words and logical, sequential thought for meaning.

Reading and calculations depend on left brain function. On the other hand, the right hemisphere responds more to visual and kinesthetic instructions, handles abstract thinking and nonverbal cues more efficiently. Creativity and philosophical thought depend on right brain function. Sophisticated assessment tools have been developed to determine "brain-sidedness;" however a quick (though not assured) evaluation is to ask "Do you remember names or faces?" A person who remembers names is usually a left brain learner, while one who remembers faces is usually a right brain learner. Other assessment checks are "Does the home care-giver do best if I give a pamphlet that highlights all the areas of care before I teach a particular area? Or does she never get around to reading a pamphlet but observes intently as I demonstrate the care?"

Using several senses during teaching allows both the left- and right-brained learner to retain information. Assessing whether a learner is "right brain" or "left brain" can help identify a preferred teaching approach. Many persons learn to use both sides of their brains and can adapt to various teaching styles while others require a specific approach for effective learning.

Principle 5. **Success in learning motivates the learner to learn more.**

Self-confidence is increased once a learner achieves a first step, thus providing motivation for the next step. Setting cooperatively developed, achievable, short-term objectives is important in order to reach more major long-term goals.

Especially when complex, technical care is required, clients and care-givers sometimes just give up if they perceive they are not making progress in some sphere. The home care-giver responsible for the ventilator-dependent client may do better if initial teaching concentrates on maintaining a patent airway. Once she feels comfortable with suctioning and the use of a manual resuscitation bag, then other areas of care can be taught.

Principle 6. **Appropriate feedback helps performance to improve.**

Meaningful, positive feedback supports desired behavior. Positively worded corrections, suggestions of alternative methods and praise encourage learners, while ridicule, anger, or sarcasm can cause withdrawal. "You're doing the suctioning very well but, if you organize all of your equipment ahead of time, you might find it to be easier. Let's develop a list as a reminder," would be positive feedback.

Principle 7. **New learning must be used and reinforced or it will be forgotten.**

Consider the many times a newly found telephone number in a phone directory is forgotten before the phone can be dialed. However, if the number is written, dialed several times, then used on an intermittent basis, it is generally available for future recall. If it is not, a quick reference to one's note brings back the information. A like situation must occur with new health information. This combination of multi-sense learning with information used and reused is more effective than "single shot learning." Most teaching carried out in the hospital needs reinforcement in the home setting. Sometimes simply a written teaching tool is needed for future reference but, many times, teaching intervention is required for self-confidence and true learning.

The home care-giver who is taught on Monday how to suction should have the procedure reviewed on Tuesday and Wednesday. This should be done until it is carried out in a correct fashion and with ease. A return demonstration and reinforcement on the initial visit is necessary if the task must be done throughout the day.

LEARNER VARIABLES

An important overlay are the many variables that each individual learner brings to the education setting. Many of these have been referred to during the health-related theory discussions. Chiefly, they are,

1. Anxiety level
2. Physical status including sensory impairment
3. Age
4. Motivation
5. Education and language
6. Life experience and style
7. Value system and cultural influences

In addition, external factors affect learning. Some of these are

1. Physical environment
2. Timing
3. Teaching strategies and tools
4. Lesson content

Adults

When asked to consider the role of teacher and learner, most persons recall their formal school experiences, where an authority-figure teacher controlled a classroom of students who sat passively while lecturing occurred. This stereotype, unfortunately, has left many with a negative impression about learning and colors even health education. Characteristics of adult learners are (Knowles 1970):

1. *Self-directing.* Their self-concept has moved from dependency toward self-direction. They see themselves as capable of making their own decisions and accept responsibility for consequences. Involve-

ment in setting objectives and the learning process is mandatory.
2. *Rich life experience.* This is a valuable resource upon which to build. Experience should be recognized and related to current learning.
3. *Role-based.* Adult learners are strongly influenced by their social roles and developmental tasks. Learning should be related in the ability to achieve as a worker, parent, *etc.*
4. *Current application.* Their time perspective is for immediate application of new knowledge. Content must be relevant for today's use.
5. *Problem-centered.* Adults are especially motivated to learn at times of crisis or when problems arise. A quick response to this need makes progress achievable toward longer term goals.

Children

The learning characteristics of children are also related to their developmental tasks; however, children are traditionally more future-oriented than are adults. Each life stage task must be considered related to learning needs.

Most teaching prior to preschool years should be directed to the primary care-giver, though even the child of three can be included in instruction. Children have a short attention span and a limited vocabulary. Schoolage youngsters should be taught directly, though much reinforcement will be required. They thrive on rules and earnestly try to follow instructions though sometimes succumb to peer pressure. Adolescents like to learn separately from parents and need to know the benefit of doing something. They are very peer-oriented and are less future-oriented than their younger siblings. They are often interested in diet and exercise as it affects them now.

Young adults straddle the children and adult line. They need independence yet rely on family and parents for confirmation of role and identity. Frequently, their "It can't happen to me" attitude influences their adherence to a medical or health regimen, especially regarding the prevention of complications.

TEACHING PRINCIPLES

Teaching is a system of activities intended to assist learning—a dynamic interaction with mutual trust and respect. There are five basic teaching principles. (Format used by Visiting Nurse Association of Allegheny County, PA, 1986, based on general information from Redman, Bloom, and Knowles).

Principle 1. **Teaching activities should help learners meet their objectives.**

Teaching should be client-centered not health professional-centered and based on a careful assessment of client learning needs. In keeping with the learning characteristics of adults, objectives should be set with the client; sometimes a "contract" approach is helpful. A contract can be used effectively with the home care-giver who desires respite assistance. With the goal of the identification of three respite care-givers qualified to care for the acutely ill client in the home, the nurse could assist but still work toward independence of the client. "You investigate these five resources and I will call five others" might be an approach.

Principle 2. **It is essential that rapport be established with trust and respect foremost.**

The home health nurse, as a guest in the home, needs to demonstrate acceptance of the client. Nonverbal communication such as eye contact and a touch of the hand can play an important part.

Principle 3. **Previous learning should serve as a base for present learning.**

Assessing where the client is with information is crucial. Because teaching is usually initiated in the hospital, the home health nurse must make a special effort to determine the learning level and build on it. Special care should be made to continue the same teaching approach. For example, if possible, the same pamphlets and/or procedures should be used to avoid confusing the client. In addition the same instructor (nurse) should work with the client whenever possible.

Principle 4. **Communication should be clear, concise, and appropriate.**

Rambling tales, mumbled words, and language at the wrong level (too simple or too complex) are to be avoided. Verbal and nonverbal communication should be congruent.

Principle 5. **Teaching activities must be oriented to the preestablished objectives.**

A carefully made educational diagnosis is the foundation for objectives and teaching activities. Most clients want to learn the information they need to know to carry out the prescribed health behaviors or procedures. Very few clients want to know all there is to learn on the topic.

TEACHING VARIABLES

1. *Time:* Clearly defined time during the home visit must be set aside for teaching. Visit time must allow for it so that neither the teacher nor the learner is rushed. The

mother of an active toddler will have difficulty with learning when she must watch her child. Teaching sessions are better timed for the child's nap or when others can supervise the child.

2. *Environment:* Having some control over the teaching setting is important. If the client's bed is in the living room, and teaching must occur there, with the family approval, the television should be "off" with attention given to the teaching.

3. *Preconceptions:* Careful assessment will avoid the danger of preconceptions, but each teacher must avoid assumptions. Reading level should not be assumed based on socioeconomic status and, likewise, food preferences should not be assumed based on ethnic background. These can provide clues but validation is required.

4. *Teaching strategies and tools:* Whether teaching is formal or informal, structured or flexible, the presentation methods and teaching supports can make all the difference in the world. Most readers have heard the reference, "He knows his material but he just can't teach." This is, indeed, an important variable.

TEACHING STRATEGIES

The formal selection of a teaching strategy is sometimes carried out only in group teaching situations; however, the same thought process should occur in one-to-one teaching. Most techniques are applicable in both settings, though some modification is sometimes necessary. Table 4-4 outlines teaching strategies by technique, advantage, and disadvantage.

TABLE 4.4 Teaching Strategies

Technique	Advantage	Disadvantage
1. Lecture or Explanation	Straightforward, efficient way to achieve learning in cognitive domain	Little influence on attitude, behavior, or readiness

Comment: Always use with discussion or question and answers to allow for expression of feeling or clarification of information and for an opportunity to evaluate learning. Never "lecture" for more than 10 minutes without varying the technique.

Technique	Advantage	Disadvantage
2. Demonstration and Practice	Teaches psychomotor skills	Requires knowledgeable teacher with sufficient time; repetition necessary

Comment: The home is the perfect setting for this approach since actual equipment is available. Should be combined with explanation and written material, thereby addressing persons who learn in different ways. A variety of teaching approaches also increases learner interest.

Technique	Advantage	Disadvantage
3. Simulation, Games, or Role Playing	Allows learner to face situation and do problem solving	Little influence on knowledge. Time-consuming

Comment: Simulation and games are more effective in group situations but role playing can be excellent in one-to-one teaching (*e.g.,* "Let's practice what you'll say the next time you go to the doctor's.").

(continued)

TABLE 4.4   Teaching Strategies (Continued)

Technique	Advantage	Disadvantage
4. Questions and Answers	Encourage clarification, help personalized information, improve knowledge.	Little influence on attitudes.

Comment: This is an imperative method for in-home teaching. Asking "Do you have any questions?" is a basic, but explanation and demonstration must precede it.

5. Modeling	Effective for the initiation of a new behavior	Little effect in changing existing behaviors

Comment: The nurse and other health workers play a crucial modeling role. Modeling can have positive or negative effects based on the role model. The nurse who says "wash your hands" but does not do it herself is not likely to be effective in her teaching of the skill. Likewise, if the home health aide doesn't wash her hands, it undermines the credibility and effectiveness of the nurse.

6. Teaching Aids	Bring variety to teaching approach, knowledge, provide reference items if in form of printed "handouts"	Preset with little individual variation. Outdated quickly

Comment: Teaching aids should be a supplement to another strategy. They need to be carefully developed and/or evaluated. Some examples are movies, film strips, video- and audiotapes, pamphlets, and teaching sheets. Programmed instruction has the added advantage of being cost-effective and allows movement at the learner's pace. Many communities have a system of prerecorded audiotapes on a variety of health topics (*e.g.,* Tel-Med).

7. Behavior Modification	Effective for motivated clients	Requires special training, must be used with caution, caring, and common sense

Comment: Based on operant conditioning or reinforcement theory, behavior modification is directed to change behaviors that are barriers to good health. It is based on the assumptions that behavior is learned and that it can be modified.

8. Self-help or Peer Groups	Helpful with adjustment to a chronic disease; effective in attitudinal domain	Time-consuming, require organizational skills and trained facilitator

Comment: Alcoholics Anonymous is the classic example. Many agencies have developed self-help groups covering disease-specific topics and life problem situations. These are an excellent adjunct to other strategies. Groups can employ strategies such as brainstorming and discussions that can affect learning in attitudinal and behavioral areas.

TEACHING TOOLS

Health professionals constantly search for the magic teaching tools to enhance their teaching effectiveness. Technology has added televisions, videocassette recorders, audiotape recorders, and various other electronic devices to the tried and true items of movies, film strips, slides, pamphlets, posters, models, and actual devices. These teaching tools are valuable supplements to other, more primary, educational strategies. They should never stand alone and they should be consistent with learning objectives.

Because of mobility and transport problems with equipment, most home health nurses use pamphlets, small posters, models, and actual devices for in-home teaching rather than films, and so forth, though videotapes with home or portable VCRs are increasingly available.

Most home health agencies purchase some teaching materials. They should be reviewed carefully so that the teaching can be accomplished in a cost-effective manner. By using evaluation criteria (such as shown below), it is possible to make appropriate decisions in selecting commercially prepared teaching tools.

Evaluation Criteria for Commercially Prepared Teaching Tools*

CONSIDER

1. *Characteristics of the audience* who will use the material (Consider age, culture, educational background, medical conditions, reading level, and other factors.)

2. *Age of the audiovisual.* (Films and printed material often become outdated in content presented or by clothing, hairstyles, and the use of slang language.)

3. *Accuracy of the content.* (Printed material can be modified and personalized by margin notes.)

4. *Amount of content.* (Too much information can increase confusion.)

5. *Length of the presentation or booklet.* (It should be long enough to cover the subject or issue concisely, but short enough to maintain interest. Motion pictures and videocassettes hold interest for a longer time than do still pictures, and anything much over 15–20 minutes in length may result in a less attentive audience. Booklets that cover all topics in subject area may be overwhelming to some patients.)

6. *Appropriateness* of the teaching aid in meeting the learning needs of the intended audience. (No one media is best. The learning objectives and setting must be considered.)

7. *The presence of* any racial, ethnic, occupational, sexual, or education slur or *insults.*

8. *The presence of advertising* of products, treatments, or opinions that are objectionable.

9. *The use of scare tactics,* violence, or gory scenes. (Fright and panic impede learning.)

10. The *clarity* of the presentation in content and concepts.

11. The *quality* of the film (*e.g.,* clear sound, picture in focus and properly developed, color appears correct and clear) or the acceptability of the layout of printed material (*e.g.,* sufficient margin space, graphics).

* Modified from Hoffer-Chatham MA, Knapp BL: Patient Education Handbook. Bowie, MD, Robert J Brady Co, 1982

Teacher-made tools are sometimes necessary although all effort should be made to find a suitable, ready-made item. It is usually more cost-effective to purchase items than to develop them from scratch. Development, printing, and distribution costs are sometimes not initially recognized. Guidelines for teacher-made tools can be useful in the event it is necessary to develop original tools. These guidelines, shown below, while targeted to the readability of printed materials, can also be used as a general guide for slide series, videotapes and even verbal presentations.

Guidelines for Teacher-Made Tools*

1. *Use the lowest reading level* appropriate for the target audience. The opposite is also fatal. "Talking down" should be avoided. Sometimes two brochures at different levels are necessary as well as brochures in several different languages.

2. *Use one or two syllable words* if appropriate (*e.g.,* use "trouble" rather than inconvenience and "make easy" rather than facilitate).

3. *Write short, simple sentences* whenever possible. Introduce one idea only in a sentence. Limit the number of new ideas on a given page. (Use only one idea to a poster or slide.)

4. *Use slogans* for increased memory (*e.g.,* "Drink a little water often" is better than "During the day, drink small amounts of water more frequently").

5. *State the main idea at the beginning* of the paragraph. Some persons skim and only read the first line.

6. *Use connectives sparingly* (*e.g.,* "consequently," "however," "in spite of", "first").

7. *Break-up long narrative* with subtitles and captions. Use headings, "bold face," effectively for the reader who skims.

8. *Use the active voice* (*e.g.,* use "was" not "shall have been"). If appropriate, a conversational style is good.

9. *Leave plenty of open white space* on the printed page. Two pages with wide margins and well-spaced printing seem less formidable than one crowded page. This method allows for personalization through margin notes.

10. *If technical terms are necessary,* add the phonetic pronunciation.

11. *Define difficult words* by context clues (*i.e.,* "Say it in other words").

12. *Summarize* important points in short paragraphs labeled as "Summary."

13. *Illustrations, cartoons, photos, and graphs* add appeal as well as important annotation. Make sure a picture can stand alone without the text since some persons look only at pictures. If it is important to illustrate what "not to do," place an "X" over it so it is clear.

14. *Develop lists.* Don't bury information in long narratives.

15. Choose a *style that is easy to follow.*
    (a) Question and answer
    (b) Share experience
    (c) Entertaining
    (d) Personal approach; refer to the reader as "you."

16. *Use large print with various type faces* for added emphasis. Readability helps to influence motivation.

17. Consider what your *final product* will look like. Selecting between in-house copy done on a copying machine and a high gloss, professional product is important. Both give the reader a message. Make sure it's one you want to give.

18. *Always give credit* to sources and follow the copyright laws.

*Adapted from Manning D: Writing readable health messages. Public Health Rep 96: 464–465, 1981

Guidelines for Use

Home health nurses must guard against being "pamphlet pushers." All teaching tools are supplements to the nurse–client–primary care-giver interactions. A careful plan for use of teaching tools needs to be developed. It should be given to clients during a teaching session and highlighted in their presence. The plan should not be disconnected from the home visit, that is, giving a pamphlet in a casual manner as the nurse leaves the room.

Follow-up should always occur. On the next home visit, the nurse should review a section of the pamphlet or allow for the client response. Did the client read the pamphlet or listen to the audiotape? Does he have questions? What does he think about a particular section? Can he now identify a particular medication side-effect and take appropriate action? This follow-up forms the basis for evaluation of the learning objectives and provides information for the next step in the care plan.

Simple teacher-/agency-made "teaching sheets" will serve the purpose. One approach is to use simple phrases with graphic supports.

The second is an activity log, which provides space to chart pulse rates (this must also be taught), distance walked, time length, and symptoms. The log can be fashioned to accommodate exercises several times a day and for an ongoing time period.

Both of these tools work well with clients who must begin to be independent in exercises. They, or variations of them, can be used for clients with the nursing diagnosis of impaired mobility due to a variety of medical reasons such as chronic obstructive pulmonary disease, rheumatoid arthritis, cardiovascular accident (CVA), orthopedic problems or any postoperative condition. In addition, similar tools are helpful with clients on special diets or who need a quick reference for medication side-effects or treatment emergencies (*e.g.,* symptoms of hypoglycemia).

Additional items can be added to each tool in order to individualize it still further. On follow-up visits, both tools are easily incorporated as evaluation measures. Affixed to the refrigerator or a bedroom wall, they serve as "reminders" to exercise as well as learning reinforcers.

READING LEVEL

Some home health nurses rely heavily on printed materials as a supplement to the introduction of new health information and as a reinforcement of teaching content. If the client is unable to read the material or if it is so simple as to insult the client, it will not be an effective teaching supplement. Studies show that at least 20% of persons living in the United States are functionally illiterate, not able to read materials written at a fourth- to fifth-grade level (Doak, Doak, and Root 1985). Most client education materials, however, are written at the eighth-grade level or above with the standard treatment consent form written at a 16th grade (college senior) level (Doak and Doak 1980). The common aspirin label requires a 10th grade reading level.

In some regions of the country it may also be important to have reading materials available in foreign languages. Many clients have a language other than English as their primary language and cannot read English with complete comprehension.

The reader is referred to McLaughlin (1969) for information on assessing readability of printed texts. This is known as the SMOG formula and gives information about the reading grade a person must have reached to understand the text being assessed.

A recent study conducted with 106 clients in an ambulatory care site (Streiff 1986) found that reported reading levels (last grade completed in school) were significantly higher (mean = 3.1 grades) than actual reading levels as determined by scores on the Wide Range Achievement Test. The readability levels of 28 commonly used client education pamphlets were evaluated with a mean readability level of 11.2 grades. The majority (54%) of the study participants read at levels that did not allow comprehension of all the study materials.

Readability tests are formulas used for determining the level of reading difficulty in written material. Most either analyze word and sentence length or compare words in a section against precalculated, standardized lists.

The three most commonly used formulae are the SMOG, Fry, and Fog methods. The SMOG formula is considered the simplest to use and one of the most accurate (Vivian and Robertson 1980 and National Cancer Institute 1982).

AGING CONSIDERATIONS

For most home health nurses, 75%–90% of their home visits are made to the elderly.

Generally, the elderly are eager to maintain their independence, although some dependence surfaces. Their lifetime of experience and problem solving skills need recognition. Physical changes with aging, however, have the potential to interfere. Both psychological and physiological considerations need to be integrated into the teaching plan.

1. *Physical changes* require
   (a) Compensation for loss of visual acuity.
      • The level of illumination should be increased but not so much as to cause a glare.
      • Pamphlets should be on low gloss, neutral colored paper. Color contrasts help. The elderly discriminate yellows and red most easily. (Yurick et al 1984). Large, easily readable print should be used.
      • Magnifiers especially with built-in lights may be required. Glasses should be worn.
   (b) Compensation for hearing loss
      • The nurse should speak slowly and distinctly in a low-pitched voice. She should directly face the client or care-giver so that lip-readers can benefit.
      • Graphics, demonstrations, and other visuals should be used to supplement poor hearing.
      • The use of unusual words should be avoided.
      • The nurse should try to control noises that interfere with hearing. (The TV or radio should be turned off.) She should be alert to facial expressions and body language that may indicate the client is not "following" the teaching.
      • Any hearing aids should be worn.
   (c) Compensation for slower reaction time and less neuromuscular endurance.

- The nurse should avoid rushing through material. Sufficient visit time needs to be planned; however, short teaching sessions may be best to adjust for attention span and aged joints. Content and time need must be coordinated.
- A comfortable spot in the home should be designated as the teaching area. The kitchen table often works best since items such as models can be placed on them. Naturally, if an abdominal wound dressing change is being taught, the bedroom works best.

2. *Psychological changes* require
   (a) Compensation for a slower rate of learning and short term memory loss (although ability to learn remains at prior levels).
      - A teaching lesson should cover one idea at a time with methods involving both sight and hearing. Main points should be repeated frequently and summarized often. Each person should have a brief review of prior content.
      - Sufficient demonstration and practice should be provided especially if there is a reduction in eye–hand coordination.
   (b) Compensation for an emerging dependence.
      - Recognition of the wealth of life experience of the elderly helps clients feel their ideas are important. Asking "How do you usually handle your injection?" both recognizes information and aids in assessment.
      - Changing long-established patterns is difficult. Allowing clients to talk about this and integrating as many of their usual routines or methods of problem solving as possible is helpful to facilitate the new behavior.

THE HOME VISIT, THE NURSING PROCESS, AND TEACHING

The basic nursing process of assessment, planning, implementation, and evaluation serves as a framework for all types of nursing in various health-care settings. It serves especially well for the nurse teaching the client at home. The process of making an educational diagnosis parallels that of making a nursing diagnosis.

ASSESSMENT

Assessment begins with the intake form or call slip. An experienced home health nurse knows her geographic territory and its cultures, resources, strengths, and weaknesses. When the nurse reviews the "intake" on a new client, step one of assessment is initiated.

Intake information varies with each home health agency and with the referral source. A referral from a home health coordinator in a hospital will be more complete than the inquiry for service received from a landlady concerned about a "boarder."

From the intake form, the nurse can begin an assessment and develop a very preliminary teaching plan. A call to the home prior to the first visit not only alerts the client that the nurse will be there but also provides an opportunity for the client to voice major problems or concerns. In addition, arrangements can be made for the primary care-giver to be present and for the nurse to anticipate equipment and learning needs.

If available on intake, the medical and nursing diagnoses, medications, treatments, and diet give major clues to potential knowledge needs. Address and "contact person" can sometimes indicate possible networks of support. The client living in Single Room Occupancy (SRO) dwellings is less likely to have care-givers who can help with complex care than is the client living in a small community where extended family members are the rule. However, all clues need further assessment.

Familiarity with referring hospitals is also a help. Knowing policies and procedures on special-care units encourages teaching continuity. Many hospitals have developed specialized pamphlets on various treatments. The home health nurse who has copies of this material, or can knowledgeably refer to them, will have a head start on teaching and will be able to decrease client confusion.

The nurse can efficiently initiate teaching on the first visit by anticipating her teaching methods *before* the visit. For example, the client discharged from the hospital with a nursing diagnosis of "urinary elimination, alterations in patterns of" with a newly inserted indwelling catheter needs to be very knowledgeable about the catheter by the end of the first visit. A sample Foley catheter, a catheter care teaching flyer, and a syringe in a demonstration kit (or paper bag) is a help.

On the first visit, the nurse should first concentrate on

1. Voiced client/care-giver concerns
2. "Need to know" information

Required care should be provided, a health history and demographic information obtained, major related physical, social, and emotional areas assessed and "need to know" information taught. Key questions are:

1. "Have you ever had any experience with a catheter? If so "tell me about it." (This identifies the level of knowledge in the area and recognizes past experience. It also serves to reveal preconceptions, fears, and misinformation.) In addition, "unwilling" care-givers sometimes take this opportunity to say "I don't know anything about them and I don't think I can take

care of it." Sometimes this is followed by "I thought that was only for nurses to do." While readiness to learn may not be present, usually a diplomatic "we'll do it together approach" works. Combined *goal setting* occurs naturally at this point.
2. "Are there any specific questions you have about the care?" This identifies concerns, provides additional knowledge-level information, and builds the nurse/client/care-giver relationship.

Before the nurse leaves, she should

1. Demonstrate with the sample catheter how and why the catheter stays in the bladder, explaining why hygienic care will not dislodge it. Demonstrate care. Give a gentle tug to reinforce that the catheter will stay in place.
2. Teach observations that indicate a free-flowing catheter, the signs and symptoms of an obstructed catheter, and methods that might alleviate it.
3. Give instructions for appropriate action if the catherer obstructs. (Who should be called? What should be done? What are the options? Is the agency available for "off hour" response? Is catheter inserted for incontinence or obstruction? Emergency room? Removal? Length of time to safely wait for reinsertion?)
4. Review and highlight the major items on the catheter care teaching flyer so that the client and care-giver have a reference item for the middle of the night—when problems usually occur. (Printed instructions are a must!)
5. Teach any specific treatments prescribed, such as bladder instillations or irrigations.

Follow-up visits should reinforce information taught on the initial visit, extend teaching to second priority items such as adequate hydration, nutrition, and hygiene, broaden the assessment to include health promotion and preventive areas, initiate bladder training if pathology permits, and allow for evaluation of teaching.

COMMON CLIENT LEARNING NEEDS IN HOME HEALTH

Common nursing diagnoses with teaching implications in home health are

Self-care deficit
Knowledge deficit
Coping, ineffective
Noncompliance
Injury, potential for

Nutrition, alteration in
Health maintenance, alteration in

All nursing diagnoses have teaching potential. For example, a fluid volume deficit may be a secondary to a knowledge deficit. Careful assessment in these areas and in those guided by the family situation and the medical diagnoses sets the foundation for the teaching plan. Table 4-5 provides information about the area of assessment and special considerations in planning a teaching strategy.

TABLE 4.5 Assessment of Learning Needs and Considerations

Area	Considerations
Nature of problem	Major body impact
	Basic definition
Potential complications	Prevention
	Identification
	Action
Emergencies	Identification
	What to do if . . . .!
	Who should be called?
Medications	Purpose
	Storage

TABLE 4.5 (continued)

Area	Considerations
	Side-Effects
	Compliance . . .
	What to do if dose skipped.
	Response monitoring (*e.g.,* pulse, blood, blood pressure, lab work)
Treatments or monitoring	Procedures
	Equipment—Care of, operation of, who to call if malfunctions, anticipate needs (*e.g.,* O₂ supply, sufficient syringes, adrenalin if self-IV, antibiotic therapy)
Diet	Normal nutrition
	Modifications and family impact
	Meal preparation
Life-style impact	Activities of daily living
	Vision, hearing impairments
	Environmental pollutants
	Energy level
	Impact
Health promotion	Anticipatory, risk factors
	Health maintenance activities
	Early identification of problems
	First aid, emergency measures

NURSING PROCESS AS BASE FOR IN-HOME CLIENT EDUCATION ASSESSMENT

1. Assessment of current or potential need for education through data collection.
   - Client and family health history, including risk factors for cancer, diabetes, hypertension, CVA, cardiac, TB, mental health, smoking, alcohol/drug use, and allergies
   - Past hospitalizations, illnesses, and injuries. Significant socioeconomic factors (*e.g.,* housing, location of bed and bath, lighting, ventilation, heating, smoke detectors, family supports, cultural influences, usual daily activities, income, unusual expenses)
   - Past admissions to home health
   - Activity with community or social service agencies (e.g., Meals on Wheels, church groups, public assistance)
   - Integument, cardiopulmonary status, mobility, food/fluid intake, elimination, reproduction/sexual, neurosensory/cognitive, family process, self concept. ADLs/home management, health practices
2. Assessment for current level of learning.
   - Awareness of diagnosis
   - Knowledge of medications and treatments, side-effects
   - Previous knowledge and experience
   - Literacy level, cognitive abilities, thought processes
   - Client demonstration of exercises, treatments, and others
3. Assessment for readiness to learn
   - Motivational level
   - Perceived need to learn
   - Developmental stage
   - Physical state
   - Health beliefs
   - Coping mechanisms

Assessment leads to the nursing diagnoses and/or the specific educational diagnosis. The defining characteristics are sometimes obvious; however, the true etiology becomes very important in making an accurate diagnosis and establishing a teaching plan.

For example, the client who does not consistently take prescribed medications (defining characteristics) may have a nursing diagnosis of "noncompliance, medications" but a careful assessment of "why" will lead the teacher to the educational diagnosis (*i.e.,* "noncompliance, medications due to. . . ." is crucial).

Depending on clues in the client situation, some helpful questions are:

"What problems do you think you might have in taking these pills?"

"What makes it hard for you to take your medicine four times a day?"

"Do you find your medicines too expensive to buy?"

"Has your daughter been able to help you take your pills?"

"Are the pills causing you to go to the bathroom at awkward times?"

"Do these medicines seem to help you?"

"Have you taken this medicine before? What was your experience with it?"

A client with a suspected diagnosis of "An Alteration in Nutrition" is best assessed by a 24-hour recall of foods eaten or a 3-day diet history. By following a similar line of questions, the nurse can then determine a possible etiology. The correct educational diagnosis allows the nurse to develop the best combination of teaching strategies and methods.

PLANNING AND GOAL-SETTING

1. Identify the involved domains of learning (cognitive, attitude, psychomotor).
2. Separate "need to know" from "nice to know" information and establish priorities based on safety and client interest and readiness to learn.
3. Set goals and objectives with client/ care-giver.

Goals are generally considered as long-term outcomes while objectives should be specific and expressed in behavioral terms. For example, a goal might be that the client will be able to return to work but an objective would be that "the client will be able to write a 24-hour diet recall consistent with a 1500 calorie ADA diet within five home visits". Another goal might be that the client remain infection-free while requiring ventilator-assisted care, but two of the objectives would be that the home care-giver will be able to "identify five possible signs of respiratory infection within the first week of care" and "initiate appropriate prophylactic care."

Contracting with clients increases client participation in and adherence to treatment programs. A variation on behavior modification, it consists of negotiating with the client and developing a written contract that includes a behavioral objective the client considers appropriate and realistic to achieve. Sometimes the formality of writing it down helps with both motivation and implementation.

This clarification, through contracting, can help alleviate the dilemma and controversy over the use of "noncompliance" as a nursing diagnosis. The term *compliance* is well entrenched in the vocabulary of health-care providers; however, its value-laden inference of client subordination makes it offensive to many. Edel, writing in *Nursing Outlook*, suggests directing efforts toward therapeutic alliances with clients through assessment and interventions directed to the cause of the behavior (Edel 1985) rather than concentrating on noncompliance. In addition, documenting client "noncompliance" with the medical regime frequently leads to denial of claims by Medicare and other third-party payers.

IMPLEMENTATION

1. Selection and utilization of teaching methods based on learning domains involved.
2. Use of media, audiovisuals and other teaching supports.

The more actual demonstration and learner participation the better! The more known about the client's life-style and daily activities the better! Implementation built on this foundation is pragmatic and more likely to be effective.

EVALUATION

Evaluation is a measurement of the client's response to the teaching process and the extent to which the objectives have been achieved. Evaluation is not an end step but a part of the feedback loop. It often serves as an assessment step for the next teaching plan. A comprehensive learning evaluation should be carried out and documented prior to patient discharge from the home-health agency. Evaluation is carried out for three reasons.

1. To assess if the goals/objectives were achieved
2. To determine that harm is not being done
3. For administrative planning

Health/client educators must resist the temptation to say that educational outcomes are intangible or unmeasurable. Very often if outcomes are unmeasurable, it is because they have not been planned, specified, or even anticipated. In today's cost-conscious world, without documented evidence of outcome measures, client education will not receive the support it must receive to be effective.

Many agencies receive denials from medicare and other third-party payers because documentation does not indicate that teaching was medically necessary or done properly.

Among words to *avoid* in documentation are the following:

Reviewed

Reinforced

Discussed

Emphasized

Noncompliant

Unwilling to learn

Among words to *use* in documentation are these:

Taught

Instructed

Return demonstration

Client demonstrated

Knowledge

Most reimbursement sources require documentation of the client's ability to perform those functions taught. Nurses not only should document exactly what teaching they perform, but also why a client/care-giver needs continued teaching (*i.e.,* slow learner, change in care-giver, change in medical regime, meds, etc . . . short-term/long-term memory deficit). However, the client/care-giver must have a capacity to learn.

In home health, visits made solely to teach the acutely ill client about care are being cost-reimbursed by most third party payers. The burden is on nurses, who do most of the client teaching, to evaluate outcomes not only in order to plan for client care, but also to support reasoning for continued reimbursement.

PLANNING FOR DISCHARGE

The nature of care provided by Medicare-certified home-health agencies is short-term, acute care. Visits are made for skilled care to the homebound on an intermittent basis. (Note: This is Medicare criteria; private insurance may not have the homebound criteria.)

For most clients the primary objectives include teaching to help the client achieve self-care independence. For a small portion of clients, care until death, through a terminal illness or hospice service, is provided. For another small group, the nurse will visit on an ongoing regular basis to perform a technical procedure that, by tradition, third-party reimbursement sources do not expect family or client to assume (*e.g.,* Foley catheter change).

On average, clients are seen for 15 to 25 visits (total all staff) per admission to service with a length of stay of approximately 60 days. As Medicare interpretation of homebound and skilled care narrows, there is third-party payment for fewer visits.

This reality mandates that the nurse begin teaching on the first visit and proceed with an efficient plan so that clients can become independent in their care and that learning reinforcement can occur. Once the client's medical condition stabilizes and there is no further documented rehabilitation or teaching progress, reimbursement ceases and practically speaking, few agencies can afford to have the nurse continue visiting.

THE READMITTED CLIENT

Just as in hospitals, clients are often readmitted to service. Long-time staff members can sometimes refer to 20 years of "active" and "discharge" episodes, especially with clients who have chronic illnesses such as the progressive neuromuscular diseases.

Each readmission should consist of the same careful assessment and complete nursing process. It is dangerous to presume "all is the same" or "she's an old diabetic, she knows about her disease." Frequently the readmission itself indicates a need for teaching in a particular area while sometimes it simply means progression of the illness.

These readmissions bring an excellent opportunity to provide learning reinforcement. Often a particular area of care can be stressed. For example, the client with diabetes who is readmitted, based on assessment, may now be more ready to learn about foot care. A specialized pamphlet on that topic alone can be used. Or if the client seems overwhelmed with all the care necessary and not able to find prior pamphlets, a simpler one can be used. Again, single sheets of paper are helpful as they can be affixed to refrigerators and walls.

Readmissions also provide the opportunity to upgrade the teaching, considering age development. Clients with juvenile diabetes received instructions appropriate to their age level. To presume they "know it all" as adults may be an error. At each developmental stage, the learning has new meaning and the teaching is approached differently. For example, the adolescent and young adult now needs to know the sexual and reproductive aspects of his illness.

AGENCY TEACHING SUPPORTS

In order for efficient and effective client teaching to occur, the home-health agency must allocate resources to and carry out program development in the area. Informal, "on the run" teaching will probably be the approach if there are no agency supports or a formal program.

1. *The client teaching program should be somebody's responsibility.* If a specific full or part-time position is not possible, sometimes a staff development instructor or a specific supervisor can be identified. Each professional staff member, of course, carries out the actual teaching, but the "client teaching specialist" should select, develop, and make available pamphlets and other teaching tools, often in cooperation with other clinicians.

2. *Teaching materials should be readily available.* Most home-health agencies quickly develop "suboffices" or multiple centers. In decentralized locations, all materials should be available. If materials need to be requested from a central location every time a particular item is to be used, usage will be low. The press of service demands make this so. This holds true even for portable videotape and filmstrip equipment, anatomical models and the like. Multiple purchases do become expensive, but they are worth it.

3. *Teaching materials should be provided as an integral cost of the visit.* Requiring purchase of low-cost items by clients is a deterrent in many situations and usually more expensive in time and collection costs. With careful selection, most printed materials can be developed at no cost or very low cost to the agency. Many pharmaceutical firms and disease-specific agencies provide materials at no cost. (See Appendices 4-B and 4-C at the end of this chapter.) Special items are another matter. For example, sometimes an agency will have "relaxation therapy" tapes or paperback books available. These often can be handled on a "loan" basis with a purchase charge as an option. Some agencies even

have audiotape recorders for loan when families do not have one.

4. *An agency-wide system of teaching resource management should be established.* Simply sending several pamphlets out to staff with a memo encouraging their use generally does not work. The tools should be organized systematically (by diagnosis, program, or developmental area usually works best), so that the desired item can be located quickly. Each item should be summarized for purpose, target population, and reading level. Areas requiring individualization should be highlighted. A numerical reorder system needs to be established to prevent periods of nonavailability. The tools should be visible in an office as a reminder to use, with new items stressed (similar to libraries and their new book sections). One system that has proved workable is a binder system. Large three-ring binders with pocket inserts can be used to hold multiple copies of each pamphlet. Each binder holds a different "diagnosis" or area (rehabilitation, cancer, maternal child health, medical diagnosis such as chronic obstructive pulmonary disease or nursing diagnosis such as comfort: alteration in). The pamphlet summary can be typed on an adhesive-backed label and affixed to each pocket. Another effective system is the tub system. Colorful milk crates can serve as file "drawers." Hanging file folders are then suspended in the tub. Each folder can hold a supply of a specific pamphlet. Each tub can hold one category area.

This system can also serve for staff education purposes. In each category "binder" or "tub," professional references can be added. Even the agency's standards, used as audit criteria, can be included.

Since teaching is so integral to home-health care, agencies should consider developing a teaching "sheet" or flyer on each topic for which there is a clinical procedure. Most of the time, the objective will be for the client or care-giver to become independent in carrying out the procedure. For example, a generic clean dressing teaching sheet is helpful, with space to fill in the particulars. Catheter care is a must. Making normal saline at home and sterilizing dressings is helpful. Close contact with hospital and special-care units is necessary. Ideally, home-care teaching flyers should be developed cooperatively.

CURRENT AND FUTURE TECHNOLOGY

Even though many teaching items are available electronically, current costs, size, weight, and complexity do not make them easy to use in home health care. Most futurists and current "hackers," however, predict that the electronics found in the workplace will soon be in the home. The home computer and VCR units will serve as the base. Indeed, some predict that not only is health care heading home but so also are medical diagnosis and follow-up primary care (Wicklein 1981). The combination of home computers, a camera, a microphone connected to a home two-way cable system on videotext is predicted to supplement the medical office visit.

Home computer systems have the potential to revolutionize health care and health education. Computer-assisted instruction for cardiopulmonary resuscitation (CPR) is already available. The teaching role will be greatly challenged but not replaced. An advantage of computer-based home learning is its contribution to the individual's perception of internal control (Watson 1983).

While the current generation of clients will probably not have access to such technology nor have a favorable response to it, the next generation, schooled in programmed instruction and computer learning, should accept it. Watson encourages current health-care providers to participate in the development of future tools.

THE HUMAN APPROACH

The individualized teaching/learning situation is, by definition, a very human approach. In order to assist the client and family, a Medication Aid Devices section (Appendix 4-A), a Problem Area Resource list (Appendix 4-B), and a Health/Patient Education list (Appendix 4-C) are included for reference. Teaching and its objectives develop from the client's perceived needs and the teacher's concern for client safety and "need to know."

> "It is the learner who determines the desired outcomes in accordance with his decisions as to which risks he chooses to avoid (or not avoid); similarly, content is learner-determined, learner preferences for educational methods are honored, and evaluation is in terms of criteria proposed by the learner." (Levin 1978)

The home is the perfect setting for client teaching. The acutely ill client who is cared for at home presents a unique care challenge. Among familiar surroundings and family care-givers, the client is truly a key member of the health-care team. During a trying period of illness, the home setting allows a very human approach that shifts control from the professional to the client and family.

References

Becker MH (ed): The health belief model and personal health behavior. Health Edu Monogr 2: 324–508, 1974

Becker MH et al: Selected psychosocial models and correlates of individual health-related behaviors. Med Care 15: 27–46, 1977

Bloom BS: Taxonomy of Educational Objectives, Cognitive Domain. New York, McKay, 1956

Craig GJ: Human Development. Englewood Cliffs, NJ, Prentice-Hall, 1980

Cushing M: Legal lessons on patient teaching. Am J Nurs 84: 721–722, 1984

Doak L, Doak C, Root J: Teaching Patients With Low Literacy Skills. Philadelphia, JB Lippincott, 1985

Doak L, Doak C: Patient comprehension profiles: Recent findings and strategies. Patient Counselling and Health Education 3: 101–106, 1980

Edel MK: Noncompliance: An appropriate nursing diagnosis? Nurs Outlook, 33: 183–185, 1985

Fink SL: Crisis and motivation: A theoretical model. Arch Phys Med Rehabil 48: 592–597, 1967

Green LW et al: Health Education Planning: A Diagnostic Approach. Palo Alto, Mayfield Publishing, 1980

Hoffer–Chatham MA, Knapp BL: Patient Education Handbook. Bowie, MD, Robert J. Brady Co, 1982

Janz NK, Becker MH: The health belief model: A decade later. Health Educ Q 11: 1–47, 1984

Knowles MS: The modern practice of adult education. New York, Association Press, 1970

Kubler-Ross E: On Death and Dying. New York, Macmillan, 1968

Levin LS: Patient education and self-care: How do they differ? Nurs Outlook 26: 170–175, 1978

Manning D: Writing readable health messages. Public Health Rep 96: 464–465, 1981

Maslow AH: Toward a psychology of being. New York, Van Nostrand Reinhold, 1962

McGuire WJ: Attitude change: The information processing paradigm. Physician's Patient Educ Newsletter 1: 7–8, 1979

McLaughlin GH: SMOG grading: A new readability formula. J Reading 12: 639–646, 1969

National Cancer Institute: Pretesting in Health Communications. DHHS Publication No. (NIH) 83–1493. Bethesda, MD, National Cancer Institute, 1982

Pohl ML: The Teaching Function of the Nursing Practitioner. Dubuque, WMC Brown, 1968

Redman BK: The Process of Patient Education. St. Louis, CV Mosby, 1984

Rotter JB: Some problems and misconceptions related to the construct of internal versus external control of reinforcement. J Consult Clin Psychol 43: 56–67, 1975

Streiff L: Can clients understand our instruction? Image: J Nurs Scholarship 18: 48–52, 1986

Suchman EA: Evaluative Research: Principles and Practice in Public Service and Social Action on Programs. New York, Russell Sage Foundation, 1967

Torrance EP, Reynolds CR, Riegel T, Bull O: Your style of learning and thinking. Gifted Child Q 21: 23–26, 1977

Visiting Nurse Association of Allegheny County (Pennsylvania): Diabetic teaching guide for patient teaching. Unpublished material developed for staff education, Pittsburgh, 1985

Visiting Nurse Association of Allegheny County (Pennsylvania): Unpublished material developed internally by education department staff and students for use in continuing education programming related to patient teaching. Pittsburgh, 1986

Vivian AS, Robertson EJ: Readability of patient education materials. Clin Ther 3: 129–136, 1980

Wallston KA, Wallston BS: Health locus of control. Health Educ Monog 6: 101–105, 1978

Watson JE: The impact of technology on the future of health/illness education. Health Educ Q 10: 95–105, 1983

Wicklein J: Electronic Nightmare: New Communications and Freedom. New York, Viking Press, 1981

Yurik AG, Robb SS, Spier BE, Elbert NJ: The Aged Person and the Nursing Process. East Norwalk, CT, Appleton-Century-Crofts, 1984

APPENDIX 4-A

MEDICATION AID DEVICES

1. Mediplanner II by Apex Medical Corp., 3505 S. Phillips Ave., P.O. Box 8008, Sioux Falls, SD 57105 has four compartments for each day with large raised bold lettering for the visually impaired and braille for the blind.)

2. Med Tymer, from Boston Medical Research, Inc., The Vendome, Suite L-10, 160 Commonwealth Ave., Boston, MA 02116, is an electronic cap that fits a standard pill vial. A flashing light and a beeping sound signal the forgetful patient to take medication.

APPENDIX 4-B

PROBLEM AREA RESOURCES

DIABETES

Periodicals

Diabetes in the News, published 6 times/year by the Ames Co. $6.00/year. Write to

Diabetes in the News
P.O. Box 3105
Elkhart, IN 46515

Diabetes Forecast, published by the American Diabetes Association, Inc. $9.00/year. Write to

American Diabetes Association, Inc.
2 Park Ave.
New York, NY 10016

For the Visually Limited:

Large print books and recorded books are usually available from the local division of Blind and Physically Handicapped Library.

Materials printed in Braille are available from

1. Local braille associations

2. Division for the Blind and Physically Handicapped

   Library of Congress
   Washington, DC 20540

Aids and Appliances for the Blind and Visually Impaired catalogue available from the

American Foundation for the Blind
15 W. 16th St.
New York, NY 10011

Organizations

American Diabetes Association
600 Fifth Ave.
New York, NY 10020

American Diabetes Association
Western Pennsylvania Affiliate, Inc.
4617 Winthrop St.
Pittsburgh, PA 15213

Juvenile Diabetes Foundation
23 East 26th St.
New York, NY 10010

The American Diabetes Association (ADA) and the Juvenile Diabetes Foundation (JDF) are national organizations with local chapters throughout the U.S.A. These associations both sponsor and encourage research. Finding a cure for diabetes is their ultimate goal.

The ADA offers a wide selection of literature on diabetes. Information is available on menus, meal planning, activity, marriage, pregnancy, and travel.

Summer Camps for Children

Throughout the U.S.A. there are about 72 summer camps for children with diabetes. Their programs include the same activities as most other camps, plus instruction in food selection, managing diabetes, and self-administration of insulin. They also devote time to building the child's confidence. A listing of these camps may be obtained from the American Diabetes Association.

STROKE

National Stroke Association (NSA)
1420 Ogden St.
Denver, CO 80218

NSA was initiated in 1984 to work with stroke survivors by providing educational materials and to encourage research. It publishes several pamphlets directed toward living at home after a stroke, as well as a newsletter. It encourages membership at $5.00/year.

American Heart Association
7320 Greenville Ave.
Dallas, TX 75231

AHA publishes several excellent, classics on stroke care: "Strike Back at Stroke," "Up and Around," "Do It Yourself Again," and "Aphasia and the Family."

Reading Reference for Clients

Episode by Eric Hodgins, A Fireside Book, published by Simon & Schuster, 1963. This is an excellent, easy-to-read book that describes a "recovery" from a stroke.

PARKINSON'S

National Parkinson Institute
1501 N.W. 9th Ave.
Miami, FL 33136

Client pamphlets and newsletter available.

CANCER

American Cancer Society
777 Third Ave.
New York, NY 10017

Newsletter, pamphlets, and self-help groups and programs such as Make Today Count, Lost Cord Club, Ostomy Society, Reach to Recovery, depending on local resources.

ARTHRITIS

Arthritis Foundation
3400 Peachtree Road, N.E.
Atlanta, GA 30326

Pamphlets, newsletter, self-help groups, and arthritis classes, depending on local resources.

CEREBRAL PALSY

National Easter Seal Society
2023 W. Ogden Ave.
Chicago, IL 60612

Pamphlets, newsletter, sheltered workshop, speech and physical therapy based on local resources.

United Cerebral Palsy Association
66 East 34th St.
New York, NY 10016

Pamphlet, newsletter, group living, social activities based on local resources.

EPILEPSY

Epilepsy Foundation of America
1828 L Street, N.W.
Suite 406
Washington, DC 20036

Pamphlets, newsletters, audiocassettes, paperbacks, and local meetings based on resources.

RENAL

National Kidney Foundation
2 Park Ave.
New York, NY 10016

Pamphlets, newsletters, and patient education workshops based on local resources.

LEUKEMIA

Leukemia Society of America
211 E. 43rd St.
New York, NY 10017

Pamphlets, newsletters, medication assistance based on local resources.

MENTAL HEALTH

Mental Health Association
1800 N. Kent St.
Arlington, VA 22209

Pamphlets, newsletters, self-help groups based on local resources.

National Association for Retarded Citizens
P.O. Box 6109
2709 Avenue E. East
Arlington, TX 76011

Pamphlets, newsletter, in-home homemaker, and training services based on local resources.

MULTIPLE SCLEROSIS

National Multiple Sclerosis Society
205 E. 42nd St.
New York, NY 10017

Pamphlets, newsletter.
Some geographic areas also have a Multiple Sclerosis Service Society that provides in-home therapy on a long-term basis.

PULMONARY

American Lung Association
1740 Broadway
New York, NY 10019

Pamphlets, newsletters, self-help groups based on local resources.

GENERAL

American Red Cross
(contact local chapter)

Pamphlets, home nursing, first aid, and CPR courses.

Reading References

American Red Cross: *Family Health and Home Nursing.* Purchase through course.
The Home Health Care Solution: A Complete Consumer Guide. By Janet Zhun Nassif, Harper & Row, 1986
Home Health Care: A Complete Guide For Patients And Their Families. By Jo Ann Friedman, Norton, 1986.

Catalogue

Comfortably Yours: Aids for Easier Living. 52 W. Hunter Ave., Department MS, Maywood, NJ 07607

APPENDIX 4-C

HEALTH/PATIENT EDUCATION

Selected Resource List

Type	Sources
1. Pamphlets, models, audiotapes, films	1. Various pharmaceutical companies (check Physicians' Desk Reference for address or hospital pharmacy for sales representative contact) Insurance companies (Metropolitan, John Hancock, etc.) Commercial companies with a product line in area of need. Pampers (Proctor & Gamble) has pamphlets on protecting infants and toddlers from being poisoned, medical equipment films, etc
2. Client and/or professional literature, films, and teaching models	2. Voluntary agencies, (*e.g.,* American Cancer Society, Arthritis Foundation, Dairy Council, Heart Association, American Diabetes Association, National Stroke Association) Department of Health and Human Services, Superintendent of Documents, U.S. Government Printing Office, Washington, DC, 20402 (free listing of selected government publications).
3. Aids for the visually handicapped	3. American Foundation for the Blind 15 West 16th St. New York, NY 10011 (free catalogue) Local "blind" association
4. Commercially prepared client education audiovisuals	4. Commercial companies such as Med Fact, Train-Aide, Robert J. Brady, Omni, etc. Spenco Medical Corporation P.O. Box 8113 Waco, TX 76710 Health Resources Kelly Communications 410 E. Water St. Charlottesville, VA 22901 (Both have a product catalogue on health education models, posters, and audiotapes). Plus many, many others.
5. General health educational materials	5. Blue Cross Association 840 N. Lake Shore Dr. Chicago, IL 60611 (The "Blues" have available [free] booklets such as "Stress," "Help Yourself," etc. Contact local Blue Cross office for current listing) Health Insurance Institute 277 Park Ave. New York, NY 10017 (Has catalogue listing many organizations and their addresses that provide health education information.)

Type	Sources	Type	Sources
	State Department of Health Varies with each state.		National Heart, Lung, & Blood Institute (DHHS) Bethesda, MD 20014 (no charge)
6. Newsletter/ Journals	6. *Baseline* A newsletter of information about the evaluation of health promotion programs. Health Services Research Center, The University of North Carolina, Chase Hall 132-A, Chapel Hill, NC 27514 (no charge).		*Physician's Patient Education Newsletter* University of Alabama – Birmingham 1016 S. 18th St. Birmingham, AL 35294 (subscription fee)
	Focal Points Bureau of Health Education DHEW Centers for Disease Control Atlanta, GA 30333 (no charge)		*The Diabetes Educator* American Association of Diabetes Educators E. Erie Street, Suite 712 Chicago, IL 60611 (Included in membership dues)
	Info Memo National High Blood Pressure Education Program		

Many of the above resources are provided free as a public service; others have a cost ranging from nominal to full retail or subscription price.

CARE OF THE FAMILY

5

Catherine Malloy

Care in the home of ill family members has always been a function of the family unit. However, the advent of recent federal legislation and advances in medical technology have created some excruciating problems for families.

Modern day medical treatment makes it possible to provide complex technical procedures such as dialysis, intravenous therapy, and ventilator support in the home setting.

Families are confronted not only with the demand to support and comfort the sick person but also to perform techniques heretofore found mainly in hospital intensive-care units.

The first section of this chapter will present the systems approach to family analysis, and will consider the impact of illness on the family and care-giver. The unique role of the home-care nurse will be incorporated. Family assessment considerations and assessment of the home environment will be highlighted.

Two major problems, family stress and care-giver burden, will be discussed in the second section of the chapter. Nursing diag-

noses specific to family, client, and care-giver will be expanded. The chapter will conclude with a case study applying the nursing process with a specific family.

SYSTEMS APPROACH TO FAMILY ANALYSIS

The systems theory approach to analyzing the family provides a structure for studying the family process and permits observation of reciprocal relationships and family patterns. Using systems theory, the family is conceptualized as a goal-directed unit composed of interacting, inter-relating individual family members (Friedman 1986). The family has structure and function with boundaries to regulate the inflow and outflow of energy to the environment. The family unit contains various subsystems that are important in defining the way in which the family functions. Examples of the subsystems are the marital, sibling, parental, individual, grandparent, and relative subsystems. The family system with its subsystems is part of the suprasystem in the environment. Changes at any system level, the family system, the subsystems, or the suprasystem, influence the entire system as well as each part. As an open system, the family continually exchanges energy with the environment and mutually influences and is influenced by the environment. For this chapter, the family system discussion will examine the interrelationship of the client's acute care needs and the care-giver's needs on family health (Fig. 5-1).

Allmond, Buckman, and Gofman (1979) conceptualized the family system as a mobile. When one thinks of a mobile, one usually thinks of it as suspended from a ceiling or from the top of an infant's crib. It is a unit composed of several parts that are arranged in relation to each other at different angles. The parts move and shift in response to environmental influences. These authors visualized the mobile as a concrete representation of the family as a system, a single unit composed of parts in mutual interaction. Think of this mobile as a set of wind chimes suspended from the ceiling on a porch. When there is no wind, the chimes hang in perfect alignment, neither moving nor shifting. When there is a wind current, the pieces move and shift in relation to each other, assuming many differ-

ent configurations based on the force and direction of the wind. In applying this model to a family, the individual pieces of the wind chimes represent individual family members. Their position in relation to each other changes in response to changes in the environment. It is useful for the nurse to have a systems conceptualization in mind when planning to assess the family. This family system mind-set allows the nurse to view the family as a unit and to focus on the interrelationships of all the members.

When acute illness strikes a family member, the entire family system responds. The need to provide care at home increases demands on the family system. Each member of the family is affected, and patterns of relating are changed to accommodate the new demands. The family unit and the ill family member respond in their own way in an attempt to maintain balance, or move to altered ways of behaving.

Quite often the family unit is placed in the role of "care-giver" without warning and without preparation. This may be due in part to escalating health-care costs and the Diagnostic Related Groups (DRG) phenomenon. Not only does the person go home "quicker and sicker" but also the equipment and the requirements for complex care go along with

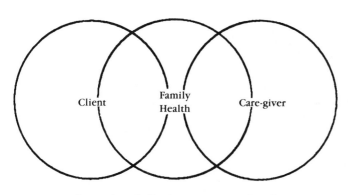

Interaction of client's acute care needs and
care-giver needs on family health

Figure 5-1. Family health.

him. This means that the family is responsible for implementing complex technologies in caring for the person at home.

While the goal of the health-care system is to provide less care in institutional settings as a way to control costs, the result often is a requirement for home care by unprepared family members. Moreover, families have little time to prepare for home care. Not all families can cope with the responsibility for this type of care. Some try and cannot sustain the effort. Others manage to provide the needed care effectively.

IMPACT OF ILLNESS ON THE FAMILY

When serious illness or disability strikes a family member and the condition requires home care, the family system receives a challenge to its very integrity. Each family responds to the impact of acute illness in a personal way. In the past, most home care was associated with caring for elderly parents or dying persons. Today, home care involves care to persons of all ages, ranging from those who have a serious illness and recover, to those who will live for many years with a chronic, progressively deteriorating condition requiring supportive care over an indefinite period of time.

In considering home care, family members must determine their willingness and ability to meet this demanding challenge. An honest exploration of the impact of the illness on the family unit and on the individuals within the family must be considered. The nature of the illness and the level of care required are important considerations in arriving at a family decision to provide home care. The task of providing care at home requires much preparation, physical and emotional.

Once a decision has been made to participate in the care of the family member at home, the family will need to acquire information about the illness with which they are dealing, as well as the type of care that will be required. Information is essential. The self-care movement in our society promotes the idea that people are active participants in the decisions affecting their health and their care. Consumer involvement and public awareness of health care means that people are better informed about their options.

A first step, then, for the family, is to learn about the nature of the illness of their loved one. The nurse can provide valuable assistance to the family by teaching them facts about the disease and by providing them with supplemental materials to read. All of this must be done in concert with an understanding of the family's readiness and ability to learn. The information should be given in sequences to permit the family sufficient time to assimilate the information.

NATURE OF ILLNESS

A variety of diseases, disorders, and health problems require home care. In many cases the individual can be supported with high-tech interventions over an indefinite period. As the acuity level subsides, the condition may assume a chronic, progressive pattern with frequent recurrences of the acute illness. Illnesses differ in severity, care requirements, and prognosis. Depending on the type of illness, the family may be able to anticipate some of the implications of providing care.

Specific conditions are discussed in the chapters in the physiologic section of this text. What is attempted here is to discuss the level of support the client will require, be it short term or long term, and the anticipated degree of the client's disability. Careful assessment of these factors may be of some use to the family members, realistically appraising them of just what providing care in the home will mean.

LEVEL OF SUPPORT REQUIRED

The circumstances surrounding the onset of illness and the need for acute care in the home are not all identical. There are differences in the nature of the illness and the degree of disability that will influence the level of care. Compare a family that is faced with caring for a person experiencing a progressively deteriorating disease with a family faced with providing support through an acute crisis in which recovery is assured. The stress is quite different. While there is an end in sight for the latter, the prospect of dealing with a chronic progressive disease can mean years, even decades of involvement. Family commitment can be short-term or long-term, depending on the health problem.

Short-Term Commitment

Many conditions treated at home today were confined to intensive-care units even a decade ago. Some of these conditions require a great deal of support for a limited period of time. Individuals across the life span, from newborns to the elderly, might require this type of home care.

In cases where recovery is expected, the demands on the family are different than with long-term care requirements. While the family might experience dramatic changes in life-style to accommodate the needs of the client, knowledge that the illness is time-limited makes the care seem manageable. Changes in family life are temporary, not permanent. Roles may be altered but not necessarily changed. In many ways the pattern and routine of family life are adjusted. Activities are postponed or revised. But there is the anticipation that there is an end in sight. Personal commitment does not seem as burdensome if recovery or recuperation are expected.

Many technical procedures can be performed safely in the home. Some require a great deal of skill but also may be limited in duration. Examples include home intravenous therapy, apnea monitors for infants, chemotherapy, and complex wound care. These interventions require a great deal of coordination and adjustment for the family while in progress, but may not require an ongoing commitment.

Long-Term Commitment

On the other hand, the client at home may need supportive care for the remainder of his life. Some respiratory and neurologic conditions are progressive and deteriorating. These situations require a series of changes as the client's condition becomes more compromised. Increased demands requiring families to make dramatic changes can be very disruptive to family health. Families respond best to progressive demands when sufficient time is available to establish new routines and to modify their usual activities. The realization that a family member has a problem that is not amenable to treatment is often devastating. Coupled with worries about possible future events, this knowledge may cripple a family emotionally. In addition, financial concerns can drain the family's energies as well as their security.

The nurse can assist the family to deal with the "here and now" aspect of the problem rather than on the anticipated disasters that might be ahead. It is often impossible to predict the course of illness. One of the most important challenges for the family is to balance the care-giving aspect of life with other priorities in the family. Doing too much for the client can leave the family exhausted, resentful, and unable to give further. It also might result in increasing the client's feeling of depression and guilt. The nurse has a pivotal role in assisting the family to deal with the realities of its situation on a day-to-day basis and to find ways to conserve the energy of the care-giver.

DEGREE OF DISABILITY; ALTERATIONS IN MOBILITY

In addition to understanding the nature of the illness and the level of commitment required over time, it is important to assess the degree of the client's disability when planning care. Functional status and alterations in mobility also need to be considered. It is helpful to focus on the client's abilities rather than disability; on what he can do rather than what he cannot do. It is important to assess ambulation. Can the client walk unaided or is an ambulation device required? Assistive devices are available to help clients improve their mobility status. Various types of walkers and canes can meet differing circumstances. The nurse can support the family in choosing appropriate devices for its particular situation. It is important to have physician collaboration to ensure that reimbursement requirements for equipment are met. In addition to physician collaboration, the nurse needs to recognize that other therapies, particularly physical, speech, and occupational therapies, can be very useful in increasing a client's ability to ambulate independently and to carry out additional activities of daily living (ADL's). One of the hallmarks of home-care nursing is the opportunity to work as an integral part of a multidisciplinary team.

Some stroke clients only have use of one hand and many assistive devices are available to enable them to be more independent. The wheelchair can be a constructive addition to the home-care situation. A wheelchair can promote a sense of mobility and independence for the client, and in that way relieves the family of the constant pressure to do things for him. As with the assistive devices mentioned earlier, wheelchairs are available in many styles and for many purposes. Accessibility to all parts of the home is of prime importance. It is necessary for the person to be able to go from one room to the other. Some clients are able to assist with food preparation, dishwashing, folding laundry, and ironing from a wheelchair while manipulating the technical equipment required for this care.

FUNCTIONAL STATUS; IMPLICATIONS FOR THE FAMILY

The family needs to be thoroughly aware of the client's ability to perform the activities of daily living. This includes bathing, oral hygiene, toileting, dressing, mobility. Can these activities be performed without assistance? Is there a need for minimal assistance? Is the client unable to perform the activity? Depending on the answers to these questions, a decision must be made to assist the family to support the client in an appropriate manner. There are many excellent functional assessment tools available and the nurse is referred to the literature for further information on this subject. But basic assessment of functional status really comes down to three questions. Is the client

1. Unable to perform task?
2. Able to perform with some assistance?
3. Independent?

The nurse can help the family to create a progress record by listing various daily activities and the amount of assistance required, such as the functional status checklist shown in Figure 5-2. Changes in status can be documented by the family, using this tool.

	No assistance	Some assistance	Unable to perform	Special hints responsible family member
BATHING				
Tub				
Shower				
Sink				
Bed				
HAIR CARE				
Shampooing				
Setting				
Hair Dryer				
Brush				
MAKEUP				
ORAL HYGIENE				
Brushing				
Flossing				
TOILETING				
SHAVING				
DRESSING				
MOBILITY				
Assistive Devices				
Wheel chair				
One-sided impairment				
Bed-bound				

Figure 5-2. Functional status checklist.

RESOURCES REQUIRED

The impact of illness changes the way a family's resources are organized. Resources include machines, equipment, supplies, and people. Many acute care clients require sophisticated technologies. These may include machines such as ventilators, intravenous pumps, nutritional pumps, diabetic monitoring devices, and apnea monitors. There may also be a need for medical supplies such as dressings, solutions, cotton balls. The most valuable resource is the human one. Family members themselves are resources for the client and for each other. The health-care team members, friends, neighbors, and individuals from various community groups are also needed to support the family in caring for the acutely ill client at home.

ROLE OF HOME-CARE NURSES

The nurse gains access to the home because a reimbursable treatment is required, and the client meets the criteria for home care: skilled care, homebound, and potential for improvement over a reasonable period of time. It is important that home-care nurses correctly interpret these criteria since payment to home-care agencies is based on the provision of appropriate service. Omdahl (1987) reported that denials for reimbursement rose from a rate of 3.5% in 1984 to 6.9% in 1987. Some areas have reported denial rates as high as 30%. These facts suggest that nurses need to be accurate interpreters of reimbursement regulations.

The Health Care Financing Administration Manual defines homebound as follows:

> Generally speaking, a beneficiary will be considered homebound if he has a condition due to an illness or injury which restricts his ability to leave his place of residence except with the aid of supportive devices such as crutches,

wheelchairs, canes and walkers, special transportation, or the assistance of another person or if he has a condition which is such that leaving his home is medically contraindicated (Manual 11, Section 208.4).

The essence of this definition is that the client seldom leaves home and if he does, considerable help is required. Skilled care means that the client requires services for the treatment of the condition. Skilled services include observation and evaluation, skilled procedures, and teaching and training activities. The definition of skilled services also applies to physical therapy, occupational therapy, and social services. The services must also be appropriate for the type of problem the client has, the severity of the problem, the client's condition, and must meet accepted standards of practice. The client must also share the potential for improvement over a predictable period of time. In other words, the client is expected to respond to the treatment plans in a defined period (Omdahl, 1987).

One of the critical responsibilities of the home-care nurse is to learn how to document services accurately and appropriately. The nurse needs to exercise considerable judgment and recognition of the reasons why denials occur.

While in the home the nurse is also alert to undetected health problems to which the family and care-giver are particularly vulnerable. Home-care nurses traditionally have focused on the family as the unit of nursing service. They have recognized that individuals are best understood in the context of the whole family. The nurse's role in family care is one of a linking pin between a variety of groups, agencies, and individuals. The holistic value prevalent in nursing today also supports the concept of family as the focus for care. By observing family members together, by reflecting on their interactions with each other, and by recognizing the many ways family members influence each other, the nurse can gain a deeper understanding of individuals.

The reciprocal nature of family health is most clearly seen when the family is conceptualized as a system. Systems concepts facilitate the nurse's intervention with the family by providing a framework in which to conduct a systematic assessment and to identify the necessary skills required for intervening with the family. The use of systems concepts as a framework enables the nurse to combine the assessment data in a meaningful way so that the needs and resources of the family can be identified accurately. Without a framework that gives direction to the nursing process, the nurse might become so overwhelmed by the amount of information that she may not be able to sort it out appropriately. The multiple variables influencing family health deem it essential that the nurse has the conceptual skills to work with dissimilar information. The use of a systems framework as a family assessment tool assists the nurse in organizing, classifying, and interpreting the enormous amount of data.

Conceptual skills are essential to synthesize the data obtained from family assessment. Critical thinking and judgment are used in the process of integrating the data. The home-care nurse must scrutinize the collected information and arrange it according to patterns in order to arrive at inferences about its meaning. These inferences serve as the preliminary nursing diagnoses. However, the tentative diagnoses must be validated with the family and must be modified or discarded as more information becomes available. The nurse must guard against insufficient data collection that leads to premature conclusions and inappropriate nursing diagnoses.

The nurse also must possess technical skills. Machinery used in the home requires specialized knowledge of equipment, and procedures. Without a competent practitioner to manage the technology, many treatments could not be provided. Home-care nurses are finding themselves in new situations. They must upgrade their technical skills and increase their competencies in order to function safely and effectively.

In intervening with the family providing acute care in the home, the nurse serves three major roles: educator, coordinator, and supervisor of care. As educator, the nurse assists the families to learn healthy behaviors and to develop skills to cope with the health problem. Self-care behavior and self-responsibility are major themes explored with the family. The nurse is the facilitator and resource person in supporting the family's capacity for self-care.

The coordinator role is a key one in home care. A sound knowledge of community resources enables the nurse to coordinate services with other disciplines so that the range of family needs is met.

The third role is supervisor of care. Since family members must learn to perform treatments in the nurse's absence, the nurse facilitates them to implement technical care. In addition, the nurse assists the family in arrangement of special alterations of the home such as ramps, removal of barriers, identification of hazards in the home.

FAMILY ASSESSMENT CONSIDERATIONS

Using the systems framework and the nursing process (Fig. 5-3), the nurse assesses the structure and function of the family. This approach provides a holistic perspective for understanding the dynamics of the family unit. Structure refers to the way the family is organized and the manner in which the members relate. Family function refers to the way the

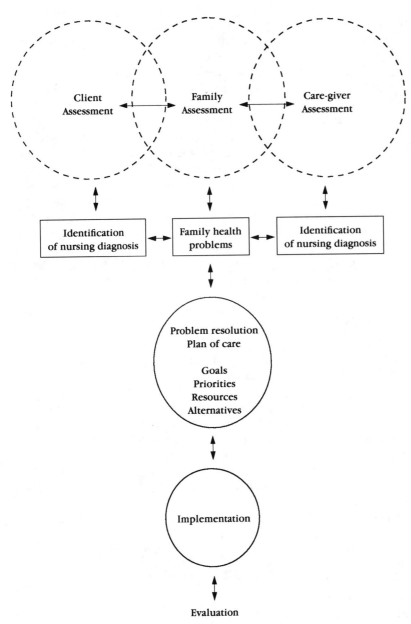

Figure 5-3. Nursing process with family providing acute care in the home.

family meets the needs of its members and itself and the way it relates to the outside community.

STRUCTURE

Roles and relationships, communication patterns, power, and values are interdependent components of family structure (Friedman MM 1986). Each will be discussed within the context of a family assessment for home care.

Roles and Relationships

Each family constellation has a set of roles established by the family in concert with the culture, sanctions, and norms of the unit. Roles define expected patterns of relating and interrelating for the family. The traditional roles of husband–father, wife–mother, daughter–sister are formal designations.

It is important for the nurse to assess both formal and informal family roles. Formal roles are explicit and derive from the individual's position within the family. Certain expectations accompany each role. Traditionally, the husband–father was responsible for earning a living and the wife–mother for caring for the home and family. Value changes in contemporary society have blurred the definition of family roles and responsibilities. Increased numbers of female-headed households and single-parent families have shifted the traditional view of the family.

The home-care nurse cannot make assumptions about family roles. There are as many configurations of roles as there are families. It is important to assess what the family's perception of its roles are, and to determine the presence or absence of cooperation and conflict. By discussing roles from a family perspective, the interrelationships of all members in role behavior will be more evident.

As stated previously, informal roles are

also important to understand in relating to the family. Since informal roles are not readily observable, the nurse will need to be particularly observant in the interactions with the family. Examples of informal roles are family mediator, jester, dominator, placator (Friedman MM 1986).

Informal roles are played to meet the family's emotional needs and needs for stability (Satir 1967). They are also useful to facilitate the performance of formal roles (Kievit 1968).

Assessment of family roles enables the home-care nurse to determine what the typical family roles are and whether the illness situation is likely to produce changes. It is quite clear that role problems can cause tension and stress within the family system. If role changes are a possibility, an assessment of formal and informal roles will enable the nurse to identify family strengths and limitations. Accurate assessment will provide the necessary data for the nurse to initiate a realistic plan with the family.

Communication Patterns

Family communication patterns refer to the ways in which the family processes information among its members. It is a network for transmitting messages, feelings, opinions, and ideas within the family. Clear communication is critical to the well-being of the family.

The home-care nurse understands that both verbal and nonverbal communication patterns are important to assess. Verbal communication has two components: content and meaning. The literal words that are spoken are not necessarily as important as the message that is intended. The words may say one thing while the actions speak of something quite different.

Nonverbal information includes gestures, body posture, facial expression, and other symbols that add meaning to the message. These behaviors provide a great deal of information. The nurse should be alert to how the family arranges itself as a group, who sits next to whom, and who interacts with whom. Body language, gestures, and eye contact all provide clues regarding the family's communication patterns. It is important for the nurse to remember that all behavior is communication (Friedman MM 1986).

In assessing the family, the nurse needs to be aware of recurring patterns of communication. It is first necessary to identify the existing pattern of communication by assessing the family as a whole as well as the set of relationships within the family. Do family members share clear statements of their needs and feelings? Are the messages congruent with their emotional expression? Are family members able to listen to each other? The nurse must be alert to the family members' ability to state their perceptions and feelings and to assess the response of family members to messages received and sent.

Power and Decision Making

Power is defined as the ability to influence or change another person's behavior (Friedman MM 1986). As with other social systems, the family has a power dimension. Knowing who holds the power for decision making is important before attempting to develop a plan of care. The nurse can ask questions to acquire this information: Who runs the family? Who ends up getting his own way? Who makes the decisions? These are the power variables. Cromwell and Olson (1975) conceptualized three areas of power: power bases, power outcomes, and power processes. The power base is the source of power. Decision making is seen as a manifestation of power outcomes. Power process is the interactional process of the family in arriving at decisions, the *how* of decision mak-

ing. The decision-making process is reflective of family power.

The nurse assesses the power variables to determine if the family is dominated by one individual or characterized by a democratic give and take, or is characterized by no actions at all. Shifts in power due to situational changes are also important to determine. Understanding the power dimension of the family providing care for an individual at home is essential in planning interventions with the family. Before effective nursing actions can be formulated, the nurse needs to know who holds the power for decision making in the family. By working with this individual, appropriate health actions can be devised.

Value System

Another interdependent structural dimension of family is its value system. The nurse needs to understand the family's value system as a beginning point of assessment. Values are a set of beliefs and attitudes that serve to shape behavior (Friedman MM 1986). Nowhere is it more incumbent upon the nurse to recognize family values than in the home. The home is the family's turf and the nurse is a visitor. To determine effective ways of working with the family, the nurse needs to understand its values. The family value system is the basis for motivation (Elkins, 1984). Before a care plan can be constructed, an assessment of what is important to the family is necessary. What is important or unimportant to the family? Do values differ from one family member to another within the family system? How congruent are family values with societal values? Are there any specific cultural, ethnic, or social class values cherished by the family that need to be considered in planning care? What is the relationship of family values and health? What is the relationship of the family to the community and community resources? The use of a value assessment tool can assist the nurse to gather accurate information about each family.

Summary of Structural Assessment

The home-care nurse has a demanding schedule characterized by serious time constraints. There are two tools that home-care nurses can use to assess the dimension of family structure quickly and accurately. These are the genogram and echomap. The genogram (Fig. 5-4) permits a visualization of the family intergenerational constellation: size, composition, order, developmental level. The echomap (Fig. 5-5) diagrams the family's external interrelating systems: religious, political, educational, cultural, health care. These two techniques enable the nurse to gather a great deal of information quickly in a visual representation that permits insight into both the internal and external dimensions of family structure.

FUNCTION

Function refers to what the family does and the purposes it serves in meeting the needs of individual family members and the family system (Friedman MM 1986). For the purpose of discussion in this chapter, three functions will be considered: socialization including personal support for members, economic, and health care.

Socialization Function

The nurse assesses the family's care and concern for each other and the signs of support

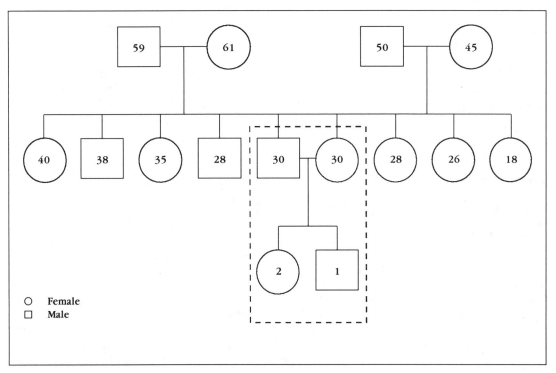

Figure 5-4. Genogram.

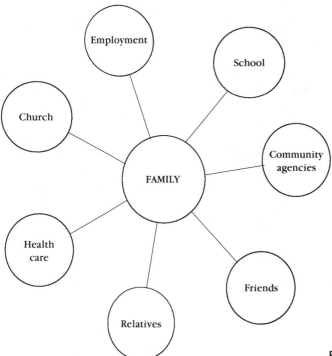

Figure 5-5. Echomap.

or nonsupport for the individuals within the family. Included in the assessment will be information about socialization, values, traditions, and education.

Economic Function

The economic function considers the family's ability to provide for the needs of its members. This is an important dimension to assess when home care is being considered. Increased expenses incurred by the family in providing complex care may drain family finances. The nurse can be a valuable resource by first assessing the family in regard to its available resources, the family's pattern of allocating resources in the past, and the potential expenses that may prove a serious threat to the family's economic security in provid-

ing home care. By obtaining this information, the nurse can plan with the family to identify appropriate resources from community agencies, if needed. Other disciplines can also be helpful to the family. A referral to a social worker within the home-health agency would be appropriate in many cases of financial hardship, or even in situations where location of resources is the prime concern.

Health-Care Function

It is especially important to assess the health-care function of the family. The nurse needs to know the past pattern of health-care practices that have value for the family. The nurse can learn a great deal by determining what resources have been used in the past: Do the family members seek care appropriately or inappropriately? Do they practice health promotion or only seek assistance in illness? Some families value privacy and self-determination to the extent that they refuse the use of community resources. By using the nursing process, the home-care nurse carefully assesses each area of family function.

Summary of Functional Assessment

By understanding the dimensions of family function, the home-care nurse can determine specific areas for assessment and can devise questions that will assist in obtaining the information. Some examples follow:

- What is the family's definition of its caring and support function?
- What is the family's definition of health care?
- What is the family's history of health-care practices?
- What effect will the financial expenses of providing care at home have on the family?
- Does the family have sufficient medical insurance?

HOME ASSESSMENT CONSIDERATIONS

Having a complete home assessment prior to providing care at home is imperative. First, the nurse should see the family in its own environment. The family's home is the environment controlled by the family, not the nurse. Before care can be planned, the nurse needs to see the home and determine what will be needed to support the care process.

Collaboration with the family is on a different level in the home setting than in the hospital. Here, the nurse is the visitor who comes episodically. The family is present 24 hours a day, 7 days a week. The interaction between family and nurse is likely to continue over a longer time span than hospital interaction and a cooperative arrangement is mandatory. In the home setting, the family will be responsible for providing the care after the nurse has given the proper instructions. One significant way the nurse can assist the family is to discuss the home environment with them, to anticipate what will be required for care and any risks that might need to be anticipated. Figure 5-6 illustrates a Home Assessment Checklist. The home is assessed by physical structure, safety features, and external systems. The use of this form can facilitate the adaptation of the home for specific care requirements and can be used to update requirements as the situation changes.

The physical structure of the home is assessed. Attention is paid to the exterior structure as well as the interior. The nurse considers potential difficulties in assessing the home. Are there any barriers to delivering equipment? If the home is built on a hill with no driveway access, arrangements to deliver large pieces of equipment must be made. The size of the doorways, steps, presence of a porch, noise level all need to be included in the assessment. As for interior assessment, space, people, and resources are carefully considered.

The number and arrangement of rooms, type of rooms, accessibility to the bathroom, adequate heating, lighting, ventilation are all important. Obstacles or barriers to providing care need to be recognized. What type of flooring is in the home? Are there scatter rugs? Is the home on one floor or several levels with stairs? Does the furniture arrangement set up obstacles to easy movement? Other factors to assess include refrigeration, water supply, sanitation, and presence of infestations. Privacy and sleeping arrangements also need to be included in the home assessment.

Safety factors in the home are determined in relation to risk of falls, fires, and poison-

POTENTIAL RISKS

Check those that apply to this family.

PHYSICAL STRUCTURE		SAFETY FACTORS	
EXTERIOR		FALLS	
Access	_____	Furniture	_____
Steps	_____	Obstacles	_____
Porch	_____	Lighting	_____
Noise	_____	Need handrails or	
INTERIOR		devices	_____
Number rooms	_____	PREVENT FIRES	
Type rooms	_____	Electrical cords	_____
Accessible bathroom	_____	Wiring	_____
Adequate heating	_____	PREVENT POISONING	
Lighting	_____	Storage	_____
Ventilation	_____		
Floors—type	_____	EMERGENCY PLAN	
Stairs	_____	Notify EMS	_____
Obstacles/barriers	_____	Electric Authority	_____
Refrigeration	_____	Phone numbers	_____
Water supply	_____	Transportation	_____
Sanitation	_____	Distance from health-	
Sleeping arrangements	_____	care facility	_____
Infestations	_____	Smoke alarms	_____
Privacy	_____	Evacuation of the	
EXTERNAL SYSTEMS		house in the case	
People	_____	of fire	_____
Support Systems	_____		
Neighborhood	_____		
Church	_____		
Health agency	_____		
Supportive Services	_____		
Need medical equipment			
Supplier	_____		

Figure 5-6.   Home assessment checklist.

ing. Attention must be directed to removing barriers and to ensuring adequate lighting. The use of certain types of mechanical equipment requires specific electrical outlets, and appropriate wiring. The nurse can assist the family in talking with the equipment supplier to see what voltage is required for the anticipated machinery.

Proper storage of medications and food supplements away from other household items will prevent accidents. Any medicinal solutions should be stored away from children and away from any food source to prevent poisoning.

Each family should have an emergency plan. Included in the plan would be the following: a list of emergency phone numbers near the phone, Emergency Medical System

(EMS) notification procedure; communication with the electric company in case of a power outage; distance from the nearest health facility and available transportation; and fire evacuation procedures.

An emergency plan should include ways of assisting the client out of the house in case of a fire. Frequently clients are bedfast and unable to help themselves in an emergency. The nurse can assist the family to make an emergency fire escape plan. The plan should include knowing two ways out of every room in the event that one way is blocked by smoke or heat. The fire department phone number should be posted on the phone. The family should also choose a place outdoors for everyone to meet. The National Fire Protection Association recommends that families practice the plan several times during the year.

When families are caring for an ill or disabled individual, the evacuation plan will need to be tailored to the particular limitations of the client. The nurse can suggest that the family confer with its local fire department to develop a specific evacuation plan based on the client's needs. In addition to the plan, the nurse can assist the family in assessing the major fire hazards in the home. Cigarettes are the leading cause of accidental multiple deaths from fires in residential properties. Fixed or portable heating equipment is the second most common cause of accidental multiple death fires. Electric fires also account for a high percentage of injury from frayed cords, overloaded outlets, and worn-out appliances. The family should inspect the home to identify possible sources of danger.

Smoke detectors can be installed and maintained in the home as an early warning device. It is recommended that there should be one smoke detector outside each sleeping area and in every level of the home. Community groups can provide individuals with help in obtaining and installing smoke detectors

in low-income housing or senior citizen residences.

Another area of home assessment includes the system *outside* the home but *interrelated* with it. Support systems in the neighborhood should be identified. Who are the individuals the family can call? What other resources are available in the community: church, health agency, support services, durable medical equipment supplier?

A thorough assessment of the home environment before care is planned is a crucial step in making sure that a realistic, workable arrangement for care is instituted.

FAMILY STRESS AND COPING ABILITIES

Families caring for an acutely ill family member at home are faced with demands that require significant family adjustments. The disruptive situation brings multiple problems for the family. Variations exist among families in their ability to adjust to the stress of providing care for a family member. Hill's (1965) theory of family stress identifies the reasons for variations in the family's response to stress. He defines crisis as *change in which old patterns are inadequate to manage the present situation.* Crises can vary from mild disruption to a serious disorganization of the family. Hill's theory considers the meaning or definition the family ascribes to the event and the family resources in terms of structure and values.

A stressor or crisis-provoking event is a situation for which the family has little or no preparation. Each family defines the event and assigns a personal meaning to it. No event is experienced in the same way by every family. Stressors become crises if the family defines them as such (Hill 1965). Hill's theory identifies *A* (the event) interacting with B (the family's crisis-meeting resources) interacting with C (the definition the family gives to event A) to produce X (the crisis). Family stress is experienced in the process of adjusting to care for the acutely ill family member. A family crisis changes many areas of family function and has the potential to produce disruptions in the usual behavior of the family.

Families vary in their ability to prevent the stressful event from becoming a crisis. Some families are more vulnerable to stress and are unable to meet the crisis constructively while other families have resources and recover from the crisis. Hansen and Will (1964) noted the concept of vulnerability as describing the family's ability to deal with stress. Some families show an amazing ability to regroup and adapt to the crisis-producing situation. The process of adapting to the changes required by caring for an acutely ill individual necessitates use of coping mechanisms by families. Families that deal with the crisis successfully find ways to strengthen their internal organization and to reach out to their support systems.

COPING STRATEGIES

Families need to use effective coping strategies to manage the requirements of home care. Coping is a way of managing stress. Coping behaviors are the crisis-meeting resources used by families in responding to the stressful situation.

When the family first encounters the need to provide home care for their acutely ill individual, there is often a period of shock and disbelief. During this period, the coping strategy used by the family unit may be denial. Denial, used for a limited time, can be an effective way for the family to step back and develop its regenerative powers. It allows the family time to gather the necessary energy to handle the disruption to the integrity of the

family system. Considerable energy will be required for the family to repattern the family system, and the temporary insulation provided by the use of denial helps the family to accomplish this.

OBTAINING INFORMATION

Once the family is receptive to acknowledging the realities of the illness and its effect on the family system, the family begins to search for information. This coping behavior assists the family to define the realities of the situation and to identify new family patterns that may be required. The acquisition of information leads to clarification and deeper understanding. Information can be obtained from many sources. The health-care team can be a valuable resource as can be social workers, spiritual advisors, extended family members and the literature.

Printed material about the disease process or the requirements of home care can provide information on what must be done to plan and deliver care in the home. An especially useful book written for the lay public deals with ways to approach home care (Friedman JA 1986). It outlines steps in the decision-making process for the family considering home care. In addition to searching for information, families search for meaning. The circumstances of the new situation threaten the family. Depending on the cultural and ethnic background of the family, illness may have a specific meaning. Some families believe illness is the result of their inadequacies or sins of the past. Religious beliefs are especially important. Some religions teach that God tests according to the abilities of the family to deal with the problem. With this philosophy, the family believes that the problem can be a way to earn more grace and faith. This belief can be a positive force in effective family coping. On the other hand, a belief that the condition is an example of divine retribution may lead to ineffective coping.

PRESERVING NORMAL PATTERNS

Another coping strategy is one directed to preserving as much normalcy in the home as possible. Whenever possible, the living arrangements in the home should not be unnecessarily disrupted. Changes in the home will need to be negotiated and typical ways of behaving will require alteration. However, these changes should be made very carefully. For example, the living room should not automatically be converted to a "sick" room. The initial efforts of the family are directed to maintaining as much as possible of the family's previous life-style. Preserving the normalcy of the family will maximize the positive adjustments of the client. The client should not be deprived of his self-reliance indiscriminately. Sometimes families react to the pain and grief of the situation by trying to do too much for the client. This is dysfunctional and promotes a dependent relationship. The use of an effective coping strategy to attempt to keep things as normal as possible minimizes the impact of the client's illness on the family system. This emphasizes the abilities of the client and the family. A focus on what is possible rather than on what is not is imperative.

IDENTIFYING SUPPORT SYSTEMS

One way to decrease stress on the family unit is to establish support systems. The family can cope more effectively by sharing its experience with others. The most critical and valuable support system is the family itself. The ability to manage the stress of the home-care situation is directly related to the ability of the family members to relate effectively and to support each other. All members of the family are important participants in the home-care process. The manner in which they communicate, assume various roles, and participate in problem solving and decision making are associated with positive or negative outcomes. When the family does not function as a support system, conflict is evident by the lack of emotional support, open communication, and tension. Cohesiveness of the family unit, on the other hand, leads to effective problem solving and management.

Other support groups outside the family can be useful adjuncts to the family system. Support groups associated with the client's specific disease, such as stroke, cord injury, head injury, and cancer, provide valuable information to assist the family in dealing with the "here and now" demands of care. These support groups bring together people who are coping with similar situations. Sharing their experience helps the family to gain additional perspectives and insights into the problems they are managing. Because the support groups are reality based, the family can express the fears, conflicts, anger, and despair openly and without fear of reprisal or guilt. The feelings of aloneness, facing an insurmountable situation, are decreased as the family learns of others sharing similar burdens.

The health-care team is also an example of a support group. The nurse as the coordinator of the team serves as a primary support, particularly in the area of information giving and in demonstrating problem solving, and ensures that other team members are used as needed.

CARE-GIVER BURDEN

Usually the major responsibility for the care of the family member falls to one member in the family, the care-giver. Literature related to the family care-giver addresses the problem of care-giver burden. Care-giver burden is defined as the social, emotional, and financial costs associated with the role (Stone, Cafferata, and Sangl 1986). While most reports in the literature are related to the role of the family in providing care to the elderly, the concepts have applicability for examining care-giver burden with acute care requirements in the home. The burden care-giving imposes on the family has been described in several studies (Brody 1981; Johnson 1983; Stoller 1983). In these studies, the data indicate that the stress of care-giving threatens the family system because of the need to provide care while also continuing to meet other family and work responsibilities. These studies suggest that care-giving for a disabled person at home is predominantly a female responsibility. Adult daughters and wives make up 28.9% and 22.7% respectively of the care-givers according to a 1986 government study (Stone et al 1986).

While the majority of care-givers are female, it is interesting to note that husbands are the oldest subgroup of care-givers and spend the most hours in care-giving activities (Stone et al 1986). Many care-givers, male and female, tend to be over 65 years of age, in the poor or near-poor income category, and report their health as only fair to poor. These data suggest that care-givers are an at-risk group for health problems themselves. Respite care and a variety of support services are needed to keep this population healthy. Because of the unique relationship of the care-giver to the client and family, the care-giver role will be addressed in terms of health implications and possible interventions.

ROLE CONFLICT

Multiple roles are necessary in the healthy development of an individual. People assume multiple roles throughout life: wife, sister, mother, teacher, and learn to balance the roles and mediate expectations and demands. Usually the complementary nature of roles in an individual's life enhances the quality of living. But sometimes the expectations and demands of multiple roles clash with each other. When this occurs, role conflict is the result.

Role conflict occurs when the care-giver is playing many roles that have competing obligations. The demands on the care-giver's time and energy are not easily reconciled. Very often, the care-giver is placed in the untenable position of trying to meet expectations and obligations of many roles simultaneously. One strategy to reduce role conflict is to reduce the number of roles. Studies show that female care-givers often quit their jobs as a way to reduce role conflict. While this does eliminate the occupational obligation, it deprives the care-giver of the stimulation provided by work outside the home.

ROLE FATIGUE

Many care-givers feel that confinement is one of the most difficult parts of the role. An increase in care-giving responsibilities leads to a restriction of activities outside the home. In their study of care-taker role fatigue, Goldstein and associates (1981) reported the negative consequences of confining one's activities to a single role. Their evidence suggests that when the individual's activities center around the single role of care-giving, and when the interpersonal interaction is chiefly confined to the ill family member, the result is role fatigue. At first, care-giving is added to other duties and roles. As time goes on, it is likely the client's condition will worsen or become more complex. Gradually, the demands of care-giving require more time and energy and become the focus of the care-giver's activities. The care-giver becomes as housebound as the client. With the technology in use today, the care-giver role may last for an indefinite period. The constant strain of care-giving along with confinement to the home can have a negative effect on the care-giver's health. The work is routine, composed of unvarying tasks with no days off and no relief in sight. Physical and mental exhaustion is not uncommon.

CARE-GIVER STRAIN

Cantor (1983) studied care-giver strain with a population of elderly clients and their primary care-givers. She found that most care-givers protect their families and their jobs but at considerable personal expense. The care-givers noted that the greatest stress occurred in the areas of personal desires, individuality, and socialization. The findings suggested that the amount of stress varies for different categories of care-givers. Children and spouses experience more stress in the care-giving role than do other relative care-givers. An overriding problem for all groups of care-givers was the emotional strain of caring for someone close. Financial strain seemed to be more of an issue of the spouse than for children or younger relatives.

Robinson (1983) developed a care-giver strain index to measure stress in informal care providers. The 13-item screening tool was devised to identify persons at risk due to stress engendered by the care-giving process. The questionnaire identified 13 stressors: inconvenience, confinement, family adjustments, changes in personal plans, competing demands on time, emotional adjustments, upsetting behavior, the client being a different person, work adjustments, feelings of being overwhelmed, sleep disturbance, physical strain, and financial strain (Robinson 1983). The author suggested the tool would be useful in primary prevention as a way to define specific care-giver populations at risk.

The care-giver role can be arduous and debilitating (Clark and Rakowski 1983). Family members who provide care often experience guilt and resentment as well as exhaustion due to the responsibilities of the role. The authors suggest education and support group programs to assist family care-givers to cope with their multiple demands.

Selected nursing diagnoses appropriate to family stress and care-giver burden will be presented as well as the assessment, implementation, and outcome for each diagnosis.

NURSING DIAGNOSES FOR HOME CARE

The next section presents selected nursing diagnoses that might be appropriate for the family in providing care at home. The diagnoses include references to the client and care-giver as well as to the overall family unit as appropriate for the discussion. These diagnoses are representative of what most families might experience when faced with the prospect of caring for the ill person at home.

INEFFECTIVE FAMILY COPING

Assessment

The home care nurse needs to identify the family's perception of the illness and the family's understanding of the specific treatments the client will require. The nurse needs to identify the family's choice and use of coping behaviors. It is especially important to assess past patterns of dealing with stressful situations. The personal characteristics of the family including age, birth order, sex, educational background, cultural beliefs, and values aid in an understanding of the meaning the stressful situation has for the family. Coping behaviors are actions used to deal with stressful events. The stress of acute illness in the home has to be dealt with to ensure family functioning. The coping strategies used by the family will influence the type of adjustment, positive or negative, the family makes.

Some families typically deal with stress by avoidance tactics. However, the avoidance may be based on fear and practiced for so long that, as a result, the family experiences increasing anxiety. Other families confront the event and feel more in control of the situation by having accurate information and an understanding of what is in store for them. The home-care nurse assesses the crisis-meeting resources of the family to identify ways in which the family can be assisted to use positive coping behaviors. The nurse must assess the family's readiness to accept more information about the home-care situation. If the family is in a period of denial, the nurse must problem solve for the family. The nurse needs to pace the amount of information shared in order to assist the family through the initial shock of the situation since they cannot absorb it. When the family is past the denial stage, the nurse intervenes by providing the needed information.

To assess coping behaviors, the nurse can ask some open-ended questions. Several examples follow:

- How has the family dealt with stressful situations in the past?
- What situations are anxiety-provoking for the family?
- How does the family deal with situations that cause anxiety?
- What are the family's actions in dealing with health problems?

The nurse also assesses the meaning of the illness/home-care situation for the family. Is it seen as part of life, part of God's plan, or punishment? Depending on the perception, the nurse will intervene in the appropriate manner. The relationship of the family members is assessed to see if they are open in their communication patterns. The nurse also assesses the family in regard to its roles and responsibilities and its process of decision making. Functional and dysfunctional aspects of relating are identified. The way in which the family relates to people and organizations outside the family is assessed. Resources available to the family are identified. The family's willingness to use support groups is explored. Is the family a closed unit with rigid boundaries or is it open and accepting of outside intervention?

The home itself requires careful assessment in terms of space, furniture, electrical supports, esthetics, and barriers to care. The nurse needs to assess the family's response to the need for an alteration in the physical surroundings of the home.

Interventions

The home-care nurse meets with the family to discuss the specific nature of the client's illness, the client's condition, and the treatment that will be required in the home. The nurse will explore the level of understanding the family has about the seriousness of the client's condition, the course of the illness, the potential problems that might arise, and the anticipated effects of home care on all aspects of family life. Anxiety caused by rumors and misinformation can be dispelled by obtaining accurate information. The nurse suggests books and articles for the family to read. J. A. Friedman's book (1986) on home care is especially useful for a family assuming the care of an acutely ill person in the home. Discussion with the family and other health-team members such as the physician, social worker, occupational therapist, physical therapist, and nutritionist are initiated by the nurse. In addition, the nurse assists the family to identify its crisis-meeting resources and coping strategies. The family is assisted in evaluating those behaviors that are effective and those that are not.

The nurse directs the family's actions to maximizing the competence of the acutely ill individual and the family system as well. By assisting the family to develop strategies to minimize the negative features of the situation and to maximize the resources and abilities of the family system, the nurse supports the family's positive coping behavior.

The nurse works with the family to determine ways of keeping the family routine and function as normal as possible. Sometimes, physical requirements for providing care necessitate modifications of the home environment. The nurse will support the family's problem-solving and decision-making process in determining the amount of restructuring required.

The nurse exhibits a nonjudgmental approach that facilitates the family members in discussing effective management of the illness. All family members are encouraged to be honest with each other about their personal needs, fears, and concerns. A discussion of expected family roles and task delineation is encouraged. In facilitating the family's need to be active agents in the home care situation, the nurse supports the family's decisions and enables them to recognize their ability to influence the environment. Through referral to appropriate sources of assistance, the nurse facilitates the family in obtaining needed services.

Adjustment to the home-care situation may take families an indefinite period of time. During this phase, new patterns of relating and interacting must be formed. Each family copes differently. By accepting the family's negative feelings in a nonjudgmental manner, the nurse helps the family to test new behaviors. When effective coping strategies are used, positive reinforcement is given. Sometimes family members can be disagreeable and even hostile. Rather than reacting to troublesome family members, the nurse attends to the necessities of treatment and care.

This focus on providing care often redirects the family's energy to constructive activity.

Outcomes

The family will reduce the ambiguity related to its situation by gaining adequate information about possibilities of home care. As a result of understanding the illness and the associated requirements for home care, the family will experience feelings of mastery and self-esteem. As the family learns more about what has to be done, feelings of anxiety will decrease. It is to be hoped that the family will gain insights through readings and discussions with others. The family begins to distinguish between which of the client's functions are affected and which are not affected to ensure as much normal living as possible.

Once potential problems are clearly identified, the family can develop a list of troubleshooting interventions that could be used in the event that a particular problem occurs. By taking positive steps to be prepared, the family will experience a feeling of mastery and competence in carrying out the demands of home care. As more experience is gained in performing technical aspects of care, the family's confidence level will increase. Reduction of uncertainty coupled with comfort in performing procedures results in the family's increasing sense of control over the situation.

Changes in family life resulting from home care are very disruptive. It is important for the family to maintain at least a portion of the previous life-style. The family is expected to make the adjustments to the demands of home care using effective coping behaviors. Improvements in daily management of care can be achieved and the progress serves to support the family's effective coping skills.

The family will see itself as a support group and be alert to support the health and growth of its members. Appropriate external support groups that might be helpful will be identified and used. As the family becomes increasingly aware of the specific requirements of its home-care situation, the resources of the health-care system will be used more effectively. The family is expected to take a long-term view of problems, and come to an acceptance of the incremental nature of finding solutions. By actively participating with the home-care nurse, a realistic workable plan for home care will be developed.

An alternate outcome is that the nurse assists the family to come to terms with the idea that the level of client care is too complex to manage and that alternate arrangements need to be made. There is a range of alternate arrangements that can be explored, depending on the individual situation, such as nursing home placement or 24-hour agency care. This is important because for many families the positive outcome is to realize the limitations on its ability to continue care at home.

DIVERSIONAL ACTIVITY DEFICIT

The degree to which an individual or family experiences an environment that is empty and unstimulating leads to diversional activity deficit (Carpenito 1984). This nursing diagnosis can be applied to the family unit, the client, and the care-giver.

The entire family unit responds to the monotony and constancy of the client's confinement. Lack of motivation and depression often result. Not only does the family as a unit experience a deficit in diversional activity, but also the family must anticipate problems the client will experience due to loss of ability to perform usual activities. Boredom is a defining characteristic of diversional activity deficit. The consequences of boredom can be feelings of oppression, anger, and hostility. In order to relieve these feelings, individuals may initiate unhealthy practices such as overeating, alcohol abuse, or drug abuse.

For the care-giver, the excessively long hours of responsibility, the lack of time to pursue former interests, and the absence of leisure activities coalesce to place her at risk of experiencing diversional activity deficit. The care-giver is especially vulnerable to restlessness and boredom, due to the constancy of the demands of home care. Prior to assuming the care-giver role, the individual may have been very active in the community or may have enjoyed recreational sports. Some care-givers, especially females, have given up jobs to be at home with the client, thereby losing the stimulation of the workplace. Day-to-day confinement to the home can lead to boredom, constant dwelling on negative thoughts and feelings, a lack of zest, restlessness, anger, and change in weight.

The client may be too ill to experience a deficit. However, even in situations where the client is severely disabled, there may be a need to provide diversional activity. The family can be assisted to use appropriate stimuli to vary the routine of care. For example, music, change in scenery, and visitors can be helpful in adding positive stimulation to the client's surroundings.

Assessment

The nurse should be careful to assess the family system as well as the client and care-giver subsystem for diversional activity deficit.

Family

An assessment of the family's diversional activity deficit due to the monotony of confinement will include observation of the family members and their interactions. Signs of boredom and ineffective patterns of communication are signals to the nurse. Questions can be directed to the family members to obtain information about their activity level prior to the client's illness. The nurse might ask

- What is the family's outlook/approach to life?
- What does the family do to have fun together?
- How does the family relate to external systems (*i.e.*, church, neighborhood, schools)?

It is important to assess the family's support system and the family's perception of assistance needed. Changes in the health status or behavior of family members are also important to assess. Weight loss or gain, insomnia, increased alcohol consumption, or the taking of over-the-counter drugs may be signs that the family system is experiencing difficulty with the monotony of care.

Client

An assessment of the client experiencing diversional activity deficit is discussed in greater detail in other chapters. The focus of the discussion here is to assist the family to become aware of potential difficulties in order to manage the client more effectively. An assessment of the client's abilities and disabilities, both physical and mental, leads to a judgment about the types of activities the client may be able to handle. It is important to assess the client's interest in hobbies. Limited mobility and compromised endurance do not close the door to diversional activity. The client may learn photography and take pictures from a window (Friedman JA 1986). Many homes have computers and if cognitive function is not impaired, the client might be able to write letters, keep a journal, assist with cataloguing household supplies, and doing the bills. Possibilities are as numerous as the creative mind can imagine.

Care-giver

In assessing the care-giver, the nurse needs to be aware of the role as it affects the specific individual. How demanding are the responsibilities? Are there competing demands for the care-giver's time? For example, many care-givers also have children who require a great deal of attention and support. Or is the care-giver primarily confined to interaction with the client? Should the activities be quiet or of a physical exercise nature? What is the care-giver's perception of the situation? Some care-givers feel overly busy with inadequate time for relaxing activities, while others feel bored and trapped and desire more recreational options. Does the care-giver experience guilt about taking time off to attend to personal needs? It is essential that the care-giver understand the need for self-care to replenish the energy necessary for the care-giver role. With the care-giver, the nurse explores the options available within the specific situation. Are there other family members, neighbors, church groups, agency personnel who can be enlisted to provide the care-giver with some time away from the home?

Interventions

For the purposes of discussion here, the nurse must intervene on three levels, the family level, the client level, and the care-giver level.

Family

On the family level, the nurse assists the family unit to recognize signs of family boredom and inertia. Encouraging the family to take the responsibility for doing something to alleviate boredom is an action that taps the inner resources of the family. Ways to reduce monotony and stimulate renewed interest are explored. Negative feelings are openly discussed and shared as a way to intervene and deal with the perception of being trapped.

Activities are redirected to increase positive stimulation in the home environment. Routines of care are varied to add diversion. Pleasant activities are chosen based on the family's desire to contribute to a cheerful environment.

Some strategies to reduce the stress and boredom of care can be employed. Use of time management techniques can be especially useful to the family. The nurse assists the family to manage time more effectively by clarifying priorities. It is helpful for the family to know what *must* be accomplished, what *should* be accomplished with delays being acceptable, and what *does not have* to be accomplished at all. Ways to restructure time and how it is spent gives the family a sense of control. There is a need to assess the "superwoman" or "superman" concept as it operates in the family system. Overcommitment to others and unrealistic expectations lead to increased frustration and irritability. Enlisting the support and participation of others in care assists the family to meet its obligations, and also increases the stimulation to the family. Families need to be supported in planning activities to increase positive experiences. Use of audiotapes to listen to a story or music while doing household tasks is a creative way to add pleasantries to everyday routines.

Client

In working with the family to alleviate the client's boredom, the nurse assists the family and client to identify manageable tasks that are within the client's physical and functional ability. Allowing the client to make as many decisions as possible supports the client's dignity and provides him with an improved quality of life.

With this nursing diagnosis, one intervention might be a referral for an occupational therapy assessment and treatment plan. Occupational therapists are trained in assisting clients to find diversional activities. A coordinated team with the occupational therapist, nurse, client, and family approach would strengthen the interventions and assist the client in realistically choosing appropriate activity.

Enjoyable activities and hobbies promote the client's self-esteem and result in a sense of satisfaction and pleasure. The pursuit of diversional activity not only lessens boredom for the client but adds meaning and purpose to his life. Together with the client and nurse, the family explores the different types of activities available. The choices are many. Photography, coin and stamp collecting, various forms of needlework, knitting, drawing, painting, chess, checkers, cards, games, crafts, and even indoor gardening are just some of the possibilities. Television can provide a diversion and be a form of recreation as long as it does not become a means of withdrawal from interaction with others. Using humor and watching amusing stories on TV or videotapes can lighten the client's mood. If a client has some physical or visual impairment, the family can participate in the hobby. This adds some zest and excitement to life and centers the attention on an activity outside the illness. Once a diversional activity is chosen, the nurse can assist the client and family to plan ahead and conserve energy. The nurse assists the client to plan for recreation as well as rest and to set priorities. Scheduling hobbies when the client is rested will result in more enjoyment than trying to encourage the activity at a time of low energy. There are many tasks that have to be accomplished. It is just as important to include those things that bring enjoyment to the client in the day's plan of care as it is to perform the tasks and procedures of care-giving.

Care-giver

In intervening with the care-giver who requires diversional activity, the nurse needs to create an atmosphere of acceptance to permit the care-giver to ventilate feelings. To plan, the care-giver should list all the tasks that must be performed each day. Then, tasks that can be delegated to someone else should be identified. The care-giver should identify ways to conserve energy by scheduling the tasks in an efficient manner. All supplies and equipment should be anticipated prior to the treatment to save unnecessary steps. A realistic time frame for the tasks and chores should be created, and a schedule should be made. The schedule should include rest breaks, recreational activities, and time away from the home. The plan should be reevaluated and modified based on the results on a routine basis. By making the requirements for diversion explicit in the planning process, the need is legitimized and the care-giver is freed from the overwhelming need to do it all. This enables the care-giver to participate in other activities such as a church choir, a community meeting, bridge, a movie, or time to read a book.

Care-givers can be assisted to reduce stress and boredom by employing relaxation techniques using imagery and visualization (Pender 1987). Recalling pleasant scenes or images promotes pleasant feelings and sensations. The nurse may suggest the following techniques:

- Have the care-giver visualize a landscape or scene focusing on the colors, shapes, and sounds.
- Have the care-giver visualize a personal room or article of clothing describing it in detail, shape, texture, and configuration.

The care-giver should also be encouraged to find time for physical exercise. This will assist in reducing stress. It will also provide a diversionary activity for the individual. One of the more effective ways to exercise is walking. It does not require expensive equipment, health club fees, or a set time. It can be worked into a busy schedule easier than more structured forms of activity such as tennis or golf or exercise classes. Whatever the choice of activity, the nurse should encourage the care-giver in devising a way to do it that is personally acceptable and achievable. The benefits are too numerous to disre-

gard. Other strategies to achieve relaxation include more formal preparation such as autogenic training, yoga, meditation, hypnosis, relaxation response.

Outcomes

Family

The family members will recognize feelings of boredom and use specific diversional activities suited to specific interests and needs of the members. Ways to modify the physical environment to increase attractiveness and cheerfulness will be employed. This may include new window shades to permit more light into the room, flowers, posters, clocks, or changing the furniture in the room. Family members will share ideas and suggestions to vary the routine and stimulate interest.

Client

The family will encourage the client to identify an activity compatible with the limitations of the specific illness. The client will plan with the care-giver and other family members to include the diversional activity at times of higher energy. Increased self-esteem and increased interest in using time for the hobby will result. The client will express an increase in the purposefulness of life. After testing the plan and schedule, the client will decide to continue, modify or eliminate the activity.

Care-giver

The care-giver will experience less hostility, boredom, and anger. Routinized boredom will decrease, and the care-giver will experience increased self-esteem from taking a constructive role in finding appropriate outlets for personal expression. As a result, the care-giver will achieve a higher energy level, decrease dysfunctional health habits, and experience more enjoyment.

FAMILY PROCESS, ALTERATION IN:

The state in which a family experiences a situation that challenges its functioning ability results in alteration in family process (Carpenito 1984). Many factors can contribute to an alteration in family process. The acute illness of a family member and change in the family member's ability to function can place burdensome demands on the usual pattern of family functioning. Add to this the need for time-consuming and expensive treatments requiring considerable technical skill, and the family process is changed. Often illness also brings a change in family roles. The illness not only influences the client but also changes the patterns of the family and alters the role relationships. The family system cannot or does not meet the physical, emotional, and psychosocial needs of its members. The family may not seek help appropriately or respond to the crisis constructively. Tension and strain often cause problems with family communication.

This nursing diagnosis is consistently appropriate for the family providing care to an acutely ill family member. The basic activities of daily living, often taken for granted, take on new meaning for the client and the family care-giver. Routines need to be adjusted and habits altered. The physical surroundings of the home may need to be modified to permit access to equipment or to allow space to maneuver a wheelchair from one room to another. Handrails may need to be added to the walls in the hallway. The kitchen and bathroom may need to be rearranged. Even sleeping space may need to be altered, as in the case of a grandparent who comes to stay with the family. A teen-age girl may be asked to share her own bedroom with grandma.

The nature of the problem, the extent of the disability, and the resources available in the home all influence the degree of adjustment required. Sometimes the need to care for an aging parent precipitates an adolescent behavioral problem. It is very clear that a change in the family system changes all members of the system. Normal family processes are interrupted by the shift in boundaries. The family responds to the new stresses and strives to maintain balance or to adapt to the situation and establish new ways of behaving.

Assessment

The nurse needs to conduct a thorough and systematic assessment of the family. Given the time constraints confronting today's home-care nurse, it is necessary to streamline the assessment process but not in a way that compromises data collection. All too often the nurse may arrive at a nursing diagnosis with inadequate information. The use of a conceptual model to provide structure for the assessment process can be an invaluable tool for the nurse.

The systems approach enables the nurse to gather information about the structure and function of the family. It is important to determine the family's usual patterns of communication and decision making. Role relationships need to be understood, and the nurse should determine whether role changes are temporary or permanent. The issue of power and control is also important to assess. The family's methods of coping with illness or stress in the past can provide information for determining how they might react to the present crisis. The belief system and values of the family provide information to assist the nurse in understanding the unique family process.

Use of a genogram to display the family constellation visually and an echomap to diagram the external relationship of the family are simple techniques that assist the nurse to conduct a systematic assessment in a deliberate and time-conserving manner.

Family assessment questions that illuminate family process might include

- What kinds of things does the family value?
- Who are the people important to the family?
- Are there adequate finances available to meet the needs imposed by this illness?
- How has the illness changed the life-style of the family?
- Which family member has been most affected by the illness?
- Who has the major responsibility for the client?
- Who generally identifies problems in the family?

Information about family patterns of daily living is a valuable source of assessment data. The nurse can acquire an understanding of the manner in which the family operates by an assessment of the following areas:

- Meal preparation
- Mealtime
- Household tasks
- Health care (dental and medical)
- Exercise
- Rest/sleep
- Leisure time
- Hobbies and recreational interests
- Interaction with friends
- Interactions with extended family
- Use of alcohol and tobacco

Interventions

The nurse assists the family to use what is known about the illness and its impact on the family and to plan for alterations in the family process. There may need to be an alteration of the home environment to accommodate the ill client. A family meeting where all members could be included in not only identifying where the changes should be made but also in deciding how to carry them out is one way to arrive at decisions. The nurse can introduce the family to a durable medical supplier for suggestions about equipment needs.

It is important for the family members to list all issues that they will be dealing with in providing care at home. The client's condition may improve or worsen, necessitating additional adjustment. The process of decision making should be clearly identified. If there is one person who typically makes decisions for the family, this should be acknowledged. If one person functions primarily as the care-giver, the nurse can assist the family to understand the requirements and strains of the role. For example, the family could reorganize roles at home to lessen the care-giver burden. Other family members or community groups such as church volunteers and neighbors can provide the family with time away from the situation.

Outcomes

The family will verbalize feelings to each other and to the nurse. Decisions will be made to care for the client in a constructive manner without jeopardizing the health of the family members or the care-giver. Recognizing the pressures on the family, mutual support and encouragement will be maintained among the family members. When appropriate, the family will seek external resources.

FEAR

The nursing diagnosis of fear is applicable for family members involved in home care. Fear is the state in which a person or family experiences an uneasy feeling that is related to a specific source perceived as dangerous (Carpenito 1984). Fear can occur in situations where the health of a family member is threatened. In situations of severe illness, long-term disability, degenerative disease, and terminal disease, the client and the family might respond with fear. The care-giver might fear the expectations of the role.

Situational factors contribute to fear when a lack of knowledge about the client's condition, a change in the significant other, invasive procedures, and the need for medical treatments are present. Characteristics found in fear include a feeling of physiological or emotional disruption related to an identified threat and feeling of loss of control. The individual, be it the client, care-giver or a caring family member may exhibit physical signs such as an increased pulse and respiratory rate and increased blood pressure, voice tremors, and perspiration.

Assessment

Families faced with the need to care for an acutely ill person are certain to experience fear to some degree. The fear is not only related to the present condition of the client but also to future changes, anticipated or expected. It is important for the nurse to assess the family unit and its perception of fear. Are all family members fearful? To what degree? Is the client fearful? To what degree? Has the family previously experienced fear of this magnitude? How has the family dealt with previous fearful situations?

It is important for the nurse to assess the coping mechanisms of the family. Has the family confronted the fearful issue or has it denied it? Which mechanism does the family use to decrease the negative sensations? It is imperative that the nurse adequately question the family for the specific characteristics of fear. It is also important to note the relationship of the fear experience with the client and other family members. What do the family members know about the illness, prognosis, and treatment plan?

Interventions

The nurse's interventions will be based on the unique circumstances giving rise to the client's care-giver's and family's fear experience. The nurse can mobilize the family as well as the client and care-giver to discuss their feelings, thoughts, and perceptions openly with each other. The act of verbalizing often helps to diminish the perception of fear. The responses to the fear should be carefully described. Family members should be encouraged to verbalize all questions. Once verbalized, they become less threatening and easier to confront. If some members are experiencing physiologic effects, the nurse can intervene with suggestions for stress management and relaxation. (A suggestion for progressive muscle relaxation is found in Chapter 8.)

The nurse can provide accurate information to the family and care-giver about the person's illness and expected course. The nurse also needs to describe the treatment plan in detail. It is necessary for the family members to understand the prescribed treatment and the expected outcome. Often knowledge about the disease can reduce some of the fear. It is easier to deal with the identifiable than to worry about the unseen problems lurking in the future. The care-giver implements the physical care of the client and manages the routines with the guidance of the nurse. The nurse can direct the family to the appropriate resources of counseling or spiritual guidance, if required. At times family members are "more afraid" than the client. What often occurs is a conspiracy of silence where the family members attempt to protect the sick person from the facts. In so doing, poor patterns of communication are established. The nurse can assist the family to identify where its processes of communication have become dysfunctional.

Outcomes

The client, care-giver and family are able to discuss their fear openly. Areas of inadequate information are clarified so that all members in the family have an accurate representation of reality. The family deals with the fear by open communication, seeking answers to problem questions, seeking support from a counselor, clergyman, or support groups as appropriate. The client and family are expected to deal with the facts of the illness constructively with a focus on the strengths rather than the limitations of the situation. Technical care is managed competently and comfortably by the care-giver.

IMPAIRED HOME MAINTENANCE MANAGEMENT

Impaired home maintenance management is a state in which an individual or family experiences difficulty in maintaining a safe home environment (Carpenito 1984). Etiological and contributing factors to this nursing diagnosis include chronic debilitating disease, injury to family member, impaired mental status, substance abuse, unavailable support system, loss of family member, lack of knowledge, and inadequate finances. Defining characteristics include difficulty in maintaining the home, difficulty in caring for self or family members at home, impaired care-giver, lack of knowledge, poor hygiene practices, inadequate support systems.

Assessment

The family's perception of its ability to maintain the home environment is very important. Very often, an elderly person is the care-giver for the elderly spouse, and is often experiencing chronic health problems of her own. The nurse can first provide an atmosphere of acceptance to facilitate an open exchange of communication. The elderly care-giver is often fearful of her ability to handle the situation.

The nurse assesses the physical, emo-

tional, and spiritual needs of the family system, including those of care-giver. Available support systems are also assessed and identified. The nurse assesses the meaning of illness to the family, and the value placed on remaining in the family home. The pattern of problem solving over the family's lifetime provides insight into how the family will think about its present difficulty. The nurse assesses the home environment in regard to safety and cleanliness.

Interventions

The nurse has a responsibility to intervene in a manner that supports the family choices but points out any serious threats to safety or health. The nurse assists the care-giver to contact resources to help with small home maintenance projects. A senior citizen center might have a program of retired carpenters, plumbers, and electricians who do odd jobs for other seniors at minimal or no cost. The nurse can inform the family or care-giver of this service and leave the phone number and the necessary information. In addition, the community often has several churches with a friendly visitor program. Arrangements could be made for a person to visit the client to give his wife some relaxation time. The nurse also informs the wife that she might contract for homemaker/home-health services to assist with the household tasks. The nurse also provides information about the cost of these services and recommends that the care-giver talk to the agency social worker to determine eligibility for designated services.

Outcomes

The care-giver will contact the senior citizen center and arrange for the needed home repairs. Arrangements will be made for a visitor to come once a week. During the time the visitor is in the home, the care-giver will rest, read a book, or engage in an enjoyable activity. The care-giver will meet with the social worker to determine if the family is eligible for any other services. It is expected that a plan will be developed to maintain the home through the use of support services available from the senior citizen center.

ALTERATION IN PARENTING

Alteration in parenting is a state in which one or more individuals experience a real or potential inability to provide a constructive environment promoting the growth and development of the children (Carpenito 1984). Families who may be at high risk for experiencing parental difficulties include parents who are terminally ill or acutely disabled and children who are physically or mentally handicapped or terminally ill. Any condition of the child or parent that increases the stress of the family unit adversely influences parenting ability. Defining characteristics for this nursing diagnosis include expressions of frustration of parental role, feelings of inadequacy, evidence of abuse or neglect, and inappropriate parenting behaviors.

Assessment

In assessing the family for alteration in parenting, the nurse must look for a history of past parental behaviors. Then an assessment of the particular health problem should be conducted with particular attention to the function of the family. The values and beliefs of the family in regard to parenting are important. Financial resources and available support systems are identified.

Another family at high risk is the one in which the parents are caring for their own parents and have less time and energy available for their children. Often conflict and guilt are the result. A situation such as this might be referred to as the sandwich genera-

tion. Care-giver parents are sandwiched between their parents and their children. They must be available to their parents and their children while dealing with their own developmental needs and managing their health and work.

Case Study

In the case of a mother who is the primary care-giver for an elderly parent and parent to five children under 14 years of age, competing demands for her time often produce exceptional stress. The mother may not have the physical or emotional energy to meet the needs of five young children. The nurse learns that the mother always attended the children's school plays and related functions but has had to miss every activity for the past year. The older children express resentment toward their grandmother for moving in with them and disrupting their lives. The husband works long hours and is not at home until 7:30 p.m. each night. The children assist with the meals but the youngest child who is five years old is becoming increasingly irritable, has frequent temper tantrums and is difficult to manage.

Interventions

Interventions related to alterations in parenting have to be carefully tailored to each individual situation. Depending on the reasons for the difficulty, the nurse's approach will be related to the problems identified in the assessment. The nurse might suggest some readings on the topic of parenting. There are many books on the market that deal with the subject and that can be useful to the family in sorting out its feelings and conflicts (Hymovich and Chamberlin 1986). In the example given above, the nurse meets with the family to determine ways the mother's energy might be conserved. The burden of physical care has been so demanding that the mother withdrew from her own role as mother. The nurse allowed her to discuss her feelings about this, and assisted her in identifying the daily tasks that were necessary. This list was carefully examined to see if other help could be obtained. A careful review of the family finances and the elderly parent's resources concluded that there was enough money to pay for some household help for the mother. The nurse suggested that the mother make a list of each child's activities for the coming month. The mother held a meeting with the children and asked them to help her to construct a schedule so that she might spend time with each one and attend at least one school or club function of each child. The husband decided to become more active with the children and to provide time for them to be together. The nurse suggested that the youngest child be seen in the health clinic by the pediatric nurse practitioner who would work with the family to devise a strategy to intervene with his temper tantrums. The parents were encouraged to accept the older girls' expression of frustration and to allow them to ventilate their feelings.

Outcomes

The family is expected to identify ways to enhance parenting behavior. The care-giver will repattern her activity to include the children. The children will become involved in some of the minimal tasks associated with their grandmother's care. The father will assume a more active parenting role. The temper tantrums will dissipate and the parents will gain confidence in being able to deal effectively with the children's problems.

POWERLESSNESS

Powerlessness occurs when there is the perception of a lack of control over events and situations (Carpenito 1984). Families experience feelings of powerlessness when confronted with the demands of home care. The family member may not wish to undertake the responsibility for home care but may feel there is no other alternative. Family reactions to loss of control vary in every family. The response may be apathy, anger, or depression. Any serious disease can contribute to powerlessness. It is all the more profound in diseases or conditions that result in an inability to communicate or to perform activities of daily living. Diseases that are progressive and debilitating such as amyotrophic lateral sclerosis and multiple sclerosis cause intense feelings of powerlessness. The disease seems relentless in robbing the person of functional ability.

Situational factors also contribute to this state. Lack of knowledge, lack of involvement in decision making regarding care, and lack of information from a health-care team are examples of situational factors. The defining characteristics present in powerlessness are the dissatisfaction over the lack of control because of the illness, the care, the recovery period. Persons react to the experience of powerlessness in many ways. Some are apathetic and resigned while others display signs of aggressive acting-out behavior.

Assessment

The family's expression of its lack of control can best be obtained by a discussion of its perceptions and feelings. The family's beliefs in regard to control and lack of control should be ascertained. If the family has been characterized by independence and self-sufficiency, the presence of acute illness can have serious consequences for family health.

The client's illness itself is perceived as a menancing threat to family integrity. The technology of the treatment modalities imposes even more of a threat. Machines, pumps, whistles, and all sorts of alien sounds are frightening enough in the hospital environment. They assume almost terrifying proportions in the home.

An assessment of the home environment must take into account the physical surroundings necessary to support the care of the client. Space, accessibility to adequate electrical supply, width of hallways and doors, and storage area for supplies need to be considered. Most families have no idea of what is involved in setting up the physical environment for home care. The nurse needs to assess what the living patterns of the family were prior to the client's illness and need for home care. An understanding of the typical use of space, leisure time, and activities of the family members can be useful in making inferences related to the diagnosis of powerlessness.

Interventions

The nurse needs to include the family in deciding areas of control. Since lack of control leads to powerlessness, finding ways to give the client and family some control over the situation will decrease those negative feelings. The nurse can teach the family about the illness, the available treatments, alternatives, and prognosis. Understanding leads to a sense of control. Effort should be made for the family unit to reinforce the client's strengths.

The nurse can assist the family to help the client resume healthy living patterns as far as possible within the limitations of the illness. When possible, the family should encourage the client to sleep in his own room or at least, in a bedroom. The nurse can discuss the disadvantages of turning a living room or dining room into a sick room for the client. The family needs to understand that the client's self-esteem will be increased by maintaining the normalcy of the home as much as possible. The family should encourage the client to wear street clothes during the day, to carry out personal grooming such as shaving if a man and use of cosmetics if a woman. Attention should be paid to hair care also. The family can support the client's interest in dressing and grooming by arranging clothing and toilet articles in an area where the individual can reach them. The nurse can assist the family to promote the client's participation in family activities. All family members can discuss possible options and offer choices that are mutually satisfactory to the client and the family.

Outcomes

The family is expected to make choices about its situation. Modifications of the physical structure of the home can be accomplished with as least disruption as possible. The client's participation in self-care will be encouraged by the family. The client care-giver and family will experience a sense of self-esteem and a decrease in powerless feelings. The family unit will continue to work together in planning care and performing treatments. Confidence in performing technical procedures will occur as the family care-giver learns how to do them and practices the techniques.

SOCIAL ISOLATION

Social isolation is a state in which the family, client, and care-giver express a desire for a contact with others but are unable to have that contact (Carpenito 1984). Social isolation can occur as a result of illness and disrupted patterns. Illness usually affects established relationships.

Social isolation is a subjective state that requires validation. Characteristics of social isolation include feelings of unexplained dread or abandonment. The perception of time passing slowly and the desire for more contact with others are common reactions. Because of these feelings the client is unable to concentrate, and experiences feelings of uselessness.

Behavioral signs can be shown in a variety of ways. Inability to make decisions is a common response. This nursing diagnosis is particularly applicable to the client and the care-giver. The client experiences the isolation imposed by the illness. The condition limits the full functioning of the person. The care-giver experiences this because of the demands of her role. Normal routine has been changed and support systems have been altered. The demands of the role place the care-giver in a very lonely situation.

Assessment

The home-care nurse assesses the entire family unit to see the types of relationships that exist. In families with limited support systems, the nurse needs to find ways to enhance family support. The nurse can serve as the counselor and coordinator for the family. With the family, the nurse can assist in identifying agencies that might provide social support. Organizations devoted to specific illnesses such as the Cancer Society, Arthritis Association, and stroke groups can be valuable resources for the client and family. It is helpful to understand the present experience of the client and care-giver by assessing the types of social contacts these individuals experienced before the illness. If the client was very active in civic affairs and attended meetings every night of the week, the change to being ill and confined to home would be even more drastic than for someone who primarily stayed at home and interacted mainly with the family. The same is true of the care-giver. The care-giver's social patterns and response to the world outside the home can be a severe loss.

Interventions

In families with supportive, caring relationships, the nurse can assist the family to mobilize energies in such a way to diminish the experience of social isolation. The nurse assists the family to establish short-term and long-term goals to reduce the feelings of isolation. The goal may be to eat meals in the family kitchen or to go outside on the porch. As the client's condition improves or stabilizes it may be possible to go to a movie or to a concert, or to a restaurant. The phone is an effective link to others. The nurse might suggest that the family encourage the client to call old friends at certain times of the day. The family could be asked to include the client in family activities such as card playing, checkers, or jigsaw puzzles.

Surround the client with the things and people that are important to him. Ask him who he wants to see. Arrange for visits according to the person's wishes. The nurse can facilitate this supportive approach to decreasing the sense of isolation. The care-giver's isolation is somewhat different. Here is a healthy person being confined to the home in order to take care of another. If there are other available family members, the nurse could call a meeting to discuss ways to increase social contacts for the care-giver.

Outcomes

The family, including the client and care-giver, is expected to find meaningful ways to decrease its isolation. The client may discover new areas of interest to engage in with friends or family. Perhaps, before the illness, the client was not interested in board games, but now finds them a pleasant diversion. The client will keep alert by watching game shows on television, and attempting to answer the questions. A game of Trivial Pursuit with the children will also include the client. For some persons, the illness is so debilitating as to preclude almost any activity. In these situations, the client will decide on a visitation schedule inviting those who are important to him.

The care-giver is expected to acknowledge the negative feelings of the care situation and to take concrete action to alleviate them. The care-giver will plan an activity with friends outside the home.

POTENTIAL FOR VIOLENCE

The potential for violence is a state in which a family or individual experiences aggressive behavior directed to self or to others (Carpenito 1984). There are physical causes that can precipitate violent behavior, but these are not being considered in this discussion. Rather, the situational determinants leading to possible violence are discussed. Situational factors include an increase in stressors over a short period of time, threat to self-esteem, fear of the unknown, poor communication patterns, response to a dysfunctional family. Defining characteristics include history of abuse, aggressive acts, paranoid behavior, perception of environment as frightening.

Assessment

The home health nurse needs to assess the family for predisposition to abusive behavior. A history of abuse to self or others as well as a history of emotional difficulties in the family would indicate a potential for violence. The level of stress due to home care requirements would also be assessed. A history of the family's ability to deal with stress in the past is important to obtain.

Clients who are very young and those who are very old are particularly vulnerable to abuse. Although physical abuse is serious, abuse on a verbal and emotional level is also serious. In assessing the interaction of family members, the nurse observes the family pattern of behavior. The manner in which the family responds to the child or elderly adult gives evidence of their treatment of that person.

The nurse should be alert to signs of mistreatment such as ridiculing comments, sarcasm, critical comments, irritation, and a lack of patience toward the client. Also signs of manipulation by the ill client should be acknowledged. Sometimes the ill person engages in difficult behavior to attract attention or to control the care-giver. It is not uncommon to hear stories of the elderly client refusing to eat, crying, throwing things, and yelling at others. This aggressive behavior can precipitate an aggressive action by the care-giver in an unstable family system.

In performing the physical assessment of the client, the nurse should be alert to suspicious markings on the body, including bruises, burns, broken bones, or other injuries. Overt aggression is only one form of abuse. Another form is neglect or indifference. Sometimes the elderly person is confined to his bed or room unnecessarily. At times families lock the door in an attempt to "protect" the client. What they are really doing is ignoring the person's needs and creating an atmosphere that leads to even more destructive behavior. If other care-givers are involved with the client it is possible that they could be involved in perpetrating abuse. Neglect also includes inadequate nutrition and withholding or overdosing on medications. The nurse also needs to be alert for these signs.

Interventions

The nurse will promote family discussion about the effects of the stressful situation on its behavior. Family members will verbalize feelings of frustration with the client. The client will be included in the discussions and will be encouraged to talk to the family about his perception of being ridiculed or chastised for having "accidents" and not handling personal care effectively. The nurse will assist the family to see how ridicule and sarcasm make the situation worse. The client's losses of self-esteem will be discussed openly. The nurse will provide information about an elder abuse support group for the family. In the extreme event that the nurse suspects overt physical violence, the appropriate authorities will be notified and family will be assisted to obtain psychiatric support. In many states the law *requires* any suspicion of neglect or abuse to be reported to the authorities.

Outcomes

The family will appreciate the client's feelings of helplessness, loss of health, and lack of control over his life. The family will seek family therapy assistance to deal with the feelings and reactions engendered by this situation. Behaviors that particularly push the family care-giver to potentially violent behavior will be identified and dealt with constructively. The client will gain an appreciation of the care-giver's feelings about the responsibility for providing care as well as worry about the ability to handle all necessary tasks. The family will attend meetings of an elder abuse support group, and will demonstrate progress in channeling its behaviors into constructive action. Abusive behavior will be reduced so that ridicule and sarcasm are not used toward the client. The care-giver will learn to recognize signs of stress on himself that are likely to result in abusive behavior.

ABBREVIATED CARE PLAN: FAMILY STRESS

Nursing Diagnosis	Assessment	Interventions	Outcomes
Diversional Activity Deficit: Client	Client's abilities and disabilities for activity Client's specific interests	Assist client to perform his own program of activity. Promote participation in family activities. Refer to occupational therapist. Tailor plan of activity to coincide with client's energy level. Use humor— watching funny stories on TV or videotapes.	Client will perform activities compatible with limitations of the illness. The family will take an active interest in the client's hobbies. The client will experience increased enjoyment in using hobbies. Client will decrease tension through laughter.

(continued)

ABBREVIATED CARE PLAN: FAMILY STRESS (*Continued*)

Nursing Diagnosis	Assessment	Interventions	Outcomes
Diversional Activity Deficit: Care-giver	Type of demands required by care Competing demands Perception of situation Attitude about self-care Outlets and supports	Help care-giver to identify ways to meet personal needs. Encourage care-giver to verbalize feelings about energy level. Employ relaxation techniques using imagery and visualization. Encourage physical exercise plan.	Care-giver will schedule activities to meet needs of rest and recreation. The care-giver will express satisfaction about scheduling tasks and rest breaks. Care-giver will achieve relaxation response. Care-giver will devise a plan for structured physical activity.
Alteration in Family Process	Structure and function of family: Patterns of communication Pattern of decision making Role relationships Power and control Values and beliefs Pattern of daily living	Identify what the family knows about the illness. Assist family members to modify the physical environment in the least disruptive manner possible. Help the family members to identify how decisions are made. Involve family members in care of the client. Encourage family to understand the requirements and stress of the care-giver role.	Family members will become informed about the client's condition and the care required. The family members will agree on the management of space, equipment, and furniture. The family will agree on a decision-making strategy to deal with changes that will occur over time due to client's condition. Family members will develop a plan to share the tasks. The family will identify supportive groups to provide respite for the care-giver.

(*continued*)

ABBREVIATED CARE PLAN: FAMILY STRESS (*Continued*)

Nursing Diagnosis	Assessment	Interventions	Outcomes
Fear	Family's perception of fear Family members' degree of fearfulness Past ways of dealing with fear Coping mechanisms of family	Encourage family to identify the factors contributing to the fearful situation. Assist family to identify effective coping patterns. Provide accurate information about illness and the care requirements. Provide situations that are predictable in the daily plan of care.	Family will distinguish real from imagined threats. Family will use effective coping strategies. Family will manage everyday events realistically. Family will experience decreased fear and increased feeling of control.
Alterations in Health Maintenance	Assess family members for physical and emotional symptoms. Presence of illness Presence of personal neglect of health	Identify the risks to the care-giver's health. Promote health behavior for all family members, especially the care-giver. Discuss methods for sharing the tasks associated with client's care.	The family members of care-givers will identify factors that increase the health risk. The care-giver will practice good nutrition and stress management. The family members will design a workable plan. The care-giver will experience decreased stress.
Impaired Home Maintenance Management	Family's perception of ability to maintain home Cleanliness and safety Patterns of problem solving Values about the family home Presence of support system	Assist the individual to identify problems in home maintenance requiring assistance. Encourage care-giver to obtain assistance for repairs.	Care-giver will acquire needed assistance. Care-giver will contact support groups to assist with household tasks.

ABBREVIATED CARE PLAN: FAMILY STRESS (*Continued*)

Nursing Diagnosis	Assessment	Interventions	Outcomes
Alterations in Parenting	Pattern of parental behaviors Values and beliefs	Work with family to find ways to conserve the care-giver's energy. Promote an atmosphere where feelings can be expressed. Suggest referral for child exhibiting behavior problems.	The care-giver will experience a decrease in competing demands between her children and the client. The family will communicate more openly. The parents will seek professional help in dealing with client's problems.
Powerlessness	Family's perception and individual members' feelings Family's beliefs and values about control and self sufficiency Living patterns prior to illness Suitability of home environment for providing care	Assist family to identify areas of care that they can control. Increase effective communication between family and the health-care team. Assist family to modify home environment to support client's care.	The family will make decisions regarding the care. The family will experience competency in performing care and seeking advice. The family will be able to adapt the home for care.
Social Isolation	Family relationships with each other and others Possible resources in community Pattern of social contacts prior to illness	Foster relationships of mutual support in the family. Arrange for visits from persons outside the family. Assist the care-giver to resolve feelings of isolation. Encourage the care-giver to increase social contacts. Engage family members, friends, neighbors to assist client.	The family will experience decreased sense of isolation. The family will contact persons to visit the client. The care-giver will verbalize feelings and frustrations. The care-giver will identify ways to decrease isolation. Client will experience the stimulation of meaningful relationships.

References

Allmond BW, Buckman W, Gofman HF: The Family Is the Patient. St. Louis, CV Mosby, 1979

Brody EM: Women in the middle and family help to older people. Gerontologist 25: 19–29, 1981

Cantor M: Strain among care-givers: A study of experience in the United States. Gerontologist 23(6): 597–604, 1983

Carpenito LJ: Handbook of Nursing Diagnosis. Philadelphia, JB Lippincott, 1984

Clark NM Rakowski W: Family care-givers of the older adults: Improving helping skills. Gerontologist 23: 637–642, 1983

Cromwell RE, Olson DH: Introduction. In Cromwell RE, Olson DH (eds): Power in Families. New York, Sage Publications, 1975

Elkins CO: Community Health Nursing—Skills and Strategies. Bowie, MD, Brady Communications, 1984

Friedman JA: Home Health Care. New York, WW Norton, 1986

Friedman MM: Family Nursing: Theory and assessment, p 121. East Norwalk, CT, Appleton-Century-Crofts, 1986

Goldstein V, Regnergy G, Wellin E: Caretaker role fatigue. Nurs Outlook January: 24–30, 1981

Hansen D, Will R: Families under stress. Cristensen HT (ed): Handbook of Marriage and the Family. Chicago, Rand McNally, 1964

Hill R: Generic features of families under stress. In Parad H (ed): Crisis Intervention: Selected Readings. New York, Family Service Association of America, 1965

Hymovich DP, Chamberlin RW: Child and Family Development. New York, McGraw-Hill, 1986

Johnson CL: Dyadic family relations and social support. Gerontologist 23: 377–383, 1983

Johnson CL Catalano DJ: A longitudinal study of family supports to impaired elderly. Gerontologist 23: 612–618, 1983

Kievit MB: Family roles. In Newart NJ (ed): Parent–Child relationships—Role of the Nurse. New Brunswick, NJ, Rutgers University Press, 1968

McCubbin H, Dahl B: Marriage and Family: Individuals and Life Cycles. New York: John Wiley & Sons, 1985

National Association for Home Care: Home Care Fact Sheet. Washington, DC, The National Association for Home Care, 1986

Omdahl DJ: Preventing home care denials. Am J Nurs 88(8): 1031–1033, 1987

Pender NJ: Health Promotion in Nursing Practice, 2nd ed. East Norwalk, CT, Appleton and Lange, 1987

Robinson BC: Validation of a care-giver stain index. J Gerontol 38(3): 344–348, 1983

Satir B: Conjoint Family Therapy. Palo Alto, CA, Science and Behavior Books, 1967

Stoller EO: Parental caregiving by adult children. J Marriage Fam November: 851–858, 1983

Stone R, Cafferata GL, Sangl J: Caregivers of the frail elderly: A national profile. Paper presented at the 32nd annual meeting of the American Society on Aging. San Francisco, CA, March, 1986

SPIRITUALITY: BELIEFS, VALUES, AND PRACTICES

6

M. Carroll Miller

Spirituality derives from the human spirit that enables persons to develop certain beliefs and values. The beliefs and values a person holds influence the choices he makes (Gordon 1987). A belief is a cognitive concept; it is something a person accepts as true by a judgment of probability rather than of actuality. When beliefs are personal and internalized, they become values, giving direction and meaning to a person's life. Beliefs and values transfer into behaviors or practices; consistent patterns of behaviors or practices reveal a person's cherished and real values (Czmowski 1974; Simon 1973).

Bodies of beliefs are formalized in institutions such as churches, governments, schools, and societies, and they are professed as worthy, desirable, and true by members of the institutions. The beliefs may be publicly claimed as creeds, constitutions, charters, or missions.

While many public beliefs are shared by groups of persons, each individual, nonetheless, holds a private belief and value system that forms the individual's spirituality. Like the human spirit, spirituality is both individu-ally unique and collectively common at the same time. It is as individual and unique as the impressions and configurations of a person's fingerprints, which are unlike those of any other person. At the same time, spirituality is common to all persons. There has never been, nor will there ever be, a human without spirituality; it is the very essence of humanity. From the moment human life begins, each person is endowed with a human spirit and is, therefore, spiritual. To be human is to be spiritual. Spirituality is vital and necessary to human life.

It is not by accident or coincidence that the vital sign long heralded as the prime indicator of the presence or absence of life, that is, respirations, is taken from the same root word as that of spirituality. The Latin root *spiritus* means breath; *spirare* means to breathe, to blow; *spiritualis* means of breathing, of wind; thus, the root, *spirit*, is defined as *an animating or vital principle, held to give life to physical organisms.* (Webster 1983).

Nurses are familiar with other terms in nursing that stem as well from the same root:

aspiration, to breathe in, to suction out; *expiration*, releasing air from the lungs, death; *inspiration*, drawing air into the lungs; *perspiration*, to emit matter through the skin. Nurses would find it difficult, if not impossible, to escape the many signs and symptoms their clients experience in this sensitive, life-sustaining or life-threatening (thus vital) dimension. When spirituality is understood in its proper context it, too, is recognized as being either life-enhancing or life-depleting to an individual.

Spirituality also needs to be appreciated as basic human spirituality, individually and uniquely incarnated from the beginning of life and developed throughout life in each person. It is generally influenced by the beliefs, values, and practices found in specific cultures, ideologies, and religions, but it may also be free from such influences in any given person. Human spirituality is an intrapersonal endowment, which means it is within each living person before, and independent of, interpersonal activity or encounter with others (van Kaam 1983).

Through interaction with others, people learn customs, facts, and socialization behaviors in the context of their cultures. Spirituality enables persons to go beyond or to transcend mere learning and to ascribe meaning to the events of life and to life itself; spirituality makes it possible for persons to embrace unique belief and value systems.

All cultures, great and small, reveal their spirituality (beliefs and values) through the art, architecture, government, institutions, laws, literature, music, technology, rites, and traditions that are both their inheritance and their contribution to the world. Individuals are microcosms of their cultures and, therefore, of its spirituality; yet each individual experiences and expresses a unique spirituality never quite duplicated by any other individual, even within the same culture.

SPIRITUALITY DEFINED

What then, is spirituality; more specifically, what is spirituality in the context of nursing? Most writers concede that spirituality is more easily described or observed than it is defined. Definitions of personally and individually incarnated realities such as spirituality tend to be more limiting than illuminating, more exclusive than expansive. Given these drawbacks, it will be helpful, nonetheless, to cite some definitions in order to lay the foundation for the meaning of spirituality as it is used in the present chapter. Friedlander, according to Colliton (1981), defines spirituality as the "life principle that pervades a person's entire being, including volitional, emotional, moral–ethical, intellectual and physical dimensions, and generates a capacity for transcendent values. The spiritual dimension of a person integrates and transcends biological and psychosocial nature, giving access to the nonphysical realms of prophecy, artistic inspiration, love, and healing actions."

Bouyer (1963) relates spirituality and dogma while defining spirituality in a generic and experiential sense by writing, "Christian spirituality (or any other spirituality) is distinguished from dogma by the fact that instead of studying or describing the objects of belief as if they were in the abstract, it studies the actions which these objects arouse in the religious consciousness." Osiek (1976) claims that spirituality is "the experience, reflection and articulation of the assumptions and consequences of religious faith as it is lived in a concrete situation." Panikkar (1973) stresses the generic sense of spirituality in defining it as "one typical way of handling the human condition." van Kaam (1983) offers the following definition of spirituality: "There is an elementary foundational spirituality, a basic style of human formation . . . not necessarily bound to any specific cultural, ideological, or religious formation tradition." Each of these definitions, although from persons and professions other than nursing, has relevance for professional nursing practice. Friedlander addresses the total person and the human capacity for transcendent values; nursing has long recognized the need to care for the whole person, not just the physical person, if care is to be effective. Bouyer centers on the study of human responses; the focus of nursing care, both by tradition and definition, is the treatment of human responses to illness or the threat of illness, not treatment of the illness itself. Osiek particularizes to each concrete situation; nursing stresses the value and importance of individualized care plans. Panikkar speaks to the commonly shared human condition; nursing provides care for the needs common to all persons, such as nutrition, rest, activity. van Kaam calls attention to a basic and distinctive human spirituality that transcends all cultures, ideologies, and religions; nursing encounters international and transcultural implications with increasing frequency as technological advances and world travel bring people from all parts of the globe closer together.

Because of the present and predictable continuance into the future of the intermingling of world cultures, with their accompanying ideologies and religions, a broad understanding of human spirituality is needed now more than ever before by nurses. Perhaps, then, van Kaam's definition is most useful to the practice of professional nursing by placing culture, ideology, and religion in *relational* positions to spirituality, thus showing that each of them contributes to, but is different from, spirituality.

Therefore, in the context of this chapter, spirituality is defined broadly as *the way a person lives out or incarnates the beliefs and values that provide meaning to a person's life*. A person's beliefs, values, and practices

may either be influenced by culture, ideology, and religion or they may be free from or even counter to such influences in any given person. A person's values may change over time as life experiences broaden and deepen.

RELIGION DEFINED

While there are many religions and a study of them may become extremely complex, the concept of religion itself is rather simple. Religion is an organized system of worship, involving a body of beliefs, rituals, and practices (Webster 1983). Globally, there are vastly different religions and it is impossible for any nurse to know the intricacies of all or even many of them.

There are differences among theists; they may believe in one God (monotheists) or in many gods (polytheists). The three monotheistic religions are Judaism, Christianity, and Islam. In America, followers of Judaism are divided into Orthodox, Conservative, and Reform styles of worship and practices. Christianity, the 2000 year old faith founded by Jesus Christ, has three major branches: Eastern Orthodoxy; Roman Catholicism; and Protestantism. Protestantism numbers many denominations. Islam is divided into two main groups: Sunni and Shi'a. It is beyond the scope of this chapter to provide in-depth information on even the major world religions. The reader is referred to *Many People, Many Faiths*, 2nd ed., by Robert S. Ellwood, Jr. (Prentice-Hall 1982) for extensive reading of world religions and their histories.

SPIRITUALITY AND RELIGION: RELATED BUT NOT IDENTICAL

Historically, nursing data base forms have provided space for a client's religion and any meaningful religious practices or activities, but the forms do not mention spirituality or any of its related concepts. Nurses, therefore, oftentimes relate a client's spirituality only with a claimed religious affiliation. By viewing spirituality so narrowly, nurses miss the broader, deeper, and richer understanding of a client's spirituality and its effects on the client's health.

Perhaps this tunnel-vision approach arises from two facts: (1) traditionally, the term spirituality has been used to indicate either a group or an individual's attachment to religious values, establishing it as being religious or church related; and (2) the term, *per se*, seldom has been addressed in nursing literature where its broader meaning could be explained. Rather, a myriad of nursing terms or concepts appear, employing the adjective *spiritual*. The list includes spiritual assessment, spiritual alienation, spiritual care, spiritual crisis, spiritual dimension, spiritual distress, spiritual growth, spiritual healing, spiritual health, spiritual integrity, spiritual need, spiritual vulnerability and spiritual well-being (O'Brien 1982). Clearly, there is a relationship between spirituality and religion. In fact, the relationship is so close that, both in thought and practice, the terms often become interchangeable. The result has been that many nurses erroneously apply the concepts cited above, which are actually subconcepts of spirituality, to a relational concept of spirituality, that is, religion. Religion relates to spirituality only when a person's significant beliefs, values, and practices are rooted in the person's religion.

When the beliefs, values, and practices that influence a person's choices and give meaning to life are not rooted in religion, the person is not religiously spiritual but is spiritual nonetheless. Nurses need a clear understanding that a relationship may exist between spirituality and religion, but the two are not the same reality. Once the relationship is understood, spiritual assessment will be more than just a religious assessment, although it

will continue to include religious data. Spiritual needs will be recognized as much more than only prayer and ritual, although these may be among a client's spiritual needs. Spiritual care will be more extensive than only religious care, and will expand to include atheists and agnostics as well as theists. Spiritual nursing care, just like physical vital signs, will rightly be an essential component of every client's plan of care.

The religious spirituality of theists differs from the nonreligious spirituality of atheists in a fundamental and obvious way: theists are believers in a creative and sustaining deity responsible for life and the world as we know it; atheists are nonbelievers in any deity. Agnostics are uncertain about the existence of a deity. Among theists the deity is named variously as God, Yahweh, Allah, or Buddha. Atheists and agnostics focus attention on human relationships and material values. They believe we are dependent only on one another for all our needs. They further believe the world is as it is because we have made it thus and we must work together to make it a better world in the future for succeeding generations of mankind.

To identify spirituality synonymously with religion is, in effect, to deny human spirituality which, by nature, is inherent in all persons from the beginning of life. In nursing, this misleading identification results in depriving atheists and agnostics of their rightful spiritual care.

NURSING PROCESS AND SPIRITUALITY

In the context of nursing process, assessment, planning, intervention, and evaluation are to be situation-specific. Since this chapter defines spirituality in broader, less traditional terms than it has usually been understood within nursing, the components of the process relative to spirituality are addressed in a general rather than case-specific manner. This approach is utilized so that the reader may gain an appreciation of the reality of human spirituality in each individual and to incorporate it in the care of each client.

Assessment

Illness in the home creates a crisis situation for all members of a household. Our homes are the showcases of our spirituality; they reflect our beliefs and values in a variety of ways. We surround ourselves with artifacts, colors, and symbols that have deep personal meaning. Generally, we open our homes with their treasured worlds of meaning and share them selectively with only invited, chosen friends. When illness strikes a member in the home, the home is visited by strangers, by professional persons carrying out professional duties. Control and routine within the home are disrupted. The nurse, who is a guest in the home, takes an active role in providing services to a member of the family. The ill family member, whose autonomy and freedom in the home are curtailed, is the receiver of care. For the nurse and the client alike there is a reversal of roles in a client's home.

Because the nurse is in an unfamiliar setting, it is important for the nurse to become oriented to the immediate environment of the client's room as well as its location relative to other areas of the house (kitchen, bathroom, stairs, etc.). The nurse has to know what household supplies and equipment are available for the client's care.

The initial responsibility of the nurse in home care, after introductions are made, remains unchanged: assessment data need to be collected. Assessment begins with the client: the client's needs, abilities, understanding, and expectations relative to the illness. Usually these data are obtainable through direct questioning. The data are needed so the nurse can formulate a beginning plan of care with the client and the primary care-giver in the home.

The days, purpose, and length of subsequent visits should be discussed and agreed upon with the client and family members. As the nurse/client/family relationship develops over time, it seems natural that many families invite the nurse to share a cup of coffee or tea with cookies, cake, or pie during a visit. This informal atmosphere can be a golden opportunity for the nurse to enrich the spiritual data base of the family. A word of caution is necessary, however; there is a danger that, because of the social nature of sharing food and drink, the nurse may forget or put aside the professional role and responsibility to the client and family. It is important that nurses learn the art and discipline of maintaining a professional relationship in the warm hospitality of a client's home.

It would seem that the spirituality of clients should be assessed easily by nurses caring for people in their homes. Clients' prized possessions are visible and readily observable, giving witness to unspoken beliefs and values. Actually, spiritual assessment is much more subtle than physical care assessment and requires the establishment of a trusting relationship before it is approached. Oftentimes, however, a client's beliefs, values and usual practices are revealed in the responses or comments offered in an initial interview. The alert nurse makes note of any value-laden remarks without becoming distracted from the primary information being sought. The nurse focuses on the meaning of remarks such as "I need to be well by the fourteenth of the month;" "Please don't move that picture on the dresser;" "Could you arrange to come either before 11 o'clock or after 2:30?" Personal meaning usually prompts such comments by the client.

In spiritual assessment the nurse seeks to

discover a client's beliefs, what holds value or gives meaning to the client's life, how these beliefs and values are lived out, and how they relate to the present health of the client. Frequently it turns out that the nurse assists the client in making the same discovery of values for himself on a personal level. Few persons take time from their healthy, busy, fast-paced lives to ponder and dwell upon values, particularly ultimate values. The world is moving too fast for most persons to dare to be still and reflect on these hidden, private matters. Reflection simply is not active enough; sometimes it is too challenging, too frightening, too threatening. Illness affords the opportunity, albeit a forced and unwelcomed one, to slow down; spiritual assessment provides the guidance for reflection. Precisely because it is so private, spiritual assessment cannot be entered into too hastily, nor can it be too prescriptive once it is begun. It may not even be openly approached or completed for several visits. Both the nurse and client need to have developed a comfort level with each other before they begin to explore the sensitive, private areas the client is asked to reveal.

The client is being asked to reveal personal values. In order to do this perhaps a values clarification process is needed. According to Raths and associates (1979), this is a process of self-discovery that helps a person gain clearer insight into his values. The nurse may select one of many strategies to accomplish this with the client. Simon and colleagues (1978) suggest three possible strategies to assist the client in discovering personal values: (1) completing unfinished values-related sentences; (2) ranking the order of values; (3) health value scale. Regardless of the strategy utilized, the goal is to have the client identify in a systematic manner the values he has freely chosen, prized, and acted upon consistently and repeatedly.

Several spiritual assessment guides have been developed over the years (O'Brien 1982, Fish 1978, and Stoll 1979). They approach the spiritual dimension from different avenues. Some are clearly focused on a theistic, religious, or faith relationship and thereby restrict the nurse's observation and interventions to religious practices and activities and to the client's relationship with his God. One guide that departs from a religion-based assessment has been formulated by Tubesing (1980). His spiritual outlook assessment poses five questions, each designed to uncover a specific, meaningful area of a person's life (see Table 6-1).

In spiritual assessment, it is beneficial for nurses to ask open-ended questions such as

TABLE 6.1 Tubesing's Open-ended Spiritual Assessment Guide

Question	Area of Life
What is the aim of life?	Life goal-related question
What beliefs guide me?	Intended to reveal the person's faith
What is important to me?	Discovery of values
On what do I choose to spend myself?	Disclosure of commitments
What am I willing to let go?	Ability to let go and receive forgiveness both from self and others

From Tubesing DA: Spiritualized Pastoral Care J: 3:17, 1980

"What does this illness mean to you? What holds the most value for you in your life? What gives you a feeling of peace? When do you sense you are most complete?" Close-ended questions that seem to be very direct, such as "Is religion important to you? Do you practice any religion? Do you believe in capital punishment? Would you defend your country in war?", are actually so slanted or intimidating that the answers they evoke may reveal little or nothing of a person's true values and meaningful relationships, which are at the heart of spirituality.

When the nurse uses the former type of questions, it is necessary to follow up on the client's responses. The nurse should seek clarification of the client's meaning in the words the *client* chooses; she should not place her own meaning on them, reflecting her values rather than the client's values. In addition to asking questions in order to gather information, the nurse also observes the environment in the client's home when doing the spiritual assessment. The furnishings and articles that surround the client may be very important and meaningful; the nurse should ascertain their importance and meaning to the client and not make assumptions about them that, again, may be based on her own values.

Family members or friends who either live with the client or visit are another rich source of data for assessment. Their interactions with the client, the mutual exchange of care and concern, speak volumes to the observant nurse. Family members should be encouraged to be present and to speak freely to the nurse during visits. The nurse needs to communicate to them that the nursing care is family centered, not exclusively focused on the client.

When religion is a strong factor in the client's life, the nurse needs to be aware of it and include it in the assessment. The absence of religion as a variable, however, does not justify omission of spiritual assessment with a client. By virtue of their being human, atheists and agnostics are also endowed with basic human spirituality or the need for beliefs, values, meaning, and purpose in life and life's events, and spiritual assessment is appropriate to their care.

NURSING DIAGNOSES

Among the accepted diagnoses from the Fifth National Conference held by the North American Nursing Diagnosis Association (NANDA) in 1982 is the diagnosis, *Spiritual Distress (distress of the human spirit)*. The foremost or critical defining characteristic of the diagnosis is said to be a patient's expression of concern with the meaning of life and death and/or belief system. (Gordon 1987)

Carpenito (1983) defines spiritual distress as the state in which the individual experiences or is at risk of experiencing a disturbance in his belief or value system that is his source of strength and hope. Both Gordon's and Carpenito's statements are compatible with the selection of van Kaam's definition of spirituality since the source of a person's belief or value system can be found in culture, ideology, or religion or any combination of the three.

Assessment is always essential before a diagnosis can be confirmed or ruled out, whether the diagnosis in question is a medical one or a nursing diagnosis. The tools used in either case are designed to be as specific as possible to the probable or suspected diagnosis. Frequently, a confirmed diagnosis that results from finely-tuned diagnosis instruments reveals not only the diagnosis but its etiology as well. Isolated identification of causative agents has proven to be immeasurably helpful in the medical treatment of a number of disease entities. Because it is concerned with the total human response to health experiences, nursing does not have the luxury, nor can it afford the risk, of being cause-and-effect oriented, as is medicine in its pursuit of cellular pathology. Total human response is so pervasive that to isolate one specific factor would be grossly misleading in establishing a valid nursing diagnosis. Rather, a cluster of relevant variables emerging from cultural, educational, health, ideological, religious, socioeconomic, and life-style aspects is needed in order to discover the scope of the human response that, in essence, is the nursing diagnosis.

NONRELIGIOUS SPIRITUAL DISTRESS

When assessment indicates the diagnosis of spiritual distress, it will undoubtedly be rooted more deeply in one aspect of the person's life, but it will be evident in other aspects as well. Perhaps a brief example will best illustrate this. The person who values freedom, independence, and privacy experiences spiritual distress when the premorbid life-style is shattered by the person's becoming ill and bedfast at home. The person is suddenly dependent on others for meals, transportation, and care. The family home is entered by strangers; the client's private life is questioned and shared. While the client's distress stems from a disturbance in life-style, it is also seen in anxiety about the fact that the individual cannot attend classes to earn the degree necessary for a promotion at work. In fact, absence from work for any length of time may result in loss of the client's job. The individual is not prepared for any other type of work. Preoccupation with such concerns makes it impossible for the client to enjoy music and literature, which previously offered relaxation and escape. The client is unable to drive in the country and take in the beauty of the changing season or he may be forced to miss the opening game of the new football season. Enforced confinement somehow makes attendance at church services

more desirable and inviting. The client is eager to vote in the coming election but may not be able to this year. The person is bewildered by a feeling of powerlessness and loss of control over his life. These worries do not permit the client to concentrate on the illness and on trying to get well. The person may have been more restless than restful and instead of eating properly, may have *skipped* more meals than he has taken. The client frequently forgets to take prescribed medications and is discouraged that satisfactory progress is not being achieved. It is not difficult to see the ever-widening involvement of all aspects of a person's life in the diagnosis of spiritual distress related to a change in life-style.

RELIGIOUS SPIRITUAL DISTRESS

When assessment interviews and observations disclose that religion is an important variable to the client, the nurse is expected to inquire about the particular religion just as she is expected to research medical diagnoses, nursing procedures, therapies, medications, and diet in planning client care. The inquiry includes a literature search, colleague and family conferences, and dialog with the client to gain a better understanding of the specific beliefs and practices of the client within the religion and how these practices may relate to the individual's health care.

The credo of a client's religion is a body of truths proclaimed as accepted doctrine by learned members of the specific religious sect. The faithful of the sect profess belief in the truths and promise to follow the practices prescribed by the rites of the church. Nurses should either contact a clergyman of the client's faith or find reliable literature that explains the major tenets of the particular religion. Nurses then need to discover the client's personal understanding and practices within that religion. Oftentimes religious beliefs and practices come under question and doubt by clients during illness.

While nurses cannot be expected to answer faith and theology questions infallibly, it is necessary for them to recognize the importance of faith concerns to clients and to allow them to voice their feelings and concerns freely. Nurses should ask clients if they want to speak with their clergyman about their concerns and then proceed according to the client's responses. The spiritual distress may be related to the client's inability to participate in important religious services or it may be related to a questioning of basic religious beliefs.

Interventions

Persons whose spiritual distress diagnosis does not include religion, will, of course, include culture and/or ideology. Therefore, they may still be guided to reveal their spirituality through the use of open-ended question such as the ones suggested earlier. These clients, too, may express concern about the ultimate meaning of life and death, and while the nurse does not have the support of religious teachings to offer them, she is still able to talk with them in an exploring, nonjudgmental way. The nurse can offer presence and honesty. It is also helpful for the nurse to assure the client that his feelings, doubts, and concerns are normal and he is not to feel guilt for having them.

Persons whose spiritual distress diagnosis focuses on religion may be assisted by the nurse to carry out certain practices and devotional exercises in the home. The nurse can arrange for desired visits by clergy of the client's faith. Prayer is frequently a source of tremendous comfort to clients. The faithful Muslim is required to pray at five specific times within a day. Other clients may request that the nurse pray with them, or for them, or read to them from scripture or any other inspirational text of their choice. Some nurses

may experience initial discomfort with such requests but will usually notice a growing comfort as they respond to the requests more frequently. Most writers are in agreement that prayer and the reading of scripture are appropriate nursing interventions. Interventions beyond these are considered by some nurses to be potentially controversial. O'Brien (1982) believes that any spiritual intervention should only be in response to a client's expressed need. Proper sensitivity in this regard should guide the individual nurse in the decision either to be the initiator or the respondent.

Some religions have dietary laws that may need to be modified during illness or, in contrast, provisions for dietary adherence may need to be worked into the parameters of the medical regimen. Dietary laws regarding fasting and/or meat prohibition are found in such religious individuals or groups as Adventist, Armenian, Black Muslim, Episcopalian, Greek Orthodox, Hindu, Islamic, Judaism, Pentecostal, and Russian Orthodox (Ellwood 1982 and Pumphrey 1977).

Medications containing alcohol or narcotics may be refused on religious grounds by persons of the Adventist, Baptist, Black Muslim, Christian Scientist, Mormon, Friends (Quakers), Mennonite, Nazarene, and Pentecostal churches (Pumphrey 1977; Ellwood 1982).

Family Members as Care-Givers

Family members are the major care-givers in the home. The opportunity for them to serve a loved one in time of illness may have deep spiritual meaning for them as well as for the client. It may be seen as a way of proving their love, of repaying a perceived debt, or of fulfilling an obligation. Any of these reasons may be of great importance to the family members and their value should not be underestimated by the nurse. Nurses should invite family members to share their thoughts about their involvement in the client's care and make sure that they are not deprived of the privilege of participation in care. Nurses must keep in mind that family members may be drained emotionally as well as physically by the client's illness and may consequently be more limited in what duties they can perform than they normally would be.

Care-givers deserve supportive feedback from the nurse. They and their work must be recognized and appreciated. They should also be encouraged to meet their own needs by taking time to renew their energies. Nurses can be instrumental in caring for the care-givers by helping them to avoid total exhaustion in service to loved ones at home. One way for nurses to do this is to help the care-givers realize their own feelings that center on service to loved ones and to dwell on the feelings they discover and the meaning of these feelings. Without this introspection and reflection the elements of home service may indeed be nothing other than psychosocial care. On the surface, there seems to be very little perceptive difference between psychosocial and spiritual care. The difference, in fact, is not surface or visible; rather it lies in the core of spiritual care, which is a reflective understanding of the present situation in relation to the ultimate value and meaning of one's life.

Evaluation/Outcomes

Spiritual distress is expressed by some clients as anger or depression over failed personal relationships. If it is a particular relationship, the nurse should encourage the client to express his feelings in greater detail in order to see if any reconciliation is possible. If it *is* possible, the client should be assisted in moving in this direction. If it is not possible, the client can then be helped to focus on successful relationships he has enjoyed. Another manifestation of spiritual distress may be the feeling that a client's illness is a pun-

ishment for transgressions. Here, again, the client should be encouraged to express feelings and then be assisted in moving on, to broaden horizons and to recall more of the positive achievements and contributions of his life.

It can sometimes be helpful when clients feel that their present illness is a punishment for past sins to have them concentrate on acts of love and kindness they have both given and received. If they persist in dwelling on the "bad" things they did and claiming that these are the reasons for their suffering, it may be helpful to remind them of the ever-puzzling reality of the suffering of innocent children, such as young victims of disease, hunger, and abuse. What "bad" have they ever done to deserve suffering and dying?

The goal (expected outcome) of interventions employed in the diagnosis of spiritual distress is that the client will experience either a decrease or a total elimination of the particular distress. Evaluation of the goal in terms of client achievement is illustrated in an abbreviated care plan at the end of this chapter.

GRIEF AND MOURNING

The ultimate meaning of life and death is addressed by all persons, especially in times of illness. To die defending a loved one or in defense of one's country is seen as a noble and courageous act. But to suffer and die from an untreated or incurable disease seems senseless. Abrupt, accidental death is equally meaningless. The age-old question of why the innocent suffer continues to puzzle and tax the mind. Theologians and scientists alike are unable to find the answer. Perhaps it remains unanswered because it is unanswerable. The Judeo-Christian tradition cites Job as the prototype of the suffering innocent. Only his steadfast faith in Yahweh enabled

Job to endure his losses and suffering. The Christian tradition offers Jesus Christ as example. For Christians, belief in the life, death, and resurrection of Christ forever changes the meaning of human life, suffering, and death. The assent to religious doctrine, however, is not necessarily incarnated so easily as it is verbalized. Many persons experience concern about the meaning of life and death in spite of their religious beliefs. In particular, they question the meaning of their own lives. They should be encouraged to express and explore their concerns in an accepting, judgment-free atmosphere. They need assurances that fear and concern are very normal human responses, as are anger and depression. In fact, according to Engel and Kubler-Ross, they are necessary responses on the journey toward death and people should not feel or be made to feel ashamed or guilty for experiencing such feelings (Engel 1964 and Kubler-Ross 1972). Nurses need to be aware of the stages or phases of suffering and dying so they can assist clients through them. They need to recognize the benefits as well as the need for a client's initial denial and not rush the client through this period before the individual is ready. Nurses need to anticipate and be prepared for the anger and depression the client will experience.

Part of the nurse's preparation will be the ability not to take the anger personally and possibly, through hurt, retaliate and close communications with the client. The client's depression is the inward direction of anger. The nurse must understand this and help the client to work through the depression. This can best be done by respecting the client's periodic need for silence and solitude. The nurse balances these times of aloneness with dependable periods of presence and assurances of willingness to listen to whatever the client may care to say. Above all, nurses should not avoid the client at this time. A nurse's avoidance well may be perceived by the client as abandonment and may cause further depression.

Denial, anger, and depression require a great deal of energy from the client. During these phases the nurse needs to make most of the decisions relative to the client's care. She must be alert to the symptoms or clues from the client that indicate he is now ready to move on and participate in both his care and decisions. The person begins to ask concrete questions such as "Why is it important for me to get up and sit in the chair?", instead of "Why bother?" or "What is this medicine for?", instead of "What's the use?" The usual "Go ahead," said with a turned away head or closed eyes, is replaced by "Can I watch you do that?" or "Show me how to do that".

QUESTIONS NOT EASILY ANSWERED

Questions not so easily answered by the nurse may also begin to be asked. Instead of "Why me?; Why is God doing this to me?", the client may turn the tables on the nurse and ask "Do you pray?; Do you believe in God?; Would you say a prayer for me?; Am I going to die?" Answers to these questions are, of course, highly individual. Nurses may find themselves unwilling or unable to answer such direct and personal questions. They may not be in touch enough with their own spirituality to be able to give thoughtful responses. The important thing is that nurses owe themselves and their clients *honest answers* to any of the questions they may choose to answer. Nurses and nursing students need to spend time reflecting on and explaining their own values and beliefs so that they will be better equipped to answer these questions.

DEATH AND DYING

Most often the ability of the client to enter into dialog on the above questions signals progression through the phases of mourning and dying to acceptance or resolution. At this time the most effective nursing intervention is the offer of support for the client. It is not necessary for a nurse to share, or even to accept, every client's religious beliefs, but it is expected that she will respect the person's right to have those beliefs.

In some religions, preparation for death and care of the body following it may require ritual acts. The nurse should be aware of the requirements and the wishes of the client. Last rites or anointing of the sick, with or without reception of Holy Communion, is a practice in the Armenian, American Buddist, Eastern Orthodox, Episcopalian, Greek Orthodox, Hindu, Judaic, Lutheran (optional), and Roman Catholic faiths. After death, the bodies of Black Muslim, Hindu, Islamic, and Jewish patients require special washing and handling, oftentimes permitted to be performed only by specifically designated persons (Ross 1981). Information of this nature should be known by all the health-care team members involved in caring for these clients.

HOSPICE CARE

Hospice care has become a popular and successful modality of intervention. Hospice was established to assist the terminally ill person. Clients in hospice receive palliative, symptomatic care rather than active, aggressive treatment. The major goal is to make the client comfortable by relieving pain but maintaining consciousness. The client's perception of pain is a prime determinant in the frequency and type of pain medication administered. The concept of hospice or, more accurately, of the hospice movement in the United States is an outgrowth of the work of the English nurse and physician, Dame Cicely Saunders, foundress in 1968 of the famed St. Christopher's Hospice in London. The National Hospice Organization (1982) expresses in its philosophy ". . . through appropriate care

and the promotion of a caring community sensitive to their needs, patients and families may be free to attain a degree of mental and spiritual preparation for death that is satisfactory to them."*

Clearly the intention is to include the family's needs as well as the client's in nursing care. The locus of hospice care may be the home or the hospice itself; the decision is made cooperatively by staff, client, and family. In both places, the freedom from hospital rules regarding visitors and any other institutional restrictions prevails. In this relaxed, homey atmosphere the nurse develops a closer, less rigid relationship with both the client and the family. The demanding schedule and pace of a hospital unit is absent so the nurse has time she and the client both need for the gift of merely being present to and with one another, without either of them feeling guilty about their time together.

Medicare now provides benefits for hospice care, making it more feasible for many families. In addition to in-patient and home care, each hospice sponsors a bereavement program of counseling and support for family and loved ones of the client after death. The grieving and mourning periods of individuals vary, but the services are available, in most instances, for at least 13 months. Both with the client and his loved ones the nurse recognizes that she cannot be "all things to all persons;" she confers with and makes referrals to clergy and other professionals when necessary. The multidisciplinary team of professionals working at hospice meets regularly to discuss and evaluate clients and their families. During the team meetings, the professionals also give and receive support from one another. Support and affirmation among colleagues are necessary to the success of team endeavors in all fields but, perhaps, no-

*For more information on hospices, the reader may contact the National Hospice Organization, 1910 N. Fort Meyer Dr., Suite 902, Arlington, VA 22209. Phone: (703) 243-5900

where are they more needed than among health-care team members. The health of each individual member is critical to the successful efforts of the team.

Nurses, who are in contact with clients and their families in times of crises and loss, cannot constantly give of their talents and themselves in those situations without renewing their own lives. Their own spiritual, mental, and physical health requires care before they can assist others. They need to assess themselves regularly, note the symptoms and diagnoses they are experiencing, and intervene to maintain or replenish their spiritual, mental, and physical strengths. If nurses do not care first for their own holistic health, they cannot be effective in meeting the health needs of their clients.

ABBREVIATED CARE PLAN: SPIRITUAL DISTRESS

Nursing Diagnosis	Assessment	Interventions	Outcomes
Spiritual Distress Related to Failed Personal Relationships	Possible sources of alienation from others Perception of guilt Furnishings and artifacts in the home	Encourage client to explore the possibility of reconciliation. Assist client to locate the significant person in the relationship. Focus on other relationships that have been successful.	Client will reestablish meaningful relationship. Client will focus on "successful" relationships.
Spiritual Distress Related to Feeling of Punishment	Relationships with family and friends Meaning of illness Beliefs about health and religion	Assist client to explore the meaning of "punishment." Encourage expression of feelings. Have client recall past experiences of punishment. Assist client to recall positive achievements and contributions.	Client will stop placing blame on self or another for illness.
Spiritual Distress Related to Inability to Participate in Religious Activities	Client's expectations about the illness Client's spiritual beliefs Past religious practices	Inform local clergy of client situation. Request clergy to visit in the home. Prepare client for visit.	Client will express acceptance of limitations.

ABBREVIATED CARE PLAN: SPIRITUAL DISTRESS

Nursing Diagnosis	Assessment	Interventions	Outcomes
		Offer to pray with or for client.	
		Provide tapes of inspirational music and/or readings for client to hear.	

References

Bouyer L: The Spirituality of the New Testament and Fathers, p viii, Ryan M (trans). New York, Descle'e & Co, 1963

Carpenito LJ: Nursing Diagnosis Application to Clinical Practice, p 451. Philadelphia, JB Lippincott, 1983

Colliton MA: The spiritual dimension of nursing. In Beland IL, Passos JY (eds.): Clinical Nursing: Pathophysiological and Psychosocial Approaches, 4th ed, p 492. New York, Macmillan, 1981

Czmowski M: Value teaching in nursing education. Nurs Forum 13(2): 192–206, 1974

Doenges M, Moorhouse M: Nurse's Pocket Guide: Nursing Diagnoses with Interventions. Philadelphia, FA Davis, 1985

Ellwood RS Jr: Many Peoples, Many Faiths, 2nd ed. Englewood Cliffs, NJ: Prentice-Hall, 1982

Engel G: Grief and Grieving. Am J Nurs 64 (9): 93–98, 1964

Fish S, Shelly JA: Spiritual Care — the Nurse's Role. Downers Grove, IL, Intervarsity Press, 1978

Gordon M: Manual of Nursing Diagnosis 1986–1987. New York, McGraw-Hill, 1987

Gordon M: Nursing Diagnosis: Process and Application, 2nd ed. New York, McGraw-Hill, 1987

Kubler-Ross E: On Death and Dying. New York, Macmillian, 1972

O'Brien ME: The need for spiritual integrity. In Yura H, Walsh MD (eds): Human Needs and the Nursing Process. East Norwalk, CT, Appleton-Century-Crofts, 1982

Osiek C: Reflections on an American spirituality. Spiritual Life 22:230, 1976

Panikkar R: The Trinity and the Religious Experience of Man: Icon–Person–Mystery, p 9. New York, Orbis Books, 1973

Pumphrey JB: Recognizing your patients' spiritual needs. Nurs '77: 64–70, 1977

Raths LE, Harmin M, Simon SB: Values and Teaching, 2nd ed. Columbus, Ohio, Charles E. Merrill, 1979

Ross HM: Societal/cultural views regarding death and dying. Topics Clin Nurs 3(3): 1–16, 1981

Simon SB et al: Meeting Yourself Halfway. Niles, IL, Argus Communications, 1973

Simon SB et al: Values Clarification: A Handbook of Practical Strategies for Teachers and Students. New York, Hart Publishing, 1978

Stoll RI: Guidelines for spiritual assessment. Am J Nurs 9:1574, 1979

Tubesing DA: Stress, spiritual outlook, and health. Spiritualized Pastoral Care J, 3: 17, 1980

van Kaam A: Formative Spirituality: 1: Fundamental Formation, p 13. New York, Crossroad Publishing, 1983

Webster's Ninth New Collegiate Dictionary. Springfield, MA, Merriam-Webster, 1983

7

CULTURE AND THE MEANING OF ILLNESS

Martha M. Skoner

We live in a complex society where economic, political, environmental, social, and cultural forces overlap, interact, and influence each other. This chapter deals with one component of this social system, culture, and, more specifically, the influence of culture on the health behaviors of individuals and groups.

CULTURE AND NURSING PRACTICE IN HOME-HEALTH NURSING

The influence of culture on client health-related behaviors is an important dimension of home-health nursing. The home-health nurse is in a unique position to observe firsthand the environments of her clients, the interactions of family members, the impact of illness on families, and the coping strategies utilized by clients and family members. Unlike the nurse in the hospital, where patients upon entry are symbolically stripped of their sociocultural identity, the home-health nurse works with her clients within their sociocultural contexts. In other words, the home-health nurse has the opportunity to examine

firsthand the culture of her clients and its impact on client response to health and illness.

In Western medicine not much attention is paid to the influence of culture on how people define and treat illness. Rather, illness is considered a clinical entity that has no relationship to culture (McElroy and Townsend 1985). This way of thinking may account for the practice in hospitals of ignoring or minimizing a patient's sociocultural identity. Today, however, people are spending less and less time in hospitals and more and more time in their homes, both being ill and recuperating from illnesses. The client's multidimensional nature is very evident in the home setting. The health professional who provides health care to the client in the home or community has to approach the client holistically if health care is to be effective.

The nurse new to home-health nursing may initially experience culture shock. From the moment she enters a client's home, the home-health nurse is faced with an array of stimuli—sights, smells, sounds, that may or may not be familiar to her. She frequently has to accommodate to unfamiliar customs and to material conditions of life to which she is not accustomed. Yet the home-health nurse must find a way to sort out and categorize her observations in some meaningful way so that they will help her in her approach to and understanding of the client. Coming from a background spent mostly in hospitals or other similar clinical settings, where infection control and cleanliness are emphasized, where supplies and support services are readily available, and where the nurse more or less dictates the how, where, and when of patient care, the nurse new to home-health care has some adjustments to make. Her contact with the client is on the client's home turf. The client does what he wants to do in his own home and the home-health nurse is limited in what she can do to intervene.

The home-health nurse frequently must convince the client that a particular treatment regime or way of doing things is in the client's best interest. Basically, she influences clients in two ways: through her interpersonal skills and through her knowledge or expertise (if this knowledge or expertise is perceived as valuable by the client), and probably interpersonal skills supercede knowledge or expertise.

The nurse who is viewed in a positive way by the client is one who shows interest in the client and who shows some understanding and acceptance of the client's point of view, even if it differs significantly from her point of view; for example, the client who prefers a weekly rather than a daily bath, and the client who insists on reusing disposable insulin syringes and needles rather than spending his money buying new ones.

The development of a positive client–nurse relationship is very important, considering that long-term support, either episodic or continuous, may be a part of what the home-health nurse provides to her clients. In summary, an understanding of cultural differences reduces fear and stimulates curiosity in the home-health nurse, reduces interpersonal distance between nurse and client, increases tolerance of differences, and facilitates the development of an approach by the nurse that is perceived positively by the client.

The purpose of this chapter is to provide a conceptual framework for the home-health nurse that will aid her in assessing cultural data and in organizing these data into categories that have meaning insofar as understanding the influence of culture on client health behaviors. The concept of culture is discussed first, following by a discussion of culture as it is used in this chapter.

AMERICAN CULTURE

Cultural diversity characterizes the United States. Our social fabric is a patchwork of overlapping cultural groups, whose basic identities stem from a variety of sources, such as ethnicity (Hispanic, Black, Indian), economic status (rich, poor), geographic location (hillbilly from the south, mountain people from the west), occupation (business, professional, blue collar, white collar), rural/urban setting (farmers, urbanites), and gender (female, male). Each of these groups has a culture that provides a blueprint for social living, helping the members of each group to define the world around them, to organize and think about life, and to cope with social problems. All Americans are products of subcultures such as those above, with all their diverse explanations about health and illness, upon which a dominant American culture has superimposed the germ theory as an explanation of illness.

THE CONCEPT OF CULTURE

Culture encompasses the beliefs, values, and behaviors of a particular group, society, population. The values and beliefs serve as prescriptions for action and are valued by members of the group (Ember and Ember 1977). These cultural components are considered right and not open to question. For example, culture determines the value we place on health, work, and relationships. Culture determines the meaning we give to health and illness and is basic to the decisions we make about seeking health care.

Culture is like a security blanket (Spradley and McCurdy 1984). It provides continuity from generation to generation, enables us to communicate with and to be understood by other group members, and gives us a sense of belonging to the group. While providing comfort and security, culture is at the same time constraining, for when we violate cultural norms, we feel uneasy and guilty. We tend to hold on to values and beliefs even when they are no longer adaptive.

ATTRIBUTES OF CULTURE

Culture is *shared*. Culture is distinct from a personal habit in that it is shared with other group members. Knowing that culture is shared helps the home-health nurse to understand the behavior of her clients toward particular health practices. Attempting to change or influence the health behavior of a client must take into account the cultural norms of the group to which the client belongs. For example, the home-health nurse may try unsuccessfully to convince a mother to have her child immunized. A cultural assessment may reveal that the mother does not believe in the germ theory of disease, hence immunizations have no value to her. Knowing this to be a cultural belief, the nurse might approach one of the leaders of the cultural group for help in interpreting to the client the necessity and value of immunizations for the child.

Similarly, we know that teen-age pregnancy is not viewed in the same way by various cultural groups. For some cultural groups, teen-age pregnancy is a disruptive event, and is considered a social problem. For other cultural groups, teen-age pregnancy is a common and acceptable life event. Accommodations are made for the young mother and baby as they have been made in generations past.

Culture is *learned*. Culture is not inherited. Culture is socially acquired through a process called *socialization* or *enculturation*. Language is crucial to the transmission of cultural information. Children learn how to get food, to avoid danger, and to secure protection against the weather. They learn what is socially acceptable behavior and what is socially unacceptable behavior (McElroy and Townsend 1985).

Culture is *arbitrary*. Culture is arbitrary in that what a child is taught in one cultural group differs from what a child is taught in another cultural group. For example, a child in one culture may be taught that children are seen but not heard, while a child from another culture is encouraged to be verbally expressive.

Culture is *integrated*. Culture is holistic, in that all of its parts are interrelated. A change in one part of a cultural system will affect its other parts (Spradley and McCurdy 1984). For example, because of improved nutrition and health care, people are living longer and surviving serious illnesses. Previously a minority group, the elderly citizens are becoming a majority. They are the fastest growing population group with a vote. This population shift is beginning to create a change in the value and status of the elderly, and will require far-reaching changes in government, housing, health care, retirement plans, work, and leisure.

Culture is *tacit*. Cultural rules are more implicit than explicit and hence are more difficult to discern. Most of us are not conscious of the cultural rules that guide our behavior.

Members of a cultural group know what to do and what to expect from others without asking. Conflict is sometimes a result of disagreement or misunderstanding related to cultural rules.

Culture is *adaptive*. People around the world have learned to adapt to their particular environments, developing patterns for organized behavior, using available resources, relating to others, and creating a meaningful life (McElroy and Townsend 1985). This capacity for adaptation has produced an array of different cultures and cultural practices. An example of an adaptive cultural practice is the long postpartum sex taboos in some tropical countries where there are limited sources of protein. Women are prohibited from engaging in sexual intercourse until the infant is weaned at the age of 2 years. This prohibition prevents the mother from becoming pregnant while nursing her infant, in which case she would have to discontinue breastfeeding, and protects the infant from protein deficiency.

CULTURE AS KNOWLEDGE

The domain of culture that is the focus of this chapter is health beliefs, or more specifically, the beliefs that persons have about illness, what causes illness, and what role the individual plays in preventing or not preventing illness.

Spradley and McCurdy (1972) define culture as *knowledge*, or what a person has to know in order to survive in the environment in which he lives. This knowledge is organized by the individual into conceptual categories that enable him to make sense of his world and to generate and interpret social behavior. Illness is a stressful life event. People try to account for illness, to understand it, and to do something about it. How persons deal with and respond to illness will be affected by the beliefs they have about illness, what causes it, and why illness occurs. In other words, given the human event of illness, how do people survive (or not survive) it? What knowledge (beliefs) do people use to deal with and to explain illness? As a way of approaching cultural data, two conceptual belief categories are proposed: beliefs about illness causation and beliefs about individual control in the prevention of illness. Using these categories as a framework in considering a cultural assessment, the community health nurse can elicit much useful information.

BELIEFS ABOUT ILLNESS

All persons have beliefs about how and why they become ill, such as exposure to a virus, stress, exposure to drafts, and even doing something wrong. Anthropologists have categorized these beliefs of illness causation into two types: naturalistic beliefs and personalistic beliefs (Chino and Vollweiler, 1986).

Naturalistic beliefs explain illness as being due to the interaction of impersonal internal or external agents, such as germs, inadequate rest, accidents, nutrition, imbalance in hot and cold bodily humors, and environmental pollution. Personalistic beliefs explain illness as being due to personal agents of which there are two types: spiritual agents, such as ghosts and deities, who employ such methods as soul loss and spirit possession; and human agents, such as witches, sorcerers, and priests, who use as some of their methods sympathetic magic, the evil eye, and curses (Chino and Vollweiler, 1986).

Some people believe solely in one or the other causes of illness. For example, Western health professionals believe that illness is caused by some organism or some physiologic or psychologic malfunction. For some, even psychologic problems are frequently believed to have a physiologic cause (Pfiffering 1985).

Some people believe that illness can be

caused by either naturalistic agents or personalistic agents, depending on the illness. This alternating belief system is referred to as eclectic (Chino and Vollweiler 1986). For example, an acute illness may be attributed to a virus, while a chronic illness, such as schizophrenia or a fatal illness, may be considered a punishment from the gods or the result of a curse.

Just as all persons have beliefs about what causes them to become ill, all persons have beliefs about why they become ill. Anthropologists refer to these beliefs as *locus of control* beliefs (Chino and Vollweiler 1986). Internal locus of control beliefs are held by individuals who believe that their own behavior determines whether they stay well or become ill. These beliefs presume that illness can be prevented through appropriate behaviors that control naturalistic or personalistic agents (Chino and Vollweiler 1986).

Individuals with external locus of control beliefs believe that their own behavior does not determine whether they stay well or become ill. These external control beliefs presume that illness is not preventable because naturalistic or personalistic agents are unpredictable and without morals (Chino and Vollweiler 1986).

When fully functional, an individual tends to "believe" the dominant cultural explanation of a phenomenon. However, when he is stressed, ill, or otherwise made vulnerable, the individual often finds subcultural beliefs coming to the surface and influencing his behaviors, feelings, and responses. For example, a mother who is very religious and whose child has a serious infection may understand and believe that a microorganism is the cause of the illness. But at the same time, she may also believe, and fear, especially when she feels most vulnerable or stressed, that the child's illness is a punishment for something that she, the mother, has or has not done.

This blending of dominant and subcultural beliefs happens to both the client and the nurse. The nurse is as much a product of enculturation experiences as is the client. Like the client, the nurse carries with her beliefs about illness that reflect her professional education as well as illness beliefs derived from family experiences in the process of growing up (Leininger 1978).

The dominant beliefs for health-care professionals, socialized in the Western medical model, is that illness is caused by naturalistic factors, and that an individual's behavior determines to a large extent whether he stays well or becomes ill. These beliefs underlie the health professional's approach to clients, who may or may not share these same beliefs. At the same time, the health professional at times of stress or illness may experience a resurfacing of less "scientific" beliefs.

It is important for the home-health nurse to recognize and examine her own beliefs about illness causation and the individual's role in preventing or causing illness, and to keep in mind that her clients may or may not share these same beliefs. In recognizing and understanding her own beliefs and in acknowledging cultural differences in health beliefs, the home-health nurse can more objectively identify and understand her client's perceptions of illness and actions taken to deal with the illness, and she can intervene more appropriately in the illness process.

Another important dimension to consider in assessing clients is the role of the client within the family context. Is the client the chief or only breadwinner? Is the client the decision-maker in the family? What effect does the client's illness have on the other members of the family, on their implicit as well as explicit roles? What adjustments have to be made to accommodate the client's illness? What role does the family play in the client's recovery?

HEALTH BELIEFS AND ILLNESS-RELATED BEHAVIOR

What a client does or does not do in relation to an illness will be influenced by his beliefs about the cause of the illness and how much control he perceives he has in preventing or doing something about the illness. Individuals who believe that illness is caused by naturalistic factors or agents would likely be receptive to remedies or treatments that act on the causal agent. For example, an individual with coronary artery disease, who believes that this illness is affected by diet and exercise, will probably comply with a diet and exercise regime that is designed to reduce the risk of a heart attack. If the individual believes that his behavior determines his health status, he will probably examine his past life-style in hopes of arresting the illness. On the other hand, if the individual attributes the cause of his illness to hereditary factors, he may feel that nothing he does will alter the status of his illness and so he does not alter his behavior.

For those individuals with naturalistic beliefs about illness causation, help may or may not be sought within the Western health-care system. These individuals are very likely to utilize the traditional health system and to seek the help of folk medical practitioners, such as an herbalist or a masseuse (or masseur). If relief is not obtained or if the illness is not cured, help then may be sought in the dominant health-care system.

An individual with an illness believed to be caused by a personalistic agent would probably seek the help of a "shaman" or priest. For example, it is not uncommon for a person suffering from depression to first seek help from a priest or minister. The dynamics of a depression include feelings of guilt for having done something wrong (frequently a fantasy or wish), something that deserves punishment. Forgiveness and absolution are sought from the priest or minister. Psychological therapy may or may not follow this action.

THE APPROACH OF THE HOME-HEALTH NURSE

Persons are not always able to articulate their beliefs about something. Frequently an individual's beliefs about something have to be inferred from his behavior. Accurate interpretation of behavior takes skill and objectivity. These characteristics are important for the home-health nurse who is a critical link between what clients do and say and her descriptive and interpretive account of these events. How the home-health nurse approaches her work with clients in the home and community will be influenced by her own enculturation experiences early in her life and later during her professional education. These experiences will color what she sees and hears and how she interprets this information (Spector 1985).

Having grown up in a particular cultural milieu, the home-health nurse has certain perceptions and beliefs about health, illness, and health-related behaviors and practices that are derived from these early experiences. As a health professional in the Western medical system, the home-health nurse has been socialized in the Western tradition. This tradition includes the belief in the germ theory of disease, the value of preventive health actions, the merits of medical technology for the preservation and prolongation of life, and individual responsibility for health maintenance and illness prevention.

Furthermore, as a result of her professional education, the home-health nurse very likely has negated or dismissed many of the folk-type health beliefs and practices that she may have learned during her early life experiences, and has become more technically advanced and abstract concerning health beliefs and practices. Just as she comes to understand her client's beliefs, the home-health nurse must objectively study her own ideas, feelings, and behaviors to identify what her beliefs are. And since one's beliefs may shift depending upon circumstances, this self study must be ongoing. The same tools can be used by the nurse to study herself as are used to study her clients.

We cannot rid ourselves completely of our cultural biases, but we can reduce the chance of selective observations and interpretations by being aware of our personal and cultural prejudices. In addition to biases, health professionals particularly are prone to ethnocentricism, or an attitude of superiority about Western medicine.

The home-health nurse wants to do what is best for the client. One of the ways she sees herself as impacting upon a health problem is educating the client about the problem, explaining why certain behaviors or practices are better than others, and teaching him the skills necessary to deal with the problem. The effectiveness of this intervention by the nurse will depend to a large extent on her understanding of the client's perspective. Educational efforts by the home-health nurse have to begin with the client.

EXPLANATORY MODELS OF ILLNESS

What have been described up to this point in the discussion of beliefs about illness causation are what anthropologists refer to as *explanatory models of illness* (Good and Good 1980). Clients as well as health-care providers use these explanatory models to give meaning to an illness experience. They represent a person's notions about his world, about himself and his environment. As mentioned earlier, a goal of this chapter is to

sensitize the home-health nurse to the existence of these explanatory models, and to provide her with a guide for eliciting information that will enable her to uncover and understand the meaning of an illness for a client so that she may appropriately intervene and assist the client.

EXPLANATORY MODELS OF ILLNESS AND COMPLIANCE

It is well known that client noncompliance is a pervasive phenomenon. Estimates are that only one third of chronically ill clients adhere correctly to their regimen, while one third are noncompliant because they adhere to a misunderstood regimen, and another third are knowingly noncompliant (Cohen 1979). Methods for increasing compliance have met with limited success; for instance, education or the provision of information about a particular condition does not alone result in increased compliance. Given the limited success of attempts to increase adherence to medical regimens, it may be of some value to examine the experience of illness from an anthropologic perspective, or from the perspective of client (and provider) explanatory models of illness.

EXPLANATORY MODELS OF ILLNESS AND NURSING INTERVENTION

Almost all health-care interventions evolve from the conceptual or explanatory model of illness of the health-care provider. The provider uses this model as a basis for assessing the client and developing a care plan, without trying to explain the meaning of an illness to the client. Client and provider may differ significantly in the meaning each attributes to an illness. In other words, in the nurse–client relationship, we are dealing with two different (and largely implicit) explanatory models of the same illness (the folk or client model and the nurse's model), and the interventions that are being proposed are based on only one model, which is the nurse's model.

Ideally, there should be recognition by the nurse that, indeed, both client *and* nurse explanatory models of illness exist, and that client and nurse need to negotiate a common understanding of the client's illness. The nurse is in a better position than the client to modify her conceptualization of the client's illness so that there is a closer fit between the client's and nurse's explanatory models of the illness. Too frequently, a client's notions about his illness are considered simplistic or false, that he is ignorant of the causes and consequences of the illness.

The nurse is guided in her approach by her professional ethics and by the appropriateness and efficacy of the nursing interventions. She must always ask herself if there is an appropriate place for her interventions within a client's explanatory model of the illness. In some cases there will be no fit between the two; that is, there will be no appropriate nursing techniques and no legitimacy for nursing intervention in these cases. For example, a client may be suffering from severe back pain for which multiple treatments have been given, with no resulting relief. A cultural assessment reveals that the client believes he had offended a spiritual being, and the back pain and resulting immobility represents a punishment for this misdeed. Does the nurse have a role in this case? It is very likely that the nurse has no role at all. There may be no intervention that the nurse can provide. Involvement, if any, by the nurse would be very limited, as there is no fit between the client's explanation of his illness and the nurse's explanation of the illness. A "shaman" would probably be the appropriate resource for the client. This idea will be developed further in the case study to follow.

GUIDE FOR CULTURAL ASSESSMENT

Cultural assessment of the client goes hand in hand with the physical assessment. This proposed cultural assessment guide is designed to assist the home-health nurse obtain information from clients about their health/illness beliefs, how they define and interpret their symptoms, what actions they take to remedy the situation, and what sources of help they utilize. The guide attempts to elicit information about the meaning of the illness to the client and to construct the client's explanatory model of the illness, taking into consideration situational and personal factors that may be relevant to the situation. Information pertaining to food and food-related behaviors, such as choice and preparation of foods and eating patterns, is important when examining culture. (Nutritional and nutritional assessment is discussed in another chapter.)

According to Ziegler and Vaughn-Wrobel (1986): "Nursing theory guides assessment by describing which client characteristics are to be assessed and how these characteristics cluster together to form patterns of behavior. Theory guides diagnosis by describing the norms against which the client's patterns of human response are compared." Similarly, Good and Good (1980) state that a model makes relevant certain data or certain aspects of reality ignored or left unanalyzed by other models, and that each model employs particular interpretive strategies for constituting the meaning of the abstracted data. The guide presented below is based on a cultural model designed to obtain data relevant to the meaning of an illness to a client.

A. *Client's explanation of present illness* (Kleinman, Eisenberg, and Good 1978; Good and Good, 1980).
   1. What do you think caused your problem?
   2. Why do you think it started when it

did? What other things were happening in your life at the time? How do you think those things are related?

3. What do you think your sickness does to you? What problems in your life have been caused by your illness? What previous experiences have you had with this illness?

4. How severe is your sickness? Will it have a short or long course? How serious do you think your illness will become in the future?

5. What problems in your life have been caused by your illness? What have you had to give up because of it?

6. Do you know others who have had this condition? What problems did it cause for them?

7. What are the most difficult or important experiences that you associate with this problem? Are such experiences especially important to you, for your family (church, ethnic group, social group)?

8. What do other people think about your having this problem? How do they react to you? How do you feel about their reactions?

B. *History of Client's Health and Illness-Related Behaviors*
1. What types of illnesses have you had in the past?
2. What did you do about these illnesses?
   a. Did you get treatment? If no, why not? If yes, from whom?
3. How long did the illnesses last?
4. What types of medicines do you take and why do you take them?

C. *Client Life-Style*
1. What is client's education? Job?
2. How does client spend his time? What are his interests? What things are important to the client?
3. What types of medicines does client take and why?

D. *Client's Health*
1. What does client look like? Overweight? Underweight? Energetic? Slow-moving? Other?
2. What worries you most about your health?
3. What do you do to keep from getting sick?

E. *Effects of Illness on Client's Roles in Family and Outside Family.*
1. Is client the principal breadwinner in family?
2. Is client the decision-maker in the family? If no, who makes decisions in the family and about what? If yes, what types of decisions does client make? Is someone else fulfilling this role during the client's illness?
3. How does client perceive his body and how it works?

F. *Family of Client*
1. How does family deal with client's illness?
2. Are family members supportive of client?
3. Are family members immobilized with client's being ill?
4. How do family members communicate with each other?
5. Is there an extended family (close relatives)?
6. Does the family have links with community groups (church, ethnic associations, others)?
7. Are there any language barriers?
8. What is the family's nationality or ethnic affiliation?
9. What is the family's socioeconomic status?

G. *Family and Health-Care Behavior*
1. What types of food are eaten in the family? How is food cooked or prepared and by whom?
2. Have family members been immunized for communicable diseases?

3. Is there a family physician?
4. Do client and family members have health insurance?

Case Study

(This example is a modified version of a case studied by Hessell 1985.)

Assessment

Mrs. M is a 62-year-old, white, married female who within the past year was diagnosed as having coronary artery disease. At that time, two balloon angioplasties were performed with successful results after coronary arteriograms revealed 90% occlusion of coronary arteries. Some of the symptoms associated with this initial episode included feeling tired and weak, a squeezing sort of burning pressure in chest, nausea, and indigestion. During her hospitalization she was instructed about diet and exercise, and prescribed medications).

Following the initial episode of hospitalization and diagnosis of coronary artery disease, Mrs. M spent a great deal of time attempting to account for why she had developed this particular condition. She expressed anger about having this disease, stating that she had always made an effort to maintain her health. According to Mrs. M's way of thinking, she should not have developed coronary artery disease, given her health-conscious life-style. She considered what she did and did not do that may have led to her contracting this illness. She did not smoke or drink, she did not eat many high cholesterol foods, and she was physically active. There was a history of coronary artery disease in the family. Her brother died of a heart attack when in his 50's but, according to Mrs. M, he abused his body by drinking, smoking, and not exercising. She concluded that the reasons she developed coronary artery disease were stress, related to the deaths of her mother and brother, which occurred close together in time, and not doing the right kind of exercise. Although she believed that she acted to prevent such an illness, she also believed that what she did was not adequate, and that, in some way, she contributed to its onset.

When Mrs. M knew of someone who had had a heart attack and either recovered or died, she would attempt to account for one or the other outcome. For example, when a male neighbor died following a heart attack, she attributed his death to the fact that he continued to smoke after having had an initial heart attack 2 years previously.

One of the most difficult things that Mrs. M had to deal with was sorting out and interpreting the various symptoms that she had, in order to distinguish between innocuous symptoms and symptoms indicating an impending heart attack. She became acutely alert to all the symptoms that she experienced, yet she could not, with any certainty, ascertain their meaning. An episode of indigestion might or might not indicate an impending attack. Coping with the uncertainty of recurrent heart problems proved to be stressful.

Mrs. M lives with her husband who is retired. Their daughter and son are married and both live with their spouses in different states. Mother and daughter are very close and talk on the phone frequently. Mrs. M attended college and has a bachelor's degree in history. She taught history in high school until a year ago. She belongs to the women's chamber of commerce and was a member of a local contract bridge club. She and her husband had season tickets to the local professional football games until this past year.

This illness episode of heart disease resulted in numerous changes in Mrs. M's life-style. She stopped working. She very conscientiously exercised and adhered to the recommended diet. She did not attend as many social functions and sports events as she had prior to becoming ill, but she did continue to have occasional lunches with her friends. She loved to read and did so whenever she could. She became reluctant to travel very far away fearing that she might have a heart attack while away, and so did not see her children as frequently as she had in the past. She and her husband adhered very closely to a low cholesterol, low sodium diet.

Despite being very compliant and doing everything she was supposed to do, Mrs. M had another episode of chest pain that resulted in her being hospitalized and having another successful angioplasty. Upon discharge from the hospital, Mrs. M was referred to the home-health nurse for follow-up. The referral on Mrs. M indicated that she was anxious about going home and fearful of having another attack of chest pain; her appetite was poor; she complained of fatigue; and lacked motivation to exercise. In addition, Mr. M was having some difficulty providing support to his wife and managing the household activities (grocery shopping, cooking, and cleaning). Prior to his retirement, Mr. M participated minimally in household activities. After Mrs. M's initial hospitalization, he did help to some extent with cleaning and shopping activities. ☐

NURSING DIAGNOSES (Gordon 1987)

Based on assessment data, the home-health nurse arrived at the following two nursing diagnoses:

1. Ineffective coping by Mrs. M due to perceived loss of control.
2. Ineffective family coping due to exhaustion of supportive capacity by Mr. M.

NURSING DIAGNOSIS ONE

Mrs. M believed that she was basically responsible for preventing or causing her illness. Yet, despite her efforts to do so following the initial episode of coronary artery disease, she was unable to forestall progression of the disease.

This realization precipitated feelings of hopelessness and powerlessness. According to Pender (1982), a person having a strong desire for control but little perceived probability of control may experience feelings of helplessness, frustration and behavior inhibition.

Interventions

In what way can the home-health nurse intervene in this case? Neither the nurse nor Mrs. M can cure or prevent the progression of coronary artery disease, despite corrective measures such as the angioplasties, and efforts made by the client, such as dietary control and exercise. Mrs. M is well informed about her illness and knows the limitations of these efforts. This knowledge has contributed to her affective state at this time. Is there a place for nursing intervention in this case? In what way can the home-health nurse impact on or help restore Mrs. M's perceived loss of control?

It is suggested that while the nurse cannot impact on the progression of the illness, she can assist Mrs. M to gain and/or to control within the context of her life as it presently is. In other words, in the cultural assessment of the client, the home-health nurse identifies the client's explanatory model of illness causation having to do with beliefs about personal control in the prevention of illness, and realizes why Mrs. M is responding as she does. The home-health nurse also realizes that the one area in which she can appropriately intervene is in assisting Mrs. M to have or gain control in other areas of her life, and to live as fully as possible within the limitations of her illness. Mrs. M taught history and loves to read. The nurse might encourage the client to get involved in a journal club, or in a group that reviews books. Some involvement in a library would be a possible activity for the client. While change cannot be made in relation to Mrs. M's illness with all its uncertainties and limitations, changes can be made in her environment or life context that will enable her to feel that she has more control of her life.

In this example, the home-health nurse identifies how the client perceives and explains her illness, and uses this information as a basis for any interventions she proposes. If the home-health nurse uses only her own theoretical or explanatory model as a guide, her interventions would probably focus primarily on health teaching related to diet and exercise, rather than on client needs stemming from the client's perceptions of the illness and its meaning to her.

NURSING DIAGNOSIS TWO

Mr. M felt overwhelmed with the responsibility of taking care of his wife and managing all household activities. He is not accustomed to participating in household activities, and had always relied on his wife to make decisions about these matters. In addition, he is very fearful that his wife will have another attack and he might not be able to assist her as he should. Nursing interventions might include the following:

(a) Arrange for housekeeper to assist with cleaning and cooking.
(b) If feasible, cooking could be a joint effort between Mr. and Mrs. M. Several meals could be cooked at the same time and frozen for later use.
(c) Encourage Mr. M to verbalize his fears.
(d) Provide him with information pertaining to symptoms of impending heart attack.

(e) Assist him with the development of a plan of action, including CPR and calling an ambulance, if this should be necessary.
(f) Encourage periodic recreation; arrange for sitter so that he is able to have time for himself.

This case example is of a typical middle-class American woman. However, the same process would be followed for a member of any ethnic group. The basic information for a cultural assessment remains the same.

Take, for example, a client who is a member of a Hmong community. The Hmong are a Southeast Asian refugee group who migrated to the United States following the Vietnam War (Hess 1985). There are a large number of Hmong living in different areas of the country. The Hmong do not have a word for health in their language. To be healthy simply means not being sick. The Hmong do not believe in the germ theory of disease, so do not understand the value or importance of immunizations. For the Hmong, illness is caused by breathing in bad air (air that is polluted), eating the wrong foods (overly seasoned, under- or over-cooked, too hot or too cold, or too much or too little), and extremes in temperature. Hot and cold food categories are based on the nature of the food rather than temperature. It is believed that illness is retained in the body with cold foods, while illness is driven out with hot foods. The Hmong also believe that some illnesses are caused by supernatural beings. Some illnesses including heart attacks, are thought to be caused by polluted air. This belief stems from the war experiences in Laos, when smoke-filled air due to heavy bombings was thought to be the cause of sudden deaths among young men (Hess 1985).

These beliefs would have to be taken into consideration by the home-health nurse if her client was a Hmong male who had coronary artery disease. Compliance with the typical medical regimen following a coronary disease episode may be very difficult for the Hmong client to achieve. He may believe that his behavior has nothing to do with his illness, and may not understand why exercise and dietary restrictions are important.

Similarly, for a Hmong family referred to the home-health agency because of a diagnosis of tuberculosis in a family member, the home-health nurse would have to keep in mind that the Hmong do not believe in the germ theory of illness and hence would have difficulty understanding immunization of family members who are well. In these cases, obtaining the assistance of a leader in the Hmong community to interpret and promote the suggested intervention would be an appropriate strategy.

References

Chino H, Vollweiler LG: Etiological beliefs of middle-income Anglo-Americans seeking clinical help. Human Organization 45(3): 245–254, 1986

Cohen SJ: New Directions in Patient Compliance. Lexington, MA, DC Health & Co, 1979

Ember CR, Ember M: Cultural Anthropology, 2nd ed. Englewood Cliffs, NJ, Prentice-Hall, 1977

Good BJ, Good MD: The meaning of symptoms: A cultural hermeneutic model for clinical practice. In Eisenberg L, Kleinman A (eds): The Relevance of Social Science for Medicine, pp 165–196. Boston, MA, D. Reidel Publishing, 1980

Gordon M: Nursing Diagnosis: Process and Application, 2nd ed. New York, McGraw-Hill, 1987

Gordon M: Manual of Nursing Diagnosis 1986–1987. New York, McGraw-Hill, 1987

Hess BL: An Ethnographic Study of Illness-related Beliefs and Practices of Hmong Refugees in the Greater Kansas City Area. Unpublished manuscript. University of Missouri–Kansas City, School of Nursing, Kansas City, 1985

Hessell JL: People with Coronary Disease: An Ethnography. Unpublished manuscript. University of Missouri–Kansas City, School of Nursing, Kansas City, 1985

Kleinman A, Eisenberg L, Good B: Culture, illness and care: Critical lessons from anthropologic and cross-cultural research. Ann Intern Med 88: 251–258, 1978

Leininger M: Transcultural Nursing: Concepts, Theories, and Practices. New York, John Wiley & Sons, 1978

McElroy A, Townsend PK: Medical Anthropology in Ecological Perspective. Boulder, CO, Westview Press, 1985

Pender NJ: Health Promotion in Nursing Practice. East Norwalk, CT, Appleton-Century-Crofts, 1982

Pfiffering JH: Cultural prescription for medicocentrism. In Eisenberg L, Kleinman A (eds): The Relevance of Social Science for Medicine. Boston, MA, D. Reidel Publishing, 1985

Spector RE: Cultural Diversity in Health and Illness, 2nd ed. East Norwalk, CT, Appleton-Century-Crofts, 1985

Spradley JP, McCurdy DW: Culture and the contemporary world. In Spradley JP, McCurdy DW (eds): Conformity and Conflict: Readings in Cultural Anthropology, 5th ed pp 1–13. Boston, MA, Little, Brown & Co, 1984

Spradley JP, McCurdy DW: The Cultural Experience: Ethnography in Complex Society. Chicago, Science Research, 1972

Ziegler SM, Vaughn-Wrobel BC: Nursing Process, Nursing Diagnosis, Nursing Knowledge. Norwalk, CT, Appleton-Century-Crofts, 1986

PSYCHOSOCIAL MANAGEMENT IN THE HOME

8

Barbara Kavanagh Haight

OVERVIEW

This chapter addresses the psychosocial needs of acutely ill clients who are being cared for at home. Often the psychosocial needs of ill clients at home are overlooked in the quest for immediate solutions to more pressing physical problems. Psychosocial problems are seldom the reason for the home visit, though they do often exist. One reason for this lack of focus on psychosocial needs is that home health care is structured around authorized services rather than involving an assessment of client needs. This phenomena in home health care, of being able to deliver authorized services only, puts the client cared for at home even more at risk psychosocially than the client in the hospital. Because of this problem, the home health nurse must be extremely cognizant of delivering holistic nursing care in all instances. Since psychosocial problems are not delineated and since the home health nurse is with the client at home for such a short time, she may fail to pick up clues of psychosocial distress in the client.

While in the home, the nurse usually focuses on the task at hand that is authorized and, therefore, reimbursable. Though psychosocial problems do not fall into an authorized service category, these problems may impact negatively on the client's ability to recover from physical illness. Thus, psychosocial problems must be addressed when planning the client's nursing care.

The psychosocial issues to be covered in this chapter are: stress, aging, reactive depression, relocation, lifestyle change. Selected nursing diagnoses appropriate to each problem will be presented as well as an assessment, intervention, and applicable outcome for each diagnosis.

STRESS

Stress is one of the most prevalent psychosocial issues for the acutely ill person at home. Because of the physical changes precipitated by stressful situations, stress needs to be monitored. Sick persons have a reduced tolerance for stress and often find anxiety in situations that presented no challenge to them in a healthier state. Because of the complications engendered by the presence of stress, stress should be considered one of the major problems facing the client who is acutely ill at home.

CHARACTERISTICS OF STRESS

Stress is defined as the nonspecific response of the body to any demand made upon it (Selye 1956). Mild stress may improve individual performance, whereas severe stress tends to impair the effectiveness of performance, suggesting that a moderate level of stress is necessary for optimal human functioning (Kermis 1986, Strauss 1984). The agent causing the stress is known as the *stressor,* and stress reactivity is the fight or flight response to the stressor causing physiologic changes in the body. These changes include increased muscle tension; increased heart rate, stroke volume, and output; elevated blood pressure; increased neural excitability; decreased saliva in the mouth; increased sodium retention; increased perspiration, change in respiratory rate; increased serum glucose, and increased release of hydrochloric acid in the stomach. The longer an individual's physiology varies from the baseline measure, the more physical difficulties are likely. Consequently, duration of stress is more significant than degree in contributing to physical illness (Greenberg 1983).

Mental stress aggravates symptoms in 50% to 90% of all hospital inpatients in the United States (Clark 1978). One can imagine the impact of increased stress on specific disease conditions such as hypertension (increased sodium retention), coronary heart disease (accelerated heart rate, increased blood pressure, and blood volume), ulcers (increased hydrochloric acid), and cancer (reduction of T-lymphocyte cells). Because of the potential

deteriorating effect of stress, it is essential, in the initial assessment, that the home health nurse be alert to clues of increased stress. Since illness itself often causes a crisis, stress is likely present in the ill client at home. It is up to the nurse to assess the degree of stress and to assess the client's ability to handle increased stress levels caused by illness.

The point at which stress becomes a health problem is different for each person; therefore, assessment of the client for stress is difficult. Tolerance to stress is individualized, and situations that may appear stressful to the nurse may be fully accepted by the client and vice versa. The way a person interprets an event is the key to the impact that event will have on the individual. To properly assess stress for each individual, the nurse must set personal values aside and assess the client's response to his own life condition. The nurse cannot interpret the impact of a stressor on the client but must rely on an assessment of the client's response. For example, a hospitalized client may be very disturbed when, on discharge and return to the home setting, evidence of neglect exists in an unmowed yard and an unclean house. The nurse may not judge the neglect an important problem, but if it is important to and upsets the client, the nurse must appreciate the impact of the stressor and the potential for comprising the client's condition. Figure 8-1 depicts a stress/illness continuum.

An ideal time to make an assessment of each stressor is at the point when the client begins to become excited or agitated in response to the stressor. The nurse needs to spend a portion of the first home visit helping the client identify those areas that have caused or are likely to cause him distress. For example, the client may be concerned about his work status. A call by the nurse or client to his place of business may be sufficient to put his mind at ease and allow him to concentrate on getting well. Other than verbalized clues

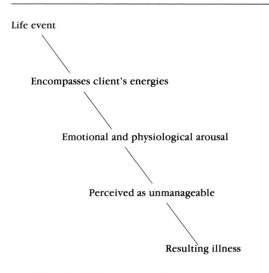

Life event

Encompasses client's energies

Emotional and physiological arousal

Perceived as unmanageable

Resulting illness

Figure 8-1. Stress–illness continuum.

given by the client, the nurse can assess those already identified physiological changes caused by stress and look for symptoms such as chest pain, rapid pulse, sighing, nausea, constipation or diarrhea, hyperventilation, perspiration, nausea, or hives. Further emotional signs of stress may appear as anger, frustration, reduced coping abilities, anxiety, tension, apprehension, overexcitedness, insomnia, uncertainty, or restlessness. As the stress becomes overwhelming, the client becomes increasingly helpless and develops additional signs of anxiety. Stress on the caregiver should also be considered and addressed since this may cause more immediate problems in carrying out the medical plan of care than the client's stress.

The ideal nursing intervention for stress is to remove the stressor or, if that is not possible, to assist the client in coping with the feelings of stress. Since home health focuses on independence for the client, the nurse should not remove the stressor personally but should assist the client in removing the

stress. Assessment, interventions, and outcomes are presented as examples under the following selected nursing diagnosis.

NURSING DIAGNOSES

ANXIETY

The client with ineffective coping skills, who is unable to manage stress, will display characteristics of anxiety. Anxiety is defined as a feeling of threat to self arising from an unidentifiable source (Stuart 1983). Characteristics present in anxiety may include fearfulness, trembling, poor eye contact, increased wariness, increased perspiration, rattled behavior, and increased urinary frequency. Additionally, the client will tend to focus on himself, indulge in extraneous movements, display facial tension, and exhibit restlessness. The client who is anxious may also participate in behaviors such as nail biting, finger tapping, foot swinging, and cheek biting.

Assessment

Persons who are ill very often experience anxiety regarding the status of their illness. In assessing the client for anxiety, the nurse must look for the above defining characteristics and related behaviors. In addition, the nurse should obtain a history of the methods the client usually uses to manage anxiety. The client's current mood should be assessed to determine if he is anxious at present and then the cause of the anxiety should be determined. Very often incomplete knowledge or misinformation regarding the client's illness can cause undue anxiety.

Interventions

Interventions are numerous and relate to the client's ability to accept them. Initially, the nurse needs to identify and assist the client and family in removing as many anxiety-causing stressors in the environment as possible. It is important for the client to help identify the anxiety causing stressors and to report past coping mechanisms that promote personal feelings of comfort. Family members may be very helpful in this assessment, providing the home health nurse with observational information. The nurse must convey caring and a willingness to listen, encouraging the client to verbalize feelings. Additionally, the nurse can reduce anxiety by seeking out and clarifying misguided information the client possesses about his illness. This is achieved by including the client in the decision-making process, and by giving clear concise explanations of events the client may not understand. In educating the client, the nurse must not create increased anxiety with an overload of information, nor make excessive demands on the client.

If the client is experiencing severe anxiety, both the client and the family may be taught modalities for management of the client's anxious behavior. Excellent management methods include relaxation techniques such as imagery, progressive muscle relaxation, and meditation. To be successful, all body parts must be involved in the exercise modality in the same manner. Progressive muscle relaxation can be self-administered and is an excellent tool for reducing stress and anxiety if the client is motivated to use it.

Outcomes

The client is expected to identify anxiety-causing experiences. After identification, the client and nurse should discuss helpful activities for decreasing anxiety, such as practicing progressive muscle relaxation techniques. Long term, with practice in the use of helpful techniques, the client is expected to live with his current illness without demonstrating severe signs of anxiety.

INEFFECTIVE INDIVIDUAL COPING

Ineffective coping is the inability to use adaptive behaviors in response to difficult life situations. Clients experiencing stress due to illness often exhibit ineffective coping mechanisms. A very graphic example is that of the client experiencing chronic pain. Unable to cope with the pain through accepted modalities, this client may turn to increased doses of medication and find himself addicted to analgesics. Another example exists in the client who is unable to accept a loss. The loss may be health, youth, or the loss of a loved one. An example of ineffective coping for this client may be an increased ingestion of alcohol because the alcohol makes the loss easier to bear.

Ineffective coping often includes the verbalization of this inability and a plea for help. Clients who cannot cope effectively are unable to problem solve or meet the expectations of others. Frequently they experience chronic fatigue as well as insomnia and are chronic worriers. Clients with ineffective coping skills exhibit a change in usual communication patterns. Frequently they display verbal manipulation with an inappropriate use of defense mechanisms. Physically, these clients experience muscular tension and irritable bowel as well as general irritability (Loxley and Cress 1986).

Assessment

The client's perception of his current situation is the key to the assessment of ineffective coping. If the client is unable to cope, the client may perceive his situation as hopeless. If this is the case, it may take time for the client to pass through several stages until the present situation seems manageable. It is essential to note the client's past problem-solving methods. If indeed he was able to cope effectively in the past, just reiterating his past actions may help him to cope again. The client's present available support systems must also be assessed. In the past the client may have been able to cope because of strong spousal support. If the spouse is no longer available, then a new support system may have to be established to assist the client in coping. Additionally, the client should be assessed for the existence of any emotional and physical impairment that interfere with coping abilities (Table 8-1). This coping assessment will provide guidelines for assisting the client to assume responsibility. Also, assessment will dictate whether and when the client can return to work and/or participate in any diversional activities.

Interventions

A primary intervention involves encouraging the client to communicate the present dilemma to the care-giver. Uninterrupted time spent with the client can be helpful in identifying the cause of the client's coping inability. In an effort to build trust, the same home health nurse should always visit the same clients. During these visits, privacy should be maintained. Initially, the client is allowed some dependency on the care-giver with a gradual increase of responsibility and independence.

As the client begins to accept responsibility for care, the client should be praised and encouraged to participate in degrees of decision making. Also, and gradually, the client is encouraged to utilize additional support systems such as the family at home. The client is encouraged to try out selected coping behaviors, to make judgments, and to provide feedback concerning the effectiveness of the behaviors. The nurse then needs to reinforce the practice of effective behaviors so they will continue. It is helpful in the home setting for the client to keep a diary of effective behaviors to share with the nurse during her weekly visit.

Outcomes

The client will become involved in planning and performing his own care in preparation for a return to a more normal life-style. Planning by the client should result in feelings of greater control over the present situation. Additionally, the client is expected to use family support systems progressively to assist in coping. After a reasonable amount of time and assistance, the client should be able to identify the need for healthful coping behaviors and demonstrate an ability to use them.

REACTIVE DEPRESSION

Yet another common response to illness is reactive depression. Most individuals who have been ill experience a temporary and reactive mood disturbance which is known as *reactive depression*. This reactive depression is normal, expected, and may occur as a result of crises (Stuart 1981). Reactive depression

TABLE 8.1 Diary of Effective Coping Behaviors

Stressor	Coping Responses	Effectiveness	Use Again	
			Yes	*No*
Noisy children in neighborhood	Turn on TV, watch movie on VCR	Good	X	
Unable to accomplish ADL tasks; therefore anxious in AM	Progressive muscle relaxation	Fair	X(Try)	

resembles a pervasive unhappiness, with an inability on the client's part to change. Also present is a feeling of lack of control and lack of power due to life's circumstances. This syndrome is particularly present in individuals who are ill and who do not have the energy to take charge of life and to function in normal capacities. In clients who have been hospitalized, early discharge (often the consequence of Diagnosis Related Groups [DRG's]) may force the client to assume self care before the client is capable of doing so.

Hospitalization provides an opportunity for dependency and gives the individual permission to be sick. Discharge, however, sends a totally different message that says it is time to resume a before-illness life-style, and to assume former responsibilities. Inability to assume these roles leads to feelings of helplessness and frustration. This syndrome can affect most adult clients: the mother who is not yet able to care for her family, the breadwinner who is not strong enough to resume job responsibilities, and the older client who has been physically compromised by his illness and is not yet able to carry out normal activities of independent daily living. The home health nurse must somehow give such clients permission to remain ill, while she helps them acknowledge that their primary responsibility is to get well.

Reactive depression is not as severe as clinical depression and differs from clinical depression in that it is only a temporary response to crises. Reactive depression presents with affective, physiological, cognitive, and behavioral manifestations (Stuart 1983). In the affective domain, clients experience a dejected mood, a decrease in life satisfaction, and decreased interest in activities they used to enjoy. Often, clients are irritable, have crying episodes, and feel emptiness. Cognitively, clients experience a slower thinking process and an indecisiveness that may be unusual for them. In the behavioral

sense, clients worry about their inability to function, hence they indulge in self-blame and self-criticism while experiencing negative expectations. Additionally, clients feel unable to cope and consequently feel guilty because they cannot cope. Clients also tend to be preoccupied with their health, feel useless, with a sense of failure, and exhibit temporary confusion and some inability to remember.

Physical symptoms include a great sense of fatigue, often a sleep disturbance, a loss of appetite, and onset of constipation. Reactive depression may lead to a decreased interest in sex and, for some, an inability to function sexually. Weight loss occurs and common symptomatic complaints are headache, backache, insomnia, indigestion, chest pain, nausea, and dizziness.

Depression may be manifested behaviorally through increased aggressiveness, withdrawal, lack of spontaneity, refusal to try new ideas, and overdependency. Characteristically, there is an increased need to escape through daytime sleep that results in an altered activity level. This also frequently causes nocturnal insomnia, further frustrating and depressing the individual. Also, there may be a complete lack of volitional activity, and the client may complain of lack of motivation to function even normally (Blazer 1982).

Several nursing diagnoses are appropriate in planning the nursing care of reactive depression.

NURSING DIAGNOSES

ALTERATION IN NUTRITION

A change in normal eating patterns resulting in body weight change defines the nursing diagnosis, alteration in nutrition. This nursing diagnosis is characterized by change in body weight of 20% less than the ideal weight, occasional abdominal pain, diarrhea, and loss of interest in food. The client often presents with poor muscle tone and pale conjunctiva and mucous membranes (Carpenito 1985).

Assessment

The home health nurse takes a nutritional history from the client to include present height and weight, the usual dietary pattern, food preparation, food preferences, financial resources, and other factors that influence food consumption. The dietary pattern should be recorded for 3 to 5 days and at least over one weekend day when dietary patterns sometimes differ. It is also helpful to explore hereditary and sociocultural influences on diet and to ask the client if there are any foods at all that sound appetizing (Roe 1983). These exploratory techniques may refresh some clients' interest in food by aiding in remembering a delicious taste of the past. The nurse should also encourage a discussion of the client's reasons for not eating. This discussion may give her some clues for appropriate interventions. For instance, the client may not be eating because the client does not like to eat alone. This problem of isolation requires a different intervention from the intervention for the client who cannot cook for himself.

Interventions

Once nutritional preferences are identified, the home health nurse should encourage the family to obtain these preferred foods. The nurse and client should plan a written schedule for eating the items in which the client has professed an interest. The nurse and the client can refer to this schedule each week to monitor progress. If the client diverts from the scheduled plan, the client should suggest a reason for the diversion and then discuss alternative plans with the home health nurse on the next visit. Family members must be an integral part of this planning process because more than likely they are responsible for the food preparation. This is not only an occasion for health education but also family members who are invested in the program will help the client comply. If some family members are at home, they may take turns eating with the client to provide sociability. The client should be weighed each week and a graph kept of the progress. Small gains will serve as further encouragement for continued eating.

At times the problem may be lack of someone (a family member) to prepare meals. In this situation the nurse may want to address the problem by assisting the client and family to arrange for home delivered meals or by recommending purchase of commercially prepared foods.

Outcomes

The client will gain a small amount of weight each week while increasing his activity level. Both client and family will communicate an understanding of the dietary plans and a willingness to participate. Nutritional counseling and planning will be ongoing until the client is functioning on his own.

SELF-CARE DEFICIT

The client experiencing a reactive depression will demonstrate a lack of interest in carrying out certain aspects of self-care. This lack of interest occurs essentially because of a feeling of apathy and general disinterest in the way one looks. An additional aspect is that the client may not be able to manage the mechanics of self-care at home, such as getting in and out of the tub. Because of the barriers to self-care, this client may neglect normal hygiene, wear dirty clothing, and become increasingly untidy as time goes on.

Assessment

The home health nurse must first make an assessment of the client's capabilities for self-care. Can the client get in and out of the tub or shower? Is there a washing machine and dryer available? When these procedural problems are solved, the nurse must then assess the client's interest in caring for himself and search for motivators to encourage self-care. Another important intervention would be to arrange short-term Home Health Aide visits to assist with personal care and bathing. Often the presence of another person motivates the client to attempt personal care. This is a service that may be covered under Medicare and Medicaid and is frequently underutilized. In an assessment of the client's recuperative life-style, the home health nurse should note if there are any occasions or reasons for the client to look well-groomed. For example, particular visitors or special dinners can be occasions for dressing up and grooming oneself.

Interventions

If the self-care deficit exists because the client is unable to care for himself due to environmental barriers, the home health nurse can help the client solve the procedural problems. For example, if the client is not bathing because the client cannot stand in the shower, the home health nurse can locate a stool or inexpensive plastic chair to place in the shower and show the client how to bathe while sitting down.

More than likely the deficit is due to neglect and apathy. In this case, the home health nurse can provide the client with occasions for socialization to give the individual a reason for wanting to be better groomed. For instance, if the client has meals delivered each day by a volunteer from a nutrition site, perhaps that individual can be encouraged to stay 5 minutes longer to visit and provide positive feedback when the client is well groomed. Very often this type of social interaction is all that is needed to supply the client with a reason for caring about his appearance. Additionally, the nurse and client should plan a program for the client's daily self-care. If the client is obligated to a plan, improved grooming will be encouraged, even when the client prefers not to pay attention to grooming.

Outcomes

The client is expected to recognize the existence of the self-care deficit and share his feelings and concerns about this deficit with the home health nurse. Also, the client is expected to carry out the planned self-care program until daily grooming becomes second nature. Eventually, the client is expected to make improved grooming a part of the normal behavior pattern.

ALTERATIONS IN THOUGHT PROCESSES

The client suffering from reactive depression may recognize an inability to process thoughts accurately and correctly. This client's response is similar to the response of an individual suffering from "overload." Often there is an inability to grasp ideas and an inability to respond quickly with clear reasoning and problem-solving ability. There may be an altered attention span and an inability to follow instructions. Memory can be compromised and there is occasional disorientation (Loxley and Cress 1986).

Assessment

The home health nurse must thoroughly assess the client's cognitive ability. Often, in older patients, symptoms of depression are mistaken for symptoms of chronic brain syndrome and the older client is incorrectly labeled senile. Use of the Mental Status Questionnaire (MSQ) shown below or the Face/Hand test is recommended to provide a distinction between the disorientation of chronic brain syndrome and that of reactive depression.

The client should also be assessed for insight. Judgment can be assessed through simple problem solving on the part of the client. For example, the client can be presented with a hypothetical situation and then given choices for managing the situation. The client then demonstrates judgment through the chosen management modality. The nurse should also explore physical causes of alteration in thought process through a close examination of the medication history, dietary history, and alcohol history. It is well known that malnutrition, alcoholism, and prescribed drug therapy can interfere with thought processes and mimic chronic brain syndrome.

Interventions

The nurse can bring order to the client's life. A daily routine and a list of expected daily behaviors such as taking out the garbage or cleaning the kitchen may be posted in a convenient spot, such as the refrigerator. If the client is slightly disoriented, a calender to cross off the days is helpful as is a large clock with black and white face making the time easily visible to the client. A structured environment is important, with belongings stored in an orderly manner and always put back in the same place so the client can find them. Drawers and closets can be labeled with signs describing their contents. The television and newspaper are also useful in maintaining orientation.

The client usually recognizes the alteration in thought processes and is disturbed by the losses, resulting in even more depressed behavior and feelings. Consequently, the client needs to be able to question the home health nurse about his confused behavior and to receive reassurances that the confusion is temporary. The client should be encouraged to increase activities each day and eventually to perform all aspects of normal living. Another helpful technique for improving cognition is to engage the client in thought-provoking games. Some card games and crossword puzzles are helpful in exercising the client's mental capabilities.

Mental Status Questionnaire

QUESTION

1. Where are we now?
2. Where is this place located?
3. What is today's date/day of month?
4. What month is it?
5. What year is it?
6. How old are you?
7. What is your birthday?
8. What year were you born?
9. Who is president of the U.S.?
10. Who was president before him?

RATING OF MSQ
FOR CHRONIC BRAIN SYNDROME

0–2 Absent or mild	3–5 Mild to moderate
6–8 Moderate to severe	9–10 Severe

Adapted from Kahn RL, Goldfarb AI, Pollack M, Peck A: Brief objective measure for the determination of mental status in the aged. Am J Psychiatry 117: 326, 1960

Outcomes

The client at home is expected to maintain orientation and to gradually assume the normal activities of daily living. More difficult tasks, those which require problem-solving abilities such as balancing the checkbook, should be assumed more slowly. The difficult tasks, however, should be assumed as soon as improvement is observed in the client. Eventually, the client is expected to become fully oriented and to regain the cognitive abilities displayed before hospitalization. In a familiar setting, with a prescribed routine, such recovery will occur more quickly.

PSYCHOSOCIAL NEEDS OF OLDER PEOPLE

The next section of this chapter addresses the specific psychosocial and emotional needs of older people who are receiving care in the home setting while recovering from the acute phase of an illness. Particularly vulnerable is the older age group, 85 years and above, known as the *frail elderly*. The people in this age group are the greatest consumers of the health-care dollar. Illness and resulting hospitalization are catastrophic events for this group of frail elderly people.

Generally, the frail elderly have little compensatory reserve for any trauma. Typically, they have suffered numerous losses. They have reduced financial assets, reduced physical strength, and fewer social contacts (Ebersole 1985). Having suffered numerous losses, they become more dependent and needy with each additional catastrophic event in their lives. The nursing plans offered in this chapter are intended to assist the home health nurse devise more effective nursing interventions for this group of frail elderly and to evaluate the outcomes of these interventions.

The Home

Often, older people choose to remain in familiar home settings at great cost to their own needs and comfort. Housekeeping and cooking become insurmountable chores because

of physical frailties yet alternate forms of living providing greater ease are not chosen. For many older people, the home represents a lifetime of memories that may be lost when the home is forfeited. Being at home provides the older person with a familiar environment, an environment in which the older person possesses space, governance, power, and autonomy. In this environment, the older person can eat, sleep, and be entertained at will. The older person manages life, with independence limited only by the degree of frailty.

Because of this common attachment to the home, the frail elderly often share one major thought on admission to the hospital: "Will I ever go home again?" Each time an older person becomes ill, he wonders if it will be the last time. For most older persons the fear of being disabled and institutionalized, thereby losing control, makes them more vulnerable than the fear of death (Burnside 1981). Many older people possess stereotypes of nursing homes as poorhouses or places where one is abandoned. Influenced by these stereotypes, older people often choose discharge to home care over discharge to an intermediate care setting.

Today, shortened hospital stays further compound the problem of home care. Many older people are discharged from the hospital to the home setting before they are physically able to care for themselves. The caregivers at home may also be elderly, and compromise their own health in an effort to care for their recovering loved ones.

Community support services exist to assist the frail elderly to return home after a period of hospitalization. Maintaining the high-risk elderly in the community both before and after hospitalization is challenging and rewarding for both clients and health-care professionals. To respond to this challenge, health-care professionals, especially home health nurses, need a basic framework in gerontology. The home health nurse should be familiar with the psychosocial and emotional changes that accompany aging. A brief description follows of psychosocial and emotional aging changes affecting the aging ill client in the home setting. Assessment and intervention modalities are included to assist the nurse in planning appropriate care.

Social Changes

Compared to younger people, the older person is much more isolated, with a decrease in support systems. Burnside (1981) illustrated such a situation in the story of an elderly woman who had outlived her family and friends and had not had a close friend in 20 years. Though a dramatic example, such scenarios are not unusual. Many aging clients endure multiple losses: the loss of a spouse, diminished financial resources, the loss of a job, some the loss of their own children. Those who have lost children and family experience a deep loneliness in the resulting lack of kinship. The importance of kinship or the existence of a confidante is evidenced in several studies on the predictors of life-satisfaction in the elderly.

Substitute support systems to make up for the loss of normal support systems must be established. One way is to inform the older person of services available in the community and to put them personally in touch with those services. The home health nurse can assist with the bureaucratic maze by helping the older client determine eligibility and make the proper contacts. Most agencies also have social workers who are skilled in assisting clients with community services. This is a Medicare-covered service.

Many communities have innovative programs, using already established services to serve the elderly. Examples of such twofold services that may be used to also check the welfare of the older person include the post-

man and others who deliver services to the home, and the neighborhood crime watch system. In one community, the sheriff's department has a list of older persons living alone in their homes, and the sheriff's men make daily stops at homes of older people. Several communities have a call system. When the older person does not answer the telephone, an investigative visit is made. There are numerous ways to expand the older person's social world, and creative planning by communities will yield new and more innovative ideas.

In addition to the social modification of isolation, the older person experiences numerous psychological transformations, some of which are caused by physical aging changes. An example of physical change causing social change is that of the older person who cannot see well, and who has lost night vision, and so becomes increasingly isolated due to fear of venturing away from home. A second example, this one of psychological change, is of the older person experiencing a hearing loss who occasionally develops paranoid behavior because he thinks the conversation is about himself and that people are talking about him. Emotional involvement occurs as the older person tries to adapt to the change and the loss, but occasionally fails. Additionally, selected precise aging changes will be addressed in the following paragraphs.

Diminished Reaction Time

Diminishing reaction time on almost any performance measure is another result of aging (Eliopoulos 1987). A consequence of this deviation is that the older person may not be able to process information as efficiently as he did earlier in his life. This slowing reaction time has implications for nursing. The nurse must adjust the nursing approach to the client. It is necessary for the nurse to speak slowly and allow time for the individual to respond. How many times does a nurse say "good morning" to a client and then rush on to another task without receiving an answer? The client may simply have been processing the good morning during the time the nurse busied herself with another chore. When the client was ready to reply, no one was there. This unfortunate incident gives the client the message that the client's response was not really important. Instead of the greeting being a positive experience, as intended, this single interpersonal event becomes a degradation of the older individual.

Decreased Problem-Solving Ability

A further debilitation for the elderly client occurs as problem-solving ability declines due to a combination of cognitive losses (Bolwinick 1985).

The older person does not organize incoming information as well as when younger, and so finds it more difficult to make a decision. Also, the older person is much more cautious in making decisions, so tends to choose the solution that is easiest, but not necessarily the best. Illness tends to emphasize these normal aging declines. Thus, a chronically ill person will find problem-solving activities more exhausting and stress provoking (Lubkin 1986). The home health nurse should refrain from asking such patients to make unnecessary decisions concerning personal care. Further, the nurse should refrain from always presenting choices to such a client until the client is well enough to indicate a desire to be in charge.

Confusion

Emotional trauma and hospitalization often result in confusion for the client discharged from the hospital to the home. The source of

the confusion is of great importance to the home health nurse because the source more than likely determines the treatment. Causes of confusion are multiple and may include illnesses other than the present illness, and the present geographic relocation. Although it is necessary to determine the cause of the confusion, it is even more important to determine whether or not the confusion is reversible. Confusion caused by one of the above mentioned factors is more than likely reversible. Nonreversible confusion is most often caused by a dementia. The MSQ, suggested as a tool earlier in the chapter, is useful for differentiation of reversible and nonreversible dementias. Although simple, the MSQ has been used extensively with the seemingly confused elderly and excellent results have been achieved. However, the MSQ is not useful for distinguishing between the dementias and depressions (Blazer 1982).

Depression is an example of an illness that causes confusion but often is misdiagnosed as dementia (Blazer 1982). An individual experiencing pseudodementia or depression is in danger of being misdiagnosed and then neglected therapeutically. Consequently, it is essential to recognize differences between the two illnesses. Table 8-2 demonstrates characteristics distinguishing depression from dementia.

Personality Type

One last important factor to consider in planning care for the older client is the individual's personality type. The client's lifetime personality will have some bearing on the individual's reaction to the crises of age and use of coping skills. There is great variations of personality styles in the aged. Neugarten (1975) defined eight personality types in old age that were actually continuations of individuals' earlier life patterns. (See the boxed

TABLE 8.2 Dementia vs Depression

Dementia	Depression
Slow onset—not connected to life event	Rapid onset—precipitated by life event
Symptoms usually of long duration	Symptoms usually of short duration
No change with drugs	Relieved with mood-elevating drugs
Improved status in the morning	Same status throughout the day
Mood and behavior fluctuate	Depressed mood is consistent
Cannot answer questions	Doesn't bother to answer questions
Client conceals disabilities	Client doesn't care
Cognitive impairement stable and progressive	Cognitive impairment fluctuate

material opposite.) Identifying patterns for individuals in the home setting might be helpful to the home health nurse in planning the client's home care. The following scenario serves as an example: An older couple was involved in an auto accident and during the course of recovery the wife died. The husband was ready to be discharged to home care. The gentleman's personality type will affect his response to this catastrophic event when discharged. If he is described as *succorance-seeking,* he has high dependency needs and will not do well alone. If he is described as a *reorganizer,* he will find other people and tasks to fill the void in his life. Although the reorganizable person will undergo normal grieving, he will have a better chance of doing well on his own at home.

Personality Type According to Neugarten

I. Integrated—well functioning with a complex inner life and a competent ego
   A. Reorganizer—competent with a wide variety of activities
   B. Focused—competent but more selective in activities
   C. Disengaged—competent and choosing a low activity level (rocking chair)
II. Armored-Defended—striving, ambitious with high defense against anxiety
   A. Holding on—aging constitutes a threat but successful. "I'll work till I drop."
   B. Constricted—defends self against aging and preoccupied with losses
III. Passive-Dependent—demonstrates recurrent needs.
   A. Succorance-seeking—strong dependency needs and seeks support from others
   B. Apathetic passivity—is a striking feature of personality (man allows wife to talk for him)
IV. Disorganized—gross defects in psychological functioning

Personality pattern is recognized and nursing care is planned according to the pattern.

Terminal Drop

Other than the normal results of hospitalization, there is a time in every older person's life when that person can no longer respond to bodily insults. This time of ineffective response is known as *terminal drop* and has been described in the literature as a harbinger of death (Bolwinick 1985). This event is characterized by cognitive losses and a general increased frailness in the older person. Terminal drop has most often been described retrospectively in the literature. Nurses who have close and continuous contact with older clients often sense an increasing frailness and withdrawal in a client experiencing terminal drop. When death occurs, the nurse often reveals that she knew the client was going to die. The nurse who works closely with older people may be able to make a diagnosis prospectively and assist the client with necessary change at the end of life.

Often at the end of life, families panic when death approaches and seek support through hospitalizing the dying client. The end of life is a time when the focus of nursing care should be on supportive measures rather than rehabilitative measures. Supportive measures by nurses at the end of life can assist the family to cope.

Many problems of older people are suitably categorized and treated by nursing diagnosis. Three key diagnoses will be presented with suggestions for assessment, nursing interventions, and outcomes.

DIVERSIONAL ACTIVITY DEFICIT

Diversional activity deficit is characterized by a decrease in the ability to utilize unoccupied time to one's advantage. Often the client will identify this state by voicing the wish that there were something to do. Older people, especially, have to adjust their recreational pastimes to fit their remaining abilities. For instance, most older people suffer from presbyopia (Ebersole 1985). Those who have enjoyed fancy needlework in the past may not be able to see well enough to continue with this kind of work. Cataracts are another common ailment accompanying aging and also interfere with the ability to do close work.

Still another category of persons experiencing diversional activity deficit in time of illness are those who have been physically active in health. People who have enjoyed participation in sports in the past must often find substitute activities when limited by physical aging changes. For example, the aging tennis player may have to settle for vicarious tennis enjoyment through tournaments on television or working with younger players.

Assessment

When assessing the client for diversional activity deficit, the nurse should examine the client in several domains. The client's physical status and functional ability often dictate the client's activity level. Mobility tolerance as well as the status of the cardiovascular and respiratory systems enter into the client's ability to perform activities he enjoyed at a younger age. Cognitive losses may also affect functioning. A vivid illustration of such a cognitive loss is presented by the Alzheimer client. The Alzheimer client is unable to sequence events and often forgets what to do next while in the middle of an activity. Hobbies, such as knitting and crocheting, not only require sequencing of events, but also require counting strikes. Consequently, these activities are often dropped as hobbies with little or no explanation for the sudden lack of interest. The Alzheimer client prefers not to call attention to his deficits.

Interventions

In treating diversional activity deficits, a suggested intervention for the Alzheimer client is to find a similar but simpler task. For example, the lady who enjoyed knitting in the past might gain a similar pleasure pulling threads from around squares of cotton to produce pretty fringed napkins. The client with visual loss who can no longer read the paper and is experiencing diversional activity deficit can certainly benefit from the television or radio news. Also, most recently, bookstores have added story tapes to their stock so that the visually impaired may still enjoy literature.

The family can be most helpful in intervening for diversional activity deficit. If the client is confined to the bedroom, the family can intervene by visiting in the client's room periodically and by setting time aside for conversation. The home setting can become quite boring for the client who is recuperating at home. There is no reason why the whole family cannot gather around the client's bed to watch television in the bedroom instead of the living room, thereby providing the client with a loving family environment.

It might also be helpful to schedule time for entertainment, creating a schedule the client can anticipate, since anticipation contributes a great deal to enjoyment. A plan is especially helpful when the client is participating in lengthy treatments, such as receiving kidney dialysis at home. If this is the case, the treatments should be scheduled to allow for adequate rest times and favorite activities. If a client's favorite soap opera is on television from 3 to 4 in the afternoon no treatment should be scheduled during this time, allowing the client an enjoyable respite and something to anticipate each day.

Outcomes

The client will express an interest in using leisure time meaningfully and in participating in a chosen activity. The client will express satisfaction with this use of leisure time and exhibit fewer symptoms of boredom. Proper planning will provide the client at home with texture to his day and meaningful

events to anticipate. Eventually, the client is expected to make decisions about the timing of treatments and leisure activities and to make his own diversional plans. Finally, the client will express satisfaction with the established schedule.

FEAR

As the older client continues to experience losses and to lose control of important elements in his life, such as work and finances, the client becomes more fearful of the future in general (Marshall 1986). This state is defined as a feeling of threat to self, arising from an identifiable source. For the older person, however, the sources are often so many that a general feeling of fear exists and the older person cannot sort out the causes. The fearful older client experiences a feeling of physiologic or emotional disruption and perceives a loss of control. Physiologically, there is an increase in the blood pressure, pulse, and respiratory rate with increased diaphoresis. The fearful older person participates in increased verbalization and increased questioning and seeks redundant information in an effort to control the fear and assuage feelings.

Assessment

Initially, the client should be asked if he is experiencing fear and if so, why. If the client is not forthcoming, then information must be gained about the client's illness experience, and the client's knowledge concerning his condition to determine if any of these factors are causing the fear. The amount of knowledge the client has about his condition will impact heavily on the element of fear. Often, the unknown is more fear provoking than knowledge of a condition. Accurate and thorough information concerning health conditions can help the client work through problem areas.

It is also essential for the nurse to assess the client's past abilities and methods of coping with fear. Information about past coping abilities is essential in making a judgment of the client's ability to handle the present predicament. Additionally, the nurse should assess for changes in behavior, appetite, and sleep pattern, as well as look for physiological signs of fear that might include increased pulse, respirations, and blood pressure.

Interventions

Often fear is present because of a lack of knowledge or because of misinformation. If the fear is seated in the present illness, it is necessary to explain all treatments and procedures surrounding the client's illness to the client, presenting information at the client's level of understanding. One should never assume that the client fully understands the situation until the client can participate in a return demonstration or recitation of the information. Here is an example of misinformation causing fear: During illness a client received blood transfusions and contracted hepatitis. After discharge from the hospital, it was necessary to give additional transfusions of plasma at home, which the client continuously refused. Because of this refusal, the client was returned to the hospital setting where he accepted whole blood. One day, quite by accident, the client revealed that he feared the plasma because of the yellow color and thought this was the reason he had contracted hepatitis. If this information had been elicited earlier, the disruptive relocation to the hospital and home again could have been avoided. Somewhere in this scenario, the nurse should have uncovered the reason for refusing blood transfusions at home by anticipating the issue and encouraging the client to share his fears.

In dealing with fear, the nurse must repeatedly orient the client to the present surroundings. At home the client often finds himself in a rented hospital bed downstairs in a dining room that has been converted to a sick room. Though the client is at home, the surroundings are unfamiliar and can cause confusion, especially if the client awakens during the night. It is helpful to have a light on as well as familiar objects from the client's own bedroom nearby, such as a radio or a bed lamp. Even with these precautionary measures, the client may become confused and needs constant reassurance that the confusion is only temporary and will clear as the client improves.

Outcomes

The client is expected to verbalize and identify sources of fear. Fear is expected to diminish or disappear as the client gains information and becomes comfortable with his condition and his environment. Long term, the client must learn to question the appropriate care-givers when there are doubts about a health condition, having learned that complete information alleviates groundless fears. Some fears such as those occurring with sensory losses may be well grounded in fact, and in this case, the client is expected to exhibit coping mechanisms that reduce fear, such as orienting himself to new environments and situations.

SENSORY–PERCEPTUAL ALTERATION

Sensory–perceptual alteration is caused by a change in the interpretation of incoming stimuli. In the aging individual, normal sensory aging changes may account for much of the misinterpretation of stimuli (Carnevali 1984). Vision is altered by presbyopia as well as a rigidity in the iris muscle, allowing less light into the eye. As a result the older person has problems discerning colors, especially blues and greens. Glare provides an additional handicap. Glare reduces the client's ability to perceive surfaces clearly, a shiny white floor may be interpreted as wet and slippery and interfere with the client's ability to maneuver within the environment.

Presbycusis develops to interfere with hearing. With presbycusis the older person can hear better in the lower auditory ranges. Vowels are spoken in low ranges and consonant sounds are in the higher ranges. Therefore the words the older person receives are garbled, for example, the words "Let's Go" may be interpreted as E O. Increased volume will not alleviate the problem, but distinct articulation will. The older person with hearing loss occasionally develops paranoia through misinterpretation of conversation. These alterations in sensory perceptions contribute to disorientation, altered communication patterns, and hallucination (Carnevali 1984).

Assessment

The nurse must obtain a complete history and physical workup to determine those losses brought about by aging as differentiated from those caused by disease processes. In assessing auditory status, it is first essential to inspect the ear canal for cerumen. Recently, a group of nursing home residents was examined by speech pathology students. Sixty percent of the residents examined presented enough clogged ear wax to warrant flushing the ears. After the ear cleaning procedure, the hearing levels of the majority of the residents improved immensely.

When one is assessing the hearing acuity portion of the sensory–perceptual status in the elderly, examination of the hearing aid should be a part of the assessment. Hearing aids should be examined to determine fit, condition of the battery, and patency of the airway between the earpiece and the receiver. In addition to the aforementioned

variables, the physical environment should be assessed for noise level and availability of adequate lighting.

In a visual assessment, it is essential to check the glasses for cleanliness and for current usefulness. Fields of vision are particularly important in a visual assessment because the older client who is recovering from stroke may be experiencing loss in selected visual fields from hemianopsia and may not be aware of the losses. Also, as the home health nurse examines the hearing and visual status, the nurse should assess for unused prostheses. Often, dentures, hearing aids, and glasses are lost in the hospitalization process or the client just refuses to use them. Absence of these prescribed prostheses contributes to even greater sensory–perceptual problems. The nurse should assess the client's ability to perform activities of daily living safely with the remaining sensory abilities.

Interventions

Interventions should first occur in the environment. Environmental noise interferes with the hearing ability of the client suffering from presbycusis and poor lighting interferes with presbyopia. Each of these environmental hazards is easily corrected. Additionally, glare from shiny floors causes additional visual impediments that are easily corrected by removing the wax from the floor. Other areas of glare occur on clocks with white faces and other objects displaying shiny surfaces. Every effort should be made to increase the safety of the client's environment. The topography should be reviewed in a walk-through with the client and scatter rugs and small furniture removed. Hard to reach items should be placed conveniently for the client's ease. Stair steps should have black strips attached to the ends to provide the older person with visual definition.

When talking to the client suffering from presbycusis, women especially should lower the voice pitch so the client can hear the whole word including the consonants. It is also helpful to speak directly in front of the client's face to facilitate lip reading. When speaking one should not sit in front of a window that creates glare and interferes with the client's vision. Further, the nurse might choose to wear bright red lipstick to define the lips and make lip reading easier. Male nurses might choose a mustache. Lastly, the stethoscope can serve as an old fashioned hearing tube when the ear tips are placed in the client's ear and one speaks into the bell.

Interventions for improvement of vision include increasing the lighting in working areas and placing lights strategically. A 25-watt light bulb sufficient for a younger person should be increased to 100 watts for an older person. The victim of hemianopsia should be taught to move his head to increase his visual field. All communities have resources for the visually impaired. The Association for the Blind provides talking books free of charge for those clients who qualify visually. Talking books are also available in bookstores. Another aid is to retype medicine labels using large letters. Finally medicines may be color coded with the correct times on a chart for easy self-administration.

Touch is an excellent intervention that may be used to include the client in the surrounding world. When speaking to the client, touch his arm to first gain his attention. Touch is extremely important to the client who is isolated by sensory losses and gives the client a sense of himself and some connection with another human being. Be aware of client withdrawal because of barriers imposed by sensory limitations.

Outcomes

The client is expected to realize that losses exist and to plan compensations with the nurse to include use of prostheses if necessary. With compensated losses, the client is expected to maintain orientation and show interest in the external environment. Additionally, the client is expected to utilize appropriate resources such as talking books provided by the Association for the Blind. The client should exhibit continued social interactions with family and friends and should express satisfaction with the adjustments in his life that have increased his adaptability.

RELOCATION

Relocation is a recurring issue for older people and one that exists naturally for ill clients as they transfer from the home to the hospital, nursing home, and back to the home setting. Generally, relocation is disruptive to an individual's life-style and requires a measure of adaptation by the client. The health-care literature in general focuses on the final location of an older person to a long-term care facility and little attention is focused on the normal relocations to smaller housing or congregate living that occur because of illness or diminishing resources. Planned relocation differs greatly from unplanned relocation in terms of the effect on the client.

Wolanin and Philips (1981) report that a relocation to a long-term care facility is not traumatic if planned, gradual, and accompanied by an orientation to the new facility. In considering the relocation of the ill client to the hospital and then to the home, one must consider that these moves are largely unplanned and, therefore, represent a crisis situation. The incidence of a crisis can be divided into stages in much the same way that grieving is divided into stages. To handle these situations of crises in general, the client's crisis stage should be assessed before nursing interventions are planned.

Relocation to the home setting upon discharge from the hospital is generally anticipated as a joyful event by both the client and the family. However, numerous problems may arise at home for which both family and client are unprepared. The client may still be dependent on the hospital system and somewhat fearful when removed from this reassuring environment. The environment at home may not be as suitably arranged for the client's recovery (Burnside 1981). For example, the client may find it much more difficult to manage walking and taking a bath on his own. If the client's significant other is working, the client may find it difficult to manage meals at home. Furthermore, social isolation takes place without significant others at home and presents a difficult adjustment for the client who is used to sickroom attention in the hospital.

The family may be hesitant to accept the burden of the client's care as well as disillusioned when the client does not resume old healthy roles. Usually, the family is not prepared for the changes that have taken place, and consequently, finds it difficult to adjust to the client as a sick person. The home health nurse, in visiting the newly relocated client at home, must be prepared to care for the family as well as the client until all adjustments have been made by all parties concerned. Three selected diagnoses will be fully addressed to include assessment, interventions, and client outcomes.

NURSING DIAGNOSES

POTENTIAL FOR INJURY

Potential for injury is described as the presence of external or internal hazards that pose a threat to one's physical well-being. The person returning to the home setting is at risk for injury because the environment is often not designed for recovery. For example, in the hospital, there are bars to hold on to near

the toilet and in the shower. Not only are these unavailable in most homes but the shower also presents further potential disaster if it is located in a tub with an edge to be stepped over. Further, if invasive techniques are continued at home and include particulars such as catheters and heparin locks, the client is further at risk for infection. The home health nurse in an effort to provide a safe environment for the client and family should make a thorough assessment.

Assessment

The environment should be examined for cleanliness. If the client and family are participating in a procedure that requires sterile technique, their ability to follow sterile procedure needs additional appraisal. In conjunction with this appraisal, an assessment is necessary of the client's and family's understanding of sterile technique, the equipment used, and signs of infection. Additionally, the environment must be examined for hazards (such as loose scatter rugs), particularly if the client is responsible for his own care during the day. The client's ability to carry out activities of daily living needs additional evaluation. If there are limitations to the client's activities, these limitations should be discussed with the client so that together the nurse, family, and client can plan alternative modes of achieving the objectives of care. The nurse should also assess the need for adaptive devices such as a bath bench, bars in the shower, or an elevated toilet seat.

Interventions

After an assessment is made of the client's abilities to care for himself, a list should be compiled of services available in the community to assist the client where he has limitations. Along with this list, an assistance plan with duties divided among family members and friends is helpful. Include arranging for assistive devices to facilitate safety if this is appropriate for the client. After daily mail delivery, a friend or a neighbor might be called on each day to bring in the mail to the client recuperating at home. This gives the neighbor a worthwhile task that does not impose on the neighbor's good nature and gives the client something to look forward to each day: a visit from the neighbor *and* the mail. This intervention also provides the client with a reason to get up and get dressed in the morning. A simple intervention like the one described sometimes accomplishes a great deal.

Another intervention is a step-wise plan for the client's recovery. This step-wise plan will encourage the client to do more each day and will also provide a viable measure of the client's progress. This plan can be patterned after the example used for goal setting in Table 8-3.

Information gained in the environmental assessment, along with the assessment of client's physical abilities, provides a blueprint for necessary environmental changes. Appropriate interventions for preventing injury include family and client teaching, particularly regarding the client's physical limitations and the limitation of the home environment. The people at home need to learn such skills as monitoring temperature changes on a graphic sheet, and hand washing before and after nursing procedures. The stage of crisis the client and family are in relative to accepting the client's disabilities impacts on their ability to learn and this issue should be factored into the teaching program.

Outcomes

The client is expected to adjust to his environment slowly and gain a little more skill in caring for himself each day. The client's fear and that of his family concerning his well-being should gradually diminish and be re-

TABLE 8.3 A Structured Task Chart for the Socially Isolated Client

Activity	Date Accomplished
Knock on neighbor's door alone, go in, and visit for 5 minutes	11/20
Knock on neighbor's door alone	11/4
Knock on neighbor's door, go in with nurse, and visit for 5 minutes	10/25
Walk to neighbor's house with nurse	10/17
Walk one block with nurse	10/14
Walk down driveway	10/8
Sit outside for 15 minutes with nurse	10/6
Walk to kitchen	10/3
Walk to living room from bedroom	10/1

placed with increasing confidence and independence. If invasive techniques exist, the client is expected to remain free of infection. Further, the client will utilize available neighborhood services that contribute to his well-being. The client will gradually regain the highest level of wellness.

SOCIAL ISOLATION

Social isolation is a particular issue for the elderly. Nursing diagnosis describes social isolation as *an imposed lack of contact without support systems* (Lubkin 1986). The client at home is unable to maintain normal social and work contacts. Additionally, the caregivers that were available in the hospital are unavailable, and if the client is in a family where all members are working, the day goes by very slowly.

Assessment

When examining social isolation it is necessary to determine the degree of social isolation and to assess the environment for support systems. If there are limited family members, then support systems in the form of community services or of church support may have to suffice. Consequently, financial resources also need evaluation. Additional support systems such as friends or business associates can exist for some individuals. For example, businessmen often encounter major social contacts on the golf course. If the client is physically unable to play golf, and cannot afford the golf fees on reduced pay, the client will be unable to maintain these social contacts. It is also helpful to evaluate the client's level of education and usual diversional activity so that acceptable substitutes may be found. An investigation of the attitudes of family members and neighborhood support systems toward the client in his new situation will add additional information.

Interventions

When the home health nurse visits such a client, she must take time for visiting. Often this type of client does not socialize well and additional socializing modalities are needed. A life review intervention is an effective way of involving the client in a relationship and in encouraging him to look back on his life and think of himself as worthy. The "Life Review and Experiencing Form" illustrated opposite lists questions helpful in structuring life review interviews with the client. This type of client might also benefit from goal setting for himself, particularly goals that will increase his social contacts. All contacts do not have to be intimate. Table 8-3 illustrates an example of goal setting for the socially isolated client.

Life Review and Experiencing Form (LREF)

CHILDHOOD

1. What is the very first thing you can remember in your life? Go as far back as you can.
2. What other things can you remember about when you were very young?
3. What was life like for you as a child?
4. What were your parents like? What were their weaknesses, strengths?
5. Did you have any brothers or sisters? Tell me what each was like.
6. Did someone close to you die when you were growing up?
7. Did someone important to you go away?
8. Do you ever remember being very sick?
9. Do you remember having an accident?
10. Do you remember being in a very dangerous situation?
11. Was there anything that was important to you that was lost or destroyed?

ADOLESCENCE

1. When you think about yourself and your life as a teenager, what is the first thing you can remember about that time?
2. What other things stand out in your memory about being a teenager?
3. Who were the important people for you? Tell me about them. Parents, brothers and sisters, friends, teachers, those you were especially close to, those you admired, those you wanted to be like.

(continued)

4. Did you go to school? Meaning for you?
5. Did you work during these years?
6. Tell me of any hardships you experienced at this time.
7. Do you remember feeling that there wasn't enough food or necessities of life as a child or adolescent?
8. Do you remember feeling left alone, abandoned, not having enough love or care as a child or adolescent?
9. What were the pleasant things about your adolescence?
10. What was the most unpleasant thing about your adolescence?
11. All things considered, would you say you were happy or unhappy as a teenager?

FAMILY AND HOME
1. How did your parents get along?
2. How did other people in your home get along?
3. What was the atmosphere in your home?
4. Were you punished as a child? For what? Who did the punishing? Who was "boss"?
5. When you wanted something from your parents, how did you go about getting it?
6. What kind of person did your parents like the most? The least?
7. Who were you closest to in your family?
8. Who in your family were you most like? In what way?

ADULTHOOD
1. Now I would like to talk to you about your life as an adult starting when you were in your twenties up to today. Tell me of the most important events that happened in your adulthood.
2. What was life like for you in your twenties and thirties?
3. What kind of person were you? What did you enjoy?
4. Tell me about your work. Did you enjoy your work? Did you earn an adequate living? Did you work hard during those years? Were you appreciated?
5. Did you marry?
   (Yes) What kind of person was your spouse?
   (No)   Why not?
6. Do you think marriages get better or worse over time? Were you married more than once?
7. On the whole, would you say you had a happy or unhappy marriage?
8. What were some of the main difficulties you encountered during your adult years?
   (a) Did someone close to you die? Go away?
   (b) Were you ever sick? Have an accident?
   (c) Did you move often? Change jobs?
   (d) Did you ever feel alone? Abandoned?
   (e) Did you ever feel need?

SUMMARY
1. On the whole what kind of life do you think you've had?
2. If everything were to be the same would you like to live your life over again?
3. If you were going to live your life over again, what would you change? Leave unchanged?
4. We've been talking about your life

(continued)

for quite some time now. Let's discuss your overall feelings and ideas about your life. What would you say the main satisfactions in your life have been? (Try for three). (Why were they satisfying)?

5. Everyone has had disappointments. What have been the main disappointments in your life?

6. What was the hardest thing you had to face in your life? Describe.

7. What was the happiest period of your life? What about it made it the happiest period? Why is your life less happy now?

8. What was the unhappiest period of your life? Why is your life more happy now?

9. What was the proudest moment in your life?

10. If you could stay the same age all your life, what age would you choose? Why?

11. (a) How do you think you've made out in life?

(b) Better or worse than what you hoped for?

12. Let's talk a little about you as you are now. What are the best things about the age you are now?

13. What are the worse things about being the age you are now?

14. What are the most important things to you in your life today?

15. What do you hope will happen to you as you grow older?

16. What do you fear will happen to you as you grow older?

17. Have you enjoyed participating in this review of your life?

Copyright 1982 by Haight BK. Derived from new questions and two unpublished dissertations: Gorney J: Experiencing and age: Patterns of reminiscence among the elderly. Doctoral dissertation, University of Chicago, 1968. Falk J: The organization of remembered life experience of older people: Its relation to anticipated stress, to subsequent adaptation and to age. Doctoral dissertation, University of Chicago, 1969

Often a visit from church members will provide the client with a feeling of caring and also provide a diversion. Planning diversional activities with the client is helpful to make the time pass. Something as simple as a jigsaw puzzle will provide an activity and something to share. Another suggestion is to give the client a responsible task such as the assigned task of working for the senior citizens call line. Each day volunteers for the call line call elderly people who are homebound to say hello and provide social contact. Such a task would give the client a feeling of self-worth and would put him in communication with other people each day.

Outcomes

As a result of the life review, the client is expected to assess his life and discover new and acceptable interventions for reordering his social situation. The client should engage in more voluntary social interactions with family members and workers with whom he has contact. Additionally, participation in meaningful diversional activity will provide the client with a purpose in life. Lastly, the client is expected to recover from the negative feelings associated with social isolation and achieve an expected state of wellness.

POWERLESSNESS

Feelings of powerlessness often accompany illness and are defined as a perception of loss of control over what happens to oneself and loss of control over one's environment. (Carpenito 1985) Often the client will verbally express dismay about having no control over the impacting events of illness and resulting changes. Occasionally, this powerlessness results in a display of apathy with an unidentified feeling of dissatisfaction toward the health care system.

Assessment

The client's perception of his own state of control may be evaluated by verbal and nonverbal displays of independence, satisfaction, interest, and calmness. The client's usual coping strategies should be analyzed to see if the present behavior is unusual. In the assessment the home health nurse must explore many issues with the client to include past experiences with the health-care system, knowledge of the present condition, and readiness to learn about the condition. An assessment of the sickroom environment is helpful and should include such items as space, privacy, noise, and equipment. A comparison should then be made with the before-illness space, to see if, in fact, the technology of health care is causing this feeling of powerlessness.

Interventions

Interventions include client education. The individual who has an understanding of the illness and the related treatments and procedures feels much more in control of the situation. Additionally the client should be provided with choices. Though the client cannot easily refuse a treatment and still recuperate as well, the client can control the time and the place of the treatment. With control over some of the environment, the client can better accept loss of control over other portions of life and will feel less powerless. If the client is in bed for a major part of the day, it will be helpful to place the telephone, television control, and reading material well within

reach so that he can care for his personal needs himself. Encourage the client to express these feelings of powerlessness and to suggest change to eliminate these feelings. It is possible that some of the annoying sick role compromises may be rearranged to be more palatable to the client.

Outcomes

The client is expected to take control over those areas that are manageable and to accept the control of other persons over those areas that are not manageable. Often, fighting the control exacerbates feelings of powerlessness, but if the situation is accepted, the client is less frustrated. The client is expected to participate in self-care activities and to plan for controllable factors in the environment and in life events. As the client becomes stronger and assumes greater charge of the environment, he can be expected to communicate a sense of reduced powerlessness.

LIFE-STYLE CHANGE

Life-style change affects those who grow older as well as those who grow ill. Being old and ill creates a state of double jeopardy for the client. One of the most important changes an older person must endure is that of a change in roles (Ebersole 1985). For the older person the role change happens on retirement and for the sick, role change occurs with the illness. The sick client not only takes on the sick role described under powerlessness, but also often must relinquish the work role. For some, giving up the work world represents a significant loss, even a loss of identity. Additional roles are lost with age. As the children grow, the role of parent is gone; as the spouse dies, the role of husband or wife is gone. The older ill client seems to have no role at all, often taking on the sick role as the only role available.

Not only is life-style affected by loss of role, it is also affected by change in income often predicated on loss of the work role. More than likely there is a decrease in financial income when illness strikes (Lubkin 1986). Those having to get along on reduced income, such as workman's compensation, find they must make other adjustments. One extremely traumatic adjustment is sale of the home because there is not enough money to maintain it.

Occasionally, forms of entertainment must also be changed. The individual with less income may not be able to afford the club dues that provided relationships in the past. The issues in role loss are addressed through several nursing diagnoses.

NURSING DIAGNOSES

DYSFUNCTIONAL GRIEVING

Dysfunctional grieving is defined as a prolongation of the normal grief response beyond the time one would expect resolution to have occurred (Loxley and Cress 1986). Grieving can be related to an object or a person and in this case is related to the losses incurred with life-style change. The amount of grieving depends upon how well the individual has accomplished the expected lifetime developmental tasks. The amount of grieving is further influenced by the individual's inner personal strength and external support systems (Ebersole 1985).

Assessment

The home health nurse must realize that illness constitutes a loss of health, money, and life-style and the illness itself may be the cause of the grieving. Therefore, in assessment the nurse must identify the client's personal perceptions of loss as a result of the present illness. Further, the nurse should assess the client's usual coping patterns for clues to his behavior. The nurse should also assess support systems within the family and within the community, such as friends and clergy. Finally, the nurse should look for any somatic problems associated with the grieving process, such as change in appetite, sleep patterns, and/or activity level.

Interventions

Verbal expression of the client's grief should be encouraged. It is also helpful for the nurse to identify the stage of grief in order to plan interventions. A life review might also be helpful to assist the client through the grieving process. Through use of the life review the client is expected to put life's disappointments in their proper place and begin living again. Also, the life review encourages clients to express themselves and to talk of their losses. Often when the entire life is examined, the present distress does not seem as great. Additionally, the nurse is able to assist clients to focus realistically on their losses and resultant changes. A realistic assessment of the present situation is the initial step in planning for the future.

Support groups in the community can provide consolation and company to grieving clients. Clubs such as stroke clubs have excellent reputations for assisting clients adjusting to losses. As clients recover, they need to begin formulating plans for new activities that further compensate for losses.

Outcomes

Initially, clients are expected to identify their losses and express feelings about these losses. The healing client will allow others to assist in management and will begin using healthful management systems. The client will begin to understand that this grieving is normal and functional. As the client begins to heal, he is expected to seek out healthful support systems and utilize such systems for continued growth and healing. Clients must allow themselves to experience this grief, alone at first, and then with family, and must begin making plans for the future.

SELF-CONCEPT DISTURBANCE

Disturbance in self-concept is best described as a *negative perception of self* that makes healthful functioning more difficult. People undergoing involuntary losses often develop poor images of themselves and think poorly of themselves. Physical and psychological changes affect body image and damage one's self-concept. Stroke clients often display symptoms of self-concept disturbance as they ignore affected body parts, such as a paralyzed arm that is limp and dangling down the side of the body (Carnevali 1986).

People with disturbed self-concept are unable to accept positive reinforcement and often indulge in self-destructive behavior. These clients often demonstrate a lack of follow-through when beginning a task. Moreover, clients with self-concept disturbance participate in defeating self-talk and seldom make eye contact (Carnevali 1986). Defeating self-talk is counterproductive to the healing process. Losses resulting from aging as well as illness can contribute to a disturbance in self-concept.

Assessment

In conducting an assessment of a client's self-concept the home health nurse must obtain information on the client's present and previous role in the family, the usual patterns of managing stress, and the client's past experiences with health problems. An occupational history and a history of the client's hobbies and interests is useful for planning nursing care. With this information, the nurse can plan compensating activities that the client can accept and perform, in spite of the new losses.

New behavioral and physiologic changes affecting the client should also be noted. Often asking the client to draw a picture of the way he views himself will provide additional insight into his perception of self. Two elderly people were asked to do this. One woman with a zest for life and a need to wear jewelry and have her hair done, despite the disability causing a need for a walker, drew herself in a positive light. In contrast, another person who seemed to be housebound with a need to remain near the bathroom and medicine chest, drew herself clothed only in a robe or slippers. Obviously, the way these individuals view themselves in old age is decidedly different.

Interventions

Suggested interventions include involving the client in discussion that will provide the home health nurse with further insights into the client's coping patterns and present state of self-esteem. The nurse must accept the client's perception of self and begin work from there. Also, the nurse should encourage the client to participate actively in performing self-care. Self-care will encourage the client to touch and look at his own body and any of its existing disabilities. In this manner the client will become more accustomed to body changes that may be a result of the illness.

Then, as the client begins to improve in self-concept, it is necessary to point out to the client ways in which bodily functions are improving and stabilizing. This positive information will provide more positive reinforcement to the client about his adaptations. Furthermore, clients should again be taught coping strategies and encouraged to provide feedback to the home health nurse about coping behaviors that seem most effective.

Outcomes

The client is expected to articulate feelings about the life changes that have occurred and to acknowledge bodily changes and a resultant decrease in body image. Eventually, it is hoped the client will be able to see how these changes have altered self-concept. With the acceptance of these changes, the client will begin to express more positive personal feelings. An ambitious long-term goal is to have the client help others through sharing the debilitating experiences as a lay counselor, or in a support group. Many women who have experienced mastectomy have demonstrated acceptance of bodily change by helping others through peer counseling. As the client continues to improve, the ability to demonstrate at least two new coping behaviors should be required.

SEXUAL DYSFUNCTION RELATED TO ALTERED BODY STRUCTURE/FUNCTION

Often after experiencing illness, clients experience sexual dysfunction. The area of sexual functioning is a basic need and is extremely important to the client. Often sexual dysfunction is not addressed in the hospital when more life-threatening measures are the issue. Consequently, on discharge, when people began to resume their normal lives, sexual dysfunctioning becomes a more pressing problem. This enigma of sexual dysfunction is most often addressed by the home health nurse because at home the nurse is the nearest authority.

Addressing the area of sexuality presents a challenge to most home health nurses. Frequently, home health nurses must reeducate themselves to dispel old myths and to be prepared to discuss the topic of sexuality knowledgeably. For example, in the past, many people thought sexual activity disappeared with old age. In fact, we now know that people may be sexually active until the end of life (Carnevali 1986) It is helpful for the home health nurse to know that a few compensations are necessary, such as additional lubrication during sexual intercourse for the woman who is past menopause. The knowledge that it takes a man longer to reach orgasm and that the orgasm is not quite as strong is also helpful when counseling an older couple. The well-informed home health nurse can impact favorably on the client's sexual adjustment to life-style change.

Most clients will not raise the subject of sexual dysfunctioning themselves. Very often clients have already made uninformed decisions about sexual functioning in an effort to return to normal living (McCarthy 1979, Stuffle 1984, Tudeman, 1981). A prime example of a poor decision regarding sexual functioning is that of the client with a heart condition who fears that sexual activity is too stressful and therefore harmful. The literature is quite clear in describing sexual intercourse as nonharmful to the recovering heart client, and recommends sexual activity with a familiar compatible partner (Giorella and Bevil 1985).

Once the client verbalizes the problem of sexual dysfunction, additional forthcoming characteristics may include an inability to achieve desired satisfaction, a change of interest in self and others, and a need for confirmation of desirability. Often the client will have conflicts involving values that may preclude the client from using alternate forms of sexual gratification and these value conflicts will emerge in discussion. A last clue to sexual dysfunction is that the client may describe an alteration in the relationship with a spouse or a significant other.

Assessment

The home health nurse must first obtain a history of the problem that caused the change in sexual functioning. Sexual dysfunction accompanies a number of medical conditions and presents different challenges for care depending on the causative medical condition. For example, sexual dysfunction may be associated with colostomy and ileostomy because of the client's altered perception of self and fear of exposing the debilitating surgery to others. Clients with colostomy often fear they are repugnant to others and find it difficult to see themselves as sexual beings, thereby limiting their own sexual abilities (Giorella 1985). Other limiting medical conditions such as spinal cord injury result in sexual dysfunction because of physical inability to perform the sexual act of intercourse. Cases such as those of clients with spinal cord injury require an altogether different approach to treatment. A thorough assessment of the client's attitude towards the loss will provide more accurate information for planning effective nursing interventions.

In assessment, it is essential to learn the client's perceptions of the personal effects of change caused by sexual dysfunction. Some people are content to give up the sexual role, while others consider sexual intercourse an integral part of life. If the client is suffering from spinal cord injury is he regretting the loss of sexual ability more for himself or for his significant other? In gathering data regarding sexual functioning, the home health nurse should collect the following information: marital status or significant other, present living arrangements, and usual sexual patterns. Further, the nurse should inquire about any sexual problems occurring prior to the present health problem. It is also important to assess the client's attitude toward modifying sexual patterns and the client's present knowledge about appropriate options to sexual intercourse.

Interventions

The initial nursing intervention is to provide a nonthreatening atmosphere and to encourage the client to ask questions and talk freely about sexuality. The client should be allowed to express feelings openly in a nonjudgmental atmosphere. Private time should be provided and specific questions answered. If the home health nurse does not know the answer to a question, she can consult an additional authority and provide the answer as soon as possible. If there are limitations imposed by the client's present physical condition, the home health nurse can provide the client and spouse with education on those limitations. Additional resources for clients to gain their own information regarding alternate forms of gaining sexual satisfaction should be included in the educational process. Clients should also be encouraged to share their thoughts with their spouses. Lastly, clients may be referred to a sex counselor, physician or other appropriate professionals for future and ongoing guidance.

Outcomes

Essentially, the client experiencing sexual dysfunction is expected to acknowledge that a problem in sexual functioning exists. Often this disclosure is most difficult to obtain, but once the disclosure is made, the client is ready to accept help. The client must also verbalize feelings about change in sexual identity and express a willingness to obtain counseling. If appropriate, the client will seek additional education on alternate forms of sexual expression. The spouse will be fully informed and will be an active partner in achieving as fulfilling a sex life as possible.

ABBREVIATED CARE PLAN: PSYCHOSOCIAL AND EMOTIONAL AGING CHANGES

Nursing Diagnosis	Assessment	Interventions	Outcomes
Diversional Activity Deficit	Physical and functional status Cognitive status Preferences for activity	Schedule treatment to allow time for entertainment. Schedule planned leisure activities. Spend time conversing with client. Encourage family and client to engage in hobbies together.	Client will express satisfaction with schedule.
Fear	Level of understanding about illness Past abilities for coping Physiologic signs Increased vital signs	Help client to identify source of fear. Explain unknown situations to the client. Orient client to situation and setting. Encourage continued verbalization of doubts.	Client will utilize support system and decrease fear.
Alteration in Thought Processes	Cognitive ability by MSQ Assess judgment through simple problem solving Possible relationship of physical problem and medications to thought process	Address client by name. Give short, simple explanations. Orient frequently to time, place, date. Help client plan quiet times. Plan a consistent routine in a structured environment. Encourage memories.	Client regains orientation and clear thought process.
Alteration in Sensory Perception	Auditory status Perceptual status Visual status	Encourage client to identify areas of loss. Supply good lighting. Reduce glare.	Client will compensate for sensory losses and adapt to present environment.

(continued)

ABBREVIATED CARE PLAN: PSYCHOSOCIAL AND EMOTIONAL AGING CHANGES (*Continued*)

Nursing Diagnosis	Assessment	Interventions	Outcomes
	Use of assistive devices — hearing aids, glasses	Give clear, concise explanations. Lower voice tone. Reduce surrounding environmental noise.	
Alteration in Nutrition: Less Than Body Requirement	Nutritional history Height and weight Cultural facts Socioeconomic factors	Determine client's food preferences and encourage family member to obtain food. Provide a pleasant environment for eating. Devise daily eating plan. Set target weight.	Client will achieve and maintain target weight.
Self-Care Deficit	Capabilities for self-care Motivating factors	Document client's cognitive ability Allow client to express feelings of inadequacy and frustration. Direct client in self-care measures using simple instruction. Provide supportive measures. Arrange for home health aide visits.	Client carries out self-care program daily.
Powerlessness	Perception of control Usual coping skills Past experience with health care Space and privacy in home	Give the client some control. Encourage the client to express feelings of powerlessness.	Client will verbalize an increased sense of control over his destiny.

References

Blazer DG II: Depression in late life, p 144. St. Louis, CV Mosby, 1982

Bolwinick J: Aging and Behavior. New York, Springer-Verlag, 1985

Burnside IM: Nursing and the Aged, pp 439, 442. New York, McGraw-Hill, 1981

Carnevali D, Patrick M: Nursing Management of the Elderly. Philadelphia, JB Lippincott, 1986

Carnevali D et al: Diagnostic Reasoning in Nursing. Philadelphia, JB Lippincott, 1984

Carpenito L: Handbook of Nursing Diagnosis. Philadelphia, JB Lippincott, 1985

Clark CC: Mental Health Aspects of Community Health Nursing, p. 52. New York, McGraw-Hill, 1978

Ebersole P, Hess P: Toward Healthy Aging: Human Needs and Nursing Response, 2nd ed. St. Louis, CV Mosby, 1985

Eliopoulous C: Gerontological Nursing, 2nd ed. Philadelphia, JB Lippincott, 1987

Greenberg JS: Comprehensive Stress Management, pp 67, 77. Dubuque, WMC Brown, 1983

Giorella E, Bevil C: Nursing Care of the Aging Client. East Norwalk, Appleton-Century-Crofts, 1985

Kahn RL, Goldfarb AI, Pollack M, Peck A: Brief objective measure for the determination of mental status in the aged. Am J Psychiatry 117: 326, 1960

Kermis M: Mental Health in Late Life: The Adaptive Process. Boston, Jones and Bartlett, 1986

Loxley T, Cress S: Nursing diagnosis cards. Nursing 86.

Lubkin I: Chronic Illness: Impact and Interventions. Boston, Jones and Bartlett, 1986

Marshall V: Later Life, The Social Psychology of Aging. Beverly Hills, CA: Sage Publications, 1986

McCarthy P: Geriatric sexuality, capacity, interest, and opportunity. J Gerontol Nurs 5(1): 20–24, 1979

Neugarten BL: Middle Age and Aging: A Reader in Social Psychology. Chicago, The University of Chicago Press, 1975

Roe DA: Geriatric Nutrition. Englewood Cliffs, NJ, Prentice-Hall, 1983

Selye H: The Stress of Life. New York, McGraw-Hill, 1956

Strauss A: Chronic Illness and the Quality of Life. St. Louis, CV Mosby, 1984

Stuffle B: Sexuality and aging. Handbook Gerontol Nurs 5(1): 20–24, 1984

Stuart GW: Role strain and depression: A casual inquiry. Psychosocial Nurs 19(12), 1981

Stuart G, Sundeen S: Principles and Practice of Psychiatric Nursing. St.Louis, CV Mosby, 1983

Tudeman K: The sexuality of the older person. review of the literature. Gerontologist 21: 203, 1981

Wolanin MO, Philips C: Confusion, Prevention and Care. St. Louis, CV Mosby, 1981

ALTERATIONS IN RESPIRATION

Barbara Hastings

Breathing is taken for granted by everyone — everyone except those who suffer from disease or injuries that depress heart and lung function. Shortness of breath causes anxiety and frustration for both patient and caregiver. Without breath there is no life. Providing persons with measures to limit and control symptoms of altered respiratory function can be a most challenging and rewarding experience for the home health nurse.

RESPIRATORY FAILURE

Although the primary purpose of the respiratory system is simple, to supply the body with oxygen and eliminate carbon dioxide, the process is complex. Respiratory insufficiency or failure result when there is a breakdown in that process so that all body systems are compromised. The three basic causes of respiratory failure are impaired ventilation, impaired gaseous diffusion, and impaired oxygen transport.

Impaired Ventilation

Paralysis of respiratory muscles or lung disease that increase the "work" of breathing result in alveolar hypoventilation. Airway obstruction, as with chronic obstructive lung disease and loss of lung elasticity due to pulmonary fibrosis, infection, and skeletal abnormalities all require more effort to expand respiratory muscles and inflate lung tissue.

Impaired Gaseous Diffusion

Destruction or removal of lung tissue, pulmonary edema, obliterative pulmonary vascular disease, or any condition that increases the thickness of the respiratory membrane results in abnormalities in ventilation due to impaired diffusion of inspired gases in the lungs.

Impaired Oxygen Transport

Abnormalities of oxygen transport from the lungs to the tissues can lead to respiratory failure. Possible causes include a decreased cardiac output and anemia.

CLASSIFICATIONS

Respiratory failure is classified as either acute or chronic. In acute failure, symptoms develop quickly and are commonly the result of acute infections, congestive heart failure, chest trauma, asthma and pulmonary embolism. In chronic respiratory insufficiency, changes are slower and progressive, allowing the body to compensate for inadequate alveolar ventilation. Clients exchange chloride and retain bicarbonate to balance the elevated partial pressure of carbon dioxide.

MAJOR SYMPTOMS OF PULMONARY DISEASE

There are five cardinal symptoms of pulmonary disease: chest pain, wheezing, dyspnea, cough, and production of sputum.

Chest Pain

Pulmonary disorders in the following structures may produce pain: chest wall, parietal pleura, bronchi, and trachea. Tracheobronchial inflammations often produce a burning or raw feeling in the pharynx and trachea that is aggravated by coughing. Pain of a fractured rib worsens with sternum depression. Investigation of the seven dimensions of pain (location, quality, frequency, chronology, setting, aggravating/alleviating factors, and associated manifestation) is useful in identifying possible causes of chest pain.

Wheezing

Wheezing is caused by bronchospasm, that is, a reduction in the size of the bronchial lumina. It may be heard with, as well as without, a stethoscope. There is a component of asthma in chronic bronchitis, emphysema, congestive heart failure, and foreign body aspiration. Wheezing is classified as mild, moderate, or severe. It predisposes an individual to retention of secretions and respiratory infections.

Dyspnea

Dyspnea is the patient's feeling of breathlessness. The sensation of dyspnea results from the sustained work of breathing necessary to try to maintain adequate gas exchange. In addition to being caused by respiratory disorders, dyspnea may be psychogenic, cardiac, or caused by anemia or obesity. It results in fatigue and anxiety. Dyspnea should be measured in degree or level, that is, lying, sitting, walking on the level less than 50 feet, walking on the level more than 50 feet, and walking up steps. In severe disease it may be measured in number of syllables spoken between breaths. Orthopnea is more indicative of cardiac disease.

Cough

The cough is the most common symptom of respiratory disease. It may be a symptom of numerous thoracic and laryngeal disorders. A chronic cough is any cough that persists for a month or longer, even if it occurs only when getting up for the day or when lying down at night. Diseases that may produce a chronic cough include tuberculosis, lung cancer, bronchiectasis, and bronchitis. A cough may indicate asthma even though there is no evidence of wheezing. Nonpulmonary disorders that may produce cough include otitis media, subdiaphragmatic irritation, congestive heart failure, mitral stenosis, gastroesophageal reflux with aspiration, and nervousness.

Sputum

Sputum is assessed for amount, color, odor, and consistency. Clients should be instructed to collect all sputum for a 24-hour period in a clear glass container for the nurse to visualize. In measuring, less than ¼ cup (60 cc) of sputum is considered scanty, between ½ cup to ¼ cup (60–120 cc) is considered moderate and over ½ cup (12 cc) is considered a large amount within 24 hours. Table 9-1 lists sputum characteristics and associated pulmonary disorders.

A review of occupational history and environmental data is important for the home care nurse to recognize continued exposure to lung allergens, and irritants (such as sulfites, pollen, dander, pigeons, fungus). A daily profile of the pulmonary client is useful in evaluating changes in activity levels and sleeping patterns. The review of the psychological system may indicate disorientation due to carbon dioxide narcosis, depression, anxiety, and numerous defense mechanisms such as denial, isolation, and obsessional traits.

AT-HOME TESTING OF RESPIRATORY FUNCTION

Portable pulse oximetry units are now available to monitor hemoglobin oxygen saturation in the home. This analysis is essential in determining a client's severity of lung function impairment, exercise capability, changes in the patient's course, and need or continued need for oxygen at home.

Ventilatory function testing at home is possible by mini peak flow meters available for less than $20 and portable spirometry units available for approximately $1200. These provide objective data for measuring a client's progress or determining the need for more intensive pulmonary care and/or continued home-care follow-up.

Lung Auscultation

Auscultation of the lungs is done by listening to air movement using the diaphragm of the

TABLE 9.1 Sputum Guide

Pulmonary Disorder	Sputum Characteristic
Abscess	Large amount/foul odor
Asthma	Stringy mucoid
Bronchiectasis	Periodic large quantities (200 cc–500 cc) in 3 layers (mucus, clear, pus)
Bronchitis/Emphysema	Very tenacious/thick/adhesive
Bronchiogenic cancer or advanced tuberculosis	Frank blood
Pulmonary edema	Frothy pink
Pneumococcal pneumonia suppuration	Rusty, prune juicelike yellow, green, or dusty gray
Pneumonia bacterial infection	Small amounts
Bronchiectasis or fistula	Large amounts
Tracheobronchitis	Mucoid

stethoscope. The tubing of the stethoscope should not be longer than 14 inches. Clients breathe slightly deeper than normal through the mouth to eliminate extraneous noise from the nose. Anything that interferes with movement of air in the lungs (that is pleural effusion, COPD, severe asthma can decrease breath sounds).

Wheezes, crackles and rubs are three types of extra sounds commonly heard in the pulmonary client. Wheezes are continuous whistling noises due to narrowed airways. Sonorous wheezes are low pitched and due to sputum in the larger airways. They are frequently eliminated or changed when a client coughs. Sibilant wheezes are high pitched and are caused by a narrowing of the smaller airways. Crackles are discontinuous sounds caused by the collapse of small air sacs (usually due to fluid) and they may be fine, medium, or coarse. A rub is a creaking noise usually heard during inspiration and expiration and caused by the rubbing of an inflamed roughened pleura. A baseline recording of the location of crackles and wheezes is helpful in assessing changes in lung status.

Voice sounds can add to the initial and ongoing picture of lung status to help supplement the pulmonary assessment. Egophony occurs when the client's spoken syllable "e" assumes a peculiar nasal quality that changes it to a hard "a" when heard through the chest with the stethoscope. Whispered pectoriloquy presents when the client's whispered word, which would normally be inaudible or muffled, is heard distinctly through the chest wall. Both egophony and whispered pectoriloquy can be heard with pulmonary consolidation. Egophony is useful in marking the level of a pleural effusion. Table 9-2 summarizes both normal and abnormal lung sounds, and Table 9-3 summarizes chest examination findings in a variety of lung conditions.

RESPIRATORY THERAPY TECHNIQUES

Techniques of respiratory therapy, if ordered, are vital to the care of the respiratory client at home. Although an area of clinical specialization in the hospital, respiratory therapy most commonly is the responsibility of the registered nurse in the home-care setting. The following text presents an overview of respiratory equipment frequently ordered, as well as information required for optimum efficiency and safety of the equipment for clients and their families.

Aerosol Therapy

In aerosol therapy, liquid or solid particles are suspended in a gas usually by means of a baffle, so that microscopic droplets can be inhaled into tracheobronchial mucosa and peripheral regions of the lungs. The three most common types of aerosol therapy used at home are intermittent positive pressure breathing (IPPB), the compressor nebulizer, and the cartridge inhaler. Their purpose is to deliver medication and humidification into the small airways of the lungs.

IPPB

Intermittent positive pressure breathing (IPPB) therapy currently is indicated in clients who can not or will not consistently take proper aerosol treatment without mechanical assistance. There is no need for IPPB therapy in clients who can inhale deeply. Research indicates there is no evidence that the chronically ill benefit more from IPPB than from a compressor nebulizer and the hazards involved with IPPB are numerous. There is the possibility of inducing a pneumothorax or pneumomediastinum, particularly with bullous emphysema. Aggravation of bronchopulmonary bleeding and production of gastric dilation are common. The pressures may

TABLE 9.2 Lung Sounds*

BREATH SOUNDS Breath Sound	Description	Pitch	Gap	Location	Diagram	Cause
Vesicular	Soft, gentle, breezy, whishing	Low	No	Normally over entire lung surface except: 1. Trachea 3. Interscapula 2. Manubrium 4. Right apex		Air in the lung normally is dissipated throughout open alveoli
Bronchial	Hollow, tubular, windy	High	Yes	Normally above the manubrium, otherwise any pathology		Compression or consolidation of pulmonary tissue facilitates transmission of sound from bronchial tree

Bronchovesicular	Harsh	Medium	No	Normally in the upper interscapula region and beneath manubrium, otherwise beginning pathology	Small degree of compression of consolidation of pulmonary tissue facilitates transmission of sound from bronchial tree

VOICE SOUNDS	Description		Cause
Egophony	Spoken syllable "e" has a peculiar nasal quality to change it to a loud "a"		The quality is often imparted by compressed lung under a pleural effusion, although it is heard above the level of the effusion. It occasionally is heard in pulmonary consolidation.
Whispered Pectoriloquy	Whispered syllables are heard distinctly		Pulmonary consolidation transmits whispered syllables distinctly, even when the pathologic process is too small to produce bronchial breathing. This is a valuable sign in detecting early pneumonia, infarction, and atelectasis.

(continued)

189

TABLE 9.2 Lung Sounds* *(continued)*

ADVENTITIOUS SOUNDS	Description	Pitch	Diagram	Cause
DISCONTINUOUS				
Fine crackles	Crackling series of discreet, soft popping sounds usually heard on inspiration	High		Separation of alveolar walls that are stuck to each other (early pneumonia, early pulmonary edema, atelectasis)
Coarse crackles	Loud series of discreet sounds with a bubbling quality to them (commonly heard on expiration)	Low		Air passing through fluid in the larger airways (post-op, pulmonary edema, bronchitis, overdose)
CONTINUOUS				
Sibilant wheeze	Continuous squeaking sound	High		Air passing through narrowed small airways (asthma, pulmonary emboli)
Sonorous wheeze	Continuous snoring sound	Low		Air passing a sputum flap which vibrates in the air stream in large airway (asthma, chronic bronchitis)

* From Maskiewicz R, University of Pittsburgh, 1976

TABLE 9.3 Abnormal Lung Conditions

	Small Consolidation	Massive Consolidation	Thick-walled Cavity	Large Pleural Effusion	Pulmonary Emphysema	Open Pneumothorax
Tracheal Deviation	Absent	Absent or deviation toward	Absent	Deviation away	Absent	Deviation away
Fremitus	Normal or increased	Increased	Normal or increased	Absent	Diminished	Absent
Percussion	Slight dullness	Dull or flat	Slight dullness	(a) Hyperresonant (b) Flat	Hyperresonant	Hyperresonant
Breath Sounds	Bronchovesicular or bronchial	Bronchial	Bronchovesicular or amphoric	Absent or decreased	Diminished	Diminished or absent
Whisper Sounds	Increased	Increased	Increased	Increased above	Absent	Absent
Egophony	Varies	Varies	Varies	Present at level of the effusion	Absent unless exacerbation	Absent
Rales	Present or absent	Present	Present	Absent	Absent	Absent
Examples	Pneumonia or atelectasis	Lobar pneumonia or atelectasis	Tuberculosis	CHF		Stab wound

cause shock by reducing cardiac output and impeding the return of blood to the right side of the heart. Hyperventilation with rapid decrease of carbon dioxide can result in coma due to respiratory alkalosis. Infections can result from contaminated equipment and hypercapnia can worsen if treatments are given with a high concentration of oxygen.

Clients and families need to know the purpose, operation, and care of their IPPB machine. They must be warned of the dangers of overuse. Treatments are given prior to meals and/or chest physical therapy. Initial supervision of administration of medications and saline by the nurse is essential. Treatments should be discontinued and the physician or nurse notified if weakness, dizziness, nausea, vomiting, palpations, pain, or increased shortness of breath occur during the therapy.

The client is instructed to sit upright in a relaxed and comfortable position during the treatment. When the machine is turned on a mist is observed at the mouthpiece. The client then closes his lips around the mouthpiece and breathes slowly through the mouth, allowing the machine to fill his lungs. He then exhales slowly through the mouthpiece. A noseclip is used if necessary. It should take a very small breath to cycle the machine and the pressure setting should be comfortable for the client. The usual pressure setting is 15–20 cm of water. The mouthpiece is removed if the client needs to cough and the machine is to be turned off during any breaks so that the medicine is not wasted. The client continues to use the machine until the medication is gone, usually within 10 to 20 minutes. Any medication remaining in the nebulizer after the treatment is discarded.

A suggested cleaning method for IPPB machines utilizing white vinegar is reviewed on this page, at right. While there are many disinfectants currently on the market, none can match the convenience and cost of white vinegar.

If the client or family have difficulty in

Cleaning Breathing Equipment

AFTER EACH TREATMENT: Disassemble all parts of the nebulizer and mouthpiece, discarding any leftover medication. Rinse all parts with warm, running water and place them on a paper towel to air dry.

AFTER THE LAST TREATMENT OF THE DAY:

1. Take apart the nebulizer, mouthpiece, exhalation assembly, and large flex tubing (part of IPPB tubing) and immerse in warm, soapy water. Use a small amount of liquid detergent.

2. SCRUB all parts with a soft bottle brush. Rinse thoroughly with warm, running water. It is suggested that all parts be completely immersed in a solution of 1 cup white vinegar and 4 cups water and soaked for at least 30 minutes. Then, discard the vinegar solution and rinse all parts with warm, running water and allow to air dry.

3. The tubing that supplies air from the compressor to the nebulizer or the two small tubings from the IPPB machine to the nebulizer and exhalation valve do not need to be washed daily. However, they should be checked for moisture after each treatment. If any moisture is visible, the tubing should be cleaned along with the nebulizer.

4. Always have two complete sets of tubing so one can be used while the other is drying. Keep clean, dry equipment in a towel or plastic bag.

WEEKLY: Wipe the surface of the machine with a clean, damp cloth. Filters need to be cleaned or changed every 6 months. Store the machine off the floor in a clean area between treatments.

operating the IPPB machine, the following checklist may remedy the problem. If not, the equipment supplier should be contacted.

- Check all tube connections and make sure they are tight.
- Check the positive pressure knob and make sure it is not turned fully clockwise.
- Check that the plug is in the electrical outlet.
- Check the exhalation balloon assembly for water, and dry if necessary.
- Make sure that the valve drum is clean of lint and dust (only in certain models).
- Look for an obstruction within the tubings, manifold, flex tube, and mouthpiece.

Compression Nebulizer

To utilize a compressor nebulizer, a client must be able to take a slow, deep breath and cough effectively. It should probably not be used by patients with a vital capacity of less than two liters or an FEV_1 of less than one liter. As with all respiratory therapy, the client and/or family need to know the purpose, operation, and care of this equipment for maximum benefit and minimum hazard at home.

There are two types of nebulizers. One is operated by a finger valve and the other is the continuous nebulizer type. The guidelines for operation of the compressor nebulizer are similar to those of the IPPB machine. Clients are instructed to take comfortable, slow, deep breaths, hold for a few seconds, and then told to exhale slowly through pursed lips or through the mouthpiece.

The cleaning procedure is similar to that for IPPB. Connection tubing on compressor nebulizers is usually easier to disconnect while the machine is on.

If saline is prescribed for breathing treatments it can be made cheaply and easily in the home setting as listed at top right.

Homemade Saline Solution Recipe

1. Add ¼ teaspoon of table salt (not iodized) or eight 250 mg salt tablets to 1 cup of distilled water in a small jar with a screw-on lid.

2. Screw lid on jar loosely.

3. Place jar in a pot of water (water level in pot should be at least ¾ the height of the jar).

4. Cover pot. Bring water to a boil and boil for 25 minutes. Allow to cool. Remove jar and tighten jar lid.

5. Store saline solution in the refrigerator. IT IS IMPORTANT TO MAKE THE SOLUTION FRESH EVERY WEEK! (Do not make more than you will use in one week.)

6. Discard any solution that has become discolored or cloudy.

(One-half Teaspoon of Solution is Approximately Equal to 2.5 cc)

Cartridge Inhaler

Increasingly popular are the hand-held, pocket-sized metered-dose cartridge inhalers. Prescription inhalers must be differentiated from over-the-counter inhalers by both nurse and client. *Overuse* and even *supplemental* use of over-the-counter inhalers without physician approval can prove dangerous for the respiratory client because treatment with those inhalers is of short duration and frequently has many cardiovascular, neuromuscular and gastrointestinal side-effects.

The purpose of the inhaler is very important. While some inhalers (metaproterenol and albuterol) are used to relieve symptoms such as wheezing, asthma attacks, shortness of breath, other inhalers (beclomethasone and cromolyn sodium) prevent the same symptoms.

Placebo inhalers, available from pharmacy representatives, are useful for instruction of clients and nurses in proper inhaler use. Good inhaler technique (listed opposite) maximizes the benefits of medications administered via this route. Swallowing instead of inhaling medication is the primary difficulty with inhaler use. This is significant because inhalation by aerosol usually results in fewer side-effects than if taken orally. Several assistive devices are now available to help clients avoid this problem (Inspirease by Key Pharmaceuticals and Aerochamber by Monaghan Medical Corporation).

There are usually 200 puffs in a full inhaler. If clients are unsure of the number of puffs left, they can put the cartridge in a bowl of water. The cartridge is over half full if the tip points downward. It is almost empty if it floats on the top of the water. The plastic mouthpiece and cap of the inhaler are rinsed daily in warm water and dried thoroughly. Because the contents are under pressure the inhaler should not be punctured or destroyed by burning, or used or stored near heat or open flame.

OBSTRUCTIVE AND RESTRICTIVE DISORDERS

CHRONIC OBSTRUCTIVE PULMONARY DISEASE

Chronic obstructive pulmonary disease (COPD) refers to a group of diseases (emphysema, chronic bronchitis, and complicated asthma) characterized by air trapped in the lungs. Although caused by different processes, airflow is interrupted in each disease.

Good Inhaler Technique

1. Shake the inhaler well and remove the protective cap.

2. Hold the inhaler upright between the index finger and thumb and breathe out fully.

3. Place the inhaler about 1 to 1½ inches in front of your open mouth.

4. As you begin to breathe in deeply through your mouth, press the metal canister down with your forefinger. Your breath should carry the particles of medication as far down into your lungs as possible.

5. Continue to breathe in deeply as long as you can.

6. Hold your breath for as long as is comfortable.

7. Slowly exhale through pursed lips.

8. If your doctor has advised you to take more than one puff per treatment, wait at least 1 minute between doses. With some inhalers you may even be advised to wait 15 minutes between inhalations.

9. Replace the cap on the inhaler when you are finished.

10. Rinse your mouth with water or your favorite mouthwash.

Emphysema

With emphysema, the walls of the lung alveoli are destroyed by smoking or other inhaled irritants or, infrequently, a hereditary deficiency of the enzyme alpha$_1$ antitrypsin. The alveoli lose their natural elasticity and remain partially full after expiration. This limits the amount of oxygenated air that can be inhaled and shortness of breath and retention of carbon dioxide become a problem.

Two types of emphysema have been identified, based on pathological findings. In the most common form, centrilobular-type tissue dilation and destruction occur primarily in the respiratory bronchioles situated toward the center of the lobules. In contrast, the panlobular affects the entire lobule. These types are often found together, especially when the emphysema is severe.

Bronchitis

Chronic bronchitis is characterized by a daily cough productive of sputum for at least 3 months each year for 2 consecutive years (Porth 1986). Repeated infections and/or irritants such as cigarette smoke may cause chronic bronchitis. The increased secretion of mucus, which initially is confined to the larger airways and eventually involves the smaller ones, hinders airflow and gas exchange and predisposes the client to mucus plugging and secondary infections. Ventilation perfusion abnormalities tend to appear earlier in the primary bronchitic (as opposed to emphysematous) client. This may explain the earlier occurrence of the blood gas abnormalities, diminished PO_2 and increased PCO_2 that set the stage for pulmonary hypertension and cor pulmonale. With both chronic bronchitis and emphysema static lung volumes may be normal but expiratory flow rates are decreased.

Asthma

Asthma is defined as *hyperactive airway disease* and is characterized by intermittent attacks of airway obstruction caused by bronchospasm precipitated by a particular stimuli. Although generally divided into two basic types (allergic and nonallergic) most clients with asthma do not fit either category. Extreme asthma (allergic) usually affects children and young adults. Stimuli commonly implicated are respiratory irritants (dust, noxious gases, cold weather), exercise, and emotional upsets. Dermal reactivity to offending allergens is significant with immunoglobulin E playing a role. Intrinsic (nonallergic) asthma usually develops in middle age. Immunologic factors have no known role in etiology and respiratory tract infection is a frequent causative factor. Status asthmaticus, a severe clinical stage of asthma, is a medical emergency and, left untreated, can result in death due to hypoxia and respiratory acidosis. Most of the 17 million individuals with COPD in the U.S. have a combination of emphysema, chronic bronchitis, and asthma.

RESTRICTIVE LUNG DISEASE

While obstructive lung disease is often compared with an inability to get air out of the lungs, restrictive lung disease prevents air from entering the lungs in sufficient quantities. It is often the result of disorders of the chest wall or lung parenchyma. Inspiration is primarily affected and breathing is shallow and rapid. Pulmonary fibrosis, obesity, neuromuscular disease, and kyphoscoliosis are the most commonly found diagnoses of restrictive lung disease found in home care.

Known causes of fibrosis include viral pneumonias, drug reactions, chemical vapors, organic and inorganic dusts, radiation, connective tissue disorders, and alveolar proteinosis. When no cause is apparent, the disease is termed *idiopathic*. Fibrotic lungs are fixed and small, mirrored physiologically by decreased lung volumes with relative sparing of the airways as noted in normal measurements of pulmonary airway resistance.

Weight on the chest wall and obstructing fat may impede thoracic movements mechanically and contribute to carbon dioxide retention. Severe kyphoscoliosis reduces the compliance of the thoracic cage and lung expansion, which results in chronic alveolar hypoventilation. There is also a limit on the capacity of the pulmonary vascular bed that may lead to pulmonary hypertension and eventual cor pulmonale.

NURSING DIAGNOSES

Care and treatment of clients with chronic restrictive and chronic obstructive lung diseases are very similar, sharing numerous nursing diagnoses. In the following pages, the nursing care of these clients in the home setting will be discussed.

INEFFECTIVE AIRWAY CLEARANCE

Clients with both obstructive and restrictive diseases may experience difficulties in effective airway clearance. In chronic obstructive disease, there is excessive production of mucus associated with narrowing of the bronchioles. Inflammation and hyperplasia of the bronchial walls may occur with any disease process, but are frequently worse with bronchitis. Airway clearance may also be decreased, due to stasis of secretions caused by impaired ciliary movement and a poor cough.

Assessment

Respiratory rate, rhythm and depth, cough, sputum, degree of dyspnea, along with chest fremitus, expansion, and adventitious sounds are assessed every visit. Chest examinations typically would reveal diminished fremitus, hyperresonance upon percussion, and diminished and/or asthmatic breath sounds. Any change could indicate a deterioration of airway clearance.

Changes in mental status may also suggest changes in oxygenation levels, reflecting difficulties in airway clearance. Forgetfulness, changes in personality, and lethargy may reflect hypoxia. Activity levels are assessed for number of words spoken with one breath, differences in distance ambulated, and performance of activities of daily living. Changes in these parameters suggest further difficulties in airway clearance and thus, hypoxia.

A common cause of deterioration in the client in respiratory failure is bronchopulmonary infection. The home health nurse assesses the client and instructs the family to observe for the signs and symptoms of upper respiratory infection. These include increased cough, changes in sputum, increased dyspnea, chills, temperature elevation, chest pain, or malaise. The physician is contacted immediately if there is suspicion of an upper respiratory infection since early intervention may prevent hospitalization for respiratory failure.

Interventions

An effective cough is necessary to remove secretions from the tracheobronchial tree. Teaching the client and family appropriate techniques for effective coughing is a major responsibility of the home health nurse. The client is taught to take several slow, deep breaths in through his nose and out through pursed lips. To maximize utilization of energy the cough reflex is suppressed until sputum is felt in the upper airways. Then the client initiates several staccato coughs to expectorate the sputum. Some clients may also need instruction in proper tissue disposal as an infection control measure.

Postural drainage may be ordered for clients with excessive amounts of sputum who are unable to cough effectively or clear the sputum spontaneously. The technique allows gravity to drain mucus from the lungs.

Some individuals will need postural drainage routinely and others will require it only with an infection. It is best done before meals, and after breathing treatments. The family also will require instruction in these techniques, since they will be assisting the client. A common postural drainage position is shown in Figure 9-1.

The various postural drainage positions may need to be modified due to differences in lung involvement or client tolerance. Each position should be held for 4 to 5 minutes and they are more effective if the hips are higher than the chest. This can be achieved in bed by placing pillows under the hips or using a triangular pillow. Clients can also be taught to use an ironing board at a 30-degree angle supported at both ends to achieve an optimum position. Postural drainage generally is most important for drainage of the lower and middle lobes. The technique may be most effective if preceded by bronchodilation and hydration.

The client should be instructed to utilize breathing retraining techniques during the procedure, followed by use of techniques to produce an effective cough. The frequency of postural drainage depends upon sputum production. Initially, it may be needed twice daily for a week. If 80 cc or more of sputum are collected within 24 hours, the procedure should be continued twice or three times a day. If only small amounts of sputum are raised the procedure may be reduced to one or two times per week. Postural drainage is not continued if sputum is not mobilized.

Postural drainage is contraindicated in a myocardial infarction, pulmonary embolism, arrhythmia, rib fracture, severe congestive heart failure, osteoporosis, obesity, seizure disorder, hiatal hernia, and pneumothorax.

Percussion and vibration aid in lung clearance by dislodging and propelling secretions into the trachea from the periphery. They should be done for 1 to 2 minutes in each of the postural drainage positions.

The hands of the individual performing this procedure are cupped so that a cushion of air is placed next to the client's chest. There should be a towel or one layer of clothing next to the client's skin to prevent irritation. The care-giver raises his hands three to four inches over the chest with elbows and shoulders relaxed, then he alternately strikes the ribs with enough force to vibrate the lungs, but not too hard to hurt the chest. Care-takers are instructed not to percuss over bony prominences. Vibration is done upon exhalation and followed by an effective cough.

Outcomes

The client will experience adequate respiratory function as evidenced by usual rate, rhythm, and depth of respirations. Dyspnea will be decreased and breath sounds improved. Mental status will return to normal for the client.

ANXIETY

The individual with chronic obstructive or restrictive lung disease usually is anxious and

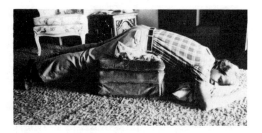

Figure 9-1. Postural drainage position. Furniture commonly found in the home can be used in positioning the client for postural drainage. (From Walsh J, Persons CB, Wieck L: Manual of Home Health Care Nursing, p 480. Philadelphia, JB Lippincott, 1987)

fearful for many reasons. He is living with the constant threat of suffocation and death. Anxiety increases dyspnea and dyspnea increases anxiety. The disease process also forces many changes in the life-style of the client and family and as such, can lead to a state of increased anxiety. Frequently clients with respiratory disorders experience a sense of lack of control over their own person and future.

Assessment

On each visit, the home health nurse will assess the client for signs of anxiety. The client may verbalize his fears or appear tense and anxious during conversations. Other physical indications of anxiety include tachycardia, restlessness, irritability, pallor, and flushing. A more subtle indication may be noncompliance with the treatment regime.

Interventions

A quiet, restful environment along with an emotional atmosphere in which the client feels comfortable expressing fears can reduce anxiety. Client education allows control over what is controllable.

Relaxation exercises can be added to breathing retraining. A relaxation guide instructs the individual to imagine that he is slowly breathing out tension with each breath. All major tension areas of the body are consciously relaxed in an effort to reduce anxiety and decrease oxygen requirements. Alternative therapies of yoga, biofeedback, foot massage, and therapeutic touch may also be beneficial.

The family can be assisted to provide support to the client at particular times. For example, the client's anxiety will most likely increase during times of respiratory distress. The family can be encouraged to stay with the client and offer support.

The home health nurse plays a major role in alleviating anxiety by maintaining a good relationship with the client and family and providing them with the information they need in order to feel comfortable with the situations they encounter on a daily basis.

If anxiety continues to be a problem for the client, the physician should be notified. At this time, mild relaxants or tranquilizers may be added to the client's therapy. The home health nurse must continue to assess the client throughout each visit. Chronic illness escalates anxiety and there will be times when anxiety is increased and will require interventions.

Outcomes

The client will experience a reduction in fear and anxiety. He will exhibit relaxed facial expressions and body movements and verbalize less feelings of fear.

INEFFECTIVE BREATHING PATTERNS

Most commonly, ineffective breathing patterns result from hyperinflation of the diaphragm, which occurs with the progress of chronic obstructive disease. Breathing patterns can also be ineffective when the client is experiencing fear or anxiety.

Assessment

On each visit, the home health nurse will want to assess the client's breathing pattern by auscultating lung sounds and performing chest percussion. The client should be assessed for symptoms such as shortness of breath, tachycardia, dyspnea, and a decrease in depth of respiration. Wheezing is one of the more common chest sounds.

Interventions

There are multiple interventions that can assist the client to achieve an effective pattern of breathing. Some clients require a comprehensive program of breathing retraining.

The basic goal for breathing retraining is the improvement of alveolar ventilation by modifying the breathing pattern and by strengthening the respiratory muscles. When teaching improved breathing habits, use simple techniques and progress slowly to minimize a client's anxiety. Breathing retraining assures maximal use of respiratory function and, of all pulmonary measures, has been the one that in this author's experience has had the most positive subjective improvement in a client's dyspnea. Although eventually the exercises should be performed on a constant basis, they are learned with practice, beginning with ten repetitions two to three times daily.

Abdominal or "belly" breathing and pursed lip breathing are the two components of breathing retraining. Before beginning the exercises, tight or restrictive clothing is removed and the mouth and nasal passages are cleared. Ingestion of a cup of hot beverage or water is suggested to mobilize lung secretions during these techniques. The procedures are initiated in a position that is most comfortable for the client. The training should not be hurried and rest periods taken as needed.

To begin, the client places one hand across the chest and the opposite hand across the abdomen. He inhales deeply through the nose allowing the abdomen to rise. He then slowly breaths out through pursed lips (lips held in a whistling position), pressing inward and upward firmly on the abdomen. The hand on the chest should move as little as possible while the hand on the abdomen moves up and down with inhalation and exhalation. Ideally, the length of exhalation should be two or three times longer than the time for inhalation. This can be demonstrated by counting out loud, "inhale for 1 and 2 and exhale for 5–6–7 and 8." Eventually the

client can adopt the breathing techniques while walking: inhale for two steps and exhale for four steps. Coaching through demonstration and encouragement greatly motivates clients to master breathing retraining.

There is some evidence that there are benefits to resistive exercises for improving the strength and endurance of inspiratory muscles. This technique involves breathing through progressively narrower bore tubes during inspiration.

Oxygen may be needed periodically by the client. The family will require the same instruction as the client in the use of this equipment. Encourage the client to pace activities throughout the day and to maintain planned rest periods. Excessive fatigue will increase problems with breathing.

Outcomes

Adverse changes in the breathing pattern will be minimized. The client will exhibit an absence of dyspnea on exertion.

ALTERATIONS IN CARDIAC OUTPUT

When lung tissue is destroyed in chronic lung conditions, pulmonary artery pressure increases and cor pulmonale or enlargement of the heart's right ventricle may result. Cor pulmonale can be present with or without overt heart failure.

Assessment

The major objective in evaluating cardiac function in the pulmonary client is early identification of alterations in cardiac status indicating cardiac decompensation. The pulse rate and quality is assessed on every visit. A blood pressure assessment is also done with a reading in both arms for at least the first visit. Periodically, the nurse will assess for a pulse deficit between radial and apical pulses. Both nurse and family monitor for fluid retention. Weight, edema, and ascites are evaluated every visit. A weight gain of 2 to 3 pounds within 48 hours is considered significant and should be reported to the physician. Fatigue, changes in exercise tolerance, jugular vein distention, and deterioration in mental status are also significant in assessing cardiac output.

Interventions

A major goal of nursing interventions is to reduce cardiac workload which, in turn, will reduce the effect of the alteration in cardiac output. The family's support in assisting the client to implement the plans developed by the home health nurse are essential. Specifically, encourage the client to maintain the fluid and sodium restrictions as ordered by the physician. Medications such as diuretics may be needed to reduce vascular congestion. During times of discomfort, the client may feel more comfortable in a high Fowler's position in bed or sitting in a chair.

Outcomes

The client will not demonstrate signs of a compromised cardiac output. Vital signs, weight, intake, and output will be within normal limits.

INEFFECTIVE INDIVIDUAL AND FAMILY COPING

Depression is a major complication of chronic lung disease. Some have suggested that it may have existed even prior to development of the disease process and may have been the reason an individual smoked. Others report it is due to the chronic anxiety of breathlessness and a feeling of being out of control and helpless (Luckmann and Sorenson 1986).

In addition to being threatened by the fear of suffocation and death, the client with chronic lung disease may fear financial ruin due to disability, and family disruption due to role reversals. Day to day there is a continual conflict of dependence and independence. Without sufficient energy to express anger and resentment these feelings go inward. Loss and grief affect every aspect of the client's life and he frequently becomes socially isolated, living in a constricted space. Clients often will exercise control over what is controllable, that is, the time and day a nurse visits and the placement of supplies on the bedside table.

Suicides among clients with chronic lung disease are often successful and every suicide threat is to be taken seriously. Another reaction to expect is a noncommittal attitude caused by the client's perception of his inability to know or control his breathing.

Assessment

An individual's ability, as well as a family's ability, to cope with chronic lung disease generally is dependent on their psychosocial assets and the number of their life-change units. Psychosocial assets include interest in life, financial resources and housing, social supports, and ability to cope with modification of the environment.

Life-change units are life events that involve significant stress and may be associated with emotional and/or physical illness. The higher the psychosocial assets and the lower the life-change units, the better the coping ability of the client and family. The lower the psychosocial assets and the higher the life-change units, the poorer the coping ability of the client and family. Evaluation of accurate coping ability is essential for the home care nurse in order to set realistic goals.

Interventions

Although the home care nurse can be helpful in assisting clients with chronic lung disease and their families to cope with the disease and its manifestations, referral to other appropriate psychosocial resources should not be delayed when severe psychosocial disruption exists.

Showing a true interest in the client and family emphasizes that they are worth the effort. With education and successful training experiences, particularly progressive exercise programs, both client and family gain control and demonstrate progress. In addition to providing hope, the home care nurse can maximize the client's psychological assets by complementing him on his knowledge or sense of humor. Most important, the client and family must learn how to accept compromise. Group interaction should be encouraged and monthly follow-up through a community support group provided.

Outcomes

The client and family will demonstrate the ability to use coping mechanisms. The client will verbalize the presence of adequate support systems.

IMPAIRED GAS EXCHANGE

Gas exchange is impaired in chronic lung disease due to a decrease in effective lung surface, associated with destruction and fibrosis of the alveolar walls. Inflammation, fibrosis, and narrowing of the respiratory bronchioles worsen the potential for gas exchange. Effective gas exchange can be hampered still further by ineffective breathing patterns and airway clearance.

Assessment

The parameters to assess for gas exchange are the same as those for breathing patterns and airway clearance. In particular, the home health nurse should observe the client's color and sensorium on each visit. The lung sounds can be auscultated frequently to determine the presence of adventitious sounds. Clinical manifestations of hypoxia include restlessness, confusion, hypotension, tachycardia and, if severe, central cyanosis.

Interventions

Oxygen therapy is needed for COPD clients if one of the following conditions exists: (1) a PaO_2 less than 55 mm of Hg; (2) cor pulmonale and congestive heart failure; (3) improvement in cognitive function with oxygen; and (4) persistent erythrocytosis.

There are four major elements of an oxygen prescription: type of oxygen system, method of administration, flow rate, and duration of use. The various types of oxygen systems are outlined in the boxed material below.

Types of Oxygen Systems

1. *Oxygen cylinders or tanks* contain oxygen gas under high pressure and come in a variety of sizes. The larger tanks, "G" and "H," are stationary because they stand about 5 feet high and weigh 150 pounds when full. "D" and "E" cylinders are also available and are smaller and more portable, weighing 15 to 17 pounds when full. Some types are constructed of a lightweight aluminum, reducing their full weight to 10 to 12 pounds. Cylinders need to be secured with a carrier or stand. If a client is using two or more cylinders manifolded together, he must be sure to turn the empty cylinder off before opening the new cylinder.

(continued)

2. *Oxygen concentrators* separate oxygen from room air and concentrate it to be medically effective. They range in size from tabletop to floor models. They are more economical for clients who utilize more than eight larger oxygen tanks per month, but they may increase the client's monthly electric bill to a degree comparable to the operation of a color television. A portable back-up oxygen cylinder should always be ready for emergency use in the event of machine or electrical failure.

3. *Liquid oxygen systems* are thermoslike containers storing oxygen that has been subjected to extremely low temperatures ($-300°F$) and has become liquid. As the liquid warms, the oxygen returns to its gaseous form. Because oxygen will escape when the unit is not in use, it needs to be kept in a ventilated area over 5 feet from flames and electrical appliances. Lightweight portable systems are refilled from a stationary home unit. If spillage occurs, the liquid must be kept away from skin, eyes, and clothing, as liquid oxygen can freeze the skin. A scale indicates how much oxygen remains and when to call the vendor for a refill.

Methods of Administration

The two most common methods of oxygen administration in the home are nasal cannula and Venturi masks. Nasal cannula or prongs offer the convenience of allowing the client to eat, drink, and talk without restraint while oxygen is in use. Flow rates are usually 1 liter to 6 liters per minute, delivering an inspired oxygen concentration of 22% to 44%. Oropharyngeal drying may occur and nostrils, cheeks, and ears may exhibit pressure necrosis with constant use.

Venturi masks fit over the nose and mouth and entrap room air with the oxygen to deliver a prescribed concentration. The manufacturer's directions must be followed precisely because of the number of models in which this mask is available. A source of humidity under 30% may not be necessary depending on the manufacturer's recommendations. The usual oxygen flow rate is 4 liters to 8 liters per minute, delivering an F_1O_2 of 24% to 40%. The mask must be removed for eating and drinking and the possibility of aspiration exists.

A humidifier is generally used with either method of administration. Clients are instructed to adjust the flow rate before putting on the cannula or mask to eliminate receiving a blast of oxygen and to check that the equipment is operating properly.

Flow Rate

Although the inspired flow of oxygen concentration is dependent on a client's rate and depth of respirations, the home health nurse can estimate the concentration by utilizing the "rule of 4's" demonstrated in Table 9-4.

Clients need to know that oxygen is a medicine and if not taken exactly as prescribed, problems can occur. Flow rates at the distal end of long oxygen tubing can be evaluated by using a liter flow meter. Defective oxygen gauges, or humidifiers, and torn or ob-

TABLE 9.4 Flow Rates and Oxygen Concentration ("Rule of 4's")

Flow Rate	Concentration
Room Air	20%
1 liter	24%
2 liter	28%
3 liter	32%
4 liter	36%

structed oxygen tubing can interfere with the delivery of prescribed flow rates.

Duration

Studies have indicated that beneficial effects of oxygen used for 12 hours daily are frequently equal to the beneficial effects of oxygen used continuously. If the oxygen is not ordered continuously, then it should be utilized during exercise, when the patient is dyspneic, after meals, and during sleep.

Clients should be instructed not to discontinue the oxygen without the physician's knowledge. Although home oxygen administration is safe, the patient and family need to be aware of the potential hazards. These are outlined in the boxes below and on the following page.

Cleaning Your Oxygen Equipment

DAILY

1. Remove cannula or mask from the humidifier and wipe clean with warm water and paper towel.

2. Remove humidifier from oxygen source. Empty water. Wash humidifier jar and lid assembly in warm, soapy (liquid detergent) water. Rinse thoroughly with warm water.

3. Refill humidifier with fresh, distilled water to proper level. Replace lid and attach to oxygen source.

4. Reattach nasal cannula or mask. Turn on oxygen to prescribed flow rate and begin using.

5. If humidifier is not to be used immediately, let it AIR DRY and then replace it on the oxygen cylinder. Fill with fresh, distilled water before using distilled water before using oxygen. (Always keep distilled water capped and refrigerated. It is best to purchase small quantities.)

NOTE: Disposable humidifiers are NOT to be cleaned with soap and water but must be REPLACED WEEKLY!

WEEKLY

1. Remove tubing and mask or cannula from humidifier and wash in warm, soapy water. Rinse thoroughly by running warm water through tubing.

2. Hang tubing up to AIR DRY. Excess water may be removed by attaching tubing to compressor to blow out water. Never attach tubing to oxygen source to dry or blow out excess water in the tubing.

3. Keep clean, dry equipment in clean towel or plastic bag.

4. An extra nasal cannula or mask with tubing should be available for use during the cleaning procedure.

5. Replace extra-long tubing MONTHLY.

NOTE: All equipment should be stored DRY when not in use to prevent bacterial growth that may lead to infection.

Filters for concentrator should be cleaned according to supplier's instructions.

**Potential Hazards of
Oxygen Administration**

1. *Infection*
It is important to keep humidifiers, filters, nasal cannula, and masks clean to prevent bacterial growth that may cause a respiratory infection. The following cleaning procedure is recommended by the Christmas Seal League/American Lung Association affiliate, Pittsburgh, in its excellent patient teaching pamphlet Self-Help: Your Strategy for Living with COPD. A daily and a weekly procedure is suggested. (See page 203.)

Oxygen cylinders should be changed when the pressure gauge reads 500 psi or ½ full to avoid inhaling irritating debris.

2. *Combustion*
Clients need to know that oxygen, although not explosive, will support combustion. The oxygen is absorbed into the client's clothing and bedding, as well as inhaled. A "No Smoking Policy" needs to be enforced within 10 feet of oxygen equipment and NO SMOKING signs should be posted. Oil, grease, and oil-based aerosols (such as room deodorizers) should be kept from coming in contact with the oxygen system. Draping the system with any material is to be avoided. There should be no open flame in the same room as the oxygen equipment. Electrical equipment should be properly grounded and electric razors and hairdryers should not be used while the oxygen is in use. Oxygen cylinders should be stored away from heat and direct sunlight. Nylon clothing and wool blankets should be avoided to prevent sparks and static electricity.

3. *Respiratory Depression*
Supplemental oxygen is prescribed by a physician after blood gas analysis and evaluation of a client's overall pulmonary condition. Clients with chronic pulmonary disease need to be informed that their breathing is controlled by lack of oxygen in the bloodstream and that excess oxygen administration over the physician's order could have deleterious consequences.

Outcomes

Client and family understand and participate in the proper use and cleaning of oxygen therapy equipment.

KNOWLEDGE DEFICIT

Client education for the individual with chronic pulmonary dysfunction is critical to obtain maximal independence in care.

Assessment

As with any chronic condition, education for the client and family will be constant. On the initial visit, the home health nurse will assess the client's and family's general knowledge concerning the disease process, treatment, and related interventions. In addition, the nurse will evaluate the client's ability to receive the information given by the home health nurse on each visit. The cooperation of the client with chronic obstructive disease is critical in assuring a desired outcome.

Interventions

Some clients with COPD believe they have a terminal illness and that after hospitalization they often go home to die. While the disease process may not be reversible, symptoms can improve and complications can be prevented with appropriate self-care measures.

A simple explanation of the respiratory system and the disease process is the first building block for instruction in self-care skills.

In addition to knowing the purpose and possible side-effects of medications, the client with chronic pulmonary disease needs to know the appropriate sequence of the medication regime. A beclomethasone inhaler, for example, is generally used *after* the albuterol inhaler.

Bronchodilators

The two basic categories of bronchodilators that relax smooth muscles around bronchial tubes are adrenergic agents and xanthine derivatives. They have a synergistic effect on one another when taken in combination. The adrenergic agents stimulate β_1 receptors located primarily in the myocardium and/or β_2 receptors located in the smooth muscles in the airways and in the skeletal muscles. Albuterol, metaproterenol, and terbutaline have a β_2 effect and are longer acting than preparations with ephedrine or epinephrine that have both a β_1 and/or β_2 effect.

Expectorants

Water is the best agent available to aid in the expectoration of pulmonary secretions. Unless the patient has a fluid restriction, 8 to 10 glasses per day are recommended between meals for adequate hydration. Humidification of air will also help to liquify sputum and relieve bronchial irritation. Many other expectorants are associated with undesirable adverse reactions.

Antimicrobials

For the majority of respiratory tract infections, tetracycline or ampicillin in doses of 1g to 2g/day is usually effective. Inappropriate and repeated use of antimicrobial agents, especially when bronchial drainage measures are neglected, may lead to superinfection with bacteria or fungi in the client with pulmonary disease. In instances where there is no response to an antibiotic, the sputum should be analyzed. Clients must be instructed to take the antibiotic for the entire time prescribed even though they may feel better in a relatively short period of time.

Corticosteroids

Corticosteroids are considered of value in clients who wheeze. Asthmatics generally tolerate the alternate day regime poorly. Undesirable side-effects of oral corticosteroids include weight gain, edema, bruising, diabetes mellitus, peptic ulcers, osteoporosis, psychosis, and opportunistic infections. Clients are instructed that abrupt discontinuation may result in withdrawal syndrome. Beclomethasone, a synthetic corticosteroid with potent anti-inflammatory activity, does not suppress the body's adrenal function and inhalation may allow for a decrease or elimination of the oral corticosteroid therapy. Side-effects include dry mouth and oral fungal infections.

Diuretics

Diuretics are utilized if fluid retention is a problem. Hypokalemia can sometimes be avoided by a combination of Aldactone or Dyrenium with thiazides in clients with COPD. Their use can sometimes cause respiratory secretions to dry out, making the secretions harder to expectorate. Clients should weigh themselves daily and should be encouraged to eat high potassium foods. They should report weakness, thirst, muscle cramps, diarrhea, and dizziness immediately to the home health nurse or physician.

Digitalis

Digitalis preparations are given to those with left ventricular decompensation but dosage needs careful monitoring because of respiratory acidosis. Clients are instructed in the symptoms of digitalis toxicity (gastrointestinal upset, pulse rate less than 55/minute or an irregular pulse and blurred vision).

Cromolyn Sodium

This medication is used prophylactically for allergic asthmatic reactions. It is inhaled through a special inhaler as a powder released from a capsule. Clients must know that it is of no benefit in an acute asthma attack.

Any over-the-counter medications taken by the client should be evaluated. Medications containing an antihistamine will cause dry, retained secretions and should be ordered only by a physician. Products containing cough suppressants or sedatives are usually contraindicated since they interfere with breathing effectiveness. Individuals with asthma or asthma symptoms may experience an increase in wheezing when taking aspirin products.

Teach the client to avoid respiratory irritants such as smoking. The most common indoor respiratory irritant is cigarette smoke. The home-care nurse can offer the client and family assistance in smoking cessation programs through education and encouragement. Any effort to decrease the number of cigarettes smoked per day should be praised. Excellent teaching materials are available from the American Cancer Society, the American Heart Association, and the American Lung Association. Other pulmonary irritants such as extremely cold or dry air, airborne allergens, aerosols such as hair spray, deodorant, and strong fumes are also to be avoided.

The client and family should be assisted in developing a schedule of daily therapeutic measures to maximize time efficiency and to monitor progress. A sample therapy cycle is shown in Table 9-5.

Because of the danger of excessive oxygen administration and the possibility of drug interactions, clients with chronic lung disease are advised to carry emergency identification such as Medic-Alert or an identification bracelet at all times.

Local groups for both education and socialization of individuals with chronic pulmonary disease are available in many communities. A supportive atmosphere is provided, in which clients can express and share pent-up fears and anxieties. It is important for the client's significant other to participate in these sessions to gain an understanding and perspective of the client's problems and to take part in resolving these problems. Pulmonary rehabilitation programs exist in both inpatient and outpatient settings.

Outcome

The client and family will understand necessary information concerning the disease process and treatment.

IMPAIRED PHYSICAL MOBILITY

Mobility is limited with chronic pulmonary disease because the lungs are unable to supply adequate oxygen for unlimited activities.

TABLE 9.5 Typical Therapy Cycle

Therapy	Time							
	8	10	12	2	4	6	8	10
Oral medications	x	x	x	x				
Fluid intake	x	x	x	x				
Inhaler		x						x
Breathing exercises		x		x	x		x	
Postural drainage	x							
Effective cough	x	x	x	x				
Rest	x	x		x				

Through a home program of physical reconditioning and rehabilitation, clients can not only control or alleviate the symptoms of pulmonary impairment, but also achieve optimal capacity to carry out their activities of daily living.

Assessment

The goal of assessment is to evaluate the client's potential for mobility despite the impairment of respiratory activity. Specific parameters to assess include the distance the client can walk without oxygen and the client's ability to climb a flight of stairs without oxygen.

Interventions

If the client experiences an alteration in mobility related to the obstructive disease, interventions are identified that will improve the client's tolerance for physical activity. A group of activities designed for this purpose are sometimes called a *pulmonary rehabilitation program.*

A pulmonary rehabilitation program is not a process that happens to the client, but rather, a process that occurs *with his help.* Such a program needs to be personalized, requires the client to see its purpose, and should be organized in approach. Because rehabilitation often requires a multidisciplinary approach, clear communication among all home-care team members is essential.

There are several aspects to a pulmonary rehabilitation program. In respiratory reconditioning a graded exercise program trains the muscles, including the heart, to use less oxygen and to use oxygen more efficiently.

An exercise prescription includes four elements: intensity, duration, frequency, and mode. Walking is one of the best exercises for conditioning pulmonary clients. A reasonable goal is set and the client's progress is evaluated every visit. When a goal in distance is achieved, the goal of the same distance in less time is set. Clients should be reminded to follow their therapy cycle daily and to allow enough time after eating for their food to digest before exercising.

While walking, slow, deliberate movements are made and long steps are taken with the shoulders relaxed. Pursed-lip breathing and abdominal breathing are used. A good walking pattern would be to have the client exhale for twice as many steps as he inhales. When walking up stairs the client inhales at rest and exhales as he climbs. If oxygen is needed the prescribed low-flow rate is utilized during the exercise program. If the client is taught to take his pulse it should be taken before the exercise, immediately after, and 2 to 4 minutes later. The count at rest should be within five beats of the count at 2 to 4 minutes after the exercise. A client is instructed to stop exercising if he experiences weakness, excessive sweating, has increased shortness of breath that does not return to normal within 2 minutes, experiences chest pain, or becomes dizzy. Once indoor goals are met, the client should be encouraged to participate in an outdoor conditioning program that includes walking in shopping malls when the weather is too hot or too cold. Short rest periods should always follow exercise periods.

In order to achieve optimal capacity, clients need to incorporate the "6 P's" of work efficiency into their activities of daily living: plan, prioritize, pace, pause, posture, and pursed-lip breathing. These activities are described in the boxed material on page 208.

Outcome

The client will experience an increased ability to perform activities of daily living.

The 6 "P's" of Work Efficiency

1. PLAN

   The best time and the best way to accomplish a task is part of planning. Steps need to be minimized and labor saving equipment, such as wagons and carts, used. Two high energy tasks should not be done back-to-back.

2. PRIORITIZE

   The most important activities are scheduled when energy levels are the highest. The time of the day may vary among individuals. There may be days when unnecessary tasks need to be eliminated.

3. PACE

   Rushing is to be avoided. A steady pace conserves energy.

4. PAUSE

   Rest periods are scheduled between activities or throughout an activity to allow for maximal utilization of energy.

5. POSTURE

   Frequently used items should be kept within easy reach. Both arms and the feet should be utilized whenever possible. Patients should be encouraged to sit whenever possible and to try to push or slide items rather than lifting them.

6. PURSED-LIP BREATHING

   Pursed-lip breathing coupled with abdominal breathing minimizes shortness of breath in performing any task. Patients should exhale slowly when performing the action part of any activity.

ALTERATION IN NUTRITION

Weight loss and anorexia are the most common nutritional problems with chronic pulmonary disease. Marked weight loss correlates very closely with a poor outlook for chronic obstructive pulmonary disease. Clients who reverse this trend become stronger and improve in physical activities. A marked increase in mental attitude usually follows. Possible causes for anorexia include hypoxia, heart failure, medications, increased amounts of sputum, air swallowing, dyspnea, and depression. Aerophagia may increase dyspnea because it results in gastric distention and pressure on the diaphragm.

Assessment

On each visit, the home health nurse will want to weigh the client and monitor any weight loss. The family will assist the client in a diet history and a calorie count can be completed. If the nurse suspects a problem in nutrition, a consultation with a dietitian may be necessary. The challenge to the home health nurse will be in determining if the dietary problems result from psychological reasons (depression), physical problems (lack of energy required for eating), or sociological problems (lack of food available or facilities/abilities to prepare food). A complete discussion of nutritional assessment can be found in Chapter 11.

Interventions

The client should be encouraged to eat five or six small-to-medium meals daily as he probably does not receive enough calories in three regular meals. This also reduces gastric acidity and minimizes gastric distention. A good nourishing breakfast and small evening meal are recommended. With this diet, the client will have adequate calories during the time of the day they are needed for activity.

The lighter evening meal will facilitate the client's ability to sleep.

The diet should be balanced and high in nutritional value. High protein supplements are usually advised. Milk and milk products cause excessive respiratory tract secretions in only a small number of select chronic pulmonary clients. Bland, nongas-forming foods prevent abdominal distention and require less energy to chew. Clients should be encouraged to eat with someone but should understand that they are not required to keep up a conversation. A 30-minute rest period prior to meals is suggested and the use of supplemental oxygen during meals may help the severely hypoxemic and dyspneic client to eat more easily.

Primary or secondary cardiac disease or corticosteroid therapy may require a sodium restriction. Foods high in potassium are recommended due to weight loss, catabolism, muscle wasting, diuretic and corticosteroid therapy. Vitamin K may need to be supplemented because of extensive antibiotic therapy. Adequate hydration is needed to liquify sputum. If reflux is a problem, fluids are taken between meals rather than during mealtime and hot, cold, and spicy foods need to be avoided.

Easy and healthful foods such as peanut butter, cottage cheese, yogurt, eggs, and ground meat can be suggested. Careful selection of food will help to provide the client with adequate calories and nutrients.

Outcomes

The client will maintain good nutritional status. Body weight will be maintained and any complications related to nutritional deficits will not be experienced.

SEXUAL DYSFUNCTION

Sooner or later the client with chronic pulmonary disease will experience dyspnea during intercourse, turning a pleasurable activity into a nightmare. Often he will experience decreased libido due to lack of self esteem, lack of communication, role reversal, and/or depression.

Assessment

While often used as a parameter for the cardiac client, the ability to climb stairs is *not* a good indicator of sexual activity for the client with chronic obstructive pulmonary disease. Dyspnea in COPD clients relates to many variables and cannot be used as a measuring stick. Therefore, the nurse must rely on other mechanisms to assist the client in determining when sexual relations may be resumed.

Once the nurse establishes a relationship with the client, it will be possible to discuss feelings about sexual relations. With an open atmosphere, the client may feel able to express his feelings to the home health nurse.

The nurse must take the initiative to allow a patient to express specific problems and fears. It is important to understand sexual attitudes, fears, preferences, and possible difficulties both before and after illness to obtain an overall picture. Sexual adjustment is also affected by the attitude and physical health of the partner.

Interventions

As a person becomes better able to exercise in a graded exercise program, he is usually able to tolerate the increased activity of normal sexual intercourse. Sexual activity is usually easier after bronchial hygiene treatments and when the client is relaxed and rested.

A bronchodilator may be used either before intercourse or as soon as sudden shortness of breath is experienced. Sexual intercourse should be avoided after a heavy meal or within 3 hours of alcohol ingestion. If even the most passive positions are too tiring for a client, inhaling low-flow oxygen may help.

Any concerns about sexual activity need to

be shared with the individual's partner. The couple needs to know that the disease process may not diminish sexual ability or capacity for enjoyment and that trained professionals are available in their community to assist them with information concerning any problems in this area.

Outcomes

The client will experience minimal disruption in sexual activities. The client and partner will be able to express their feelings and concerns about their sexual relationship.

POTENTIAL FOR INFECTION

Clients with COPD have an increased likelihood for the development of infections. As their respiratory disease progresses, the client's ability to withstand exposure to infectious agents without becoming infected is limited.

Assessment

On each visit, assess the client for signs of infection. These will include a productive cough, that is, a cough producing more sputum than would normally be the case. Instruct the family to assist by monitoring the client for signs of infection such as fever, malaise, increased cough, change in sputum, increased dyspnea, chills, temperature elevation, chest pain, and increased pulse rate.

Interventions

Avoidance of risk factors for upper respiratory infection is of prime importance for the client with chronic pulmonary disease. He should avoid close contact with persons having infections and, if possible, avoid crowds, especially in areas of poor ventilation. The client should discuss with his physician the need for both Pneumovax and influenza vaccine.

Instructions concerning measures to increase resistance to infection, that is, adequate rest, well-balanced diet, and avoidance of temperature extremes, are needed. The client or family should be taught to recognize early signs and symptoms of an upper respiratory infection and to contact the physician immediately if these symptoms occur.

Outcome

The client will be free of respiratory infection.

SLEEP PATTERN DISTURBANCE

Clients may complain of insomnia or restlessness at night. This may be due to anxiety, depression, hypoxemia, hypercapnia, shortness of breath, or a combination of these conditions.

Assessment

The most effective assessment for sleep patterns is to discuss the client's sleep habits. Reports of difficulty sleeping or not feeling rested in the morning are good indicators of difficulty. The family may also be able to provide good evidence of problems in the client's sleep pattern.

Interventions

Sleep aids such as sedatives, analgesics, tranquilizers, and alcohol are respiratory depressants that could increase sleep disturbances. The client and family should be warned of the potential problems from use of these drugs. Orthopnea and paroxysmal nocturnal dyspnea are associated with cardiac disease and may interfere with sleep. Oxygen should be administered during the night if these conditions exist. Clients may be more comfortable sleeping with the head of the bed elevated or on two or three pillows.

Discussion of fears should be encouraged. Some clients fear suffocation during sleep and will have difficulty sleeping because of this fear. Relaxation techniques should be taught and practiced. As the client progresses on a reconditioning program during the day, there is usually a decrease in wakefulness at night.

Outcome

The client would be expected to have a restful sleep pattern.

MECHANICAL VENTILATION

Ever since the poliomyelitis epidemic of the 1950's, persons who require mechanical ventilation as a means of life support have been successfully managed in the home. The numbers of these clients have recently significantly increased in the United States, due to a number of factors.

The federal government has taken vigorous efforts to control and limit health-care costs and there are pressures to transfer ventilator clients out of acute care settings. There are relatively few nursing homes that will accept ventilator clients. Respiratory equipment has become more portable and simplified and community support services have increased so that transfer to the home setting is a viable option. In addition to extending life, long-term ventilator care can and should enhance the quality of life whether required continuously or for predetermined periods of time during the day and/or night.

There are several mechanical aids for breathing that are sometimes used to avoid the need for mechanical ventilation. These include rocking beds, phrenic nerve pacemakers, and pneumobelts. These aids should be evaluated in an inpatient setting, if appropriate, before the client becomes a candidate for chronic ventilatory support in the home.

Ventilators utilized at home are either of the negative or positive-pressure types. Negative-pressure ventilators apply negative pressure around the thorax for inspiration and include the iron lung, chest cuirass, and plastic wraps (Fig. 9-2). The positive-pressure ventilators (PPV) are more common and apply above-atmospheric pressure to promote inspiration (Fig. 9-3). A PPV may be either pressure or volume controlled and operated in the control or the assist/control operating mode. The control mode is for the individual with no spontaneous respiratory efforts. The assist/control mode allows the patient to control the respiratory rate.

Many factors are critical in selecting a client for long-term home mechanical ventilation in addition to disease process and clinical stability. The desires of the client, the desires of the family, the cost, and the availability of resources in the home must all be taken into consideration.

The discharge of the ventilator-assisted client to the home requires a comprehensive education program for him, for his family members, and for all home care-givers. It is most beneficial for all immediate care-givers, both professional and nonprofessional, to care for the client independently and obtain "hands-on" experience while the client is in the acute care setting. Teaching methods include lectures, discussions, written materials, audiovisual aids, demonstrations, simulations, and repeated practice. Overnight trips home may be useful in identifying problems before final discharge. Electrical requirements and safety considerations are evaluated.

NURSING DIAGNOSES

In the following pages, nursing diagnoses specific to the care of the client undergoing

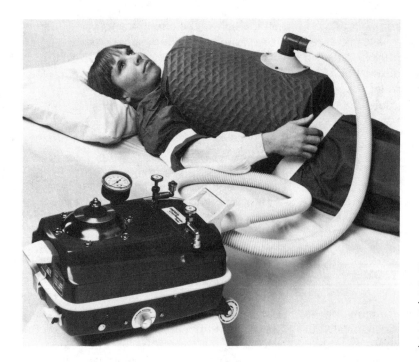

Figure 9-2. Negative pressure ventilator. (From Walsh J, Persons CB, Wieck L: Manual of Home Health Care Nursing, p 505. Philadelphia, JB Lippincott, 1987)

home mechanical ventilation will be discussed. Despite the underlying medical diagnosis, these nursing diagnoses should remain the same.

INEFFECTIVE AIRWAY CLEARANCE

Clients undergoing mechanical ventilation may experience ineffective airway clearance for many reasons. With the presence of an artificial airway, clearing of the airway may be difficult. Depending on the disease process involved, the client may have copious respiratory secretions, causing problems in clearance of the airway.

Assessment

The home health nurse will need to work with the family to assure their understanding of techniques for suctioning and clearing of

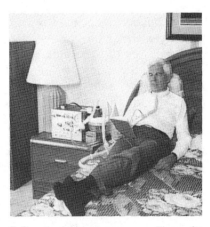

Figure 9-3. Positive pressure ventilator. (From Puritan-Bennett. 2800 Portable Volume Ventilator)

the airway. On each visit, the home health nurse must evaluate the client's breath sounds for the presence of adventitious or extra sounds. Other parameters indicating potential problems in airway clearance include dyspnea, shortness of breath, poor color, and tachypnea.

Interventions

All the interventions for tracheostomy care and tracheal suction techniques listed under the Airway Management section (page 218) are to be followed for ventilator-dependent clients requiring artificial airways. In addition, care-takers need to demonstrate proper use of the manual resuscitation bag. Effective cough technique, postural drainage, and proper use and cleaning of both aerosol and oxygen equipment are also included in a ventilator home-care program. The client and care-givers need to demonstrate ventilator checks, practice ventilator circuit assembly and equipment cleaning and must understand ventilator maintenance and trouble-shooting.

Outcome

The client and family will demonstrate the ability to maintain a clear airway for the client.

IMPAIRED VERBAL COMMUNICATION

With mechanical ventilation, the client will experience an inability to communicate, due to the presence of the artificial airway.

Assessment

Once the client is intubated, the ability to communicate verbally is lost. However, the client may be able to utilize nonverbal techniques to communicate needs and desires. If these techniques are ineffective, the client will experience anxiety and frustration. If the difficulties are prolonged, the client may even become withdrawn and angry.

Interventions

A wide range of communication systems is now available to assist the ventilator-dependent client. If there is a sufficient leak around the tracheostomy tube, a finger can occlude the tracheostomy during exhalation when the client is off the ventilator. Speaking cuff tracheostomy tubes, eye-scanning and audible alarm systems are also available. A speech pathologist should be consulted to evaluate a person for assistive communication devices. Enthusiastic encouragement from all care-givers and significant family members is essential in motivation for speech therapy.

Outcome

The client will be able to communicate needs and desires successfully.

INEFFECTIVE INDIVIDUAL AND FAMILY COPING

Care of the client undergoing mechanical ventilation in the home is a process that involves the entire family. Depending on the group, the stress of caring for this individual can cause the family to grow closer together or farther apart. The home health nurse plays a vital role in assessing the responses of the client and family and assisting them as they make the many transitions during this difficult time.

Assessment

On each visit, the home health nurse will assess the client and family for signs of anxiety and response to the disease process. The nurse may also be able to identify the relationship between the family and client and how the stress of mechanical ventilation may have supported or interfered with that relationship.

Interventions

Family members of the ventilator client make a commitment to the home-care program prior to the client's discharge. All efforts are made to promote family strengths and to minimize stressors and conflicts. Being able to manage the client at home can be a very positive experience but care-givers and family need to understand and even anticipate psychosocial problems. The client often needs encouragement and support in achieving goals for independence in some aspect of care, or education for employment opportunities.

Care-giver needs change and should be evaluated frequently. Dividing and sharing responsibility for a client's care and utilizing respite options all help in relieving the family of the tremendous "burden of care" associated with the home care of a ventilator patient.

Outcome

Both client and family should demonstrate effective use of coping strategies.

POTENTIAL FOR INJURY

There are several causes of injury for the client on a home ventilator. Malfunction of the equipment may occur due to several factors including electricity, tubing malfunction, and machinery malfunction.

Assessment

A respiratory therapist will visit the home periodically to assess the ventilator tubing and functioning. The specific areas to check include the ventilator settings, alarm settings, and all connections of the ventilator.

On each visit, the home health nurse will assess to assure that the client is receiving the correct tidal volume and any other parameters specified by the physician. The respiratory therapist can assist if any problems are identified. Periodically, the home health nurse will analyze the oxygen concentration the client is receiving and will assure that all of the alarms are functioning correctly.

Interventions

The portable positive pressure ventilators used in the home are usually electrically powered and should have an internal battery with an operating capacity of at least 1 hour. External batteries with a capacity of 24 hours should be provided for emergency use. An adaptor to an automobile battery is important for travel.

Monitors with alarms are needed to provide adequate safety for the client on a home ventilator. The positive pressure ventilator is generally equipped with a low-pressure disconnect alarm and a high-pressure alarm. Apnea and oxygen concentration monitors may also be necessary.

On each visit, the home health nurse will assess the ventilator for correct functioning. While demonstrating the technique to the family, the nurse can drain condensation from all tubing of the ventilator system. Drain the tubes into a bucket or other receptacle, rather than back into the humidifier. Research indicates that draining fluid back into the humidifier can increase the possibility of infection. Only distilled water should be used in the humidifier.

Outcome

The client will not experience any injury related to performance of the mechanical ventilator.

POTENTIAL FOR INFECTION

Clients undergoing mechanical ventilation experience the potential for infection because of two major reasons. With the institution of an artificial airway, the normal filtering system (the nose) is bypassed. For that reasons, bacteria ordinarily trapped by the mucus blanket in the nose will travel through the respiratory system with the potential for initiating infection.

Repeated suctioning may also increase the probability of infection. Clients and family must use careful aseptic technique while suctioning to decrease the potential for infection. Finally, improper care of the ventilator circuitry may also increase the potential for infection.

Assessment

Care-givers need to recognize changes in respiratory status to include respiratory distress, tachycardia, sputum color change, edema, diaphoresis, and lethargy for early detection and treatment of pulmonary infections. The presence of a fever may also indicate infection.

Interventions

Two to three ventilator circuits are generally provided for home care and they are changed daily. Circuits not in use are cleaned with soap and water and then soaked in disinfectant as recommended by the equipment vendor. Clean technique is utilized and all circuits should be allowed to dry thoroughly.

Suctioning and stomal care should be completed, utilizing aseptic technique. These procedures are outlined in the boxed material below and on pages 216 and 217.

Outcome

The client will not experience infection.

Suctioning Procedure

1. Check the operation of the suction machine.
2. Wash hands.
3. Pour clean tap water in a fresh, disposable bathroom cup.
4. Attach the connecting tubing to the suction machine. Attach the Y-connector to the connecting tube.
5. If supplemental oxygen is available, administer to the client for a few minutes before suctioning.
6. Select a catheter and attach it to the Y-connector. Perform blind endotracheal suctioning or suction the artificial airway as indicated.

   BLIND ENDOTRACHEAL SUCTIONING (ETS)

   1. Place the client in a sitting position.

Lubricate the tip of the catheter with sterile lubricant.

2. Insert the catheter at a downward angle through the nostril and into the nasopharynx.
3. Advance the catheter slowly. Stop at any sign of obstruction.
4. When the catheter is in the oropharynx, ask the client to take a slow, deep breath.
5. Ask the client to continue to take deep breaths through the mouth while slowly advancing the catheter as far as possible. Withdraw the catheter 1 cm to 2 cm.
6. Withdraw the catheter slowly while rotating it between the fingers and applying intermittent suction.

(continued)

7. If secretions are tenacious, instill approximately 5 ml of sterile normal saline through the catheter.

8. Suction for 10 to 15 seconds only.

9. Allow the client to rest before repeating the procedure. Give supplemental oxygen if appropriate.

10. Rinse the catheter by suctioning a few milliliters of water between attempts, if necessary.

11. Suction the oropharynx and mouth after the tracheal suctioning is complete, if necessary.

12. Suction water through the catheter and connecting tubing to rinse. Disconnect the catheter and soak it in a soap and water solution.

13. Turn off the suction machine. Leave the connecting tubing and Y-connector attached to the suction machine, and coil conveniently for future use.

SUCTIONING A TRACHEOSTOMY OR LARYNGECTOMY

1. Disconnect the ventilator (if appropriate). Place the connector on a clean towel on the client's bed or on his lap if the person is seated.

2. Introduce the catheter into the tracheostomy or laryngectomy tube.

3. Use sterile water-soluble lubricant to moisten the catheter tip if insertion is difficult.

4. Withdraw the catheter slowly while rotating the catheter and applying intermittent suction.

5. Apply suction only while withdrawing the catheter.

6. Instill approximately 5 ml of sterile saline into the airway if secretions are tenacious.

7. Limit suctioning attempts to 15 seconds.

8. Reconnect the ventilator if the client is being ventilated. Suction a few milliliters of water to rinse the catheter.

9. Repeat the procedure if necessary.

10. Rinse the catheter and suction the mouth and pharynx if necessary. Rinse the tubing with water.

11. Turn off the suction machine. Disconnect the catheter from the connector and place it in soap and water to soak.

12. Coil the tubing conveniently for future use.

Tracheostomy Care

1. Place the client in a semi-Fowler's position.

2. Wash hands thoroughly.

3. Assemble the equipment on a table or TV tray convenient to the client. Pour hydrogen peroxide and saline or distilled water into two receptacles.

Open the paper bag to receive soiled articles.

4. Suction the tracheostomy before giving tracheostomy care.

5. If the client is on mechanical ventilation, disconnect the ventilator and place the connector on a clean towel.

(continued)

6. Remove the inner cannula. Place it in the peroxide and clean it with the brush or pipe cleaners. Rinse it in the saline or distilled water.

7. Replace the inner cannula, taking care to lock it into the correct position.

8. Reconnect the ventilator if the client is being ventilated.

9. Using a 4×4 gauze pad soaked in peroxide, gently remove exudate from around the stoma. Rinse the area with saline or distilled water, using a 4×4 pad.

10. Pat the area dry with a 4×4 gauze pad. Note the condition of the skin.

11. Unless excessive amounts of exudate are a problem, leave the area open.

12. If secretions are a problem, cut a slit in a 4×4 gauze pad and place it around the tube.

13. A small piece of Telfa (nonadhesive dressing) can also be used to dress the stoma.

14. Remove the tracheostomy ties and replace them with clean tape. Knot the ties rather than tieing in a bow to prevent them from accidentally becoming untied.

15. If the cuff is inflated, suction the airway. Deflate the cuff and suction again before reinflating the cuff.

16. Perform tracheostomy care on a daily basis, or more often if managing secretions is a problem.

17. Manipulate the tracheostomy tube as little as possible during the procedure to prevent discomfort to the client, irritation to the stoma, and the introduction of bacteria.

18. Discard soiled articles in the paper bag.

19. Wash hands.

ALTERATION IN NUTRITION

Without adequate nutrition, ventilatory muscle strength and endurance is reduced as is the resistance to pulmonary infections. With the presence of an artificial airway, the client may experience a decrease in nutritional substrates. Occasionally, the situation can be worsened by the addition of stress ulcers and the potential for gastric bleeding.

Assessment

Dietary intake and weight require ongoing evaluation. The home health nurse may need the assistance of the family in constructing a nutrition history of the client. The caloric intake must match the expected caloric expenditure. As the client is in a stage of repair, the metabolic requirements may be increased, requiring an increase in calories. A further discussion of nutritional assessment can be found in Chapter 11.

Other parameters to assess include bowel sounds, abdominal distention, and the presence of abdominal tenderness. If gastrointestinal bleeding is suspected, the stool and any vomitus should be hematested.

Interventions

In many cases, the client will require nutritional supplements. For the client requiring mechanical ventilation only at specific times of the day, nutritional supplements such as Magnacal or Ensure may be appropriate. If the client requires continuous mechanical ventilation, parenteral or enteral feedings may be indicated. To prevent any gastrointestinal complications, antacids may be administered.

Outcome

The client will maintain good nutritional balance.

KNOWLEDGE DEFICIT

Although there are many aspects to the care of the home bound client on a mechanical ventilator, the need for appropriate teaching for the client and family is critical. The teaching will begin in the hospital before the client is discharged. Similar teaching will take place in the home setting and will be reinforced on each visit.

Assessment

There are many ways to assess the client's and his family's knowledge of the care required for the client on mechanical ventilation. If the client or family exhibits signs of anxiety or asks multiple questions, they may need additional teaching. Their perception and understanding of mechanical ventilation will be important.

Interventions

One of the primary interventions will be to allow the client and family to express their feelings and to offer them the opportunity to ask further questions. Specifically, they should be taught to develop a daily routine for care of the client. This includes a daily routine for checking the ventilator, techniques for maintenance of the ventilator and oxygen equipment, and safety precautions.

The family must be taught to troubleshoot the ventilator and know how to place the client on back-up systems while adjusting the ventilator. They should be encouraged to contact the home health nurse immediately if problems develop with the equipment. It would also be appropriate to contact the respiratory therapist who represents the company supplying the ventilator. Techniques for managing the artificial airway, including postural drainage, percussion, vibration, and suctioning should be taught.

The family should be encouraged to report any symptoms of respiratory infection including purulent sputum, dyspnea, or an elevated temperature. Irritants can be removed from the air through the use of air conditioners or humidifiers.

Outcome

The client and family will possess the knowledge needed to care for the client on a mechanical ventilator.

AIRWAY MANAGEMENT

EMERGENCY AIRWAYS

The home care nurse must be prepared to recognize and manage an obstructed airway in the home setting since it is a clinical emergency. In addition to being trained in cardiopulmonary resuscitation and obstructed airway techniques, the nurse should include a resuscitation mask in her nursing bag. The home health nurse should always carry disposable mouthpieces in the event mouth to mouth resuscitation is needed.

TYPES OF TRACHEOSTOMY TUBES

Tracheostomy tubes are made of silver, stainless steel, or synthetic materials and range in price from $14 to $100. Generally more durable, the synthetic tubes have the advantage of greater pliability and comfort. Tubes may be cuffed or uncuffed. A cuffed tube is usually used to prevent aspiration of gastric or naso-pharyngeal secretions into the lungs or to provide adequate positive-pressure ventilation when inflated. It forms a seal between the trachea and tracheostomy tube.

Tracheal cuffs can be detachable or integral. A hazard with a detachable cuff is that it can slip down over the end of a tracheostomy tube and occlude a patient's airway. Most integral cuffs are of the low-pressure variety and require 5 cc to 7 cc of air to be inflated. Tracheostomy cuffs can be inflated either continuously or intermittently, depending on the needs of the client. Tracheal tubes for infants and young children are usually uncuffed.

Tracheostomy tubes generally consist of three parts. The outer cannula holds the air-way open and is angled to fit into the neck opening and down into the trachea. The inner cannula fits into the outer cannula and locks into place, providing an easily removable tube to allow for cleaning. Disposable plastic tubes under size 4 do not have an inner cannula. The obturator is a guide that is inserted into the outer cannula with the inner cannula removed when the tracheostomy tube is inserted.

A fenestrated tracheostomy tube has an opening between the flange and the distal tip of the tube, allowing for air exchange between the lungs and upper airway. It is used to begin weaning form mechanical ventilation and/or to allow a client to talk when the tracheostomy tube is plugged (Fig. 9-4).

Several cuffed tracheostomy tubes are now

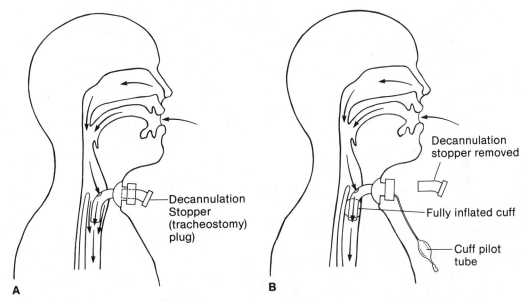

Figure 9-4. Fenestrated tracheostomy tubes. When the inner cannula (not shown) is removed, air from the upper airway is able to pass into and out of the lower airway. When the decannulation stopper or tracheostomy plug is inserted into the outer cannula, normal ventilation occurs (A). Fenestrated tracheostomy tubes may also be cuffed (B). If a decannulation stopper is used, the cuff must be deflated, otherwise air movement or respiration are insufficient. (From Luckmann J, Sorenson KC: Medical–Surgical Nursing: A Psychophysiologic Approach, p 752. Philadelphia, WB Saunders, 1986)

available that facilitate speech by directing an external air supply into the upper airway while the cuff is inflated.

Tracheostomy buttons protrude only slightly past the anterior tracheal wall and, when plugged, cause less resistance to airflow than tracheostomy tubes. They are held in place by an expansion lock and are useful in maintaining the tracheal opening (Fig. 9-5). Frequently the tracheostomy client with sufficient scar tissue or the laryngectomy client with a stoma will do well without wearing a tracheostomy tube.

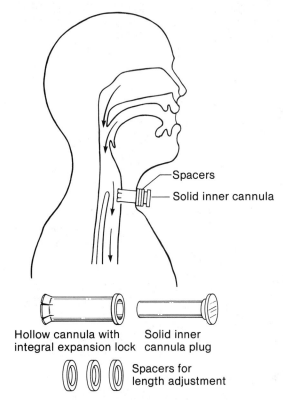

Hollow cannula with integral expansion lock

Solid inner cannula plug

Spacers for length adjustment

Figure 9-5. Tracheostomy button to be used when weaning a patient from a tracheostomy. (From Luckmann J, Sorenson KC: Medical – Surgical Nursing: A Psychophysiologic Approach, p 757. Philadelphia, WB Saunders, 1986)

Suctioning

The primary goal of suctioning is to maintain a patent airway by clearing secretions from the tracheostomy. Cannula suctioning should be based on need and should not be done routinely. It is indicated if secretions build up and cannot be cleared by coughing, if the client demonstrates signs of respiratory distress, and prior to deflating the cuff when a cuffed tracheostomy tube is used. Suctioning is unnecessary if the client can cough adequately by reflex or with a reminder.

To prevent oxygen deprivation during suctioning the pressure setting of the suctioning machine should be checked for accuracy. The usual suction pressure for adults is 12 cm to 15 cm of water. In addition, suction catheters should not be larger than the inside diameter of the tracheostomy tube. Suctioning should be discontinued if bradycardia or moderate to severe tachycardia develops. Cardiac arrest from vagal reflex or anoxia can occur.

Meticulous clean technique coupled with good handwashing is utilized for tracheostomy suctioning in the home. Emphasis is placed on preventing situations where organisms can multiply. A clean, unwaxed paper cup filled with distilled or tap water is used to lubricate the suction catheter and to rinse the catheters and tubing. For very tenacious mucus, a saline or sodium bicarbonate solution (½ teaspoon in 1 cup) can be utilized for clearing suction catheters.

Homemade or commercial eye drop solutions of sterile saline can be utilized to help liquify pulmonary secretions. Up to 3 cc of solution can be instilled with a clean dropper or syringe with the needle removed to help liquify sputum.

Suction catheters are inserted gently 4 inches to 5 inches into the tracheostomy tube, with the vent open. Deep tracheal suctioning requires a specific physician order.

When applying suction, the catheter is withdrawn in a rotating motion. If the client coughs or resistance is felt, the catheter should be withdrawn slightly with the vent open. The catheter should not remain in the client more than 10 seconds for the adult or more than 5 seconds for a child. Three minutes' rest is allowed before reinserting the catheter if the client is not bagged for 3 to 10 breaths. These breaths should be synchronized with inspiration between suctionings. Disposable gloves are worn if secretions are excessive or infectious.

After the suctioning session(s), the catheters are flushed well with detergent water, rinsed, dried with a clean cloth, and reattached to the suction machine, which is turned on to help dry the inside of the catheter. For smaller lumen catheters, it is recommended that one catheter be used per day and then discarded. Catheters with larger lumens can be reused unless cracked or unclear. Clean catheters are wrapped in a clean cloth or paper towel and left beside the suction machine. The insides of ziplock bags are sterile and are an excellent container in which to store suction catheters. The suction bottle and tubing should be cleaned once daily. A small amount of detergent solution should be kept in the bottom of the suction container at all times. The procedure for suctioning is outlined on pages 215 and 216.

Changing the Outer Cannula

The outer cannula of a tracheostomy tube is changed in the home setting after it has been changed without problems in a supervised setting. In most cases there will be very little danger of tracheal collapse with the outer cannula removed. The tract usually becomes well established 4 to 5 days after surgery. Caution and close collaboration with the physician is indicated if there is tracheal stenosis, new growth at the tracheal opening, a tracheal–esophageal fistula, or bleeding from the tracheostomy.

It is advisable to have a Trousseau dilator handy for the first few changes. This instrument can be inserted into the tracheostomy opening in case of collapse. Although bleeding may occur with this procedure due to trauma to superficial blood vessels, it can be minimized by being gentle. Reentry of the outer cannula should never be forced. Occasionally it is difficult to reinsert the tube because of muscle spasm. Inserting the new cannula as soon as possible after removal of the old sometimes prevents this. Removal of a cuffed tracheostomy tube may be more difficult than removal of an uncuffed tube. The cuff must be completely deflated prior to removal and a steady, even pull should be exerted. A clean cuffed tube should be inflated to check for leaks and then deflated completely prior to inserting. No additional force is required to insert a cuffed tube if adequate water-soluble lubricant is used. It is best to have the client sitting or well supported in bed for the outer cannula change. If the client is to be taught the procedure, he should be seated in front of a mirror. With his head bent slightly forward, the client takes several deeper than normal breaths and then holds his breath. This usually prevents coughing during the cannula change.

The old cannula is removed with one hand and the new cannula with obturator and twill ties is inserted with the other hand, using a smooth motion that follows the curve of the throat. With a firm hold on the outer flange the obturator should be quickly removed as it obstructs the airway. The tapes are then tied at the side of the neck and knotted in three places, allowing for introduction of one finger under the tapes with the neck slightly flexed.

Frequency of tube changes varies according to client needs. A laryngectomy client may need to change the tube only monthly. Frequent changes will usually reduce the incidence of infection and prevent tissue granulomas around the stoma. The client or caregiver should be trained to change the tube as soon as possible so that they may appropriately intervene if the tube comes out inadvertently. Every client with a tracheostomy should be discharged from the hospital with at least one spare identical tracheostomy set.

Cleaning the Tracheostomy Set

The inner cannula is cleaned as often as necessary in order to keep the tracheostomy tube patent. A twice-daily cleaning is usually adequate for clients at home. If inspired air is adequately humidified, the cannula will probably not need to be cleaned as frequently. Humidification can be provided by a vaporizer, a steam kettle, allowing steam from a hot shower to build up in the bathroom, or by placing a washcloth or gauze moistened with water directly over the tracheostomy. Secretions can build up in the outer cannula, so it is best not to have the inner cannula out for longer than 10 minutes.

The inner cannula and outer cannula should be allowed to soak for 5 minutes in a cool detergent solution or a 1 : 2 solution of hydrogen peroxide and water. They should then be scrubbed with a small bottle brush and rinsed well. The cannula can be held up to the light to look for all secretions. Metal tubes can be held up to the light to look for all secretions. Metal tubes can be boiled for 5 minutes, drained, cooled, and dried thoroughly. Plastic tubes should never be boiled. Cleaned equipment can be stored in a plastic bag or boiled jar with lid.

Deflation and Inflation of a Cuffed Tracheostomy Tube

When a tracheostomy cuff is being deflated, secretions that have pooled above it are sucked downward into the lower airway. Prior to deflation the pharynx is suctioned first with one catheter and then the trachea is suctioned with another catheter simultaneously with deflation. The cuff is deflated by withdrawing air, using a 10 cc syringe attached to a one-way valve on the fine bore tubing. A deflated pilot balloon indicates cuff deflation.

When inflating a cuffed tracheostomy tube, just enough air should be injected to seal the trachea (minimum seal). The client should be unable to talk and there should be no leaks of air from the nose, mouth, or around the tracheal opening. After a certain number of cubic centimeters have been established as a sealant, this amount should be used as a guide for reinflation. No more than 10 cc of air should be used in a low-pressure, high-volume cuff unless there is a specific physician order. A minimal leak seal occurs when ½ cc of air is withdrawn after a minimum seal is obtained. This allows the client to speak. Not all clients can tolerate this technique.

Cuffs can leak or rupture. A cuff is probably defective if the pilot balloon does not remain inflated, large amounts of air do not seal the trachea, or no resistance is met in injecting air. Pilot balloon inflation indicates that the cuff is inflated but gives no information about the degree of cuff inflation.

When a cuff is inflated continuously there must be daily evaluation of cuff pressure to prevent tracheal necrosis. The effectiveness of periodic cuff deflation is controversial but may be ordered. Cuff pressure can be monitored using a sphygmomanometer and a three-way valve or a cuff pressure monitor.

Pressure should not exceed 15 mm of Hg or 21 cm of water.

If the cuff is inflated during meals a minimum seal is formed. The client should be in the sitting position with the neck flexed to minimize any occurrence of aspiration. The cuff inflation should be maintained for at least 30 minutes after a meal.

Skin Care Around the Tracheostomy

The skin surrounding the tracheostomy can be cleaned with a mild soap and water, using a clean washcloth or with hydrogen peroxide and a Q tip. Care must be taken to prevent soap, peroxide, or the Q tip from entering the tracheostomy opening.

If the skin around the stoma is reddened or slightly irritated, vaseline or an antibiotic ointment can be used judiciously. Ointments should not be used routinely as there is danger of macerating the tissue and causing local sensitivity or a lipid pneumonia. Danger of tissue maceration is reduced by applying a thin film of ointment and wiping it off after 2 minutes. The skin should be cleaned and dried between applications. Betadine solu-

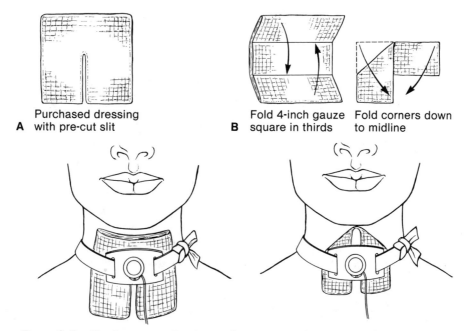

A Purchased dressing with pre-cut slit

B Fold 4-inch gauze square in thirds   Fold corners down to midline

Figure 9-6. Tracheostomy dressings. These are not always used. If there is significant bleeding or tracheal secretion, cleaning the skin and changing the dressing frequently may prevent infection and skin breakdown. *(A)* Manufactured dressing with pre-cut slit has no fine threads that could unravel and enter the stoma. Place dressing around the tracheostomy tube with the slit downward (as shown) or upward. *(B)* 4 × 4 gauze pad folded and placed under tracheostomy tube. Do not have any cut edges that could unravel. (From Luckmann J, Sorenson KC: Medical–Surgical Nursing: A Psychophysiologic Approach, p 754. Philadelphia, WB Saunders, 1986)

tion should be used with caution as it may lead to tracheal scarring if it comes in contact with mucous membranes. Crusts around the stoma caused by dried secretions and blood can be softened with a 4 by 4 gauze pad dampened with half-strength peroxide and removed with tweezers.

The Tracheostomy Dressing

If secretions are not a problem, a dressing may not be needed. Nothing should be used for a dressing that has lint or strings that are likely to come off and be aspirated. There is no need to cut a 4 by 4 pad for use as a dressing (Fig. 9-6).

Tracheostomy ties should be changed, depending on how quickly they become soiled. Several sets of ties should be prepared in advance. It may be more convenient to use a single length of tie and thread it through the flange openings. Cotton ties absorb moisture and secretion while synthetic ties do not. The techniques for tracheostomy care are outlined in the boxed material on pages 216 and 217.

An assessment of the home for the client undergoing alteration in respiration is outlined in Table 9-6.

TABLE 9.6 Assessment of the Home

Access	Assess stairways and number of steps to reach building. This can be a significant problem in a multifamily structure. If appropriate, can ramps be installed and doorways widened?
	There are often monies available for structural changes for an individual's residence, to accommodate hospital beds, wheelchairs, etc. To investigate the possibilities, a social worker consultation should be considered.
	For a long-term, compromised patient, senior citizen complexes are designed and built with elevators, and apartments and common rooms are designed for wheelchairs and walking aids.
Bedroom	The patient should not feel isolated, but should have the option for privacy. This is a necessity for patients establishing a new bowel and/or bladder routine.
	The bed should be positioned to enable client to observe who enters the room.
	The family members need privacy and need to maintain as "normal" a life-style as possible.
	The room size must accommodate any needed machinery, *i.e.*, ventilators, O_2, feeding apparatus, etc. The room must be large enough to permit transfer to and from wheelchair, bedside commode, etc., when appropriate.
	The room should be pleasant and lend itself to accommodating the client for extended periods of time when indicated. (Include some of the client's favorite possessions.)

TABLE 9.6 Assessment of the Home *(continued)*

	The room should have access to the bathroom.
	Consider the position of internal stairways to allow for ease of movement.
	Availability of electrical outlets for support machinery is important. The information concerning wattage and voltage can be obtained through the equipment supply company. Also consider the financial burden the client and/or family may incur, due to increase in utility bills.
Kitchen	Assess what foods client has in refrigerator and cupboards.
	Assess ease of access to refrigerator, stove, sink, hot plate, etc.
	Does client understand and can he afford prescribed dietary changes? Possibly consult with nutritionist to work with client and/or support person to incorporate low-cost dietary modifications with family meals when applicable.
	Explore possibility of Meals on Wheels.
	Redesign kitchen, if appropriate, to conserve client's energy during meal preparation.
Bathroom	Large enough and accessible to patient in wheelchair, walker? If patient is wheelchair-dependent, is bathroom large enough to permit transfer?
	Are there handrails next to sink, toilet, tub to aid client?
	Skid grips or mats in shower and/or bath?
	Elevated toilet seat if indicated?
Safety Measures	Assess for scatter rugs (skid-proof), toys, heaters, furniture or any clutter that could impede a wheelchair, walker, or client with cane; do they pose a potential safety factor?
	For clients suffering from a visual impairment, assess home for hanging objects that could be a safety threat.
	For clients suffering from impaired sensation to heat and cold, lower temperature of water heater to prevent accidental scalding. Reinforce that a family member/care-taker should pretest bath water and assess if client is dressed appropriately for inside/outside weather conditions. Shoes should always be worn to prevent accidental injury to the feet. Heating pad, heat lamps, hot water bottles, electric blankets, etc., pose safety threats.
Poor Tissue Perfusion; Tissue Breakdown	For clients at risk for decubiti, assess and teach support persons to assess pressure point areas. Reinforce keeping linen dry, wrinkle-free, gentle massage, turning frequently, etc., in accordance to client's needs. Reinforce that client becomes a high risk during periods of incontinence. Use of air mattresses, lambs wools, etc., when indicated.
	If O_2 is in use, smoking, heaters, fireplaces, furnances should be recognized as potential hazards and precautions should be taken.

(continued)

TABLE 9.6 Assessment of the Home (*continued*)

Assess client's skills in ambulating safely, *i.e.*, transfer, turning, good body mechanics. This includes support persons also.

Assess condition of ALL equipment (used or in the home for use by the client).

The utility companies should be notified as to what kinds of apparatus are being used in the home, *i.e.*, ventilators, O_2, etc.

Emergency telephone numbers for doctors, EMS, supply companies should be in plain view.

Support personnel should be comfortable with CPR and other applicable procedures.

ABBREVIATED CARE PLAN: CLIENT UNDERGOING HOME MECHANICAL VENTILATION

Nursing Diagnosis	Assessment	Interventions	Outcomes
Ineffective Airway Clearance	Breath sounds Dyspnea Shortness of breath Color	Instruct family and client in tracheostomy care. Assure client and family knowledge of ventilator care.	Client and family will demonstrate the ability to maintain a clear airway for the client.
Impaired Verbal Communication	Anxiety Frustration Nonverbal techniques	Utilize speaking cuff tracheostomy tubes as appropriate. Consultation with speech therapist as needed.	Client will be able to communicate needs and desires.
Ineffective Individual and Family Coping	Anxiety Response to disease process	Assist family in techniques to divide responsibility for client care. Support client	Client and family demonstrate effective use of coping strategies.

ABBREVIATED CARE PLAN: CLIENT UNDERGOING HOME MECHANICAL VENTILATION (*continued*)

Nursing Diagnosis	Assessment	Interventions	Outcomes
Potential for Injury	Ventilator settings Alarms Connections	Monitor strength of backup. Check monitor alarms. Drain condensation as needed.	The client will not experience any injury related to performance of the mechanical ventilator.
Potential for Infection	Respiratory distress Tachycardia Fever	Change circuits daily Suction as needed.	Client will not experience infection.
Alteration in Nutrition	Dietary intake Weight Bowel sounds Bleeding	Add nutritional supplements. Administer antacids as needed.	The client will maintain good nutritional balance.
Knowledge Deficit	Anxiety Perception and understanding of mechanical ventilation.	Allow client and family to express feelings. Develop daily routine for care. Report symptoms of infection immediately.	The client and family will possess the knowledge needed to care for the client on a mechanical ventilator.

References

Banaszak EF, et al: Home Ventilator Care. Respiratory Care 26(12): 1262–1268, 1981

Brown B, Campbell B, Scott J: Infection control guidelines for home respiratory therapy. Dimens Health Serv 62(8): 38–39, 1985

Brunner LS, Suddarth DS: The Lippincott Manual of Nursing Practice, 3rd ed. Philadelphia, JB Lippincott, 1982

Chalikian J, Weaver TE: Mechanical ventilation. Where it's at; where it's going. Am J Nurs 84(11): 1372–79, 1984

Christmas Seal League of Southwestern Pennsylvania: Self Help: Your Strategy for Living with COPD. Palo Alto, Bull Publishing, 1983

Continuous or nocturnal oxygen therapy in hypoxemic chronic obstructive lung disease. Ann Intern Med 93:(3): 391–398, 1980

Escarrabill J, Estop`a, R, Huguet M, Manresa R: Letter: Domiciliary oxygen therapy. Lancet 2(8458): 779, 1985

Flenley DC: Long-term home oxygen therapy. Chest 87(1): 99–103, 1985

George RB: Long-term hospitalization of ventilator-dependent patients. Can we afford it? Arch Intern Med 145(11): 2089, 1985

Glover DW, Glover MM: Respiratory Therapy. St. Louis, CV Mosby, 1978

Goldberg AI, Faure EA, Vaughn CJ, Snarski R et al: Home care for life-supported persons: An approach to program development. J Pediatr 104(5): 785–795, 1984

Goldberg AI, Faure EA: Home care for life-supported persons in England: The responaut program. Chest 86(6): 910–914, 1984

Goldberg AI, Faure EA: Home care for life-supported persons in France: The regional association. Rehabil Lit 47(3–4): 60–64, 103, 1986

Gower DJ, Davis CH, Jr: Home ventilator dependence after high cervical cord injury. South Med J 78(8): 1010–1011, 1985

Govoni LE, Hayes JE: Drugs and Nursing Implications 4th ed. East Norwalk, CT, Appleton-Century-Crofts, 1982

Guyton, AC: Textbook of Medical Physiology, 4th ed. Philadelphia, WB Saunders, 1971

Guenter CA, Welch MH: Pulmonary Medicine, 2nd ed. Philadelphia, JB Lippincott, 1982

Haas A, Pineda H, Haas F, Axen K: Pulmonary Therapy and Rehabilitation Principles and Practice. Baltimore, Williams and Wilkins, 1979

Howe J, Dickason EJ, Jones DA, Snider MJ: The Handbook of Nursing. New York, John Wiley & Sons, 1984

Hudson LD: Management of COPD. State of the art. Chest 85(6 Suppl): 768–818, 1984

Indihar FJ, Walker NE: Experience with a prolonged respiratory care unit—revisited. Chest 86(4): 616–20, 1984

Johnson DL, Giovannoni RM, Driscoll, SA: Ventilator Assisted Patient Care. Rockville, MD, Aspen Publishers, Inc., 1986

Kahn L: Home care wrap-up—patients. Ventilator-dependent children heading home. Hospitals 58(5): 54–5, 1984

Kopacz MA, Moriarty-Wright R: Multidisciplinary approach for the patient on a home ventilator. Heart Lung 13(3): 255–62, 1984

Long-term domiciliary oxygen therapy: Editorial: Lancet 2(8451): 365–367, August 17, 1985

Luckmann J, Sorenson KC: Medical–Surgical Nursing: A Psychophysiologic Approach. Philadelphia, WB Saunders, 1986

Make BJ: Letter: Home care for ventilator-dependent individuals. Chest 87(3): 412, 1985

Netter FH: The CIBA Collection of Medical Illustrations. Vol 7: Respiratory System. Summit, NJ, CIBA Pharmaceutical Co, 1980

O'Donahue WJ, et al: Long-term mechanical ventilation guidelines for management in the home and at alternate community sites. Chest (Suppl) 90:1, 1986

Ostrow DN: Managing chronic airflow obstruction: Part II. Geriatrics 40(3): 51–53, 56–59, 62, 1985

Petty TL, Nett LM: Outpatient oxygen therapy in chronic obstructive pulmonary disease. Arch Intern Med 139: 28–32, 1979

Porth CM: Pathophysiology: Concepts of Altered Health States, 2nd ed. Philadelphia, JB Lippincott, 1986

Providing Respiratory Care: Nursing Photobook. Springhouse, PA, Intermed Communications, 1979

Selecting a home care equipment vendor. Am J Nurs 84(3): 349–50, 1984

Sexton DL: Chronic obstructive pulmonary disease: Care of the Child and Adult. St. Louis, CV Mosby, 1981

Smith AP, Gunawardena KA: Nebulisers in domiciliary practice: Letter: Lancet 2(8414): 1281–1282, 1984

Votava KM et al: Home care of the patient dependent on mechanical ventilation: Home care policy development and goal setting using outcome criteria for quality assurance. Home Health Care Nurse 3(2): 18–25, 1985

ALTERATIONS IN CIRCULATION

Nancy Pratt

The circulatory system is a continuous circuit that serves to deliver oxygen and remove metabolic wastes from the body tissues. In this chapter, some of the conditions that impair this system are discussed. Particular focus is placed on the management of clients with cardiovascular disease in the home setting.

PROBLEMS RELATED TO CORONARY BLOOD FLOW

The coronary system supplies the myocardium with blood flow from which the heart extracts oxygen. Normally, there is flexibility in both the supply of this oxygen and the demand from the heart. With an increase in activity such as exercise, excitement, or stress, there is an increase in myocardial oxygen demand. The coronary arteries dilate to increase perfusion and therefore oxygen supply. In disease states of the coronary system, this delicate supply–demand ratio is upset. Ischemia results when oxygen demand exceeds supply.

PATHOPHYSIOLOGY

Angina pectoris is the intermittent chest pain or discomfort (often felt as pressure or chest tightness) that occurs as a result of myocardial ischemia. One of the most common causes of angina is atherosclerotic narrowing of the coronary arteries. This occurs as a result of fatty deposits in the lumen of the arteries. The condition may progress until the vessel lumen is completely occluded.

In the absence of plaque build-up within the coronaries, any condition leading to limited oxygen delivery to the myocardium can lead to angina. Oxygen delivery can be limited by such factors as anemia and hypoxemia. It can also be limited by circulatory problems such as severe hypotension, arrhythmias, hemorrhage, and the Valsalva's maneuver. Aortic stenosis or insufficiency can also decrease flow to the coronaries since the origin of these arteries is at the cusps of the aortic valve. In addition, angina may occur in the presence of excessive metabolic demands such as hyperthyroidism or extreme tachycardias.

Finally, a cause of angina that has been receiving more attention recently is arterial vasospasm in the coronary system. The angina of vasospasm is often referred to as *variant angina* or *Prinzmetal's-type angina*.

Conditions that lead to an increase in the workload of the heart can lead to angina, especially when combined with atherosclerotic narrowing of the coronary arteries. Examples of situations that increase myocardial work are diastolic hypertension and excess catecholamine excretion, such as in exertion, excitement, or the adrenal tumor, pheochromocytoma.

Although it may occur without chest pain, angina more often presents as a squeezing or pressurelike pain felt beneath the sternum. The pain may radiate down one or both arms or up the neck and jaw. Angina often occurs during physical exertion and may be relieved by rest. Variant angina, or that caused by vasospasm, typically occurs during rest and is therefore not relieved by cessation of activity. Nitrates are the first drug of choice for the treatment of acute angina, regardless of its etiology. Medical therapy for the underlying cause follows.

If angina is not treated promptly and aggressively, the prolonged ischemia to the myocardium results in an infarction. Whereas the pain of ischemia can be likened to a muscle cramping from lack of oxygen, an infarction results in loss of function to the affected muscle. The portion of the heart muscle that sustains an infarct becomes scar tissue and does not contribute to the pumping function of the heart. Angina is treated to prevent its progression to an infarct. Myocardial infarction is treated to limit its size.

Included in this discussion of clients with angina and myocardial infarction are clients who have received invasive medical therapy for these conditions such as angioplasty and coronary artery bypass grafts (CABG). Angioplasty is a relatively recent medical intervention in which a balloon-tipped catheter is inserted into the coronary artery and inflated, pressing a large and identifiable occlusion against the artery walls. This opens the narrowed area, permitting increased blood flow. In CABG surgery a section of the saphenous vein is sewn to the root of the aorta and to the coronary artery distal to the occlusion, resulting in increased blood flow past the narrowed area. Another surgical technique involves sewing the distal end of the internal mammary artery to the coronary artery distal to the occlusion.

Since clients with angina, myocardial infarction (MI), angioplasty, and CABG surgery all have problems with coronary blood supply, they will be discussed as a group.

NURSING DIAGNOSES

There are several nursing diagnoses for the client with problems related to coronary perfusion. For each of the following diagnoses, assessment, planning, interventions and outcomes will be discussed.

DECREASE IN CARDIAC OUTPUT RELATED TO ISCHEMIA/ARRHYTHMIAS

As the heart muscle is deprived of oxygen, the ischemic area ceases to function. This area of muscle that no longer contracts compromises the overall efficiency of the heart as a pump. The result is that less blood is ejected from the ventricles with each systolic contraction. This decrease in cardiac output may be transitory, as the ischemic muscle may recover, or permanent if an infarction ensues.

Ischemia can also affect the conduction system of the heart, leading to arrhythmias. In premature beats and very rapid beats the ventricles have had inadequate time for diastolic filling and therefore can only eject a small volume of blood. Again, the result is a decrease in cardiac output.

Assessment

Assessment of cardiac output includes evaluation of the heart rate and regularity of the rhythm. Blood pressure measurement, strength of peripheral pulses, and heart sounds should be evaluated. These data should be compared with historical information on the client as they may reflect the degree of compromise in cardiac output the client is experiencing. Other assessment criteria are adequacy of urine production and level of consciousness. These measures indicate adequacy of perfusion of the kidneys and brain.

The home-care nurse should be aware of the client's cardiac history and patterns of angina. It is prudent to assess for the presence of chest pain. The client's subjective report of chest discomfort is critical information. One method of quantifying this discomfort is having the client report the degree of pain on a scale of 1 to 10 with 10 being excruciating and 1 being slight pressure. Related complaints that accompany ischemic pain are nausea, diaphoresis, epigastric burning, fatigue, and feelings of impending doom. Ischemic pain should be differentiated from sternal incision discomfort in the CABG client.

Interventions

Interventions are aimed at improving oxygen delivery to the myocardium and decreasing myocardial oxygen demand, thus preventing a deterioration in cardiac performance. This is accomplished by having the client rest and administering nitroglycerin sublingually if the pain persists. For unrelieved chest pain, nitroglycerin (NTG) may be administered every 5 minutes for a total of three doses. Angina unrelieved after three doses of NTG represents a serious problem and the client's physician should be contacted immediately.

Significant changes in heart rhythm and rate or the absence of peripheral pulses should be described to the client's physician. The client should be warned that nitroglycerin may cause headaches.

NTG works by causing vasodilatation, which decreases venous return and the workload on the heart, and by causing coronary vasodilatation, which increases myocardial oxygen supply. Decreasing the workload on the heart is also facilitated by positioning the client in a semi-Fowler's position. Lying down increases venous return to heart, increasing myocardial muscle wall tension and oxygen consumption. Therefore, if the client is alert, maintaining a "head up" position is preferable.

If arrhythmias are suspected, the physician may order a Holter monitor. This device records the client's cardiac activity over a 24-hour period. The use of this monitor is displayed in the boxed material below. In certain conditions (*i.e.*, severe bradycardia or heart block) a permanent pacemaker may be needed. A description of this procedure appears on page 233. A teaching plan for the client can also be found on page 233.

Procedure for the Use of Holter Monitors

Equipment

Holter recorder	Electrode-retainer clip
Battery	
Recording tape, new or cleanly erased	Belt or shoulder strap
	4 × 4 gauze pads
Hypoallergenic tape (1 inch)	70% isopropyl alcohol
	Felt-tip pen

(continued)

Benzoin

Patient diary

Electrodes

Adhesive overlays
(to secure
electrodes)

Extension cable

Fine sandpaper
(6/0 or 220 grit)

Razor

Empty take-up reel

Magnetic tape head
cleaner

Cotton-tipped
swabs

Procedure

1. Load tape into the recorder following the manufacturer's instructions. Record 3 to 5 minutes of calibration pulses at the beginning of the tape.

2. Prepare the skin and apply electrodes:
   • Defat the skin with alcohol and 4 × 4 pads. Allow the skin to dry thoroughly.
   • Locate the bony sites for electrode application by palpation.
   • Mark the electrode sites with a felt-tip pen.
   • Dry shave the hair from the electrode sites.
   • Gently abrade the skin, using fine sandpaper, until the skin is slightly pink.
   • Using a cotton-tipped swab, apply benzoin to the skin that will be covered by the adhesive portion of the electrode.
   • Apply the disposable electrodes.
   • Remove the paper backing from the adhesive overlay and press the overlay over the electrode. Secure the overlay to the electrode and the surrounding skin.

3. Connect the snap leads to the electrodes and the extension cable. Connect the extension cable to the recorder at the proper location.

4. Insert the battery into the recorder. Se-

cure the recorder to the client's torso with the belt or shoulder strap.

5. Following the manufacturer's instructions, test the client–electrode interface and the recorder before beginning the recording:
   • Connect the test cable to the scanner or ECG machine as directed by the instructions.
   • Obtain real-time write out from the ECG machine or scanner.
   • Observe the tracing for a minimum of 0.5–m V amplitude on at least one channel.
   • Gently tap each electrode with an index finger and observe the appropriate channel for artifact.
   • Replace the electrode if artifact is observed.

6. Secure the lead wires together with tape to reduce movement.

7. Prepare the recorder to begin recording, and set the clock on the recorder.

8. Enter the time when the recorder was started and the recorder serial number into the client's diary.

9. Check that the recorder is functioning correctly:
   Is the clock reading the correct time?
   Is the tape being properly wound on the take-up reel?
   Is the tape still moving and the motor still operating?
   Is the pinch wheel still closed?

Adapted from Walsh J, Persons CB, Wieck L: Manual of Home Health Care Nursing. Philadelphia, JB Lippincott, 1987

Procedure for Client with a Permanent Pacemaker

1. Teach the client to check pulse daily.

2. If requested by the cardiologist, place a magnet over the pacemaker generator before taking the pulse.

3. Perform a telephone pacemaker check as required:
   - When the pacemaker clinic calls, place the electrodes on the skin.
   - Turn on the ECG transmitter.
   - Place the mouthpiece of the telephone over the transmitter's audio output (this usually makes a beeping sound).
   - If requested by the technician, place the magnet over the generator. The client may lie down and place the magnet over the generator if unable to hold it.

4. Use the radio test to determine the rate of pacemaker stimulation:
   - Turn on the transistor radio and tune it to 55 or 550 AM.
   - Lie down and place the magnet over the generator.
   - Listen for clicks on the radio.
   - Check the pulse at the same time. Each click should correspond with a heartbeat.
   - Contact the cardiologist if the pulse rate with the magnet decreases by 5 or more beats per minute.
   Alternative:
   - Use the telephone transmitter to count the pulse.
   - Turn on the transmitter and connect the electrodes to the body in the same manner that is used for telephone transmission.
   - Count the beeps.

Adapted from Walsh J, Persons CB, Wieck L: Manual of Home Health Care Nursing. Philadelphia, JB Lippincott, 1987

Teaching Plan for Clients with a Permanent Pacemaker

1. Expect minimal incisional discomfort following pacemaker insertion. This can be relieved by acetaminophen or a similar oral pain medication. Chest pain may occur just the same as before the pacemaker insertion. Follow the physician's instructions for treatment of chest pain.

2. Stay on bed rest, with the head no higher than 30 degrees, for 48 to 72 hours after pacemaker insertion to prevent dislodging the electrode. After 72 hours, enough tissue will have formed around the electrode to secure it to the endocardium.

3. Report any signs of infection of the subcutaneous pocket (*e.g.*, redness, drainage, or an unusual amount of pain)

4. Limit vigorous movement of the arms for 6 weeks following surgery to prevent electrode displacement. Resume all previous activities after 6 weeks. Discourage contact sports that could result in chest trauma. Swim, bathe, and shower as desired once the wound has healed. The generator will be watertight.

5. Check the pacemaker function daily by taking the pulse. Do not be concerned if the rate changes slightly from day to day. The pacemaker might be required more on some days than others. The rate should not drop below the present pacemaker rate.

6. Avoid close exposure to sources of electromagnetic interference (EMI), such as heliarc welding equipment, radar installations, malfunctioning electrical appliances or tools, dental treatment devices such as drills and

(continued)

ultrasonic cleaners, internal combustion engines, and microwave ovens with faulty shielding. These can affect pacemaker function. Certain radio frequencies used by ham radio operators and citizen's band radio can affect pacemaker function. The most common frequencies that affect pacemaker function are 3.5 MHz and 28.5 MHz. Internal combustion engines, such as snowmobile engines, car engines, or lawnmower engines, are safe unless the person leans up against them. Hospital devices such as diathermy or electrocautery can affect pacemaker function.

7. Electronic metal detectors used by airport security personnel or libraries will not affect pacemaker function but will set off the alarm. Living near a radar installation such as an airport will not affect pacemaker function. If any device interferes with pacemaker functions as indicated by dizziness or fainting, move away from the source.

8. Check the information received when the pacemaker was inserted to determine whether the pacemaker meets the standards established by the Association for the Advancement of Medical Instrumentation (AAMI). Most pacemakers meet these standards, and the client can be reasonably sure the EMI will not affect pacemaker function.

9. Wear a Medic-Alert bracelet or neck chain. Carry a card that has details of the type of pacemaker.

10. Be prepared for battery replacement at a future date. The leads do not necessarily have to be replaced at the same time. Mercury-zinc batteries last 3 to 5 years, lithium batteries last 7 to 15 years, and nuclear pacemakers last 15 to 20 years.

11. Teach the client that sexual activity can be resumed in 6 weeks.

12. The pulse generator can be easily covered by wearing appropriate clothing. Tight clothing that might put pressure on the incision should be avoided (*e.g.*, tight bra straps).

Adapted from: Walsh J, Persons CB, Wieck L: Manual of Home Health Care Nursing. Philadelphia, JB Lippincott, 1987

In summary, positioning, administration of NTG, and notification of the client's physician are key interventions in dealing with an acute decrease in cardiac output related to ischemia. Careful assessment for signs of a slow loss of cardiac function are indicated for the nonacute state.

Outcomes

Successful interventions will result in an absence of acute angina and signs of an adequate cardiac output.

INEFFECTIVE BREATHING PATTERNS

The relative decrease in oxygen available to the tissues caused by inadequate cardiac output excites a reflex mechanism that sends a message to the brain to increase the rate of respirations. The vasomotor center, which controls heart activity and peripheral vasoconstriction, is also closely related to the respiratory center in the brain. Any factor that increases activity in the vasomotor center also has some effect on increasing respirations. Therefore, clients with myocardial ischemia typically have "shortness of breath."

For clients who have had bypass surgery, breathing often causes incisional pain, especially with deep inspirations. These clients often breathe rapid, shallow respirations to ease this discomfort.

Assessment

The rate and depth of respirations should be assessed. The symmetry of chest wall motion, use of accessory muscles, and adequacy of ventilatory effort are also important. The client's subjective statement regarding whether he is "getting enough air" provides insight into whether his effort is adequate. Breath sounds should be ascultated and absent or adventitious sounds noted.

Interventions

Since the etiology of the ineffective breathing pattern is different for medical and surgical clients, they will be discussed separately.

The client experiencing chest pain with shortness of breath should have oxygen administered via nasal cannula, if available. This intervention simply makes more oxygen available should the client be hypoxemic. Positioning in a semi-Fowler's or high-Fowler's position also facilitates ventilation. Constrictive clothing around the neck or chest should be loosened. Pain relief with NTG is a high priority in this situation.

For the client with a sternotomy incision, interventions are aimed at pain relief and continued ventilatory exercise. Clients should use analgesics prescribed after discharge from the hospital if they are unable to do deep breathing exercises because of incisional discomfort. This is generally a short-term problem and resolves as the chest heals.

Breath sounds, if abnormal, require similar interventions. For both types of clients rales suggest fluid overload. If they are increased over the client's baseline examination the nurse should evaluate the medicines the client is taking and *whether* these medications are being taken. If the client is not on any diuretic therapy and has increased rales on examination, the physician should be consulted.

Outcomes

The interventions should result in adequate ventilation as evidenced by a normal rate and depth of respirations and absence of severe "shortness of breath," rales, or use of accessory muscles of respiration (trapezius, sternocleidomastoid).

ALTERATION IN COMFORT: PAIN

As described earlier, the chest pain of angina is a result of oxygen demand in excess of supply to the heart muscle. For the surgical client with a sternal incision, chest pain may be incisional in nature, although he may also experience angina.

Assessment

Differentiating incisional pain from angina may be accomplished by having the client describe the pain. Terms such as "crushing," "tightness," "takes my breath away," and "radiates to the shoulder, neck, or jaw" suggest ischemia. Clients may describe incisional pain as occurring on deep breaths only and often are able to differentiate it from "heart pain." Taking a history of the pain including precipitating factors, methods of relief, and associated symptoms is useful. Angina may be quantified as described earlier on a scale of 1 to 10. This scale is useful for evaluating whether interventions are helping to relieve the pain.

Interventions

Angina is best relieved with rest, positioning as described earlier (either sitting or maintaining a head-up position), and administration of NTG at 5-minute intervals for three doses. Intervention is also aimed at prevention of angina. Determining the precipitating factors with the client and identifying strategies to prevent their occurrence may be effective. This may require significant changes in life-style that the client may or may not be willing to make. (This will be discussed further under *noncompliance*.)

If the chest pain is an evolving MI, the client will need further interventions, including hospitalization. In this case NTG administration alone may not resolve the pain.

For incisional discomfort in the CABG client, analgesics as prescribed should be administered. In order to prevent severe discomfort, the administration of analgesics may precede breathing exercises.

Outcomes

The goal of nursing therapy is the absence of anginal chest pain. For the surgical client, steadily diminishing incisional pain until it is absent is the objective.

ACTIVITY INTOLERANCE

Activity in clients with coronary artery disease (CAD) may be limited due to the client's lack of understanding, frequent precipitation of angina, or as a result of immobility imposed by hospitalizations. The effects of prolonged bedrest include decreased physical work capacity (hypoventilation and decreased cardiac reserve), diminished vasomotor reflex, increased potential for thromboembolic events, nitrogen and protein loss from muscle disuse, and loss of skeletal muscle mass and strength. Physical activity minimizes these deconditioning effects, may minimize anxiety and depression, and may enhance body image.

Clients who have had a simple MI are typically on bed rest with or without bedside commode use for 48 hours. Clients who have had CABG surgery are usually on bed rest for 24 hours and only out of bed in a chair for the next 24 hours. Activity is progressed throughout the hospital stay so that by discharge both types of clients are generally ambulating about the room and corridors and performing personal hygiene activities.

Assessment

Assessment of activity tolerance may be accomplished by discussing with the client what activities he can and cannot do. This may be contrasted with the client's activity level prior to a recent MI or surgical procedure. Data may be obtained by observation, such as, does the client get short of breath while talking on the telephone, coming down the stairs or eating a meal? Family members may have valuable and objective input on changes in the client's activity tolerance. Depending on the client's response to his illness and possible grief response he may or may not be able to identify changes in his level of activity.

Exercise tolerance can be monitored by pulse and blood pressure measurement (BP) before and after exercise. If the BP drops by 20 mm Hg or more, the pulse increases by 20% of the resting rate (or climbs higher than 120), or chest pain develops, the activity level is decreased. These criteria demonstrate that the client's cardiovascular system is not yet ready for the activity.

Specific activities are graded on cardiac rehabilitation charts in terms of energy expenditure. The client's current level of activity may be identified within the framework of a cardiac rehabilitation chart in order to identify progress as interventions are made.

Interventions

Interventions generally are directed at promoting the maximal level of activity achievable given the client's disease state. This maximum activity is different for every client. Therefore, increasing levels of activity should be monitored, guided by common sense on

Activity Guidelines

1. Just after discharge from the hospital, personal hygiene activities such as shaving, bathing, using the toilet, and getting dressed should be acceptable activities.

2. Avoid activities that require the arms to be raised over the head for prolonged periods, such as curling the hair.

3. Plan periods of rest and relaxation with specific amounts of time.

4. Activity should take into account the weather and location of activity (*e.g.*, whether the surface is level or hilly).

5. Avoid extremes of temperature. For example, during winter, walk in the shopping mall.

6. Know how to evaluate fatigue.

7. Encourage quiet recreational activities such as taking short rides, watching television, and reading.

8. Sexual intercourse may usually be resumed as soon as the client is able to climb a flight of stairs or accomplish 5 METS of work on the exercise stress test. (Additional information on this is presented later in the chapter.)

9. Returning to work should be guided by the cardiologist.

10. If travelling, the client should carry a medical summary and sufficient medication.

the part of the client, and done in consultation with the physician. If the client is not in a supervised cardiac rehabilitation program, specific information should be provided by the physician regarding pulse limits, specific activities, and precautions. Some general guidelines for clients are shown below.

Interventions should facilitate assimilation of these guidelines into daily activities on the part of the client. The client should be encouraged to live as fully as possible.

After a CABG procedure the client's potential exercise tolerance is generally improved over the preoperative state once the client has recovered from surgery. Some activity restrictions are imposed on postoperative clients during the early convalescent period (about 4 to 6 weeks). Examples of these are outlined in the box below.

Outcome

Evidence of successful interventions is demonstrated by a client who maintains the maximal possible activity level within the limits imposed by his cardiac function.

Activity Restrictions

1. Avoid driving for 4 weeks to allow time for the sternum to begin healing. The risk of traumatic injury from a steering wheel in the event of an accident is serious.

2. Avoid lifting, pushing, or pulling anything heavier than 10 pounds.

3. Take time climbing stairs.

4. Activities such as working at the computer, dusting, doing dishes are acceptable.

SELF-CARE DEFICIT

If a client with coronary artery disease is ill to the extent that a self-care deficit exists, it is often due to the repeated effects of ischemia on the ventricular muscle. This results in a loss of functional muscle mass and a decreased ejection fraction (normal is about 60%). This type of client lives with some chronic degree of ventricular failure and will be considered in the next section on ventricular dysfunction.

DISTURBANCE IN SELF-CONCEPT: ROLE PERFORMANCE

Clients who develop angina, have a "heart attack," or who have "open heart surgery," are at high risk for disturbed self-concept. These conditions are known to be life-threatening and the client may find himself confronting his own mortality at a relatively young age. Such a client often has a difficult time adapting to his medical condition and may experience grief in response to his perceived loss of youth, health, or function. His perceptions of himself in his respective roles as parent, spouse, worker, or financial supporter are often changed. Family members and friends as well may respond differently to the client. These changes in outlook may or may not accompany significantly decreased physical capacity.

Although the client may appraise his situation realistically, make appropriate life-style changes, and receive tremendous support from his family, quite often this is not the case. There may be complete denial, outbursts of anger, feelings of inadequacy, or depression.

Assessment

Assessment of factors contributing to this problem begin with establishing and maintaining a relationship with the client and family. The client's sentiments regarding the illness may be elicited during individual client education sessions as he describes his current health status. The client's feelings are likely to surface if asked about life-style changes that are planned or have been implemented, or how his family is responding to his illness.

The assessment should be guided by a realistic appraisal, in consultation with the physician, of the client's physical capacity. Changes in role function may be necessary; however, a disturbed self-concept does not have to accompany them.

Interventions

Interventions are directed towards assisting the client in adopting to appropriate life-style changes and fostering a strong sense of self-worth. There are many approaches that are useful in this situation. For example, persons often tend to see only the negative side of change that is forced upon them. Assisting the client and family in identifying positive outcomes, areas of progress, or alternate ways of fulfilling specific role functions are some strategies. Just providing an opportunity for the client to express frustration is effective. These interventions are predicated on having established a positive professional relationship with the client and family.

Outcome

The objective is to assist the client in maintaining or developing self-esteem in the face of real or potential changes in role function.

ANXIETY

Anxiety may be present in clients with CAD as a result of a recent change in their health status (such as a recent MI) or due to a perceived threat of death. It may be related to a lack of knowledge about their illness or a perceived loss of control over their life.

Assessment

Anxiety is difficult to assess objectively and is therefore more likely determined by the client's report of having vague feelings of uneasiness or concern. These feelings are more likely to be reported to the health professional with whom the client has a continuous trusting relationship and only if given the opportunity.

Interventions

Relief of anxiety may be accomplished by mutually identifying the underlying cause of this uneasiness. If the client is anxious about his ability to care for himself, specific review of his daily needs and what he is able to do may relieve this anxiety. Anxiety from the threat of death may reflect a lack of understanding of the disease process and medical interventions. Strategies to deal with this situation are discussed under "knowledge deficit." If the threat of death is a realistic concern, consulting a professional counselor may be indicated. Some families deal with their anxiety by obtaining training in cardiopulmonary resuscitation and establishing contingency plans in the event of an emergency. The home health nurse should encourage the family to participate in these classes.

If the basis of the client's anxiety is related to a perceived loss of control over his life, interventions should be directed toward identifying areas where he does have control. For example, although there is no cure for CAD, the client does have control over several of its risk factors. (See the following discussion of cardiac risk factors.)

Outcomes

The objective of these interventions is to decrease the client's anxiety by identifying the cause(s) and giving the client tools with which to alleviate his concerns.

KNOWLEDGE DEFICIT RELATED TO PATHOPHYSIOLOGY OF DISEASE STATE AND CARDIAC RISK FACTORS

Clients receive varying amounts of information during their hospitalizations and are in varying states of readiness to receive this information. Therefore, their retention of the facts regarding their disease state and how to care for themselves should be evaluated in the home setting. There is, quite often, a gap between what the client understands and what health-care providers want him to understand. The subjects for education include the pathophysiology of the disease state, cardiac risk factor modification, and drug therapy.

Assessment

Assessment of the client's current understanding may be accomplished when he is rested and motivated to participate in such a discussion. There has to be readiness to learn on the part of the client or interventions are ineffective. Another area that should be evaluated prior to education is the client's intellectual level. This will influence the approach the nurse takes in giving information (such as the use of audiovisual aids, written pamphlets, etc.).

Interventions

Interventions are designed to educate the client about coronary artery disease, cardiac risk factor modification, and the medications currently prescribed for them. This includes instruction on coronary blood flow, atherosclerosis, angina, and myocardial infarction. Progression of CAD and interventions such as cardiac catheterization, balloon angioplasty, and CABG procedures should be discussed. Education on cardiac risk factor modification includes uncontrollable risk factors such as family history, gender, and age. The controllable risk factors should be discussed at length including smoking, hypertension, elevated serum cholesterol and triglycerides, diabetes, obesity, lack of exercise, and stress. The client should identify his risk factors and develop a personal plan to modify them where appropriate (see standard teaching plan on cardiac risk factors). When dietary modifications are discussed it is important for the person who prepared the meals to clearly understand the information. Diet planning is facilitated by the use of printed instructions or guidelines. Literature is often available in local communities that assist in this area. The local chapter of the American Heart Association has excellent literature that can be beneficial to the client and family. A consultation with a dietitian may be indicated.

Instruction on the client's current medications, including their purpose, dose, time, and side-effects, should be given. There are commercially produced cards that include this information and that can be used to aid in this instruction. The client keeps the cards and can review them whenever necessary. Some medicines require that additional skills be taught such as pulsetaking with digoxin.

The presence and inclusion of the spouse or significant other is very important as lifestyle changes usually affect family members as well as the client. Some guidelines that facilitate the learning process in client education for adults are shown in the box at right.

Outcomes

Goals include the client having a clear understanding of his disease process, a plan to modify his controllable risk factors, and the knowledge to administer his own medica-

---

Client Education Principles

1. Allow the client to be in control of his own learning, including WHEN, HOW FAST, and HOW MUCH.

2. Give information for which the client has USE.

3. Build on his PRIOR EXPERIENCE.

4. Allow him to PARTICIPATE.

5. Acknowledge his CURRENT KNOWLEDGE.

6. Make sure he is COMFORTABLE.

---

tions correctly, including those on a "p.r.n." basis.

NONCOMPLIANCE

Probably one of the most costly and frustrating problems in health care is noncompliance. It is difficult to understand why a client continues to do something he knows will harm him or not do something he knows will help him. What health care providers view as a single choice in complying with medical therapy is actually many choices that the client must make daily.

It is helpful to deal with this problem with an understanding of the factors influencing the client's decision to follow medical therapy. One simple model that logically addresses this problem is the Health Belief Model. It is based on the following four points.

1. *Susceptibility*: The client must believe he has the disease or is susceptible to it.
2. *Severity*: The client must feel the disease is potentially harmful to him; he must feel a sense of vulnerability.

3. *Benefits*: The client must believe that the medical therapy is beneficial and will help him.
4. *Costs*: The disadvantages of following the medical therapy must not outweigh the benefits. (See Chapter 4 for a more complete discussion of client education and health teaching).

Some specific components of the "costs" of following medical therapy have to do with how complex the therapy is, how accessible it is, how long the therapy must be continued, what side-effects accompany the therapy, and whether a whole new pattern of behavior must be developed.

Assessment

In assessing the client who has an identified problem with compliance, the nurse should determine what the client knows about his illness. This eliminates knowledge deficit as the source of the problem. Determine the client's daily routine to identify changes he would have to make to follow the therapy. This helps identify the "costs." The nurse may ask the client whether he intends to follow the therapy. The questions can follow the four points in the health belief model to find out what is influencing the client so he will not comply.

If the client is in denial, a response that is frequently seen, he does not believe he is "susceptible." He may think he has a very minor case of angina and therefore may decide not to follow the diet. This suggests the "severity" component has not been satisfied. Some clients do not believe that a low-fat diet will make any difference in their disease. The "benefits" component has not been satisfied and the client probably will not follow the diet. A client may continue to smoke cigarettes even though he has CAD and knows that smoking is dangerous. For these clients,

perhaps the "costs" of adopting a different behavior pattern outweigh the benefits.

If an assessment is done along the format of this model, the specific reasons for non-compliance may be identified.

Interventions

Interventions should be directed at whatever component is not satisfied in the Health Belief Model. The nurse can support, encourage, and instruct the client. Community resources can be used in referral, such as smoking cessation clinics, dietitian consultations, and exercise physiology consultations. The client's health status can be reviewed, the severity of the disease state underscored, the benefits of medical therapy reinforced, and strategies to decrease the obstacles to compliance discussed. Ultimately, it is the client's decision whether or not to comply with the treatment prescribed. The health-care provider should communicate her respect for this fact to the client.

Outcomes

Interventions are directed at facilitating compliance with the prescribed medical regimen. This includes activity guidelines, diet, medications, avoidance of stress and smoking, weight loss if necessary, diabetic control, and attendance at follow-up appointments.

SEXUAL DYSFUNCTION

There is a substantial incidence of sexual dysfunction, such as impotence, orgasmic difficulties, and decreased libido among men and women who have cardiac disease. These problems are infrequently due to organic problems or drug therapy. For many clients with CAD, sexual dysfunction is related to anxiety, depression, avoidance, lack of knowledge, and poor self-esteem. This situation is exacerbated by a lack of adequate instruction by health-care professionals on resumption of sexual activity after infarction or bypass surgery.

The cardiac client's concerns include (1) fear that intercourse will lead to sudden death; (2) fear that medical advice will preclude sexual activity; (3) fear that sexual performance will be inadequate; (4) concern that sexual activity may cause another infarction; (5) concern that illness signals aging and diminished sexual ability. These concerns are unabated by discharge instructions that include extensive information about diet restrictions and when to take medications. The absence of specific instruction on resumption of sexual activity can inadvertently suggest to the client that this activity is risky.

Physiologically, martial coitus has been compared to activities such as climbing a flight of stairs, walking briskly, or performing usual work activities associated with many occupations. It was also felt to be equivalent to 5 METS of work on the exercise stress test. This comparison was made based on research that measured mean peak heart rates in the 120s and blood pressures of up to 162/89 mm Hg at orgasm. Participation in an exercise training program was found to decrease the peak measures of cardiovascular stress during coitus. The physiologic cost of sexual activity differs in individuals and counseling should take into account concurrent illnesses, drug therapy, and other physical limitations. There is no information about the physiologic cost of extramarital coitus.

Regarding drug therapy, there are sexual side-effects of some drugs commonly prescribed for cardiac clients, most notably the antihypertensives. There is great variability in drug effects from person to person. This is related to factors such as body weight, dose, rate of absorption and excretion, interaction with other drugs, and compliance with a medication schedule. Much of the available information on sexual side-effects have been studied in men.

Some drugs that have been implicated in causing impotence, decreased libido, impaired arousal, or retarded ejaculation include thiazide diuretics, spironolactone, alpha-methyldopa, guanethidine, and furosemide. (Specific difficulties associated with specific drugs are beyond the scope of this text and the reader is encouraged to consult the references at the end of the chapter.) Antihypertensive drugs that have been reported to be relatively free of sexual side-effects include hydralazine and propanolol.

Assessment

Advice on return to sexual activity should be given with some knowledge of previous sexual patterns of the client. If a client had difficulty with sexual functioning prior to his MI, this must be considered in giving suggestions after an MI. The subject should be handled nonjudgmentally, as a normal physical activity. There should be an ongoing professional relationship in which rapport and trust have been developed. Advanced age should not preclude this discussion; with advancing age sexual response may become slower but there is no physiologic reason for it to stop.

Interventions

When giving information on return to sexual activity the client's partner should be included. This hopefully will prevent the partner from feeling sexual activity should be avoided in order to "protect" the client. The partners are subject to the same fears as the client.

For the client who has had an MI or cardiac surgery that was not complicated with cardiac failure or arrhythmias, and who can sustain a heart rate of 110 to 120 beats per minute without having angina or shortness of breath, sexual activity can be resumed. This advice should be given in consultation with the physician. For many clients post-MI, this means return to sexual activity may safely occur about 2 to 4 weeks after discharge from the hospital.

Gradual increases in activity should take place over time. The nurse, client, or significant other can do pulse checks before and after activity such as climbing a flight of stairs to check heart rate response to physical exertion. The nurse can also advise the client of the guidelines shown opposite.

In dealing with the fears and concerns identified earlier, interventions should be directed at creating an atmosphere in which the client can express concerns and receive factual information. With appropriate information much of the client's anxiety can be eliminated or prevented. It is possible that problems with sexual function are significant and warrant counseling by a professional trained in this area. If so, referral should be made.

Outcomes

Client goals include resumption of sexual activity to the maximum physical capacity and satisfaction of the client and partner. Excessive concern and fear related to sexual activity are minimized.

PROBLEMS RELATED TO PERIPHERAL CIRCULATION

Peripheral vascular disease is a term that applies to several medical diseases in which perfusion of blood and oxygen to an extremity is inadequate. One of the most common causes of arterial occlusive disease is atherosclerosis. This condition involves a thickening of the intimal lining of the affected artery,

---

Guidelines for Resumption of Sexual Activity

1. Resumption of sexual activity should proceed gradually, in comfortable positions. Positions that require isometric muscle contraction should be avoided since these positions cause a greater increase in heart rate.

2. The client should avoid sexual activity immediately after meals or alcohol consumption. Alcohol decreases cardiac output and meals cause a diversion of blood flow to the gut.

3. If symptoms of chest pain occur during intercourse, the client should slow down or stop the activity. This can be discussed further with the physician.

4. The client and his spouse should be encouraged to speak freely and directly with each other about their feelings regarding sex to avoid misconceptions that commonly occur in this situation.

5. Resumption of sexual activity is least stressful in familiar surroundings with the client's usual partner. Caressing and foreplay help prepare the heart gradually for the activity.

---

along with the accumulation of fibrous tissue and deposits of lipids and calcium. The vessel becomes less elastic and the lumen progressively narrowed. Mechanical stress exacerbates this problem by leading to platelet aggregation at the site.

The effects of this occlusion depend on the location of the vessel, extent of its occlusion, adequacy of collateral circulation, and the degree of associated arterial spasm.

(Text continues on p 247)

ABBREVIATED CARE PLAN: PROBLEMS RELATED TO CORONARY BLOOD FLOW

Nursing Diagnosis	Assessment	Interventions	Outcomes
Decrease in Cardiac Output Related to Ischemia	Heart rate Regularity of rhythm Blood pressure Peripheral pulses Urine output Level of consciousness	Have patient rest. Administer NTG sublingually q 5 minutes X 3 for persistent pain. Position patient in semi-Fowler's. Loosen restrictive clothing. Monitor pulse and BP for signs of compromise.	Adequate cardiac output: strong peripheral pulses, normal heart rate, regular pulse, absence of chest pain, alert and oriented
Ineffective Breathing Patterns	Rate, depth of respirations Symmetry of chest wall motion Use of accessory muscles Adequacy of ventilatory effort Patient subjective indication of adequacy of ventilation Breath sounds	Monitor ventilatory status for increasing fatigue. Administer oxygen by nasal cannula. Position in semi-Fowler's. Loosen constrictive clothing. Auscultate breath sounds for presence of rales. Treat chest pain.	Adequate ventilation: normal rate and depth of respirations, absence of severe shortness of breath, rales or used accessory muscles
Alteration in Comfort: Pain	Pain history Precipitating factors Methods of relief Use scale of 1 – 10	Differentiate angina from incisional pain. Administer NTG, position in semi-Fowler's for angina. Administer analgesics as ordered for incisional pain. Identify strategies to decrease frequency of anginal episodes.	Absence of angina; absence of severe incisional discomfort

ABBREVIATED CARE PLAN: PROBLEMS RELATED TO CORONARY BLOOD FLOW (continued)

Nursing Diagnosis	Assessment	Interventions	Outcomes
Activity Intolerance	Current level of activity Expected level of activity per M.D.	Identify with patient activities that can be resumed safely (see guidelines page). Encourage patient to be as active as he is able. Facilitate participation in regular exercise.	Maintenance of maximal possible activity level within limits of cardiac function.
Disturbance in Self-concept	Readiness for discussion Patient's view of life-style changes related to illness	Establish environment that facilitates sharing of patient concerns. Assist patient and family in identifying positive outcomes. Identify alternate methods of fulfilling roles.	Maintenance or development of self-esteem in light of real or potential changes in role function
Anxiety	Patient feelings of uneasiness or concern	Assist patient in identifying cause of anxiety. Educate patient on disease process. Refer to counselor if indicated. Identify areas patient has control over, i.e., risk factor modification.	Decrease anxiety
Knowledge Deficit re: Pathophysiology of Disease State, Cardiac Risk Factors	Patient's current level of understanding Intellectual level Readiness to learn	Educate patient on coronary artery disease. Give specifics on atherosclerosis, angina, and MI. Give information on risk factors: family history,	Clear understanding of disease process, modification of controllable risk factors, self-administration of medicines

(continued)

ABBREVIATED CARE PLAN: PROBLEMS RELATED TO CORONARY BLOOD FLOW *(continued)*

Nursing Diagnosis	Assessment	Interventions	Outcomes
		gender, age, smoking, hypertension, elevated cholesterol and triglycerides, diabetes mellitus, obesity, lack of exercise and stress.	
		Educate patient on drug therapy.	
		Include spouse, significant other, or family in education.	
Noncompliance	Knowledge deficit	Determine how patient's behavior fits the Health Belief Model.	Compliance with medical regimen including activity, diet
	Evidence of noncompliance		
	Patient report of noncompliance	Susceptibility	Follow-up appointments
		Severity	Medications
		Benefits	If necessary; stress avoidance; smoking cessation; weight loss; diabetic control
		Cost	
		Instruct, support, encourage patient.	
		Make community resources available.	
		Communicate respect for fact that it is the patient's decision.	
Sexual Dysfunction	Patient/partner satisfaction	Consult with M.D. on specific restrictions.	Resumption of sexual activity to capacity and satisfaction of patient and partner.
	Current sexual function	Include partner in education.	
	Previous patterns of sexual activity	Create atmosphere that facilitates patient's expression of concern, receipt of facts.	
	Current drug therapy		
	Patient/partner knowledge on resumption of sexual activity	Give information on resumption of sexual activity.	

Risk factors associated with the development of arterial occlusive problems include male gender, middle age, hyperlipidemia, hypertension, cigarette smoking, and diabetes mellitus.

Aside from atherosclerosis, there are many other medical diseases that cause problems with peripheral circulation such as the use of birth control pills, vessel trauma, inflammatory diseases, and hypoperfusion states. These diseases share in common a detrimental effect on tissue perfusion. It is from the perspective of inadequate tissue perfusion that these peripheral vascular diseases are presented.

NURSING DIAGNOSES

In the following pages, the nursing diagnoses related to alterations in peripheral circulation are discussed.

ALTERATION IN TISSUE PERFUSION

Assessment

Acute occlusion from the build-up of a thrombus associated with the narrowed area or from an arterial embolus is manifested by coldness, pain, paresthesia, cyanosis, and absence of a pulse in the affected extremity. Another presentation of this problem is worsening claudication over a period of several hours, coolness, numbness, weakness, and eventually absence of sensation. This latter presentation can progress without the sensation of pain.

Chronic atherosclerotic arterial occlusion may cause pain at rest that is dull and aching (often worst at night) along with coolness, numbness, and ulcer formation in the extremity. Lower leg ischemia is associated with thin, dry skin, muscle atrophy, the absence of subcutaneous fat, coolness to touch, and toenail changes (thick, brittle, or ridged toenails). The presence of blisters, flexion contractures of digits, skin swelling, or gangrene may accompany this problem.

If the client at home has been diagnosed to have a disease that interferes with arterial circulation, progression of the symptoms identified may be documented. (Development of acute arterial occlusion is a medical emergency and the client should be referred to a hospital emergency room.)

Interventions

Nursing care of the affected extremity is guided by maximizing conditions that favor development of collateral circulation, maximizing vasodilatation, and minimizing vasoconstriction. Vasodilatation is enhanced by positioning the affected extremity in a position 15 degrees below the level of the heart. Placing shock blocks under the head of the bed to raise it 12 to 16 inches places the legs in a dependent position for sleep. With occlusive disease in the lower aorta, iliac, or femoral region this position facilitates blood flow by gravity to underperfused legs. Maintenance of a warm environment (80°–85°) favors vasodilatation.

Vasoconstriction is caused by drugs (such as beta blockers, *i.e.*, propanolol) and cigarette smoking. Interventions to enhance tissue perfusion include counseling the client on the effect of cigarette use. The primary physician should be consulted to resolve any questions regarding drug therapy. Other activities that interfere with perfusion include crossing legs and wearing restrictive clothing or shoes. The nurse can counsel the client on avoidance of these activities, if indicated.

In some types of arterial occlusive disease, such as microemboli, nitroglycerine ointment is placed topically to enhance circulation. This measure is not universally effective with all types of peripheral vascular disease.

Vasodilator therapy is not generally useful in chronic peripheral atherosclerotic disease.

The affected extremity should be washed in lukewarm water with nonmedicated soap. Lanolin is applied to prevent the development of skin fissures. Strong antiseptics should be avoided. This care is designed to minimize potential trauma to tissue that heals poorly due to poor perfusion.

If there is skin breakdown, cleansing may be done with hydrogen peroxide or povodine iodine solution and the site covered gently with sterile dressings. Pressure areas should be padded and collouses or corns should not be trimmed. Infections of lesions on the extremity should be referred promptly to the physician for antibiotic therapy and debridement of necrotic or purulent material.

Many clients have surgical interventions for peripheral vascular disease, including sympathectomy to prevent vasoconstriction and to minimize pain at rest. Reconstructive procedures either replace the diseased artery with a vascular graft or bypass the diseased area to generate blood flow distal to the occlusion.

Interventions for postsurgical clients include monitoring for signs of inadequate tissue perfusion as described in the assessment. Pulses may be documented as strong, weak, only present by Doppler sound, or absent. This framework minimizes subjective interpretation of the quality of a pulse. Care of the extremity is as described earlier, as the aim continues to be promoting vasodilatation and preventing vasoconstriction. The physician may or may not want to continue use of shock blocks to tilt the bed.

Finally, collateral circulation is enhanced by exercise. A regular exercise program creates increased metabolic demand in the tissues distal to the occluded site. Regular stimulation of this sort encourages dilatation of nonoccluded vessels and enrichment of capillary beds. Central to this concept is the regularity of exercise. Exercise should not be overdone so as to cause significant discomfort to the client. Rather, the client should perform activity that is comfortable and effective. Brisk walking is an example of exercise conducive to perfusion of the legs. Referral to cardiovascular rehabilitation services may be indicated. Activity should be designed in consultation with the physician. A referral to physical therapy may also be needed.

Outcomes

Assisting the client in developing collateral circulation, enhancing vasodilatation, and avoiding vasoconstriction are the client goals. Avoidance of trauma to the affected extremity is included as impaired perfusion interferes with tissue healing. Successful interventions are evidenced by arresting the progression of signs or symptoms of ischemia and prevention of tissue breakdown.

ALTERATION IN COMFORT: PAIN

Pain in the affected extremity usually accompanies peripheral vascular disease. The discomfort is related to inadequate oxygen delivery to the muscles in the extremity. Physical activity often stimulates the pain that may be relieved with rest. However, as the disease progresses and the arterial lumen narrows still further, the client may experience pain at rest.

Assessment

Gathering a profile on the client's pain is helpful in developing strategies to deal with it. Muscle pain from ischemia varies in intensity, frequency, quality, and activities that cause it. It is described as dull and throbbing, or very sharp. Some clients experience this muscle pain most often at night, while others have more difficulty when walking.

Interventions

Many of the interventions discussed in the previous section on altered tissue perfusion apply to this problem as well. Interventions are guided by improving perfusion to the extremity as one method of relieving pain.

Analgesics may be prescribed by the client's physician. The nurse may assist the client in deciding how to manage the pain. For example, if the pain is worst at night and the bed has already been placed on shock blocks, analgesic administration before sleep may be indicated. However, if the pain is worst when climbing stairs, perhaps altering the frequency of this activity or the speed with which stairs are climbed would diminish the discomfort.

Outcomes

Improving circulation to the affected extremity, use of analgesics and modifying physical activity are all methods to achieve the goal of pain relief. Depending upon the individual client and the extent of disease present, absence of ischemic pain, fewer episodes of pain, or arresting the progression of pain are goals for consideration. Obtaining a full night of uninterrupted sleep is an appropriate goal for clients who lose sleep as a direct result of pain from impaired perfusion.

SENSORY–PERCEPTUAL ALTERATION: TACTILE

As arterial occlusive disease progresses, clients may develop paresthesias such as tingling, burning, or numbness. Eventually, impaired perfusion of the nerve supply to the extremity may cause partial or total loss of sensation.

Assessment

Sensation may be assessed in an organized manner from the distal end of the extremity moving proximally until "normal" sensation is achieved. Complete sensory examination may include testing for touch, pressure, movement, vibration, pain, or temperature.

Interventions

Once a deficit in sensation is detected interventions are identified to protect the affected extremity from trauma and infection. Some measures that may be suggested to the client are listed in the boxed material below.

Outcomes

The objective is to prevent traumatic injury to the underperfused extremity. If injury does occur, it should be cared for as described in the section on altered tissue perfusion.

Interventions to Protect Extremity from Trauma

1. Avoid use of concentrated heat.

2. Wear foot coverings to avoid unintentional trauma.

3. Examine extremity for signs of trauma.

4. Prevent excess pressure from bedsheets.

5. Footwear should be well fitted, nonconstrictive.

6. Use common sense in preventing injury to extremity.

SEXUAL DYSFUNCTION

Vascular disease that interferes with blood supply to the penis can interfere with the vasocongestive changes necessary for erection in the male. Although the study of sexual dysfunction in the female with similar occlusive disease is not described, it is likely that the engorgement of the pelvis that leads to vaginal lubrication may also be affected.

Clients with vascular occlusion at the bifurcation of the aorta are at risk for sexual dysfunction. They are typically also symptomatic for vascular insufficiency in the lower extremities. Surgical repair of such a lesion may resolve the dysfunction. However, the surgery may interfere with the nerve supply to the sex organs, creating sexual dysfunction. Organic sexual dysfunction such as that encountered in clients with peripheral vascular disease should be referred to a physician trained in this area.

Assessment

In clients with signs of arterial occlusive disease in both lower extremities, the nurse may assess for sexual dysfunction during an interview. The client may describe difficulty with arousal, erection, ejaculation, vaginal lubrication, or orgasm. This discussion should occur after a trusting professional relationship has been established. The client or partner may bring up the issue with the home-care nurse.

Interventions

Referral should be made promptly to the client's primary physician. If the dysfunction is not organic and is related to some other cause, the nurse may intervene as described in the section on coronary artery disease or refer the client to a certified sex therapist.

Outcome

Normal sexual function is ideally achieved. With organic disease, hopefully satisfactory sexual function is achieved.

PROBLEMS RELATED TO VENTRICULAR FUNCTION

In a cardiovascular system that functions normally, the heart serves as a pump to transport oxygen to the tissues. The heart's effectiveness as a pump relies on a healthy myocardium, proper hydration, functional valves, and the absence of significant resistance to systolic ejection. There are several disease states that can result in failure of the heart to meet the body's metabolic needs.

PATHOPHYSIOLOGY

Cardiomyopathy is a disease state in which cardiac muscle cells are dysfunctional. The causes of cardiomyopathy are either ischemic or idiopathic. Clients with coronary artery disease and a history of myocardial infarctions may have eventually destroyed enough muscle to render the heart an ineffective pump. Idiopathic cardiomyopathy is believed to be caused by viral disease or some other unknown cause. The results are similar in that the diseased muscle cells cannot contract effectively and cardiac output is diminished.

Regardless of the cause, the client's ejection fraction (percent of ventricular volume ejected with each beat) is decreased and perfusion of vital organs is adversely affected. As blood accumulates in a ventricle unable to eject its volume, pressure begins to build. Increased pressure in the left ventricle interferes with emptying of the left atrium. As pressure builds in the left atrium with blood that can not move into the left ventricle, pulmonary blood flow is affected. Blood accumulates in the pulmonary vasculature, disrupting pressure relationships there that guide the flow of fluid. This "back-up" of blood favors extravasation of fluid into the pulmonary interstitium as the lymphatic system is overtaxed. The result is pulmonary edema and impaired diffusion of oxygen and carbon dioxide between alveoli and pulmonary capillaries. If allowed to progress, the dysfunctional pulmonary perfusion creates increased work for the right ventricle, which is not accustomed to dealing with elevated pressures. This can result in right ventricular failure and accumulation of fluid in the right ventricle and right atrium. Central venous engorgement follows and may be identified by jugular engorgement, hepatojugular reflux, and right upper quadrant tenderness from liver engorgement. Increased venous pressures result in disrupted fluid flow in the capillaries with a net extravasation of fluid into the interstitium. Peripheral edema is often noted, especially in the lower extremities.

This situation is exacerbated by poor perfusion of vital organs from low cardiac output. The kidneys, experiencing low perfusion pressures, begin conserving fluid. The increased fluid load worsens the situation because the heart is unable to deal with the fluid with which it has already been presented.

Valvular dysfunction can also lead to ventricular failure. As the aortic valve becomes stenotic, it creates tremendous resistance to ventricular ejection. The ventricle hypertrophies in order to overcome the resistance but eventually fails in response to this excessive work.

In aortic insufficiency, blood finds its way back into the left ventricle after it has been ejected through the aortic valve. The cusps fail to approximate allowing leakage that can be significant in volume. The excess fluid load in the left ventricle causes dilatation of the chamber as a compensatory mechanism. Eventually systolic function deteriorates and left ventricular pressure rises. The ensuing picture of congestive failure occurs as described above.

Mitral regurgitation creates similar problems in that a portion of the left ventricular volume is ejected back to the left atrium instead of to the aorta. The left atrium dilates with the elevated pressure and volume load. Again, progression to congestive heart failure occurs as described earlier.

Hypertension can also lead to ventricular failure. With high diastolic pressures the heart must generate significant wall tension to build pressure high enough to open the aortic valve and eject blood. Over a prolonged period of time this excessive afterload (resistance to ventricular emptying) results in left ventricular failure. Left-sided failure may progress to right-sided failure, again as described earlier.

Congestive heart failure (CHF) can result from any of the pathologic conditions described above. Ventricular function is impaired, fluid tends to accumulate in both pulmonary and peripheral interstitial spaces, gas exchange is impaired, and vital organs are underperfused. While untreated failure eventually leads to death, clients may live with varying levels of compensation for their ventricular dysfunction.

NURSING DIAGNOSES

The nurse's approach to the client with ventricular dysfunction is similar, regardless of etiology. Therefore, clients with ventricular failure from valve disease, cardiomyopathy, and hypertension will be considered together.

CARDIAC OUTPUT RELATED TO VENTRICULAR FAILURE

Assessment

Clients with ventricular failure exhibit physical signs consistent with the "back-up" of fluid in the cardiopulmonary system. These include increased heart rate, respiratory rate, orthopnea, and elevated jugular venous pressure. Heart rate is increased in an attempt to increase cardiac output. Respiratory symptoms are discussed under "altered gas exchange."

Blood pressure should be evaluated as well as peripheral pulses. As the ventricles fail, blood pressure decreases and pulses become weaker. Urine output is diminished and the client's level of consciousness is decreased. These symptoms represent the underperfusion of vital organs. Cool temperature of the skin also suggests poor perfusion.

The presence of peripheral edema and whether it is pitting are important. Pitting edema has been associated with large volumes of excess fluid. Ascultation of heart sounds is done to identify the presence of an S3 (or gallop), which is one sign suggestive of congestive failure. This sound is produced by turbulent blood flow during rapid diastolic filling in a noncompliant ventricle.

Interventions

The objectives in dealing with a poor cardiac output from congestive failure are to decrease the work of the heart and optimize its performance. This is accomplished by careful fluid management, decreasing resistance to systolic ejection, decreasing cardiac demand, and supporting contractility if necessary.

In congestive failure, there is a relative fluid volume excess so diuretics are typically ordered by the physician along with a salt-restricted diet. Fluid restriction is practiced in the acute care setting and may be carried over in the home setting. Monitoring of intake and output as well as daily weights facilitate effective fluid management.

Rest is important in diminishing metabolic demand. Clients typically need extra pillows when resting due to the orthopnea created by excess pulmonary fluid. Blood pressure control is important to decrease the resistance against which the heart has to pump.

Inotropic drugs to enhance the contractility of the heart are often used in congestive failure. Digitalis preparations are frequently ordered by physicians to support contractility.

Outcomes

Goals for the client with ventricular failure include maintaining peak cardiac performance within the physiologic limitations of his cardiac function. This includes maintaining strict fluid control, optimizing cardiac output with drugs and rest periods, and prevention of episodes of failure.

ALTERATION IN GAS EXCHANGE

The accumulation of fluid in the pulmonary interstitium interferes with the diffusion of oxygen (O_2) and carbon dioxide (CO_2) across the alveolar–capillary membrane. Excess CO_2 and inadequate O_2 in the blood along with excess pulmonary water excite the respiratory center of the brain to increase the rate and depth of respirations. The vasomotor center, sensing a decreased blood pressure from ventricular failure, further stimulates the respiratory center. Clients feel short of breath and usually demonstrate measureable changes in their arterial blood gases.

Assessment

The presence of excess fluid in the lungs is typically heard on auscultation as inspiratory rales. The lungs should be auscultated from apices to bases and the level at which rales present should be noted. Increasing rales suggest that the degree of failure has increased or that fluid has not been adequately controlled. Respiratory rate and the use of accessory muscles of respiration should be assessed. These give the nurse information on the degree of pulmonary compromise.

The color of the skin and mucous membranes give clues about the adequacy of oxygenation. However, cyanosis only occurs when there is marked desaturation of hemoglobin and therefore is not a very useful tool. By the time a client demonstrates bluish discoloration of the skin and mucous membranes many other physical signs have already demonstrated themselves.

Interventions

Optimizing gas exchange and ventricular function guide interventions in caring for the client with pulmonary edema secondary to ventricular failure.

Lessening the fluid load on the heart is done by positioning the client in high-Fowler's position and administering diuretics as ordered. For the client with chronic congestive failure body position is routinely of concern. While sleeping, multiple pillows are used to ease shortness of breath. Lying flat is often uncomfortable. Gravity favors movement of fluid from dependent areas into the circulation and eventually into the lungs, causing difficulty breathing.

Oxygen administration, if ordered for use at home, improves respiratory symptoms by increasing the diffusion of oxygen into the blood. Administering oxygen during exercise or activity may facilitate client comfort. Adherence to dietary salt and fluid restrictions also provides for control of respiratory symptoms.

Other than fluid management and the administration of oxygen, nursing interventions to resolve the gas exchange problem are closely linked with those directed at improving cardiac output.

Outcomes

Episodes of congestive failure and pulmonary edema should be avoided or resolved quickly. Respiratory rate should be within normal limits and shortness of breath should be absent at rest and during light activity.

ALTERATION IN FLUID VOLUME: EXCESS

Fluid accumulates in the client with congestive failure largely due to poor perfusion to the kidneys. With a low cardiac output the glomerular filtration rate is decreased. The kidney senses this as hypovolemia and starts conserving sodium and fluid in an attempt to raise glomerular filtration. As fluid is conserved it accumulates in dependent interstitial spaces as described earlier.

Assessment

Excess fluid is easily documented with daily weights. It can also be seen in pitting edema, especially about the lower legs or dependent areas. Excess fluid can be heard on ascultation of breath sounds as rales.

Interventions

Management of fluid volume excess is closely tied to interventions described earlier regarding cardiopulmonary problems. Use of diuretics, dietary restriction of sodium and water, and improving renal perfusion by optimizing cardiac output all help to decrease excess volume.

An upset in the client's balance of fluids should be carefully assessed. Interventions are guided by the cause, be it failure to adhere to sodium and water guidelines, worsening ventricular function, or need for increased doses of diuretics. Clients may develop renal failure from consistent underperfusion of the kidneys. This would require prompt medical intervention, underscoring the value of monitoring intake and output.

Outcome

Avoidance of fluid overload is the goal in caring for this client.

ACTIVITY INTOLERANCE

Poor tissue perfusion from ventricular failure produces fatigue in clients. Their capacity for physical work is decreased and often their desire for activity is diminished. The client's level of activity should be determined in consultation with the physician. Clients with ventricular failure may have an exercise prescription from an exercise physiologist or may be involved in a cardiac rehabilitation program. The client's functional ability is influenced by his ejection fraction and presence or absence of symptoms of ischemia with activity (if he has coexisting coronary artery disease).

Assessment

Identifying the client's current physical capacity can be determined by interviewing the client and spouse or significant other. Observation for shortness of breath while visiting the client gives information concerning the level of exertion he can tolerate. Assessment should include a discussion with the physi-

cian to determine the optimal level of activity the client can tolerate based on preserved cardiac function.

For clients with ventricular dysfunction, limitations in activity tolerance often develop insidiously, over a longer period of time than with the client who has a myocardial infarction, for example. Therefore, the client has generally had more time to adjust to the changes in his life.

Interventions

Similar to clients with coronary disease, clients with ventricular failure should be encouraged to be as active as possible within their functional ability. This should be guided by the physician and in consultation with cardiac rehabilitation staff if ordered. The guidelines listed for clients with CAD apply to clients with ventricular dysfunction as well. Interventions should facilitate the use of these guidelines and a common sense approach by the client. Regular activity should be emphasized as a method to improve cardiovascular efficiency, decrease blood pressure, and manage stress.

Outcome

The client should maintain the maximal level of activity possible given the limits of his disease state.

ALTERED TISSUE PERFUSION: RENAL

When cardiac output fails due to poorly functioning ventricles, all major organ systems are affected. One system which suffers from decreased perfusion and as a result worsens cardiac failure is the renal system. As described earlier, underperfusion of the kidneys leads to fluid retention. Below a critical point, underperfused kidneys become ischemic and fail. Once renal failure has occurred there is no homeostatic mechanism to remove fluid from the body with the exception of sweat glands. Fluid can therefore accumulate with rapidity and exacerbate congestive failure.

Assessment

Monitoring of intake and output gives the nurse vital information on renal function. The absence of adequate urine output suggests underperfusion of the kidneys. Clients should have ½ to 1 cc of urine per kilogram of body weight per hour. For a 50 kg person this corresponds to about 1200 cc of urine per day. A minimum urine output for adults is about 750 cc for 24 hours.

Interventions

Nursing actions are guided by the underlying cause of the oliguria. Interventions may be directed at improving ventricular function, identifying whether the client is complying with diet restrictions and drug therapy, or educating the client on aspects of the medical regimen. If the client has developed renal failure, the physician should be consulted promptly.

Outcome

Adequate urine output as an indicator of adequate renal perfusion is the goal. An adequate volume must be identified for each client, based on body weight.

SEXUAL DYSFUNCTION

The client with ventricular failure is subject to many of the same problems with sexual function as the client with coronary disease. His physical work capacity is often more lim-ited than the client with CAD. Fatigue can decrease libido, even in very healthy persons. The assessment, interventions, and goals identified in the section on problems with coronary blood flow also apply to clients with ventricular dysfunction. The major difference between these two groups of clients is that the latter group is more limited in its physical work capacity. Therefore, specific guidelines should be identified in consultation with the physician to assure that the physiologic costs are acceptable for each individual client. Clients who are unable to tolerate the moderate cardiovascular work required for sexual activity are often so fatigued that their libido is very low. Improving physical work capacity through a cardiac rehabilitation program may resolve both issues simultaneously. This assumes there is some cardiac function to be rehabilitated.

ALTERATION IN SELF-CONCEPT: ROLE DISTURBANCE

Clients with impaired ventricular function are at risk for developing altered self-concept as a result of activity intolerance and their perception of how the illness affects their lives. Decreased physical capacity may prevent the client from fulfilling formerly held roles. If the client develops ventricular dysfunction over the years as infarctions decrease the working myocardium, the client may have had time to adjust to life-style changes. However, acute valvular disease may occur from an infectious process. Idiopathic cardiomyopathy can cause congestive failure in a few months in a previously healthy person.

Although time to adapt to change is usually beneficial it does not assure positive adjustment. The assessment, interventions, and goals appropriate to this problem are detailed in the section on problems with coronary blood flow.

KNOWLEDGE DEFICIT RELATED TO VENTRICULAR DYSFUNCTION AND DRUG THERAPY

One of the reasons it is important for clients to have a clear understanding of their disease process is to facilitate informed decision making regarding compliance with medical therapy. For those clients who have developed ventricular failure as a result of CAD, or who have coexisting CAD, knowledge deficit is covered in the section on CAD. For clients who have developed ventricular failure as a result of valvular disease or idiopathic cardiomyopathy, a discussion of the nurse's approach to knowledge deficit follows.

Assessment

Identifying the client's current level of understanding may be accomplished by simply asking him what he knows or has been taught about his medical condition. This discussion should take place when the client is rested, alert enough to participate, and motivated to learn. Assessment of the intellectual level of the client and other family members participating in the discussion helps the nurse formulate an effective educational program.

Interventions

Content areas that concern self-care and a broad understanding of the disease state should be included in the education session. This includes education on medications, the pathophysiology of heart failure, and activities that influence cardiac performance. Although all the risk factors of CAD do not necessarily apply to clients with ventricular failure, several of them do apply.

The discussion on drug therapy should include indications, dose, appearance of the drug, how it should be administered (with or without food, etc.), and adverse effects. This follows what would be taught to any client who is given a prescription medicine.

Explaining the meaning of ventricular failure is valuable in that it may encourage client compliance and it enables the client to fully participate in his own care. The client should understand the cardiopulmonary response to failure, that tachycardia, hypotension, increased respiratory rate, and shortness of breath accompany this syndrome. The facts that rest, managing hypertension, controlling fluids, and using drugs to enhance contractility are methods to manage failure should be made clear to the client. This insight may influence the method in which a client gets out of bed in the morning, climbs a flight of stairs, or cleans laundry. Knowledge of the effects of poor organ perfusion helps the client understand what to tell the home-care nurse during visits. A very low urine output may be overlooked by a client who does not understand its importance.

Risk factors that are appropriate in this context include smoking, hypertension, obesity, lack of exercise, stress, and diabetes mellitus. Instead of concentrating on dietary cholesterol, emphasis may be placed on dietary sodium. (Controlling dietary cholesterol and fat is prudent anyway.)

An outline for client education regarding ventricular dysfunction is shown on page 257.

Guidelines for effective teaching (page 240) are applicable for this group of clients.

Clients who have had surgical replacements of diseased valves should understand antibiotic prophylaxis that is recommended prior to dental care. This is to prevent seeding the valves with bacteria that obtain entry to the body via dental work. This regimen is ordered by their attending physician. If the client recently had surgery he may require education on incisional care.

Educational Needs for the Client with Ventricular Dysfunction

1. Effects of ventricular failure:
   - Fluid accumulation in lungs
   - Development of venous engorgement and peripheral edema
   - Underperfusion of vital organs, effects on kidneys, brain

2. Signs of worsening cardiac function:
   - Tachycardia
   - Increasing shortness of breath
   - Altered mentation

3. Activities that increase cardiac work:
   - Stress
   - Extreme temperatures
   - Exercise (discuss monitoring of activity)

4. Methods to enhance ventricular function:
   - Diuretics
   - Fluid and sodium restriction
   - Normal blood pressure
   - Drugs that enhance contractility (*i.e.*, digoxin)
   - Rest
   - Exercise (explain)

5. Drug therapy
   - Indications, dose, time schedule, appearance
   - Administration, adverse effects

6. Risk factors/ life-style
   - Smoking
   - Hypertension
   - Obesity
   - Lack of exercise
   - Stress
   - Diabetes

Outcomes

Successful interventions result in a client who is knowledgeable about cardiac failure, activities that influence cardiac performance, self-care, and medication administration.

NONCOMPLIANCE

Clients with ventricular dysfunction are at as much risk of being noncompliant as any other group of clients. Assessment, interventions, and goals for these clients are as presented in the section on problems with coronary blood flow (see page 229).

ANXIETY

See the discussion on anxiety under problems with coronary blood flow (page 238).

References

Becker MH: The health belief model and sick role behavior. In Redman BK (ed): Patient Teaching. Rockville, MD, Aspen Publishers, Inc., 1978

Cummins RO, Eisenberg MS, Bergner L, Hallstrom A et al: Automatic external defibrillation: Evaluations of its role in the home and in emergency medical services. Ann Emerg Med 13(9): 798–801, 1984

Curtis P: Letter: Treating myocardial infarction at home. JAMA 253(3): 344–45, 1985

Gloag D: Rehabilitation of patients with cardiac conditions. Br Med J (Clin Res) 290(6464): 617–20, 1985

Guyton AC: Textbook of Medical Physiology. Philadelphia, WB Saunders, 1986

Hilgenberg C, Crowley C: Changes in family patterns after a myocardial infarction. Home Healthcare Nurse 5(3)d: 26–35, 1987

Kion MS, McFarland GK, McLane AM: Pocket

Guide to Nursing Diagnoses. St. Louis, CV Mosby, 1984

Kolodyn RC, Musters WH, Johnson VE, Biggs MA: Textbook of Human Sexuality for Nurses. Boston, Little, Brown & Co, 1979

Liddy KG, Crowley C: Do MI patients have the information they need for the recovery phase at home? Home Healthcare Nurse 5(3): 19–25, 1987

Niskala H: The role of community health nurses in cardiac rehabilitation. Home Healthcare Nurse 5(3): 10–15, 1987

Porth CM: Pathophysiology: Concepts of Altered Health States, 2nd ed. Philadelphia, JB Lippincott, 1986

Redman BK: The Process of Patient Teaching in Nursing, 4th ed. St. Louis, CV Mosby, 1980

Rippe JM, Irwin RS, Alpert JS, Dalen JE: (eds): Intensive Care Medicine. Boston, Little, Brown & Co, 1985

Rowley JM, Hampton JR, Mitchell JR: Home care for patients with suspected myocardial infarction: Use made by general practitioners of a hospital team for initial management. Br Med J (Clin Res) 289(6442): 403–6, 1984

Sanderson RG, Kirth CL: The Cardiac Patient: A Comprehensive Approach. Philadelphia, WB Saunders, 1983

Smith J: Home is where the heart is. Nurs Mirror 159(11): 24–25, 1984

11

ALTERATIONS IN NUTRITION

Linda E. Evans and Carol Jean DeMoss

Nutritional care is a necessary part of total client care. The responsibilities of the home health nurse in regard to food and nutrition are very different from the responsibilities of the nurse in the hospital. In the hospital, the nurse's primary function is to assure that a tray arrives and that she has physically prepared the client to eat. In the home setting, the nurse needs to assure that food is in the home. This may include helping the client identify who can do the shopping or making a referral to a food bank or social agency for emergency food supplies. The major area of responsibility, though, is instructing the client and family in ways to improve food intake. Since many physicians are not prepared in the area of nutrition and most home health agencies do not employ registered dietitians to provide client and family teaching, the responsibility for nutrition care belongs to the nurse. Techniques for integrating nutritional care into the client's plan of treatment through oral, enteral, or parenteral modalities will be discussed in this chapter.

NUTRITIONAL ASSESSMENT

For the client who has an alteration in nutrition, be it less or greater than body requirements, a nutritional assessment must be performed by the nurse. The assessment includes overt factors affecting nutrition such as height and weight and current food and fluid intake plus assessment of other areas that indirectly affect nutrition.

The components of nutritional assessment are

1. The meaning of food
2. Client's diagnosis and prognosis
3. Health history
4. Current food and fluid intake
5. Height and weight
6. Biochemical data
7. Family and community resources
8. Food preferences and practices
9. Medications
10. Assessment of gastrointestinal function

11. Learning abilities of client and family
12. Previous special diets
13. Food quackery and/or nutrition myths

MEANING OF FOOD

Determining the meaning of food for the client and care-taker is essential. Some persons live to eat, others simply eat to live. It is much easier if both the client and care-taker are in the same category. If both simply eat to live, the interventions must reflect methods to increase or decrease food and/or nutrient intake. With families who live to eat, food is an expression of love, caring, and nurturing. When restrictions are required or the client can no longer eat, both the client and family must learn that altering food patterns is not altering love. Learning that love can also be expressed by not providing foods that are harmful needs to be emphasized by the home health nurse. Many care-takers feel that by reducing the food intake through a low calorie diet or a lipid-reducing diet they are depriving the person who provided so well for them for many years. The nurse's interventions include explaining how food volume can remain high through the use of salads and two vegetables at a meal, while still adhering to the diet.

Conversely, if the care-taker lives to eat and the client is not interested in food, compromises need to be made. Teaching the care-taker to give only one fourth the regular portion size and no more than two food items at a time is helpful; concurrently, the nurse also encourages the client to try and eat the smaller quantity of food. The home health nurse must reinforce that if the client does not eat, it is not because he is trying to hurt the care-taker, but that he is just not able to eat. When the client does not eat the hospital food, the family rationalizes that it is because he does not like it, or it is cold, or not prepared the way his wife cooks.

If he does not eat at home, families often feel it is because he does not love them enough to eat. If the client can not eat solid food the emphasis can be switched from foods to fluids. The care-taker is providing some nourishment and the liquids are something the client can ingest, therefore both parties are accomplishing something positive.

Before concurring that the client is unable to eat, be certain that he has not just decided to stop eating. Not eating could be a means of asserting control or "getting even" for past conflicts. The decision not to eat can also mean that the client has given up hope of becoming well and has chosen, whether consciously or unconsciously, to die. The home health nurse must distinguish between the person who can not eat and the person who has chosen not to eat. During hospitalization neither the client nor family has control of the environment or the treatment plan. After discharge to home, even though acute care is still required, control switches to the client and/or family. Often both client and family need help in dealing with the new control.

KNOWLEDGE OF DIAGNOSIS AND PROGNOSIS

The nurse must determine if the client knows the medical diagnosis and its nutritional implications. The client's prognosis strongly affects nutritional teaching by the home health nurse. The caloric goal for a person who is expected to return to normal health is much higher than the goal for the client with cancer who is being treated palliatively. For the restorative client, the protein, calorie, vitamin, and mineral intake must be great enough for healing and rebuilding. Comfort and preventing secondary complications such as decubiti and infection would be the goals for the palliative client. The intake of protein, calories, vitamins, and minerals is less for preventing secondary problems than for restoring health.

When developing food intake goals with the client and family, it is important to remember that many persons equate food with life. If the food intake becomes very small the reality of dying becomes greater. The health care provider needs to encourage food when food intake can make a difference. When this is no longer true, the nurse must take an active role as a client advocate and assist the family to understand that the client can no longer eat and should not be constantly asked to eat when life expectancy is measured in days. If the care-taker continues to focus on food intake, quality time between client and care-taker will be lessened.

HEALTH HISTORY

The collection of biographical data includes age, occupation, marital status, and smoking and alcohol habits. The nurse must know high-risk factors to decide if preventive teaching is indicated. Past illness and surgeries, especially related to the gastrointestinal system, are pertinent. For example, a gastric resection performed years before may be the cause of persistent pernicious anemia if vitamin B_{12} has not been replaced through injections. Obtain information about past history in relation to use of enemas and if the client is a chronic laxative abuser. Also explore health crises that occurred in the past and how they affected food intake. A family health history will provide background information and will allow the home health nurse to look for diseases with nutritional implications. The nurse must also have the client identify his chief problem or complaint. Sometimes the client will have extensive pathology but will identify the chief problem as something "simple," such as constipation. Until the home health nurse modifies or eliminates what the client sees as the prob-

lem, additional learning will not occur. If the chief complaint is pain, ask the client where and when it occurs, any relationship to dietary intake, and have the client describe the pain and rate the pain on a scale of one to ten. This knowledge will provide the nurse with a baseline from which to evaluate interventions to control the pain and increase the food intake.

FOOD AND FLUID INTAKE

Obtaining a valid 24-hour food and clear fluid recall is another dimension of the assessment process. The home health nurse must not make assumptions when evaluating food intake. If the client says he ate a small piece of meat, have him define "small." To some people that may be 5 to 6 ounces of meat while to someone else, it may be 2 ounces. Conversely, a large piece of chicken may mean a chicken wing or a leg and thigh. Be very specific about foods, methods of preparation, and serving sizes. Avoid such terms as "breakfast" or "lunch" because some people munch all day and will tell you they did not eat anything for lunch.

To help evaluate meat portion sizes, 1 ounce of meat is about as large as the palm of the hand and one fourth inch thick. Another frame of reference is that the regular McDonald's hamburger is about 1½ ounces and a chicken leg or a thigh is usually 2 ounces. Always differentiate between what the client was given to eat and what was eaten. Many care-takers will say they made the client a sandwich, a bowl of soup, and ice cream. But when asking the client what he actually ate, it was 2 bites of the sandwich and 1 sip of the soup, and 1 bite of ice cream. The two versions are quite different. During the food history reassure the care-taker that you are not judging what she gave to the client but obtaining a frame of reference from which to plan nutrition interventions.

A food recall determines only what food has been ingested. It does not reflect if the body can properly utilize the food. The two are very different. One is food intake, which the home health nurse can determine. The other is nutritional status and needs to be determined by laboratory tests not available in the home or even sometimes in small hospitals.

In addition to the short-term food recall, determine if the client has had an adequate food intake in the recent past. Was the patient N.P.O. for several days in the hospital? Were meals often missed because of tests and various procedures?

Clients and families often believe that adequate nutrition was obtained if intravenous fluids were given during hospitalization. They need to know that the standard intravenous fluids contain no protein and few calories. If the intravenous was 1000 mililiters of 5% dextrose, the client received only 200 calories. The following calculation can be used to determine the caloric content of intravenous solutions:

1000	Total fluid
× 5%	Strength
50.00	Grams of carbohydrates
× 4	Calories per gram of carbohydrates
200	

If three intravenous solutions were given in a day, the total caloric intake would have been only 600 when the requirements may have been 3000 calories. That caloric deficit along with the protein deficit must be made up after the client is discharged.

As part of the food history, question the client if there have been problems associated with any foods, such as abdominal pain or distention following ingestion of milk. If so, he may be lactose-intolerant, a condition caused when the body cannot break down lactose, the carbohydrate component present in milk. It is relatively common in the healthy negro and Oriental population and in the ill population at large. Lactose intolerance is characterized by cramping, bloating, and diarhea following ingestion of milk.

Some clients with lactose intolerance can drink milk in very small quantities but not more than ½ cup at a time. To assist these clients in digesting milk, an over-the-counter product called Lactaid can be added to milk before drinking. The Lactaid breaks down the lactose, making the milk better tolerated by some of the lactose-intolerant population.

Before finishing the food recall inquire as to what medicines are taken with food. Sometimes clients consider certain foods as "medicines." A client may not mention the banana or the glass of orange juice he has daily since the doctor told him to take them for potassium replacement. The client may not realize how important this information is. For example, a diabetic with hyperglycemia may need to include high potassium vegetables that will not affect the blood sugar, rather than the orange juice or banana.

Always end the food history on a positive note. The nurse may need to look very hard to find something positive. More than half of home care is motivating the family to carry through your instructions, so be honest but also look for positive things.

Nutritional assessment is important not only for the client, but also for the family or care-takers. Occasionally, the many responsibilities of the care-takers may make it difficult for them to achieve adequate nutritional balance. Therefore, in addition to the client's food recall, sometime during the second or third week a food recall should be done on the care-taker(s). Often they skip meals or do not take time to eat balanced meals. If they are skipping meals, early intervention may help prevent care-taker illness. Since the unit of care in the home includes the client and his family, interventions must be planned for both to give comprehensive home health care.

The basic four is an eating guide for healthy individuals and the servings listed are for adults (Table 11-1). Higher nutrient intake is required during and following an acute illness. If the client is underweight and has nutritional deficits to overcome, one and a half or two times the basic four may be required but this increase will have to be gradual and meeting the basic four intake may be the first step. The home health nurse must also understand the individual nutrients

(Table 11-2) and vitamins (11-3) necessary for good nutritional balance.

When a fluid restriction is not ordered, clear fluids should be totaled separately from full liquids. Milk and milk products contain protein and minerals, solutes that need to be excreted. Since full liquids carry a renal solute load, they should not be included in the total fluid intake. If a fluid restriction is required, all fluids, clear and full, must be calculated along with such foods as jello, ice cream, sherbet, and any other foods that are liquid at room temperature. When a fluid restriction is not indicated, daily clear fluid intake should be 8 cups. If dehydration, temperature elevation, and/or thick secretions

(Text continues on p 270)

TABLE 11.1 Basic 4 Food Groups

Food Group	Servings	Serving Size	Nutrients Provided
Milk	2	1 cup	Calcium Riboflavin (B_2) Protein Carbohydrate Vitamin D if enriched Fat unless skimmed
Meat	2	2 ounces	Protein Niacin Iron Thiamin (B_1) Fat
Fruits/Vegetables (Food high in vitamin C daily and food high in vitamin A 3 or 4 times a week)	4	½ cup or one individual piece	Vitamin A Vitamin C Fiber or cellulose
Grain (Whole grain, fortified, enriched products)	4	½ cup or individual piece	Carbohydrate Thiamin, Iron, and Niacin if fortified, enriched whole grain, fortified or enriched. Some provide fiber and cellulose.

TABLE 11.2 Nutrient Summary

Nutrient	Function	Digestion	Absorption	Storage	Food Sources
Carbohydrate	1. Quick energy—4 calories/g 2. Major source of energy for the central nervous system 3. Protein sparing—provides energy so protein can be used for building and repairing instead of for energy 4. Indigestable forms provide fiber 5. Necessary for fats to be broken down from ketones to carbon dioxide and water 6. Bowel regulation	Mouth: Salivary amylase (very weak enzyme) Small intestine: Pancreatic amylase Intestinal disaccharidase	From small bowel through wall of intestine To portal vein To liver to be formed into glucose To systemic circulation	Limited amts. glycogen in liver and muscles	Sugar milk, cereals, grains, pasta, potatoes Cellulose—fresh fruits/vegetables

Protein				
1. Necessary for muscle, nerve, skin, and bone cell structure. Needed to build, repair, and maintain body tissues and red and white blood cells	Mouth: none Stomach: gastric protease Small intestine: Pancreative protease Intestinal protease Intestinal dipeptidase	From small bowel through wall of intestine. To portal vein To liver To general circulation after excesses removed	No. The nitrogen is detoxified by the liver and excreted by the kidney. The remainder is used as energy and stored as fat.	Complete proteins (contain all the amino acids the body cannot produce): Meat, fish, poultry, milk, eggs, cheese except cream cheese.
2. Necessary component of enzymes, antibodies and some hormones				Incomplete proteins are missing one or more of the essential amino acids: Nuts, dried beans, peas
3. Provides essential amino acids or base				
4. Regulates water balance through albumin				
5. Regulates acid/base balance because it can act as acid or base				
6. Energy if insufficient carbohydrates and fat intake				

(continued)

TABLE 11.2 Nutrient Summary *(continued)*

Nutrient	Function	Digestion	Absorption	Storage	Food Sources
Fat	1. Stored energy 2. Concentrated source of calories —more than twice the level of protein or carbohydrates—9 calories/g 3. Provides and carries fat soluble vitamins 4. Provides essential fatty acids 5. Provides satiety by delaying gastric emptying. Protects body organs from trauma by providing padding 6. Acts as body insulator to help maintain body temperature	Mouth: none Stomach: none Small intestine: liver–gallbladder Bile not a digestive enzyme but emulsifies fat (breaks into smaller particles) Pancreatic lipase Intestinal lipase	Long-chained fatty acid: from small bowel through wall of intestine→sub→clavian vein → systemic circulation Medium-chained fatty acids: from small bowel through wall of intestine→ portal vein→ liver→ systemic circulation	Yes — as adipose tissue or body fat	Saturated fats: butter, cream, hard shortenings, hard margarines, coconut oil Monounsaturated fats: olive oil Polyunsaturated fats: liquid corn oil, liquid safflower oil

From Robinson H, Lawler R: Normal and Therapeutic Nutrition, 16th ed. New York City, Macmillan, 1982; Williams SR: Nutrition and Diet Therapy, 5th ed. St. Louis, CV Mosby, 1985; Lewis C: Vitamins and Minerals—Sodium and Potassium. Philadelphia, FA Davis, 1978

TABLE 11.3 Vitamin–Mineral Summary

Nutrient	Function	Storage	Food Sources
Vitamins **Vitamin A** **(Retinal)** Fat soluble	1. Necessary for building and maintaining skin mucous membranes and epithelial cells 2. Necessary for healthy eye tissue and adaptation to changes in light and color vision 3. Necessary for formation of connective tissue	Yes—in the liver. May be toxic in excessive amounts.	Liver, dark yellow vegetables such as carrots and winter squash, dark green vegetables such as spinach, greens, and butter, fortified margarine, and whole milk
Thiamin (B₁) Water soluble	1. Essential for energy metabolism 2. Promotes normal appetite 3. Required for normal functioning of nerve tissue (at synapses)	Very limited	Lean pork, nuts, and fortified cereal products
Riboflavin (B₂) Water soluble	Essential for energy metabolism	Very limited	Liver, milk, poultry, fish, and fortified cereals
Niacin Water soluble	1. Essential for fat breakdown and synthesis 2. Required for utilization of carbohydrates 3. Required for normal functioning of nervous tissue	Very limited	Liver, meat, poultry, fish, and peanuts
Folic Acid **(Folocen)** Water soluble	1. Required for maturation of red blood cells 2. Required for synthesis of DNA and RNA	Probably not	Meats, deep green leafy vegetables, eggs, and whole grain cereals
B₁₂ Water soluble	1. Required for synthesis of DNA and RNA 2. Necessary for function of mature red blood cells	Limited	Meats, seafood, eggs, and dairy products. Note: deficiencies have been found among vegetarians when no animal foods are consumed
Vitamin C **(Ascorbic Acid)** Water soluble	1. Necessary for formation and maintainence of collagen in connective tissues	No	Oranges, grapefruit, fresh strawberries, cantaloupe, broccoli, Brussels sprouts, green peppers

(continued)

TABLE 11.3 Vitamin–Mineral Summary *(continued)*

Nutrient	Function	Storage	Food Sources
	2. Necessary for maintaining capillary walls 3. Catalyzes conversion of folic acid to folinic acid 4. Enhances iron absorption 5. Necessary for amino acid metabolism *NOTE:* Cigarette smoking alters the utilization of vitamin C and results in a slightly increased need. Doses of 3000 mg to 5000 mg are given to patients with indwelling catheters to help acidify urine.		*Note:* Vitamin C is rapidly destroyed by exposure to heat and light.
Vitamin D (Calciferol) Fat soluble	1. Required for calcium and phosphorus absorption 2. Helps maintain correct concentration of calcium in extracellular fluids 3. Required for mineralization of bone 4. Required for muscle contractions 5. Maintaining nerve irritability	Yes—may be toxic in excessive amounts	Fortified foods such as milk
Vitamin E (Tocopherol) Fat soluble	Prevents oxidation of polyunsaturated fatty acids	Not to any extent	Vetetable oils, nuts, legumes
Vitamin K (Mendadione) Fat soluble	Required for liver formation of prothrombin	Yes	Green leafy vegetables *Note:* Half of vitamin K is produced by microflora in gastrointestinal tract. Long term antibiotic use may kill microflora and decrease vitamin K production
Macronutrients: Calcium	1. Helps to provide structure and strength to bones and teeth 2. Activates enzymes, especially those concerned with fat 3. Required for nerve transmission 4. Functions in normal muscle contraction and relaxation	Yes. If taken in excess with large doses of vitamin D, will be laid down in soft tissue, which is not desired	Milk, yogurt, cheese, cottage cheese, clams, oysters, shrimp, and greens

TABLE 11.3 Vitamin–Mineral Summary *(continued)*

Nutrient	Function	Storage	Food Sources
	5. Required for clotting of the blood		
Magnesium	1. Necessary for protein synthesis 2. Necessary for activation of specific enzymes (ADP →ATP) 3. Required for transmission of nerve impulses 4. Required for muscle contraction 5. Required for carbohydrate, protein, and fat metabolism	Yes	Dairy products except butter. Flour and cereals, meat, legumes, beef, lamb, pork
Phosphorus	1. Required for linkage of DNA and RNA 2. Regulates transport of solutes in and out of cells 3. Required for absorption of sugars 4. Assists calcium in bone and teeth development 5. Required for energy transfer within body cells 6. Necessary for buffer system	Yes. If taken in excess with large doses of vitamin D, will be laid down in soft tissue, which is not desired.	Milk, yogurt, cheese, cottage cheese, whole grain cereals, and flour
Micronutrients or Trace Elements: Copper	1. Required for taste sensitivity 2. Required for maturation of collagen 3. Required for formation of hemoglobin 4. Essential for utilization of iron 5. Constituent of many enzymes	Yes	Oysters, liver, nuts, dried legumes, raisins, and cocoa
Iron	Necessary for formation of hemoglobin, which acts as a carrier of oxygen from the lungs to the tissues.	Yes. No mechanism for excretion after it is absorbed	Liver, red meats, and some enriched cereals

(continued)

TABLE 11.3 Vitamin–Mineral Summary *(continued)*

Nutrient	Function	Storage	Food Sources
Zinc	1. Required for activity of many enzymes 2. Required for synthesis of protein 3. Required for synthesis of RNA and DNA 4. Essential for mobilization of vitamin A 5. Essential for formation of insulin	Yes, but not readily available	Oysters, liver, whole grain cereals

From Robinson H, Lawler R: Normal and Therapeutic Nutrition, 16th ed. New York City, Macmillan, 1982; Williams SR: Nutrition and Diet Therapy, 5th ed. St Louis, CV Mosby, 1985; Lewis C: Vitamins and Minerals—Sodium and Potassium. Philadelphia, FA Davis, 1978.

are present, the total needs to be higher. Simply asking the client or care-taker to recall the number of cups of water, coffee, tea, juice, broth, and soft drinks consumed daily is an easy means of obtaining the total clear liquid intake.

A teaching tool similar to "What's Your Nutrition Score" (Figure 11-1 *A* and *B*) may be helpful for ongoing evaluation of the client's and the care-taker's food intake. When the tool is being used in the home, the client and care-taker complete the front portion (Figure 11-1*A*) and the home health nurse completes the back portion (Figure 11-1*B*) with them on the following visit.

To use the tool, score the foods eaten in the previous 24 hours as indicated in the credits column. If the client drank one half cup of milk, he would earn five credits. If he drank two cups of milk he would earn 20 credits. If three cups of milk were consumed, the total credits would still only be 20 because the maximum credits in each category cannot exceed 20. Each of the six categories would be scored in the same manner.

When marking the grain group emphasize that only the whole-grain or enriched foods can count. The fluids category is the only one where a food can be counted twice. Fluid and/or vegetable juices can be included in both the fruits and vegetable group and the fluid group.

After scoring each of the six groups, turn the paper over to document the areas needing improvement. If the client had consumed only one half cup of milk, you would indicate the need to increase the milk one and a half servings. You would then discuss other food sources such as pudding and yogurt. Discuss all of the areas that did not receive a score of 20.

A scoring guide could be: 95–100 credits, balanced food intake; 80–90 credits, needs improvement; 75 and below, poor.

HEIGHT AND WEIGHT

The person's height and weight should be obtained. Measure height if the client does not know his height or if the nurse feels his

WHAT'S YOUR NUTRITION SCORE?

Directions: Carefully recall all the food you ate and/or drank in the past 24 hours. Score the food according to the food groups and the credit points indicated.

FOOD	CREDITS	SCORE	
		Day 1	Day 2
MILK			
One cup of milk	10		
Second cup of milk	10		
FRUITS AND VEGETABLES			
One serving of dark green or deep yellow vegetable	5		
One serving of citrus fruit, tomatoes, or broccoli	5		
Two or more servings of other fruits and vegetables including potato	10		
GRAIN (BREAD AND CEREALS)			
Four servings of whole-grain or enriched bread, cereal or grain products (each serving counts 5 points)	20		
MEATS (PROTEIN)			
One serving of egg, meat, fish, poultry, cheese, nuts, dried beans, or peas	10		
One or more additional servings of egg, meat, fish, poultry, or cheese	10		
IRON			
At least two servings of red meat, egg yolk, deep-green leafy vegetables, or whole-grain or enriched bread or cereals (May include same food as counted above)	10		
FLUIDS			
Eight cups of fluid daily including coffee, tea, juice, water (May include same food as counted above)	10		
TOTAL			

Figure 11-1A.   Teaching tool—"What's Your Nutrition Score?"—front page. (Used with permission of Visiting Nurse Association of Allegheny County, PA. Copyright 1986)

answer is inaccurate. This is especially important with the elderly client since height decreases with age. Note any changes in weight within the year prior to illness. A pre-illness weight, a current weight, and the highest and lowest weights within the last year are helpful.

It is important to assess the client's weight goal. The physician may want the client to weigh 120 pounds but if the client feels 150 pounds is the least she can weigh and be healthy, there will be difficulty in reaching the goal. In this case, the nurse must first work within the client's goals unless the goals are potentially harmful. After the client and family gain confidence in the nurse, then the nurse may be able to help the client revise the weight goals.

When recording weight, be aware of any edema and indicate in the record its absence or degree. This helps differentiate between fluid weight and gain in body mass. There

TO HAVE YOUR FOOD INTAKE REFLECT THE BASIC 4 RECOMMENDED DAILY PATTERNS, YOU NEED TO:

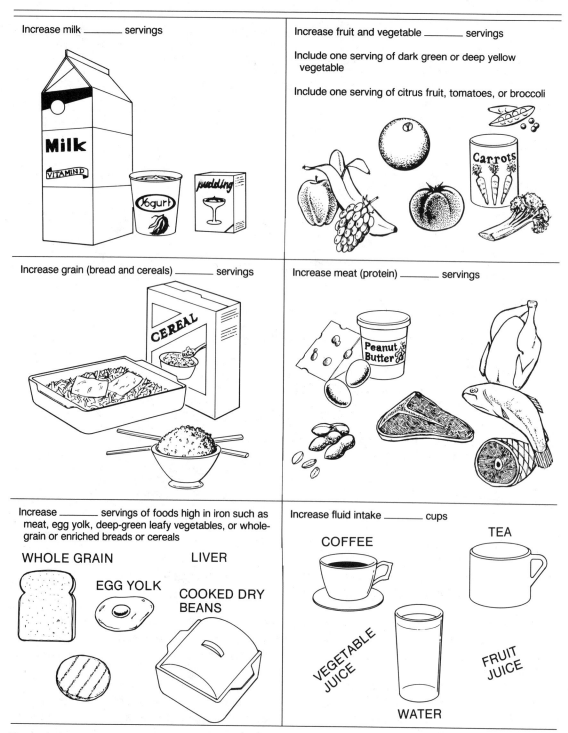

Increase milk _____ servings

Increase fruit and vegetable _____ servings

Include one serving of dark green or deep yellow vegetable

Include one serving of citrus fruit, tomatoes, or broccoli

Increase grain (bread and cereals) _____ servings

Increase meat (protein) _____ servings

Increase _____ servings of foods high in iron such as meat, egg yolk, deep-green leafy vegetables, or whole-grain or enriched breads or cereals

WHOLE GRAIN   LIVER

EGG YOLK   COOKED DRY BEANS

Increase fluid intake _____ cups

COFFEE   TEA

VEGETABLE JUICE   FRUIT JUICE

WATER

Figure 11-1B. Teaching tool—"What's Your Nutrition Score?"—back page. (Used with permission of Visiting Nurse Association of Allegheny County, PA. Copyright 1986)

may be a 3 pound weight loss between visits. Knowing that the edema present on the first visit is absent on the next visit identifies the loss as fluid. Using a tape measure to measure size of ankles, calfs, and mid-thigh can be more helpful in determining edema than the subjective assigning of "one to four plus edema." If the upper extremities have edema, measure at the wrist and mid- and upper arm.

The home health nurse should have a scale in case the client does not have his own. To weigh the client, find a level, noncarpeted area within the patient's walking range on which to place the scales. Weigh yourself first to ascertain the accuracy of the scales. Then weigh the client. For the client who is unable to stand long enough for an accurate weight, a scale is now available that is placed on a chair; the client then sits on it, and her weight is recorded. Scales may vary. What should be observed is a change in weight on the same scale. Strongly encourage the client to be weighed regularly as a means of monitoring weight. If the client is overweight and sensitive about it, reassure him that the weight will be helpful in showing the positive results of his efforts.

If obtaining a weight is not possible, measuring the client's mid-upper arm, bust, waist, hips, and upper leg is a means of monitoring.

If the client is emaciated and there are no goals to gain weight, it may be wise not to weigh him. Why confront the client with the fact that he only weighs 87 pounds when there are no interventions planned to increase the weight because of an advanced terminal illness? Never put the client through procedures that do not have a correlating intervention.

There are numerous height/weight charts available for determining ideal body weight. See the boxed material opposite for a simplified method of determining ideal body weight.

Method for Determining Ideal Body Weight

Female — 100 pounds for the first 5 feet and add 5 pounds for every inch over 5 feet.

Male — 106 pounds for the first 5 feet and add 6 pounds for very inch over 5 feet.

Ten percent should be substracted for small frame and 10% added for large frame. Many people try to convince themselves and you they are large-framed. Frame size may be estimated by placing thumb and middle finger around the wrist. If the thumb and finger meet, the person is average frame. Overlapping finger and thumb indicates a small frame and if finger and thumb do not touch the persons is large-framed.

BIOCHEMICAL DATA

Current laboratory data is a part of nutritional assessment. Today, most home health nurses perform venipunctures or their agency has made arrangements with a medical laboratory for home phlebotomies. This provides an added dimension to the assessment and ongoing management. It also provides the nurse with added responsibility. In most cases, the nurse is responsible for the initial interpretation of the results and then contacts the physician for changes in the plan of care. The nurse must also rely heavily upon observation skills to detect possible signs of abnormal laboratory data since it may be necessary to obtain orders for additional blood work.

Specific laboratory tests with nutritional

implications include hemoglobin and hematocrit, serum iron binding capacity (SIBC), sedimentation rate, and transferrin and albumin levels.

Hemoglobin readings can be obtained in the home immediately for both adults and infants with a hemoglobinometer. If the iron is low, an iron binding capacity (SIBC) is necessary to determine if iron is not available or if there is a problem with its utilization.

FAMILY AND COMMUNITY RESOURCES

The family's resources must be assessed before formulating a nutritional care plan. Resources include money, time, facilities to prepare and store food, and persons available to help the client. All too frequently, the home health nurse will find clients who are poor, live alone, have no family or friends, and live in a single rented room. The care for this most challenging client is very different from the person who can afford convenience foods to heat in a microwave oven and have friends and family to help with the care.

Interventions for the client who does not have access to a kitchen may include placing a cold lunch in a lightweight cooler. Warm food can be placed in several wide-mouthed, thermos-type containers. High protein, high calorie drinks can be placed in the thermos-type containers that are made to be used with a flex-straw and the client can sip on them during the day.

Meals-on-Wheels are often an answer for many homebound clients. Inform clients that if they do not eat the hot meal immediately, it must be placed in the refrigerator until it is reheated. Many elderly clients place the meal in the oven and let the pilot light keep the food warm. This promotes bacterial growth that can be harmful, especially to the elderly and the ill. Some elderly people think it is unsafe to place warm food in the refrigerator because in the past the warm food would melt the ice in the old fashioned icebox. Encourage the Meals-on-Wheels staff to date the hot food container and stress to the client that the hot meals should not be kept longer than two days.

On each visit, look in the client's refrigerator and assess its contents. It may be empty or if the client is on Meals-on-Wheels you may find six to ten containers each with a small portion of food. Reinforce that discarding food is not wasteful. It is healthful.

If the client and spouse went to a senior citizen nutrition program for lunch before the illness, try to arrange for the home health aide to come at lunchtime so the spouse can continue attending the lunch program. This may take much encouraging but the spouse can have a short respite once or twice a week while the client is homebound. Lunch and socialization programs should be available in most communities through Area Agency on Aging (AAA) or the local government through Title 3 funding.

Often an elderly client moves in with his adult child. If finances are a problem, encourage the family to see if the client's grandchildren are eligible for half-price or free school meals. If there is a grandchild under the age of five with a medical problem such as a low hemoglobin, hematocrit, or body weight, encourage the family to contact the Women, Infants and Children (WIC) nutrition program. If accepted into the program, the family will be provided with monthly vouchers through WIC for the purchase of specific foods for the child. Adding one or two persons to the household may make the extended family eligible for the food stamp program. If there is a social worker available, additional information regarding these programs and assistance with referrals, may be obtained. If not, the nurse must help the family with referrals.

Other community resources that help with finances/food purchasing are disease-specific organizations such as the Cancer Society and Multiple Sclerosis Society. In some cities, nonprofit home health agencies can belong to local "food banks." With this membership, the agency can provide food to the needy clients. Churches, nationality organizations, or men's and women's social organization such as Rotary, Moose, Elks, Eastern Star, Pithany Sisters, Kiwanis, or St. Vincent de Paul Society are often overlooked as community resources. Even if the client is not a member of the organization, it may help by providing small durable medical supplies, helping with babysitting, providing care-taker relief, or donating small amounts of money. One of the special aspects of home care is that it is family care and what helps one person usually helps the family. Helping to meet family expenses in one area may help to make money available for the purchase of food or help to decrease family anxiety. Much can be said for the generosity of many small communities and organizations when they are approached for help. The home health nurse must become familiar with the various community resources available.

FOOD PREFERENCES AND PRACTICES

Food likes, dislikes, and practices must also be considered when formulating the plan of care. Food preferences and religious and cultural food practices must be respected and incorporated into the plan of care. For example, it is inappropriate to ask a vegetarian to eat meat. Instead, work within the client's limitations, using soy products, legumes, nuts, whole grain cereals, and complementing vegetables, and stress that food quantities must be increased. If the client has never eaten breakfast, do not discuss the attribute of eating breakfast. Encourage the client to try a

bowl of cereal or even a glass of milk in the morning. Foods that are enjoyed at another time of day, such as cold pizza, a sandwich or even a piece of pie with milk, can be suggested as normal nourishment for the morning meal.

MEDICATIONS

The nurse must determine what prescriptions and over-the-counter drugs the client is taking that affect nutrition.

Durgs can affect the supply of nutrients by changing the appetite, changing the sense of taste or smell, or causing the side-effects of nausea and vomiting. Medications can also decrease absorption of nutrients by changing gastrointestinal motility or body secretions, inactivating enzymes, changing mucosal cells, and forming drug nutrient complexes. Some medications affect the diet by producing large amounts of unwanted or restricted substances such as sodium. One example is the laxative Sal Hepatica that contains 1000 milligrams of sodium per dose. Laxatives such as citrate of magnesia and milk of magnesia are contraindicated for most renal patients because of the magnesium they contain.

Medications also affect the time when food can be eaten. If a patient is on an antibiotic every 6 hours, which must be taken 1 hour before meals or 2 hours after a meal, mealtimes are certainly limited and eating six or seven small meals daily is almost impossible. See the box on page 276 for selected medications that affect or are affected by food intake.

ASSESSMENT OF GASTROINTESTINAL FUNCTION

Assessment of the gastrointestinal tract should be a component of total assessment for all clients whether their illness is end-stage renal disease, cancer, bulimia,

---

Selected Medications That Affect or Are Affected by Food Intake

Anti-inflammatories such as aspirin, Bufferin, and Indocin make the person prone to bleeding, gastritis, and ulcers.

Dilantin frequently results in gingival hyperplasia, nausea, vomiting, and constipation.

Antihypertensives such as Aldomet and Catapress cause edema of salivary glands and diarrhea.

Iron causes constipation or diarrhea and black stools that may disguise gastrointestinal bleeding.

Antineoplastics have many gastrointestinal side-effects including stomatitis, nausea, vomiting, anorexia, and diarrhea.

Digoxin's side-effects include nausea, vomiting, anorexia, and diarrhea.

Mineral oil, that is taken frequently by the elderly as a laxative, results in chronic nutrient deficit. The mineral oil binds fat soluble vitamins and causes them to be excreted in the stool. If the client insists on taking the mineral oil, advise him to take it as long as possible after a meal.

Antacids decrease the availability of iron, calcium, and B_{12} because these nutrients are best absorbed in an acid medium. The current trend of obtaining calcium in the form of certain antacids needs to be evaluated. If calcium supplementation is needed, clients should be instructed to take over-the-counter calcium preparations.

---

pulmonary disease, or a disease of the gastrointestinal tract. Percussion, auscultation, observation and palpation are performed to detect deficits in the process of food ingestion, digestion, absorption, and excretion in order to formulate appropriate nutritional interventions.

If the problem affects food *ingestion*, interventions are appropriate that will cause a change in food consistencies or in the entry point for food such as insertion of nasogastric feeding tube. However, if the problem affects *digestion*, interventions planned should include the use of elemental feedings. Elemental products require no digestion because the feedings contain simple sugars, amino acids, and fatty acids that are the end products of digestion. Absorption problems are also treated with elemental products or by hyperalimentation.

Another important consideration includes decreased or altered excretion due to changes in the gastrointestinal tract. For example, surgically forming a new exit point for stool, such as a colostomy or an ileostomy, creates water and electrolyte losses so the client needs to be carefully monitored, especially when it is a new ostomy.

CLIENT'S ABILITY TO LEARN

There may be no correlation between a client's educational preparation and his ability to learn nutrition information. Too often the assumption is made that since the client is a college graduate, teaching will be easy and require little time. Factors such as stress, fatigue, illness, change in life-style, and financial problems affect learning ability, so nutrition teaching and interventions must be planned accordingly.

PREVIOUS SPECIAL DIETS

Adult clients may have participated in many different diets throughout their lifetime.

What was a beneficial nutrition practice 5 years ago may not be correct today. If a person had diverticulosis 10 years ago, he was told to follow a low residue diet. Now the proper diet is a high fiber diet avoiding seeds and nuts. If the intervention is to include eating eggs daily, the client and the client's wife may become very upset because he has been on a low cholesterol diet for years. For clients who have been in weight reduction diets for many years, it may be hard to convince them to increase caloric intake. The home health nurse must understand the client's previous diet in order to assure successful implementation of a new dietary program.

FOOD QUACKERY AND/OR NUTRITION MYTHS

Always be aware of food quackery and nutritional myths. Even the very intelligent and well informed may follow nutritional myths and/or adhere to quackery. If the quackery or myths are dangerous to the client, deal with them early. If the consequences are not harmful but are a financial stress to the family, they can be dealt with later after rapport has been established and teaching is less extensive. Deal with the quackery remembering that you may not be able to make a change but you can provide the information needed so that change can occur.

ENTERAL AND PARENTERAL NUTRITION

A complete nutritional assessment as already described is the first step in working with the client. The next step is to determine the client's nutritional needs. If the client is unable to obtain adequate nutrition through oral feedings, enteral or parenteral feedings may be required.

ENTERAL FEEDINGS

Enteral nutrition is the treatment of choice for many nutritionally compromised clients. The critically ill or chronically ill client who is nutritionally compromised can benefit from enteral feedings often as much, if not more so, than from hyperalimentation. Moreover, it is less invasive and less expensive. While the home health nurse does not decide which form of nutrition to use, information should be provided to the physician about which method is more suitable to the individual client, based upon assessment of the client, environment, and financial status. The nurse must know the principles of each technique and be equally skilled in both delivery systems.

Indications for enteral feedings include dysphagia, gastrointestinal fistulas, malabsorptive syndromes (*i.e.*, Crohn's disease and short gut syndrome), anorexia nervosa, and/or malnutrition. It is often an adjunct to chemotherapy. Enteral feedings can be used preoperatively to improve nutritional status for the client with cancer. The feedings can also be used in conjunction with therapy to overcome iatrogenic malnutrition, frequently associated with massive radiation and chemotherapy.

Sometimes, there is a delay in starting enteral nutrition at home. If concerted efforts to increase food intake have not been successful in stopping weight loss, enteral feedings must be considered. It is the responsibility of the home health nurse to alert the physician to the continuing weight loss and encourage the physician to prescribe home enteral feedings.

Advantages of enteral feedings over parenteral include no need for an inpatient admission to start the procedure, less cost and a procedure that is relatively simple. The disadvantages include slower results since the feeding must start slowly and must be titrated. Enteral feedings cannot be used if there is any obstruction in the bowel since the feedings require functioning of the gastrointestinal system. Administrative problems, such as the tendency of some feeding tubes to clog, may occur. A final disadvantage to enteral feedings is that clients may experience feelings of fullness and discomfort, especially when the feedings are first started.

Financial Considerations

The monthly cost for enteral nutrition, including feeding pump, IV pole, 30 administration sets, and 2000 calories a day of Isocal can range from $700 to $1100. Sometimes the difference in cost may reflect a difference in service from the various suppliers. Comparative shopping is especially important if there are caps on the insurance policy. When doing comparative shopping consider the services provided. Delivery, assembling, and servicing the pump, 24-hour telephone availability, and third party direct billing should be the minimum services. Additional supplier services may include providing a nurse to help teach and evaluate the tube feeding procedure.

Robert Martin, vice president of Keystone Medical Supplies in Pittsburgh, states that billing Medicare for enteral supplies and nutritional products is done under Part B. The diagnosis of the client determines eligibility for payment. Some of the diagnoses that Medicare will accept are dysphagia, aphagia due to CVA, a comatose condition, inability to swallow due to paralysis, brain tumor with neurological deficit, lack of gag reflex, and impaired gag reflex. In other words, there must be a nonfunctioning of one or more of the structures that normally allow food to reach the digestive tract.* Medicare pays 80%

*Keystone Medical Suppliers. Pittsburgh, PA. From Parenteral and Enteral Nutrition Manual prepared by Blue Cross/Blue Shield of South Carolina

of the cost. If the patient has a major medical policy, it will pay the remaining 20%.

Coverage by private insurance carriers and HMO's varies widely. Some cover 100% of the cost while others have the same coverage as Medicare. Some cover the equipment only and none of the nutritional products, while still others cover nothing. Sometimes by enlisting the help of the physician, some insurance companies can be persuaded to cover part or all of the cost. If faced with a hospital bill (*i.e.*, for enteral or parenteral feedings in the hospital) and offered an alternative of home care, many insurance companies will "make an allowance" and choose to pay for home care.

Welfare is state-regulated and coverage varies from state to state. Generally coverage is nonexistent or minimal, including only the feeding tube and possibly the administration sets. Before enteral feedings and equipment are ordered, payment sources must be investigated because the client is responsible for uncovered costs. This is done most efficiently by the company from whom the supplies will be ordered.

Feeding Tubes

The home health nurse needs to be knowledgeable about the various types of feeding tubes, how to insert them, and the advantages and disadvantages of each. The specific tube that was used in the hospital may not be the most appropriate at home.

Nasogastric/Nasoduodenal (Nasoenteric) Tubes

The use of traditional Levin tubes for gastric feedings should be discouraged. If a Levin tube is ordered, the nurse should pursue the possibility to using the new small-lumen flexible tubes. Most physicians do not object to another type of tube as long as the client receives the designated nutrients. The advantages and disadvantages of the traditional levin tube are shown below. If the Levin-type tube is used, insert the smallest size (12F and 14F) that will permit flow of the home-prepared feeding.

Within the past few years there has been a revolution in the development of nasogastric and nasoduodenal tubes. The tubes are small-bore (8F), silastic, very flexible, weighted at the tip with mercury and, most recently, tungsten. The many advantages and disadvantages of these tubes are shown in the boxed material opposite.

If the tube was inserted while the client was in the hospital, the nurse, prior to visiting, must become familiar with the type of tube, its care, and the technique for changing the tube. In some instances, the home health nurse will be inserting the nasogastric tube and initiating the feedings. The nurse must be knowledgeable and confident in order to reassure the family they are capable of providing the client's care. In addition to order-

---

Advantages and Disadvantages of the Levin Tube

DISADVANTAGES

1. The tube can be uncomfortable.

2. The tube may undergo chemical changes in the presence of gastric fluids.

3. Clients with a Levin tube are at high risk for aspiration and gastric reflux.

4. There is an increased chance of bacterial growth from the blenderized diet usually prescribed with these tubes.

ADVANTAGES

1. Home prepared formulas may be used.

Advantages and Disadvantages of Silastic, Flexible Tubes

ADVANTAGES

1. Tubes generally are more comfortable.

2. Oral ingestion with the tube in place is possible.

3. The tube does not undergo chemical changes from contact with digestive fluids.

4. Use of the tube can prevent reflux esophagitis.

DISADVANTAGES

1. The tube has a tendency to clog if the client/family do not follow irrigation guidelines specifically.

2. Very slow formula administration is required, due to the small lumen of the tube.

3. If using a feeding pump, the client is usually connected for 12 to 24 hours and requires commercially prepared formulas.

---

ing initial supplies, the home health nurse must order an extra tube to be kept in the home for unscheduled changes. When a tube has been removed, the family cannot incinerate the tube if it is weighted with mercury because the vapors are harmful.

Each tube is prepackaged with specific directions for insertion but there are general guidelines for inserting, each of the two distinct categories—carrier tubes and stylet tubes.

Carrier Tubes

The most commonly used carrier tube is a Duotube. For ease of insertion it consists of a large, clear, stiff polyvinyl outer tube and a small white silastic inner tube (most common size, 8F) that is weighted at the tip with mercury or tungsten and remains in the client. These tubes are passed in the "traditional" method: measure first for approximate distance; lubricate with K-Y jelly; then pass through the nares into the stomach with the client swallowing as the tube advances.

After the tube is inserted, using the bulb syringe packaged with the tube, insert the end of the bulb syringe into the end of the feeding tube. This will inject air and separate the tubes. At the same time, listen with a stethoscope in the left upper quadrant for air, which indicates proper placement. If you hear air, fill the bulb syringe with water and attach it to the feeding tube. Again, using quick, forceful squeezing action, inject the water. Repeat one or two more times. The inner tube will no longer be visible as it has been passed into the stomach. The final step is to pull out the clear tube until the connector is visible and the small white tube is out about 4 to 6 inches from the nares. Cut off the clear tube distal to the connector. Secure the tube on the client's cheek with a plastic occlusive dressing. These tubes will pass spontaneously into the duodenum within 24 hours without further interventions by a nurse.

Stylet Tubes

There are many brands of small bore feeding tubes that use a stylet for insertion. Most of the tubes are weighted with tungsten and the usual size for an adult is 8F. Brands include the Flexiflo, Dobbhoff, Entriflex, Keofeed, Vivonex, and CorSafe tubes. See Table 11-4 for specific characteristics of small-lumen feeding tubes.

TABLE 11.4 Specific Characteristics of Small-Lumen Feeding Tubes

Tube	Use	Lubrication	Flow-thru Stylet	Special Direction/ Characteristics
Carrier Tube Duotube	Nasoduodenal	K-Y Jelly	—	Small 8F silicone tube inside a 12–14F PVC tube for ease in placement. External tube is withdrawn after placement and "freeing" the silicone component with water. Older tubes have mercury tip
Stylet Tubes CorSafe	Nasogastric and Nasoduodenal	Dip tip in water	Yes	Inject 10 cc water with stylet in place prior to inserting tube to aid removal of stylet.

(continued)

TABLE 11.4 Specific Characteristics of Small-Lumen Feeding Tubes *(continued)*

Tube	Use	Lubrication	Flow-thru Stylet	Special Direction/ Characteristics
				Manufacturer claims anti-clog exit port in tip. Multiple types of tubes available. Some tubes may be passed without stylets (see packaged literature)
Dobbhoff	Nasoduodenal	Hydromer-lubricated Activate tip by dipping in water	Yes	Inject 10 cc water into tube to activate hydromer coating prior to inserting stylet. Aspiration may be done with stylet in place to help confirm placement
Entriflex	Nasogastric	Activate tip by dipping in water.	Yes	Inject 10 cc water into tube to activate coating prior to inserting stylet. Some tubes weighted with mercury. Aspiration may be done with stylet in place to help confirm placement
Flexiflo	Nasogastric or nasoduodenal	Dip entire tube into water	Yes #8F prepackaged with stylet	Feeding ports are in the bolus. Available three sizes/styles: #8F prepackaged with stylet #8F without stylet #12F: 36-inch length for nasogastric use only; may be inserted without stylet
Keofeed	Nasogastric or nasoduodenal	Lubricate tip with K-Y jelly. Inject 1 cc water (packaged	No	Do not use more than 5 cc water as this will cause

(continued)

TABLE 11.4 Specific Characteristics of Small-Lumen Feeding Tubes *(continued)*

Tube	Use	Lubrication	Flow-thru Stylet	Special Direction/ Characteristics
		with tube) into tube lumen with stylet in place		difficulty removing stylet. Literature with feeding tube states to partially remove when tube has passed to the 50 cm mark. May then continue tube passage into duodenum to 75 cm mark. Most are weighted with mercury.
Travasorb Duo-port	Nasogastric (3 g bolus) and nasoduodenal (5 g bolus)	Lubricate tip only	Yes	Comes with insertion kit that includes lubricating jelly. Has slide ring on tubing for a reference to check for tube migration. Prelubricated tube; no need for water
Others				
Vivonex	Nasogastric or nasoduodenal	May lubricate tip with K-Y jelly.	No stylet	For nasoduodenal feeding, pass tube into stomach (first single black line), then pass at 2- and 4-hour intervals to the double black line

Most product literature of newly manufactured tubes say aspiration is possible with the small-lumen tubes. Sometimes gastric fluids are not obtained and tube may still be in proper location.

The major advantages of these weighted tubes include comfort and decreased possibility of regurgitation and reflux esophagitis. Most tubes have a hydrophilic polymer coating on the tip, inside the lumen, and on the outside of the tube to facilitate insertion of the tube and stylet and removal of the stylet. Most tubes have flow-thru stylets. K-Y Jelly is not required except for the Vivonex tube.

While the principles of insertion for each tube are basically the same, it is helpful to read the specific instructions that are packaged with the tubes. Most of the tubes require injecting water into the lumen to activate the coating. A few tubes are dipped into water. The nurse must feel free to review literature packaged with the tubes even with the family present since changes occur frequently. Tell the family you are reviewing the directions to be certain no changes have been made re-cently in the product. The general directions for inserting small-lumen weighted tubes are outlined in the box below.

The home care nurse assumes responsibility for teaching the client and family and for "troubleshooting." Teaching must be basic, simplified, and continually reinforced until the client, family, and nurse are confident the

---

Insertion of Small-lumen Weight Feeding Tubes with Stylet

1. Measure from tip of earlobe to nostril and to xyphoid process. If the tube is to be placed in the duodenum add 6 to 8 inches.

2. Prepare tube: Inject water inside tube or dip in water, depending on brand. Dip tip of catheter into water.

3. Insert stylet into tube, being sure end is positioned against the weighted tip. Be careful that the stylet does not perforate the tube.

4. Insert tube gently into nostril. Direct tube down and back toward the ear.

5. Have client bend head slightly forward if possible. This may help close epiglottis and make it easier to avoid entering the trachea.

6. After the tube is in the pharynx, have client swallow if able, and pass the tube further with each swallow. Taking sips of water will help the client swallow. Stop when tube has been inserted to the premeasured place.

7. Using 50 cc syringe, draw up 30 cc air and attach syringe to tube.

8. Place stethoscope over left upper quadrant and quickly and forcefully inject the air. You should hear the air immediately and then will know the tube is in the stomach.

9. Additional tests for placement include the following: a. Ask the client to hum. If the tube is in the trachea he cannot hum. b. Place the end of the tube in water and observe for continuous rhythmic bubbles, indicating the tube is in the lungs. Remove tube and reinsert tube if tests do not indicate tube is in the stomach. Many physicians require an x-ray film to check placement of the tube (for tubes with mercury). Most major towns and cities have a portable x-ray service and if ordered by the physician, this cost is generally covered by insurance and Medicare.

10. Remove the stylet when proper placement has been verified.

11. Secure the end of the tube to the face with plastic occlusive dressing. If tube is to enter duodenum, tape very loosely and leave slack on tube. Change tape when slack is gone. Continue until tube no longer advances for up to 24 hours.

12. If there is any reason that the client should not have any feeding into the stomach, such as a gastric fistula, do not start the feeding for 24 hours so tube will have time to advance into the duodenum.

feeding is being given safely. Even after extensive teaching there can still be problems. Questioning, continually reviewing technique, and reobserving the client/family technique seems to be endless. Do not assume the family can transfer learning, that is, they may know they should not disconnect the feeding without irrigating the tube but may think that disconnecting and not irrigating the tube while the client is in the bathroom for 10 to 15 minutes is acceptable. Most agencies have an RN on call 24 hours a day to assist clients and their families with "troubleshooting" problems.

Guidelines for small-lumen feeding tubes that can be used for teaching the client and family are displayed in the boxed material below.

Guidelines for Small-Lumen Feeding Tubes

1. Never place crushed or powdered tablets down the feeding tube. All medications must be in liquid form.

2. An infusion pump should be used. If gravity feedings are necessary, give the feedings very slowly.

3. Irrigate the tube any time the feeding is interrupted and at least every 8 hours with 30 cc water. Once a day or more often if indicated, irrigate with 30 cc Coke, which decreases the possibility of clogging. (Check with the manufacturer for specific recommendations.) Follow Coke with 30 cc water to rinse the stickiness from inside the tube.

4. Never use a syringe smaller than 50 cc. (Some tubes can be irrigated with 30 cc but 50 cc is safe for all tubes.) If giving small amounts of medications, add water to increase volume.

5. Always follow medications with 50 cc water.

6. Enteral nutritional products designed for tube feedings (*i.e.*, Isocal, Osmolite, and Compleat B) should be used whenever possible. The consistency is appropriate for the small-bore tubes and is well tolerated by clients.

7. If the tube comes out partially (8 to 10 inches or less), *do not* remove the tube. The weighted tip permits the tube to return to the desired position. Leave tube untaped if possible or allow slack and retape periodically until tube returns to measured mark on tube.

8. Check tube placement prior to each feeding by placing a stethoscope over the upper left quadrant and rapidly injecting air. A rumbling or bubbling sound should be heard if tube is positioned correctly. And one of the following should be checked:
   (a) Aspiration: Aspirating for gastric contents may be unreliable due to small bore of tube. Some tubes collapse when aspiration is attempted. Some product information inserts say aspirating is permitted but lack of gastric contents does not indicate tube is incorrectly placed.
   (b) Place end of the feeding tube in glass of water and observe for bubbles. If rhythmic, continuous bubbling is seen the tube is probably not in the stomach. Do not give feeding. Remove and reinsert tube.
   (c) Ask the client to hum. If tube is in correct position he will be able to hum.

Feeding Pumps

The use of an infusion pump helps eliminate many of the problems associated with too rapid formula administration, such as diarrhea, abdominal cramping, and a feeling of excessive fullness. The small lumen feeding tubes allow using formulas (*i.e.*, Enrich, a fiber-containing formula) that have a thicker consistency and will not flow through the small tubes by gravity alone. The current pumps are compact and simple to use. Minimal teaching by the home health nurse will result in the client/family becoming proficient and comfortable in their use.

The operation is basically the same for all pumps. All have audible alarms while some have both audible and visible alarms. All pumps have alarms to indicate when the feeding bag is empty and when the line is occluded. Most can be operated by battery for 1 to 6 hours and these have an alarm warning when the battery charge is low. A few can be operated from a car cigarette lighter outlet with a converter obtained from the supplier. Some pumps can be set digitally in 5 cubic centimeter increments from 5 to 295 cubic centimeters. For pediatric use, a few pumps can be set in one to two increments for lower volumes and then in 5 cubic centimeter increments. Still others have 5 to 15 preset flow rates from which to choose. Some pumps have alarms that are activated if there is a change in flow rate while the pump is operating to prevent an accidental change of flow rate.

Another feature of some pumps is an indicator showing the volume of feeding administered during the time the pump has been running. Whenever the pump is stopped the volume starts again at zero. The plug for most pumps is three prong and must be used with a converter if the house does not have a three-prong receptacle. See Figures 11-2 and 11-3 for illustrations of feeding pumps.

Teaching includes filling the feeding bag,

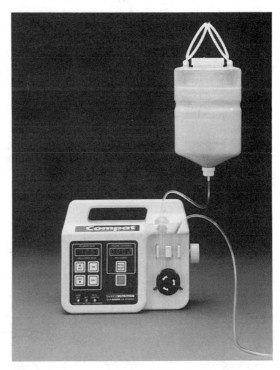

Figure 11-2. Sandoz Compat enteral delivery system. (Courtesy Sandoz Nutrition Corporation, Clinical Products Division, Minneapolis, MN)

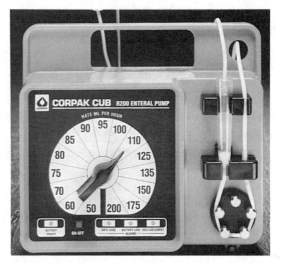

Figure 11-3. Corpak Cub enteral pump. (Courtesy Corpak, Inc., Wheeling, IL)

priming the tubing, threading the tubing around the drive mechanism, and setting the desired rate of administration which is in cubic centimeter per hour. The home health nurse must be familiar with several product lines and if some equipment is difficult for the client to use, a substitution must be made. For example, if a client/family member experiences difficulty filling tube feeding bags with flexible openings, the nurse should recommend feeding bags with a firm opening. Currently most bags from one manufacturer can be used with pumps from another manufacturer. This convenience is nearing an end since, with new pumps, only the manufacturing company's bags can be used.

The procedure for enteral nutrition by a feeding pump is shown on page 287.

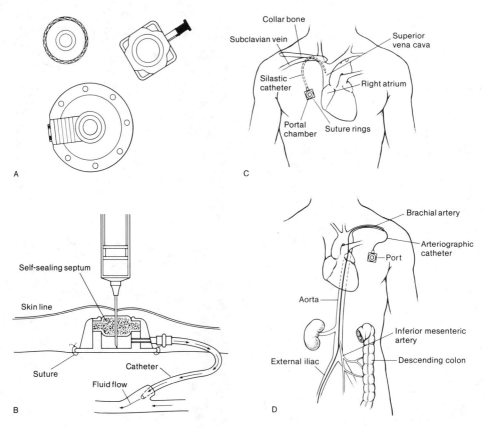

Figure 11-4. Vascular access devices. *(A)* Three VADs and their self-sealing silicone septums encased in ports and attached to silicone catheters. *(B)* A needle puncture through the skin into the port allows drugs, fluids, and blood to be administered. *(C)* For systemic drug and fluid delivery, the catheter is placed in the subclavian vein. *(D)* Port catheter is attached to an arteriographic catheter inserted percutaneously. (Reprinted with permission from Oncology Nursing Press, January 1988)

Procedure for Enteral Nutrition by a Feeding Pump

1. *Purpose:* The feeding pump ensures accurate volumetric nutrition via enteral tube feedings. It may be used for nasogastric, gastrostomy, nasoduodenal or jejunostomy feedings.

2. *Equipment:*
   Feeding pump
   Administration set—bag with tubing
   Formula or nutritional product
   Polar pack or ice if using bag with pocket for ice IV pole
   Three-way converter if outlet is only two-way
   Procedure:
   (a) Obtain the pump, administration set, pole and formula.
   (b) Secure the set to the IV pole or place on flat, stable surface near the client.
   (c) Plug the power converter into wall outlet. If at all possible, avoid using an extension cord and do not use the other outlet of the extension cord.
   (d) Set the desired flow rate (if the client has not been receiving tube feedings or p.o. feeding start feedings at 50 cc/hr or closest setting).
   (e) Check the placement and patency of the feeding tube by using a 50 cc syringe to inject 30 cc of air into the tube and auscultate over the left upper quadrant. A swishing sound will occur if the tube is in the stomach. Also use one of the following methods.
      (1) Aspirate the tube to check for stomach contents unless a weighted nasogastric tube is used. Omit this step for some weighted tubes.
      (2) Place the end of the tube in a glass of water. Continuous rhythmic bubbles will appear if the tube is in the trachea or bronchus.
      (3) Ask the client to hum. He will not be able to hum if the tube is in the trachea.
   (f) Place the client in a semi-Fowler's position.
   (g) Using 50 cc syringe, introduce 30 cc of water into the feeding tube.
   (h) Close clamp on feeding tube and fill the feeding bag with the desired amount of formula (usually an 8-hour feeding) and close bag.
   (i) Fill the ice pocket with ice or a polar pack.
   (j) Hang feeding bag higher than feeding tube entry point.
   (k) Open clamp on tubing and slowly allow the formula to fill the entire line with fluid. Close clamp.
   (l) Thread the administration set around drive mechanism.
   (m) Connect the administration set to the client's feeding tube.
   (n) Open clamp.
   (o) Start the pump.
   (p) Stop the pump every 8 hours and irrigate the feeding tube with 30 cc to 60 cc water.
   (q) Once a day or more often if indicated, irrigate feeding tube with 30 cc coke. Follow coke with 30 cc water. See manufacturer's recommendations).
   (r) If reusing the feeding bag and administration set several times, change the bag and set every 8 hours to prevent continuous pressure on and splitting of tubing. If

(continued)

not reusing, change bag and administration set every 24 hours.

(s) If reusing bags, rinse the used feeding bag and administration set with a cleaning solution of one teaspoon vinegar to one pint water. Allow to air dry.

3. General Information:

(a) Cleaning: The exterior of the feeding pump can be cleaned with a cloth or sponge, lightly dampened with warm, soapy water or alcohol. Care should be taken that no fluid gets inside the pump since damage to the electronic components could result. The cloth or sponge that is used to clean the pump should be as dry as possible.

(b) Irrigations should never be forceful.

Adapted from Walsh J, Persons CB, Wieck L: Manual of Home Health Care Nursing. Philadelphia, JB Lippincott, 1987

Another major responsibility for the home health nurse is to assist the client and family in coping with problems related to the feedings. A guide to troubleshooting is shown in Table 11-5.

When feedings are started it is important to titrate the formulas for optimum tolerance, comfort, and prevention of GI disturbances. See Table 11-6 for tube feeding rates and formula concentration.

Gastrostomy Tube Feedings

The initial placement of a gastrostomy tube requires a surgical procedure that can be performed on an outpatient basis in the one day surgical unit. Stoma care is very simple — keeping the area clean and dry. If irritation does develop from leakage, Skin Prep may be used as a barrier. The feeding tube is usually a large Foley catheter with a 30 cubic centimeter bag. But there are specific gastrostomy feeding tubes with a disc shield that rests against the outside of the abdomen and prevents the tube from entering the duodenum. When changing the tube, the family is taught to insert the feeding tube 6 to 8 inches into the stoma, inflate the balloon, and then pull back on the tube and secure the tube to the abdomen.

If leakage occurs around the feeding tube, instruct the client/family to pull the tube secure so that the balloon rests snug against the opening and to have the client lie down 30 minutes after feeding. Decreasing the amount of feeding being given at one time and increasing the number of feedings are also interventions that may decrease any leakage.

A gastrostomy feeding tube is not considered skilled by Medicare for payment of Skilled Care Facilities admission but Medicare will cover costs of feedings and equipment as discussed under enteral feedings. Usually a pump is not necessary for gastrostomy feedings because the tube is larger and the receiving receptacle, the stomach, is larger. Other advantages of the gastrostomy tube are listed on page 290.

Jejunostomy Feeding Tubes

Insertion and changing of a jejunostomy tube requires a surgical procedure. When food

TABLE 11.5 Guide to Troubleshooting

If this problem occurs:	Try this solution:
1. Empty/Occluded Alarm • Feeding container empty • Feeding tube or feeding set occluded	Hang new container. Locate the point of occlusion and correct. Occlusion may occur distal or proximal from the pump.
• Control clamp closed • Tubing kinked • Bubbles in the drip chamber • Drip chamber full • Alarm comes on after filling • Drip chamber is placed incorrectly	Open control clamp. Straighten tubing. Clear bubbles, clear chamber. Reread instructions and correct. Prime the tubing to clear the air from tubing. Check to make sure drip chamber is properly locked in pump positioning bar.
2. Drip chamber walls are coated with feeding.	If formula cannot be removed from inside walls of chamber via chamber anipulation, replace set.
3. Sensors in drip chamber bracket have become inoperative due to spillage on unit.	Remove any deposits on sensors by using cotton swab dampened with warm, soapy water.
4. Low Battery • Battery has been run down below point of maintaining accuracy of pump.	Plug pump power converter into 110V AC wall outlet.
5. Rate change • Pump flow rate has been changed with pump running.	Check flow rate to make sure rate selected is correct for patient. If the flow rate needs to be changed, set correct flow rate. Start pump.

TABLE 11.6 Tube Feeding for Adults: Rates and Formulas

Tube Feeding Rates	Formula Concentration at Continuous Drip
50 cc/hr	One fourth (¼) strength formula for 12 hours
If tolerated:	One half (½) strength formula for 36 hours
If tolerated:	Three quarter (¾) strength formula for 48 hours
If tolerated:	Full strength for 24 hours
60 cc/hr	Full strength for 24 hours

If tolerated: Increase speed 10 cc an hour each day until 100 cc per hour is reached. If client expresses concern about an increased rate, explain 10 cc equals 2 teaspoons

---

Advantages of the Gastrostomy Tube

1. It is easier to change. If the tube is not sutured the client or family can be taught to change the tube. (As with the nasogastric tube there should always be an extra gastrostomy tube in the home.)

2. It rarely becomes occluded.

3. Aesthetically it is more acceptable. People cannot see the gastrostomy tube, which helps the client have a more positive body image.

4. Blenderized foods can be given because of increased tube size.

---

enters the jejunum, most areas of digestion are bypassed; consequently, an elemental nutritional product should be used.

Jejunostomy tube feedings are harder to manage because the reservoir where the food enters is even smaller than the duodenum. These clients require a pump because the rate needs to be very slow to prevent overload that could result in abdominal cramping and diarrhea. Clients should lie flat for at least one half hour after the feeding to decrease transit time.

Types of Enteral Nutritional Products

There are several types of nutritional products available. These include, soy and caseinate products such as Isocal, Osmolite, and Resource; feedings formulated from food, such as Compleat; elemental products such as Precision, Vivonex, and Vital; and disease-specific products such as Trauma Cal, Pulmocare, and Isotene.

The elemental products are more costly because they are prepared with simple sugars, amino acids, and fatty acids, nutrients that are more expensive than caseinate. If elemental products are ordered and there is no pathophysiology necessitating them, it is the home health nurse's responsibility to contact the physician, inquire if another supplement could be substituted, and familiarize him with the cost. Most physicians are not aware of the cost of the supplements and will react positively if given rational reasons and factual information. (For specific information about selected nutritional products, see Table 11-7.)

HOME PARENTERAL NUTRITION

The administration of total parenteral nutrition into the central venous system has been possible in USA hospitals since the 1960's. Shortly after this time, Broviac developed a permanent indwelling silastic catheter that permitted the administration of home parenteral nutrition. Modification of the catheter by Hickman included increasing the lumen size, improving the catheter's durability and lessening the incidence of clotting. Other improvements in the delivery system and fluids have changed the focus of parenteral nutrition from use for the short-term, acutely ill hospitalized patient to include clients with advanced chronic nutritional disorders and potential or actual iatrogenic illnesses.

Until recently, the use of home parenteral nutrition was associated with large university hospitals. Only a very select group of hospital nurses were taught the "complex" procedure so that they could provide the care and teach a few very carefully selected, highly intelligent clients. Presently parenteral nutrition is a treatment found in almost every hospital and it is being taught successfully to motivated, emotionally stable clients of average intelligence with average dexterity who are discharged on short- or long-term therapy.

Most clients who are discharged to the home on home parenteral nutrition (HPN) have been taught either by a hospital Total Parenteral Nutrition team or by a nurse who is a representative from a medical supply company such as Travenol or Volunteer Hospital Services. The nurses from these companies are available for consultation, home visitation, and advising patients. They normally cover a large geographical area and cannot be physically present each time a problem arises or each time a change is necessary.

The home health nurse and the medical supply nurse must work cooperatively in order to provide the best care possible, meet the client/family needs, and avoid confusing the client with conflicting instructions. Usually it is the responsibility of the home health nurse to reinforce teaching, assist the client and family to individualize the techniques, and assess the ability or desire to comply with the interventions.

Other roles of the nurse include teaching the client/family the complications of parenteral nutrition, and to be alert for any problems or early signs of complications. If for any reason the client is unable to do the HPN himself, because of physical deterioration, for instance, the home health nurse will be expected to initiate teaching to a family member. It is generally best if a family member becomes familiar with the procedure very early to avoid a crisis if debilitation of the client occurs.

Access to the vascular system for parenteral nutrition is either by tunneled catheter such as a Hickman or Broviac catheter or more recently through an implantable infusion device such as a Medi-Port, Infuse-a-Port, or Port-a-Cath, (Figure 11-4). Both methods have their proponents. The apparent evidence of fewer systemic complications from the infusion devices and the fact that they are

cosmetically more acceptable is responsible for their increased usage. The disadvantages are a need for daily needle punctures and needle access is generally limited to less than 2000 punctures. The implantable infusion devices are a silastic catheter attached to a portal made of an inert metal, such as stainless steel, with a self-sealing silicone diaphragm. The portal is implanted totally under the skin and attached to the fascia. The end of the catheter is inserted into the central venous system.

The Hickman catheter consists of a long silastic catheter that is tunneled subcutaneously under the chest wall into the subclavian vein with the tip entering the superior vena cava (Figure 11-5). Both the Hickman and Broviac (most often used for children) have a dacron cuff that, after 4 to 6 weeks, adheres to the fibrous tissue, sealing off the catheter and providing a bacterial barrier. Because of the cuff, sterile procedure is not necessary after about 6 weeks from insertion and clean technique can then be used. The home health nurse will be responsible for teaching the client to alter the procedure from asepsis to clean technique. Remember, sterile technique is still necessary for any infusion or injection, but not for site care.

(Text continues on p 298)

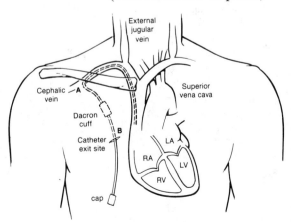

Figure 11-5. Hickman catheter.

TABLE 11.7 Nutritional Products

Product	Manufacturer	Form	Major Protein Source	Major Fat Source	Major Carbohydrate Source
Citrotein*	Sandoz	Powder	Egg white solids. 41 g	Partially hydrogenated soybean oil. 1.6 g	Sucrose, maltodextrin. 122 g
Compleat	Sandoz	Liquid	Beef, nonfat milk, 43 g	Beef, corn oil. 43 g	Hydrolyzed cereal solids, fruits, vegetables maltodextrin lactose. 128 g
Compleat modified	Sandoz	Liquid	Beef, calcium caseinate. 43 g	Beef, corn oil. 37 g	Hydrolyzed cereal solids, fruits, vegetables. 141 g
Criticare HN	Mead Johnson	Liquid	Enzymatically hydrolyzed casein, free amino acids. 38 g	Safflower oil. 3g	Maltodextrin-modified corn starch. 222 g
Enrich	Ross	Liquid	Sodium and calcium caseinates, soy protein isolate. 39.7 g	Corn oil. 37.2	Hydrolyzed corn starch, sucrose soy polysaccharide. 162 g
Ensure*	Ross	Liquid	Sodium and calcium caseinates, soy protein isolate. 37.2 g	Corn oil. 37.2	Corn Syrup, sucrose. 145 g
Ensure Plus*	Ross	Liquid	Sodium and calcium caseinates, soy protein isolate. 54.9 g	Corn oil. 53.3	Corn syrup, sucrose. 200 g
Isocal	Mead Johnson	Liquid	Calcium, sodium caseinates, soy protein isolate. 34 g	Soy oil, MCT.† 44 g	Maltodextrin. 133 g

From Your Source Chart. Minneapolis, Sandoz Nutrition, 1985
*Preferred for oral use.
†MCT = Medium chained triglycerides, more easily absorbed fat.
‡Osmolality (mOsm/ky) is the concentration of a solute in a solution per unit of solvent.

Calories/ ml	Osmolality‡	Calcium	Iron mg	Potassium g	Potassium mEq	Sodium g	Sodium mEq
0.66	480 (Punch)	1.06	37.8	0.71	18.2	0.71	31
1.07	405	0.67	12	1.4	35.9	1.3	56.5
1.07	300	0.67	12	1.4	35.9	0.67	29.1
1.06	650	0.53	9.5	1.32	34	0.63	27
1.1	480	0.719	12.9	1.564	40	0.845	36.8
1.06	450	0.528	9.5	1.564	40	0.845	36.8
1.5	600	0.706	12.7	2.113	54.1	1.141	49.6
1.06	300	0.634	9.5	1.32	34	0.53	23

(continued)

TABLE 11.7 Nutritional Products *(continued)*

Product	Manufacturer	Form	Major Protein Source	Major Fat Source	Major Carbohydrate Source
Isocal HCN	Mead Johnson	Liquid	Calcium, sodium caseinates. 75 g	Soybean oil, MCT. 91 g	Corn syrup. 225 g
Isotein HN	Sandoz	Powder	Delactosed lactalbumin. 68 g	Partially hydrogenated soybean oil, MCT. 34 g	Maltodextrin, monosaccharides. 156 g
Magnacal	Chesebrough-Pond's	Liquid	Calcium, sodium caseinates. 70 g	Partially hydrogenated soybean oil. 80 g	Maltodextrin, sucrose. 250 g
Meritene Liquid*	Sandoz	Liquid	Concentrated sweet skim milk. 57.6 g	Corn oil. 32 g	Lactose, corn syrup solids, sucrose. 110 g
Meritene Powder* (prepared with whole milk)	Sandoz	Powder	Nonfat milk. 69 g	Milk fat. 34 g	Lactose, sucrose, corn syrup solids. 119 g
Osmolite	Ross	Liquid	Sodium and calcium caseinates, soy protein isolate. 37.2 g	MCT, corn oil, soy oil. 38.5 g	Hydrolyzed corn starch. 145 g
Precision Isotonic Diet	Sandoz	Powder	Egg white solids. 29 g	Partially hydrogenated soybean oil. 30 g	Glucose, oligosaccharides sucrose. 144 g
Precision LR Diet	Sandoz	Powder	Egg white solids. 26 g	Partially hydrogenated soybean oil. 1.6 g	Maltodextrin, sucrose. 248 g
Pulmocare	Ross	Liquid	Sodium and calcium caseinates. 62.6 g	Corn oil. 92.1 g	Sucrose, hydrolyzed corn starch. 106 g
Ross SLD*	Ross	Powder	Egg white solids. 37.5 g	—	Hydrolyzed corn starch, sucrose. 137 g
Sustacal*	Mead Johnson	Liquid	Calcium caseinates, soy protein isolate, sodium caseinates. 61 g	Partially hydrogenated soybean oil. 23 g	Sucrose, corn syrup. 140 g

Calories/ ml	Osmolality‡	Calcium	Iron mg	Potassium g	Potassium mEq	Sodium g	Sodium mEq
2.0	690	0.67	12	1.4	36	0.80	35
1.2	300	0.56	10.2	1.07	27.4	0.62	27
2.0	590	1.0	18	1.250	32.1	1.00	43.5
0.96	505 (Vanilla)	1.2	14.4	1.6	41	0.88	38.3
1.0	690	2.2	17.3	2.8	71.8	1.1	47.8
1.06	300	0.528	9.5	1.014	25.9	0.634	27.6
1.0	300	0.64	11.5	0.96	24.6	0.77	19.7
1.1	530 (Vanilla)	0.58	10.5	0.88	22.6	0.70	30.4
1.5	490	1.056	19.0	1.902	48	1.310	57.0
0.82	550	0.83	15	0.833	21	0.833	36
1.0	625	1.0	17	2.08	53	0.94	41

(continued)

TABLE 11.7 Nutritional Products *(continued)*

Product	Manufacturer	Form	Major Protein Source	Major Fat Source	Major Carbohydrate Source
Sustacal HC*	Mead Johnson	Liquid	Calcium and sodium caseinates. 61 g	Partially hydrogenated soybean oil. 58 g	Corn syrup solids, sugar. 190 g
Travasorb	Travenol	Liquid	Sodium caseinates, soy protein isolate, calcium caseinates. 35 g	Corn oil, partially hydrogenated soy oil. 35 g	Sucrose, corn syrup solids. 136 g
Traumacal	Mead Johnson	Liquid	Calcium and sodium caseinates. 82.5 g	Soybean oil, MCT.† 68.5 g	Corn syrup, sugar. 142.5 g
Twocal HN	Ross	Liquid	Sodium and calcium caseinates, soy protein isolate. 83.4 g	Corn oil, MCT. 90.5 g	Hydrolyzed corn starch, sucrose. 216.4 g
Vital HN	Ross	Powder	Protein components (partially hydrolyzed whey, meat soy), free amino acids. 41.7 g	Safflower oil, MCT. 10.8 g	Hydrolyzed corn starch, sucrose. 185 g
Vivonex Standard	Norwich Eaton	Powder	Free amino acids. 20.4 g	Safflower oil. 1.5 g	Glucose, oligosaccharides. 231 g.
Vivonex T.E.N.	Norwich Eaton	Powder	Free amino acids. 38 g	Safflower oil. 3.0 g	Maltodextrins, modified starch. 206 g

Calories/ ml	Osmolality‡	Calcium	Iron mg	Potassium		Sodium	
				g	mEq	g	mEq
1.5	650	0.85	15	1.48	38	0.84	37
1.06	488	0.527	9.5	1.266	32.5	0.738	32
1.5	550	0.75	9.0	1.4	36	1.2	52
2.0	740	1.06	19	2.316	59.4	1.052	45.7
1.0	460	0.667	12	1.333	34.1	0.467	20.3
1.0	550	0.556	10	1.172	30	0.468	20.4
1.0	630	0.50	9	0.782	20	0.460	20

Usually there is only one catheter but there are times when a double-lumen or even a triple-lumen catheter is in place. The double-lumen is actually a Broviac and a Hickman catheter that have been fused together. The triple-lumen consists of three fused catheters. If there is a multiple-lumen catheter in place, always use the same lumen for the HPN.

Dressings for the catheters are at first sterile and then clean. If the client does not have an occlusive dressing, the home health nurse should initiate the use of a plastic occlusive dressing such as Tegaderm, Op-Site or Ensure, and teach the client its use. The use of the occlusive dressing is preferred at home and enables the client to shower. It also decreases possible contamination from surface bacteria and only needs to be changed 1 to 2 times a week.

The use of a self-sealing cap for the catheter is also a must for the client at home since it lessens the possiblity of bleeding into the catheter and chance of contamination. Individual preference determines if a Hickman clamp is also used but it is not necessary. The caps will need to be changed at least weekly and are one-time use only. Caps that are punctured frequently may leak and require more frequent changing. The technique for connecting HPN solution to the cap is very simple. After preparing the HPN solution, cleanse the cap with two alcohol wipes and two Betadine wipes. Insert the needle into the center of the cap, tape in place and start the infusion. When the client is out of the home, an extra sterile cap and a clamp should be carried in case of leakage from around the cap. This is a rare occurrence if the cap has been screwed on firmly.

The solutions administered by total parenteral nutrition provide all the nutrients necessary for life. The composition of the solutions vary according to needs of the body. Frequent blood studies must be performed to evaluate the appropriateness of the solution and the client's biochemical status. Usually the frequency of blood studies following discharge from the hospital is once a week, then tapered to once a month. Monthly blood values should continue as long as HPN is received.

Several parameters are considered in determining needs for parenteral hyperalimentation. These needs include fluid, protein, calories, glucose, lipids, vitamins and minerals.

NEEDS FOR PARENTERAL HYPERALIMENTATION

Fluid

In determining fluid needs, obligatory renal loss, insensible loss, and gastrointestinal losses must be replaced. If the total fluid is not restricted by cardiovascular problems, up to 1000 milliliters over the losses may be given.

Protein

Protein is administered in the form of amino acids. Different combinations of amino acids are used depending upon existing medical conditions. If the client has liver disease, high-branched chain and low-aromatic amino acids will be used. If the client has renal disease, the essential amino acids will be used. In stress, high-branched chained amino acids are used. This is often referred to as therapeutic alterations in protein quality.

The maximum concentration of amino acids is 10% but lower dilutions are usually prepared. The adult requirement for anabolism is 1½ grams of amino acids per kilogram of body weight. (To determine protein, multiply amino acids by 6.25.) Since actual body weight is being used instead of ideal body weight, the protein requirement will need to be recalculated periodically when weight increases (Smith 1986).

Calories

Adult requirements when anabolism is occurring are 30 to 40 kilo calories per kilogram of ideal body weight. In stress, it is even higher but the body probably cannot use a caloric intake greater than 3500 calories, so that should be the highest level provided. It was previously thought that if enough insulin were given to allow the glucose to enter the cell, it would be used by the body. We now know that during periods of stress, glucose utilization decreases while fat and amino acid utilization increases (Treat 1986).

Glucose

In stressed clients, dextrose can provide at least 80% of the basal energy requirement. Glucose in 50% concentrations is most commonly used. In clients with COPD, the glucose load should be kept as low as possible because of the increased CO_2 production from carbohydrates.

Lipids

Fat emulsions can provide up to 60% of the client's total caloric needs. They cannot be used if the client has an egg allergy. Lipids are needed in very small amounts to meet the essential fatty acid requirements (about 4% of total calories). Commonly, lipids are available in dilutions as high as 10%. The disadvantages of a high lipid solution include development of Type I and Type V hyperlipidemia. Other concerns are acute pancreatitis associated with hyperlipidemia, severe liver disease, and thrombocytopenia. In most cases parenteral lipids are given once or twice a week (Smith 1986).

Vitamins and Minerals

Vitamins should be added to the HPN solu-tion just before administration since studies have shown that vitamin A is quickly oxidized in plastic and/or glass and therefore inactivated.

Electrolytes and trace elements must be individually determined by current blood values. Generally speaking, zinc is the most common trace element deficiency with copper being the second most likely deficiency (Howard 1986).

Parenteral nutrition is delivered by one of the many infusion pumps. All pumps work on the same principles and permit a continuous, electronically controlled flow of solution. Each pump is equipped with alarms to warn of problems such as air in the line, in-line obstruction, infusion completed, or low battery. If the client does not have an infusion pump that automatically tapers the beginning and ending flow rate, he must set the pump manually to increase the flow rate after the first hour of infusion and decrease the flow rate by one half the last hour. The tapering on and off of the flow rate will prevent reactive hyperglycemia and hypoglycemia. The HomePro pump (Figure 11-6) available from the Travenol company automatically adjusts the flow rate. It starts with a rate of 60 cubic centimeter and increases to the desired rate within 1 hour. During the last hour of infusion it tapers off the flow rate to 40 cubic centimeters.

When at all possible the in-home infusin should be periodic, preferably at night (*i.e.*, 7 PM to 7 AM) to permit the client more mobility and to allow a more normal life.

Intralipids

While final in-line filters for HPN are usually used to lessen the hazard of particle, air, or microorganism contamination, Intralipids cannot be filtered due to their large molecular size. Lipids may be hung piggyback by using the Y tubing that has the filter in the

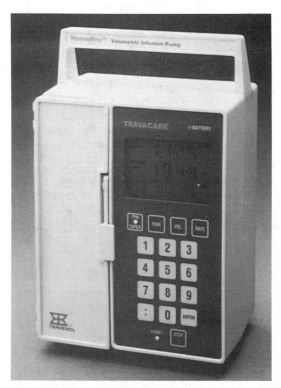

Figure 11-6. HomePro volumetric infusion pump. (Courtesy Travenol Laboratories, Deerfield, IL)

proximal tubing. This is convenient for the client at home, especially if the infusion is given during the night. If the client is able to take oral food, essential fatty acids may be provided by ingesting one teaspoon of corn oil daily. The side-effects of Intralipids are rare but must be taught. Side-effects may include nausea and vomiting, headache, flushing, perspiration, insomnia, vertigo, fever, and chills. If side-effects do occur, instruct the client to slow the infusion rate. Usually the client will be able to tolerate the infusion at a slower rate and the lipids will not need to be discontinued.

Costs

The cost of HPN ranges from $100 to $300 per day with the average cost being closer to $200 to $250 per day. This cost includes formulas and ancillary supplies. The amount of lipids given each week accounts for the range. Reimbursement for parenteral feedings is similar to enteral feedings. There appears to be better reimbursement from welfare for HPN than for enteral feeding. HCFA guidelines used for determining reimbursement say that daily parenteral nutrition is considered reasonable and necessary for a patient with severe pathology of the alimentary tract that prohibits the absorption of sufficient nutrition to maintain weight and strength commensurate with the client's general condition. The guidelines are more diagnosis-specific than for enteral nutrition and mention Crohn's disease, short bowel syndrome, radiation enteritis, and pancreatitis.[16] When selecting a provider for HPN, the same considerations should be examined as discussed with enteral supplies.

While there are benefits of HPN there are possible complications from its administration. While complications are rare, the client/family must be aware of the potential problems so they can detect any early signs or symptoms and prevent a major problem.

The Oley Foundation is an excellent resource for professionals and clients. Established in 1983, it is affiliated with the clinical nutrition program of Albany (New York) Medical College and it is designed for clients and professionals involved in home total parenteral and enteral nutrition. The foundation's goals include research, training, and education. The main component of education is the publication of the bimonthly "Lifeliner Letter." The publication is informative for both patients and professionals. It is mailed to clients at no charge and to professionals for a minimum yearly fee. The address is The Oley Foundation, 214 Hun Memorial, Albany Medical Center, Albany, NY 12208

NURSING DIAGNOSES

There are several medical diagnoses that may cause the client to experience a need for nutritional support. These causes include ulcers, ulcerative colitis, Crohn's disease, and liver disorders.

Stomach ulcers or extensive gastric diseases may interfere with the client's ability to absorb nutrients. Pernicious anemia will occur if the client has over 50% of the stomach removed.

Liver disease may cause many nutritional changes. The liver participates in metabolism of carbohydrates, fats, and proteins, storage of iron and vitamins, manufacture of bile, storage of glycogen, and production and storage of specific coagulative substances. Disease of the liver can affect any of its functions and, depending upon the extent of the disease and dysfunction, can have multiple nutritional ramifications. Clients with moderate to severe liver disease may also experience episodes of hyperglycemia and hypoglycemia because of delayed formation of glycogen from glucose and glucose from glycogen.

Finally, diseases of the colon may also cause the need for nutritional support. Any inflammatory disease of the intestine affects absorption. The intestines contain microscopic villi that are fingerlike projections along the gastrointestinal tract; absorption occurs along the entire villi. When the bowel becomes inflamed, the villi swell together and only the small top portion is available for absorption. This results in a much smaller absorptive surface, substantially reducing absorption.

Therefore, the client experiencing any of these disorders will be at risk for the need for nutritional support. In the following pages, the nursing diagnoses related to clients requiring nutritional support will be presented. If the reader requires additional information on the various gastrointestinal diseases discussed, please refer to a text on medical–surgical nursing.

ANXIETY

Both client and family may experience anxiety related not only to the disease process but also the therapy. Use of either enteral or parenteral therapy may be very threatening to the client.

Assessment

Assess the client and family for signs of anxiety. For example, if they ask multiple questions and have difficulty listening to instructions, the home health nurse may suspect anxiety. Friction between the client and family members may also be an indication of anxiety.

Interventions

Providing the client and family with complete information concerning the disease process, treatment, and related care is one of the most effective interventions in decreasing anxiety. The home health nurse will want to provide opportunities for the client and family to express their feelings and concerns. The nurse will be very instrumental in supporting and encouraging the client and family as they work through their feelings about the existing situation.

Outcome

The client and family will not experience episodes of increased anxiety.

POTENTIAL FOR INFECTION

Clients receiving enteral or parenteral nutrition are at risk for the development of infections. Due to the amount of glucose in the solution, parenteral nutrition, is an excellent medium for the growth of bacteria.

Assessment

On each visit, assess the client for the traditional signs of infection including fever, tachycardia, and malaise. It is also important to monitor the administration set-up procedures for possible breaks in technique that would endanger the client.

Interventions

Assist the client and family as they work to maintain an aseptic system. The solution or feedings should be evaluated carefully for the presence of any contaminants.

The catheter or tube should be carefully dressed to decrease the chance of further infection. Dry, sterile dressings should be maintained. Antibiotic therapy may be required if infection becomes a problem.

For the client undergoing hyperalimentation, special considerations for prevention of infection are needed. The client can be taught to use either clean or sterile technique in preparing the solution and equipment for infusion. Stress the need for adequate handwashing whenever working with the solutions or equipment. Stress the need for adequate soap and water, using friction and washing for 2 to 3 minutes.

Outcome

The client will not experience infection.

INEFFECTIVE INDIVIDUAL OR FAMILY COPING

The need for nutritional support may cause problems for the client or family as they attempt to cope with the many changes necessitated by the illness and treatment. A major role for the home health nurse is to assist the client and family as they develop mechanisms for coping with the problems.

Assessment

On a continual basis, it is necessary to assess the client and family for their ability to cope with the changes imposed by the disease and treatment.

Interventions

Assisting the client/family to cope with the client's limitations and helping to meet the emotional needs is a very vital role of the home health nurse. It is after hospital discharge that the full impact of the dependency for life upon home parenteral nutrition and "a machine" is felt by the client and family. The restriction of the client's life-style and the responsibility of self-care may be overwhelming.

If nursing support proves to be inadequate to assist the client in coping, a consultation with a psychiatric clinical nurse specialist or other counselor may be necessary.

Outcome

Client and family are able to utilize effective coping strategies.

ALTERATION IN BODY IMAGE

Clients who have experienced changes in body weight or who have had an acute illness often experience disturbances in body image. The client who is undergoing nutritional support may also experience an alteration in body image, often precipitated by the presence of life-sustaining equipment.

Assessment

Explore the client's feelings about current body weight and body image. Do the reactions seem within normal limits? If not, can the incorrect feelings be explained by the client's weight history or illness? The client may say that when he was healthy and worked 10 hours a day 7 days a week, he weighed 185 pounds at 5 feet 8 inches tall. Since he has been sick he weighs 160 pounds but thinks he looked much better at 185 pounds. What he is doing is equating his former health with his former weight. Reinforce that his current weight may be foreign to him but it appears adequate, he looks good at that weight, and should consider not regaining more than 5 pounds.

If a person was obese, then his weight became normal before the illness and he then lost more weight during the illness, the client's own body image may still be that of being overweight. If the nurse discusses interventions concerning gaining weight, the client will not want to implement the suggestions. If the assessment reveals the disturbance in body image, teaching should be directed towards replacing nutrient losses instead of weight. If a client is 5 feet 7 inches tall, weighs 105 pounds and states she is fat, consideration must be given that the patient may have anorexia nervosa requiring immediate psychiatric evaluations and not merely nutritional interventions.

Interventions

Encourage the client to continue to express feelings about himself. The home health nurse may be able to provide support as the client attempts to adopt a more positive attitude towards himself. Recommend that the client become as involved as possible in routine family activities. If these interventions fail, it may be necessary to refer the client to additional psychological support.

Outcome

The client will begin to verbalize acceptance of body image.

ALTERATION IN NUTRITION

Clients may experience an alteration in nutrition that includes less than body requirements or more than body requirements. Overweight is not a problem to be corrected during the early recovery phase following an acute illness. Interventions to promote weight loss should be started after the acute phase and may include having the client weighed weekly and follow a weight-reduction diet. The diet should include progressively fewer calories. Expected nursing care for this client is outlined in Table 11-8.

More commonly, however, clients experience an alteration in nutrition of less than body requirements.

Assessment

Nutritional assessment was discussed in detail at the beginning of this chapter. Please refer to that discussion.

Interventions

When nutritional intake is inadequate, individualized aggressive attempts should be made to increase intake orally by "power-packing" foods and/or using supplements. Power-packing means increasing the protein and/or caloric content of a food. Examples follow:

1. Add a jar of strained meat to soup (example: strained chicken to cream of chicken soup).
2. Gradually add dry skim milk powder (up to 4 tablespoons) to a cup of milk.
3. Add powdered or fluid milk and/or cheese to scrambled eggs. Two eggs

TABLE 11.8 Nursing Interventions for Clients with the Nursing Diagnosis of Alteration in Nutrition: More Than Body Requirements

Parameter	Intervention
Calories	1. Dietician to evaluate calorie intake of 3 day diet history. 2. Assist client to establish weight loss goal. 3. Instruct client/family on 1500 calorie reduction diet. 4. Identify high calorie food client is eating. 5. Suggest low calorie alternative. 6. Identify high calorie and low calorie vegetables. 7. Stress need to reduce meat intake to total of 5 ounces daily.
Sodium	1. Instruct client/family on 2 g sodium diet. 2. Identify high sodium foods client is eating. 3. Suggest alternatives for lunch meat, natural, nonprocessed cheese, home made meat loaf, meat from previous evening meal. 4. Discuss cooking with spices and herbs. 5. Stress need to avoid foods such as ham and bacon, except for the low salt brands of ham and bacon.
Potassium	1. Identify high potassium foods client is eating. 2. Instruct client concerning high potassium foods. 3. Instruct client not to use potassium containing salt substitutes. 4. Identify reasons potassium intake must be decreased.
Fat-Soluble Vitamins	1. Stress need to reduce intake of fat soluble vitamins to 100% of R.D.A. 2. Discuss the side-effects of vitamin toxicity. 3. Explain that R.D.A. for vitamins are higher than minimum requirements. 4. Identify food sources where client is obtaining vitamin A such as egg yolk, fortified margarine and whole milk.

scrambled do not look as large to a client as two poached or soft-cooked eggs.

4. Add an egg and/or ice cream to milk, making an eggnog or egg milkshake. (If the client is immunosuppressed, do not use raw eggs; instead use egg substitutes such as Egg-Beaters or Egg Scramblers).

5. Heat chocolate Carnation Instant Breakfast and serve it as hot chocolate.

6. Add powdered milk to instant or cooked puddings.

7. Add an egg and/or ice cream to Carnation Instant Breakfast.

8. After a flavored gelatin is set, whip in the same or a complimenting flavor of yogurt.

9. Cook dry cereal in milk instead of water.

10. Add a beaten egg to a broth soup while it is boiling.

11. Make high protein, high calorie drinks in a blender.

Recipe I	*Recipe II*
1 cup orange or orange/pineapple juice	1 egg or egg substitute
1 egg or egg substitute	⅛ teaspoon vanilla
1 tablespoon sugar	1 tablespoon sugar
¼ cup instant dry skim milk	½ jar (¼ cup) pureed fruit
	¾ cup milk
	2 teaspoons lemon juice

12. Use margarine, butter, cream cheese and/or mayonnaise whenever possible. (Example: put butter on crackers, put margarine and jelly on toast instead of jelly alone).

If protein needs to be increased, calories must also be increased to assure the protein will not be used for energy. Whenever carbohydrates are increased, B-complex vitamins must be increased. If food odors cause nausea the food can be prepared in a microwave or slow cooker in another part of the house or on another floor. Cold food is less odoriferous than hot foods.

If supplements are used, see Table 11-7. To add variety use both soy/milk based supplements and egg-based supplements. Some clients/families want to use supplements because they helped the client in the hospital or because of previous experiences. Others want to prepare their own power-packed foods. Families require constant reassurance that adequate nutrition can be obtained from liquids whether they are power-packed or commercial supplements.

Outcome

The client will maintain adequate nutritional balance.

KNOWLEDGE DEFICIT

Almost all clients and family members have a knowledge deficit of nutrition. In some situations it may be a severe deficit while in others it may be mild and the teaching can be completed in two to three visits. Nutrition misinformation requires more teaching than lack of information.

If nutrition teaching is not started early or the nurse does not regard it as an important part of care, the patient and family will not regard it as important, either. Teaching requires more time than doing the activity itself but the client and family must be motivated to change unsound or inadequate practices. For established practice to change, the information provided must be correct, relevant, presented in a positive manner with confidence, and include client and family input.

Assessment

Initially, the home health nurse will assess client and family for their understanding of the disease process that initiated the need for nutritional support. On each visit, further evaluation of their knowledge of the treatment and projected outcomes is required.

Interventions

Instructions should be concise and simply stated. All of the diet sheets prepared by the author are limited to one page front and back if at all possible. Adapting information to the client's learning ability through a variety of teaching sheets can be shown by the diabetic teaching tools of the Visiting Nurse Association of Allegheny County. The nurse can select from five different diabetic teaching sheets. Examples of Level One and Level Three are included below (Figures 11-7 and 11-8). Teaching by the nurse must accompany the tools. Showing an overwhelmed client the foods to avoid and telling him to eat protein (meat, milk, eggs, or cheese) at each meal may result in better compliance than using the exchange lists.

The diet is only one of the many things the patient and family need to learn during the first few weeks of service. Simple, specific directions expedite learning.

Interventions to increase the knowledge of the family and client about parenteral nutrition are many.

The home health nurse must assist the client/family with organization skills. Prepar-

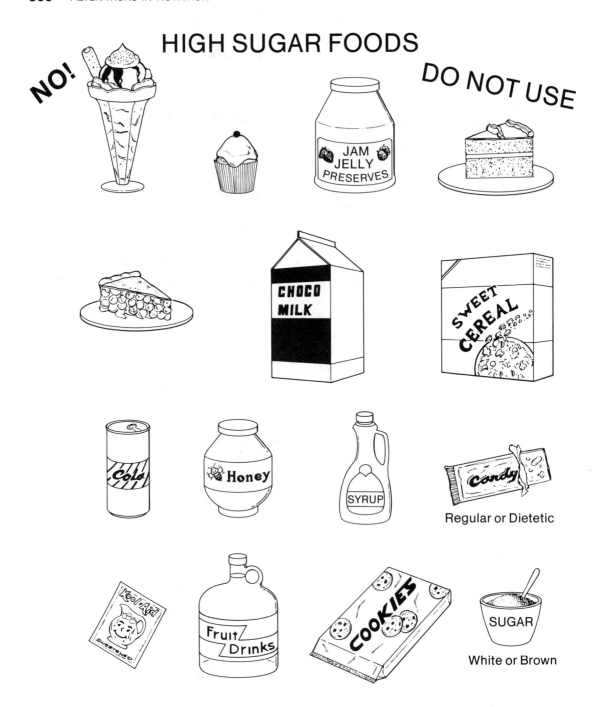

Figure 11-7. Level I: High sugar foods. (Used with permission of Visiting Nurse Association of Allegheny County, PA. Copyright 1986)

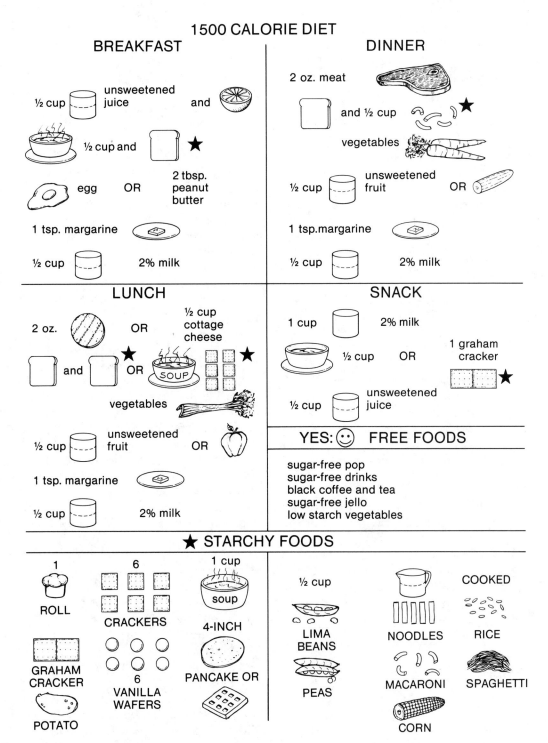

1500 CALORIE DIET

BREAKFAST

½ cup — unsweetened juice — and

½ cup and — □ ★

egg — OR — 2 tbsp. peanut butter

1 tsp. margarine

½ cup — 2% milk

LUNCH

2 oz. — OR — ½ cup cottage cheese

□ and — OR ★ — SOUP — ★

vegetables

½ cup — unsweetened fruit — OR

1 tsp. margarine

½ cup — 2% milk

DINNER

2 oz. meat

and ½ cup — ★

vegetables

½ cup — unsweetened fruit — OR

1 tsp. margarine

½ cup — 2% milk

SNACK

1 cup — 2% milk

½ cup — OR — 1 graham cracker

½ cup — unsweetened juice — ★

YES: ☺ FREE FOODS

sugar-free pop
sugar-free drinks
black coffee and tea
sugar-free jello
low starch vegetables

★ STARCHY FOODS

1 — ROLL

6 — CRACKERS

1 cup soup

4-INCH PANCAKE OR

GRAHAM CRACKER

6 VANILLA WAFERS

POTATO

½ cup

LIMA BEANS

PEAS

NOODLES

MACARONI

COOKED

RICE

SPAGHETTI

CORN

Figure 11-8.   Level III: Instructions for a 1500 calorie diet. (Used with permission of Visiting Nurse Association of Allegheny County, PA. Copyright 1986)

ing and administering home parenteral nutrition is very time consuming and unless the client is well organized and has the support of the family, there will be no time to do anything else. Help the client identify a storage area where the multiple supplies can be kept and organized and to select a permanent area in the home for the preparation of HPN. Refrigeration of the solution is required. If refrigerator space is not available, the client must purchase/rent a small refrigerator for the fluids. Some infusion companies provide the client with a refrigerator as part of the service. This may be checked prior to choosing a service. For the first few days at home, preparation will be lengthy. The directions for preparing and administering the HPN are most convenient for the client if they are taped to the wall above the preparation table. The nurse must have patience to sit and observe the client do the procedure. The nurse should assist only if client starts to make a major error or if the client becomes totally confused and cannot proceed. This is much more time consuming than giving each direction or actually doing the procedure. The goal is for total independence of the client and this goal must be kept in mind during all teaching.

There are many excellent patient teaching guides written by the companies that provide HPN supplies. These are useful both for the lay person and the professional and it is really not necessary for the home health agency to write its own instruction booklets. If the agency does feel obligated to have a specific guide, the authors suggest that the agency adapt a specific booklet/guide that includes simple, concise, easily understood instructions.

Special problems encountered in the home include inadequate storage, presence of children or grandchildren who may play with supplies or try to "adjust" the pump when adults are not looking, lack of cleanliness, as well as disposal of equipment.

The preparation area must be away from heavy traffic and inaccessible to small children and pets. The simple use of "baby gates" provides privacy for almost any area. If the HPN is given during the night, a spare room near the bedroom or even part of the bedroom is an ideal preparation area.

Although rules regarding the HPN supplies and equipment must be set for children/grandchildren, the nurse must be certain that the client does not begin to feel isolated. After the client feels comfortable with the home procedure, allow the children to watch so they do not fear or resent this procedure and consequently the parent. It is most suitable if another adult is present to be sure the children do not totally distract the person preparing the infusion. Children's reactions to HPN do vary but some generalities may be made. Most often younger children will readily accept the HPN and should be encouraged to play "HPN" with their dolls and friends. Older children who want peer support may have problems since they want to be accepted by their peers and they want everyone to believe they have a "normal family."

Self-monitoring should be carefully performed and accurate daily records should be kept for the home health nurse and the physician. Parameters for which the client is responsible include monitoring intake and output, weight and urine reductions. Some clients who are diabetic or who have frequent episodes of hypoglycemia and hyperglycemia will be required to obtain blood sugar values routinely. Using the self-blood glucose monitoring machines such as the Accu-Check or Glucometer is convenient and the use is easily learned. A record of all oral fluids as well as intravenous fluids should be kept.

Clients need to include in the fluid total the foods that are liquid at room temperature. Weight should be obtained and recorded three times a week. The client must weigh at the same time of day, placing the scales at exactly the same location, and wearing approximately the same attire. Urine reductions provide information concerning the body's utilization of the high glucose concentrations. Tes-tape is a convenient test for urine glucose levels and should be done twice a day when first discharged and then, if stable, once a day. Urine results of 2+ or greater for three consecutive readings should be reported to the physician so the HPN can be adjusted.

A summary of teaching instructions about problem solving for Home Parenteral Nutrition can be found in the boxed material below.

Home Parenteral Nutrition: Problem Solving for the Client/Family

While you are receiving hyperalimentation at home or HPN, you need to be alert for complications that may occur as a result of this procedure. The complications are rare and it is unlikely any of them will develop. While the home health nurse is providing service to you, contact her if you suspect any of the following complications unless the problem is an "emergency" and then you should try to contact your doctor and proceed to the hospital.

METABOLIC COMPLICATIONS: The following complications may occur due to an imbalance in the body chemistry:

1. *Hyperglycemia* is a high level of sugar in the blood stream. The condition may occur if the body is unable to use all of the glucose that is given or if the solution is infused too rapidly.
   Symptoms: Nausea
   Weakness
   Excessive thirst
   Excessive urination
   Headache
   Prevention: Slowing infusion rate to one half the usual rate of flow for the first hour of feeding may help.

   Detection: Urine reductions with Tes-tape will show excessive sugar since sugar "spills" into the urine. If urine reductions are 2+ or above on three consecutive tests or if any of the above symptoms are present, notify your physician. Additional insulin may need to be added to the solution.

2. *Hypoglycemia* is a low level of sugar in the blood. The conditions will occur after you have received your infusion if the body continues to release insulin in large amounts into your blood.

   Symptoms: Sweating
   Pallor or paleness
   Nausea
   Headache
   Irritability or nervousness
   Blurred vision
   Unexplained drowsiness

   Prevention: Slow infusion rate to one half the usual rate during the last hour of feeding.

   Treatment: Eat a carbohydrate food (jello water or candy) followed by a protein food (milk, Ensure, Sustacal, or cottage cheese). OR
   If unable to take any food by mouth, restart an infusion.

   (continued)

MECHANICAL COMPLICATIONS:

1. *Infection at catheter site*

   Symptoms: Local:
   Redness
   Swelling
   Tenderness
   Thick, yellow drainage
   General:
   Fever
   Chills
   Sweating
   Lack of energy

   Treatment: Notify the home health nurse or physician.

   Prevention: Careful handwashing. use of aseptic technique.

2. *Damage to catheter.* This is a rare problem that may occur after long-term use of the catheter.

   Treatment: Immediately pinch catheter closed. Then clamp it with a hemostat. The catheter will have to be replaced so it is necessary to go the hospital.

3. *Other metabolic complications.* There are several other metabolic complications that may occur as a result of too much or too little fluid, sodium, potassium, or magnesium in the blood.

   Symptoms: Extreme weakness
   Nausea or vomiting
   Muscle cramps
   Tingling of toes or fingers
   Muscle twitching or cramps
   Swelling of feet or ankles
   Diarrhea
   Decrease in urine output
   Flushing of the skin
   Abdominal cramps

If any of these symptoms occur, contact your physician. Blood tests may be ordered to determine the specific problem.

   Prevention: Do not clamp catheter in exactly the same place each time. Do not keep catheter bent at a sharp angle.

4. *Blood backing up into tubing:* This may occur if the cap is not attached properly, if the pump malfunctions, or if you forget to turn on the pump.

   Treatment: Turn off pump if connected. Clamp catheter with hemostat. Irrigate catheter with heparin. Change cap if leakage has occurred around cap.

   Prevention: Replace cap carefully. Turn pump on immediately after connecting. Do not turn pump off until ready to disconnect the tubing from the catheter. Maintain adequate battery charge on pump or keep plugged into electrical outlet.

5. *Clotting:* Occasionally blood will clot at some point in the catheter and you will not be able to get a blood return. This may occur if you forget to irrigate your catheter or if blood backed up into the catheter and was not detected.

   Treatment: *Gently* irrigate the catheter with heparin. If you meet resistance, do not continue. Replace the catheter cap and notify
   (continued)

your physician.

Prevention: Heparinize your catheter immediately after infusion is completed.

6. *Air in blood stream.* This can occur if the cap was removed without clamping the tube or if the tubing comes apart during the infusion.

Symptoms: Shortness of breath
Chest pain
Coughing

Treatment: Heparinize the catheter to prevent catheter blockage. Lie on your left side. The symptoms should go away in 10 to 20 minutes. If symptoms continue, notify your physician and go to the hospital emergency room.

7. *Clot in vein where catheter was inserted.* On rare instances the vein that is used for HPN becomes blocked with a blood clot.

Symptoms: Swelling of the neck or arm on the same side as the catheter. Enlargement of neck veins on same side as catheter.

Treatment: This requires immediate treatment. Contact your physician and go to the hospital emergency room immediately.

Outcome

The client and family will possess adequate kowledge about nutritional care in the home.

For the nurse, details to be considered in assessing the client's home can be found in Table 11-9. A Care Plan for Home Nutritional Support is on the following page.

TABLE 11.9 Assessment of the Home

Financial	Ascertain what the feedings will cost and the percent reimbursable.
	Support groups in the community? Food banks?
	Homemakers to do shopping?
Room for Client	Have a scale.
	Room large enough for necessary feeding equipment?
	Does the room provide the necessary privacy?
	Are necessary electrical outlets available?
	Exact specifications are available from supply company.
Kitchen	Sufficient refrigeration for feeding solutions?
	Sufficient storage for feeding solutions?
	Sufficient ice supply if needed?
	Overall cleanliness for preparation and cleanup?
Safety	Utility companies notified concerning equipment in the home?
	Emergency telephone numbers for physician, EMS Supply Co., etc.?

ABBREVIATED CARE PLAN: HOME NUTRITIONAL SUPPORT

Nursing Diagnosis	Assessment	Interventions	Outcomes
Anxiety	Number of questions asked Friction between client and family	Provide complete information. Provide opportunities to express feelings. Provide support.	Client and family will not experience episodes of increased anxiety.
Potential for Infection	Fever Tachycardia Malaise	Maintain aseptic system. Carefully dress catheter. Use sterile or aseptic technique.	Client will not experience infection.
Ineffective Individual or Family Coping	Ability to cope	Provide support Refer as necessary.	Client and family are able to utilize effective coping strategies.
Alteration in Body Image	Feelings Weight	Encourage expression of feelings. Encourage client to become involved in family activities. Refer as necessary.	Client will begin to verbalize acceptance of body image.
Alteration in Nutrition: Less than Body Requirements	Total nutritional assessment	Increase oral intake. Increase calories. Utilize supplements as necessary.	Client will maintain adequate nutritional balance.
Knowledge Deficit	Disease process Treatment Projected outcomes	Keep instructions simple. Assist client and family to organize for HPN. Utilize teaching aids as necessary. Teach self monitoring.	Client and family possess adequate knowledge about nutritional care in the home.

References

Adams MM, Wirschion RG: Guidelines for planning home enteral feedings. J Am Diet Assoc 84(1): 68–71, 1984

Curtiss RF: Letter: New Medicare guidelines for home nutrition. Am J Hosp Pharm 41(10): 1190, 1992, 1984

Dahlstrom KA, Strandvik B, Kopple J, Ament ME: Nutritional status in children receiving home parenteral nutrition. J Pediatr 107(2): 219–24, 1985

Dzierba SM, Mirtallo JM, Brauer DW, Schneider PJ, et al: Fiscal and clinical evaluation of home parenteral nutrition. Am J Hosp Pharm 41(2): 285–91, 1984

Finn SC, Zola EM, Sheridan JF: Issues facing nutrition support teams. Drug Intell Clin Pharm 18(10): 826–28, 1984

Hopper SV, Miller JP, Birge C, Swift J: A randomized study of the impact of home health aids on diabetic control and utilization patterns. Am J Public Health 74(6): 600–02, 1984

Howard L: Lecture delivered at eight annual Frontiers in Nutrition presented by School of Medicine, Medical College of Georgia, 1986

Lewis C: Vitamins and Minerals—Sodium and Potassium. Philadelphia, FA Davis, 1978

Ralston CW, O'Connor MJ, Ament M, Berquist W, et al: Somatic growth and developmental functioning in children receiving prolonged home total parenteral nutrition. J Pediatr 105(5): 842–46, 1984

Reese P: Kid Stuff. Lifeline Letter: July/August, p 3, 1986

Robinson CH, Lawler R: Normal and Therapeutic Nutrition, 16th ed. New York, Macmillan, 1982

Smith K: Lecture delivered at eighth annual Frontiers in Nutrition presented by School of Medicine, Medical College of Georgia, 1986

Swoboda RJ: Home health care: Bane or boon for hospitals? Am J Hosp Pharm 41(10): 1990, 1992, 1984

Treat C: Lecture delivered at eighth annual Frontiers in Nutrition presented by School of Medicine, Medical College of Georgia, 1986

Williams SR: Nutrition and Diet Therapy, 5th ed. St. Louis, CV Mosby, 1985

Alterations in Elimination

Nancy L. Bohnet

Elimination of the body's waste materials—urine and feces—is an essential process. Interference in normal patterns of elimination due to disease or trauma pose a tremendous threat to normal, healthy existence, mandating that alternate patterns of elimination be established. The assessment, interventions, and expected outcomes in the home setting that are associated with the vital process of urinary and bowel elimination will be the focus of this chapter. Its purpose is to provide an overview of the care of the client with renal failure and alterations in bowel elimination. In addition, the techniques of home hemodialysis and peritoneal dialysis will be discussed.

ALTERED URINARY ELIMINATION

The ability to manufacture and excrete urine normally via the proper functioning of the kidneys, ureters, and bladder is an action that can easily be taken for granted in a healthy individual. Even a slight disruption of normal elimination patterns, however, can result in a dramatic change of life-style. Not only does such a change affect the normal activities of daily living, but its potential for damaging the integrity of one's self-esteem is great. For the most part, care of the renal client at home will require specific attention to the complex needs that arise. The needs are both mechanical and psychosocial in nature. They will best be met by a nurse who is equipped with the clinical expertise, and the astute sensitivity required in caring for the renal client at home.

PATHOPHYSIOLOGY OF RENAL FAILURE

Kidney function centers on the maintenance of normal composition, volume, and pH of body fluids. The kidneys produce urine that may be very concentrated or very dilute. This ability to adjust the reabsorption or secretion of water means that the kidneys play a vital role in the body's water balance maintenance. In addition, the amount of inorganic salts excreted by the kidneys (for example,

ted by renal func-
's also have the
a ia and to sub-
st. helping to
ma. of the body.
Cons. lly impor-
tant in xcreting
wastes, re to the
plasma, ana is (Chaffee
1974).

The filtration fu. of the kidney serve to remove end products of metabolism, excess fluid and electrolytes, and certain drugs. Disruption of normal renal function can result from many causes, such as infections, diabetes, hypertension, and neoplasia. Irreversible renal damage will require either peritoneal dialysis or hemodialysis unless kidney transplantation is an option. Chronic renal failure can be caused by several different conditions, including glomerular nephritis, nephrosclerosis, or polycystic kidney disease.

Chronic renal failure due to glomerular nephritis or pyelonephritis is the result of an infection that results in a decrease in the number of functional nephrons. (Porth 1986) Typically, glomerular complications are the result of a streptococcal infection elsewhere in the body (scarlet fever, throat, tonsils, or skin). Antibodies and antigens react at the site of infection, producing a precipitate that the kidneys are unable to excrete. In such cases, the precipitate becomes entrapped in the glomerular membrane, causing a severe and harmful inflammation of the glomeruli (Porth 1986). In the final stages of the disease, total blockage occurs when normal glomeruli are replaced by fibrous tissue. Pyelonephritis is an inflammation of the renal pelvis that eventually leads to an inability to concentrate urine. The consequences of severe infections may be permanent destruction of kidney function (Guyton 1986).

Adequate oxygenation of all body tissues is essential for optimal functioning. When such oxygenation is compromised, the result is ischemia caused by sclerosis. Nephrosclerosis is a hardening of kidney tissue usually caused by renal hypertension (Guyton 1986). Glomerulosclerosis is one of the complications associated with adult-onset diabetes mellitus.

Polycystic kidney disease is a condition in which normal kidney tissue is replaced by clusters of cysts. These cysts cause compressions of normal surrounding tissue, thereby destroying nephrons and causing progressive fibrosis of interstitial tissue. Eventually, renal failure occurs.

Whatever the immediate cause, the consequences of renal failure are the same. In the home health setting, it is likely that the nurse will be caring for a client with an acute attack of chronic renal failure. Chronic renal failure usually occurs in three separate stages. The first stage is that of diminished renal reserve, where renal function is impaired, but metabolic waste products do not accumulate (Porth 1986). Correspondingly, the blood urea nitrogen (BUN) is normal. At this stage, there are only minor symptoms such as polyuria, nocturia, and polydypsia.

The second stage is that of renal insufficiency where metabolic wastes accumulate in the blood and the BUN begins to increase (Price and Wilson 1986). The final stage of chronic renal failure is uremia. In this stage, the kidney looses its ability to maintain homeostasis. Electrolyte balance is disturbed, urinary output is decreased, and nitrogenous waste products accumulate.

Uremia can also occur with acute renal failure. During this stage, the disease process has extended to the point where there is an imbalance between the client's metabolism and the ability of his kidneys to excrete wastes and regulate fluid and electrolyte concentrations (Porth 1986).

Several changes occur simultaneously with the onset of uremia. Since protein metabolism is impaired in renal failure, the end product of protein metabolism, urea, which is formed in the liver and excreted by the kidneys, increases. Creatinine, the end product of the metabolism of creatine, an amino acid present in the body tissues and concentrated in the muscles, is increased in uremia. Uric acid, the end product of the metabolism of purine, is also increased. Potassium levels are also high in the serum because, when protein is broken down, excess potassium is liberated into the system.

Serum sodium levels may increase, particularly as urinary output is decreased. Calcium levels are decreased, usually in association with increased levels of phosphate. Magnesium levels increase due to the decreased ability of the kidney to excrete magnesium. Chloride levels may be decreased due to loss from nausea and vomiting. Finally, sulfate levels may be increased. Metabolic acidosis occurs because of a decreased ability of the kidney to excrete acid and to reabsorb bicarbonate.

DIALYSIS

The client with renal failure resulting from any of the previously discussed conditions will require dialysis to remove the body's harmful waste products. Dialysis is a substitute for the body's normal filtration system, using the process of diffusion. Diffusion is the passage of particles from an area of high concentration to an area of low concentration, across a semipermeable membrane. In dialysis, waste products and fluids move across a semipermeable membrane by the process of diffusion into dialysate. There are two types of dialysis available for the client with renal failure.

Hemodialysis requires that the blood leave the body and travel through a series of chan-

nels surrounded by dialysate (Chambers 1981). Once cleansed, the blood is returned to the client. This process requires the placement of a permanent arterial–venous fistula, lines that transport blood from the body to the machine and back into the body, a mechanical pump, and a dialyzer containing dialysate, where diffusion occurs. Generally, hemodialysis is necessary at least 3 times a week and requires the client to be immobilized for up to 6 hours at a time during the procedure (Kirkby 1982).

Peritoneal dialysis is based on the same principle of diffusion of waste across a semipermeable membrane. The difference, however, is that the client's own peritoneum serves as the membrane for the process. Peritoneal dialysis requires the placement of a catheter into the peritoneum. A local anesthetic is given to numb the area. A small midline incision is made into the lower half of the abdomen, and the catheter is then inserted into the peritoneal cavity. Special tubing and bags of specially prepared dialysate are utilized during dialysis. Peritoneal dialysis may occur intermittently by the use of a machine ("cycler") that automatically cycles the dialysate through the peritoneal cavity. This is usually done at night while the client sleeps.

More recently, an alternative method known as Continual Ambulatory Peritoneal Dialysis (CAPD) has been developed. This method requires the infusion of a 2-liter bag of dialysate containing dextrose, sodium, chloride, calcium, and magnesium. The solution flows into the peritoneal cavity within 10 to 15 minutes. The catheter is then clamped until time for the next infusion occurs, from 4 to 9 hours later. The dialysate, now containing waste products, drains out, the bag is discarded, and a new bag is attached for the next cycle. The procedure is repeated 3 to 6 times a day (Johnson 1981, Stansfield, 1985). Peritoneal dialysis has several advantages: minimal dietary and fluid restrictions, freedom from a machine, and better control of uremia (Wilson 1983). The procedures for home hemodialysis and continuous ambulatory peritoneal dialysis are described in the boxed material that follows.

Procedures for Home Dialysis

HEMODIALYSIS

A. For clients with an external arteriovenous shunt, prepare the machine as indicated and fill with dialysate as prescribed by the physician.
1. Assemble sterile equipment
   3 drapes
   shunt-care tray containing:
   gloves
   4 × 4 gauze pads
   2 bulldog clamps
   20 cc syringe
   stainless steel cup
   2 shunt adapters and test tubes
   Betadine solution
   nonallergic tape
   1500 cc heparin (1000 u/ml)
   250 cc normal saline
   5 cc syringe with #21 needle
2. Explain procedure to client. Obtain weight and vital signs, wash hands.
3. Drape shunt around client's arm.
4. Pour saline into cup, add 1500 cc heparin; put on sterile gloves.
5. Place gauze pads on skin between cannula exit sites. Fill a 20 cc syringe with heparinized saline solution.
6. Apply bulldog clamps to shunt near insertion site. Separate shunt cannula, leaving the connector attached to one of them.
7. Place a sterile adapter into the cannula without the connector.
8. Attach the 20 cc syringe to the adapter and flush. Insert the second adapter over the connector that remains on the end of the other cannula. At this time, remove top from test tube, place cannula inside test tube, unclamp, and allow the tube to fill if blood sample is to be obtained. Flush the cannula with heparinized solution.
9. Grasp the arterial blood line on the dialysis machine. Attach to adapter on the end of the arterial shunt. Remove bulldog clamp. Turn on machine and set for flow rate of 80–120 ml/minute.
10. Before the blood reaches the machine's venous blood line, attach it to the adapter on the client's venous shunt. Remove all clamps.
11. Remove gloves, tape shunt junctions. Remove drapes, 4 × 4's, dress and wrap client's arm in order to secure and protect shunts during dialysis.
12. After dialysis has been completed, remove dressing from arm, turn off machine, reclamp shunt cannula and put on sterile gloves. Disconnect machine blood lines and reconnect the shunt blood lines one to another with the shunt connector between them.
13. Clean shunt and its site with Betadine. Remove Betadine with alcohol. Apply dry dressing to shunt.
14. Weigh client and obtain vital signs.

B. For client with an arteriovenous fistula prepare the machine as indicated and fill with dialysate as prescribed by physician.
1. Assemble the following sterile equipment:
   2 tube-occluding clamps
   gloves
   #25 needle
   TB syringe filled with lidocaine
   10 4 × 4 gauze pads
   2 fistula needles with

(continued)

2 attached 20 cc syringes filled with heparinized normal saline solution
2 cotton-tipped applicators
Test tube for blood sample
Betadine solution
nonallergenic tape
Betadine ointment
Tourniquet
Blue pad

2. Explain procedure to client. Obtain weight and vital signs. Wash hands.

3. Flush fistula needles with heparinized saline solution; set aside, if necessary, to obtain blood sample; flush the needle only after sample is withdrawn.

4. Clean fistula site with Betadine solution covering a three-inch-wide area. Remove excess Betadine with dry 4×4.

5. Place tourniquet above fistula site (proximal to heart). Put on gloves. Anesthetize site with lidocaine if prescribed.

6. Insert fistula needle into vein 1 inch above fistula in direction of blood flow.

7. Release tourniquet, flush needle with heparinized saline solution. Use tube-occluding clamp to clamp tubing.

8. Secure needle with tape.

9. Insert arterial needle a few inches distal to first needle, keeping tip pointed away from fistula. Repeat Steps 7 and 8.

10. Apply Betadine ointment with applicators to needle insertion sites. Firmly secure needles with additional tape.

11. Uncap and attach machine's arterial bloodline to client's arterial needle tubing after removing syringe from tubing.

12. Tape junction and repeat procedure for venous lines.

13. Unclamp venous and arterial needle tubings, set flow meter to 5 L/minute. Remove machineline's clamps and turn on pump.

Adapted from Walsh J, Persons CB, Wieck L: Manual of Home Health Care Nursing. Philadelphia, JB Lippincott, 1987

Procedure for Peritoneal Dialysis—CAPD

1. Gather equipment.
   (a) 2 L bag dialysate
   (b) 2 outlet port clamps
   (c) CAPD prep kit
       Betadine swabs
       4×4 gauze pads
       mask
       nonallergenic tape
   (d) IV pole

2. Warm dialysate in sink of warm water; keep wrap on bag.

3. Open CAPD prep kit.

4. Instruct client to remove empty dialysate bag from inside clothing. Place below abdomen.

(continued)

5. Open clamp on drainage tubing allowing solution to drain for 15–20 minutes.

6. While old solution is draining, prepare new solution for infusion. Check for cloudiness, leaks, and proper concentration.

7. If medications are to be instilled, add to bag via injection port.

8. When drainage is complete, place the old bag and new bag side by side on a flat surface. Allow tubing to hang free over the edge. Put on mask.

9. Place clamp on the outlet port of new bag to keep it stable during spike insertion.

10. Remove cover from outlet port of new bag.

11. Remove spike from old bag, taking care not to contaminate. Insert into outlet port of new bag.

12. Unclamp outlet port on new bag and hang on IV pole.

13. Open clamp on tubing and allow dialysate to drain into abdomen for about five minutes.

14. Fold bag and tubing and place inside clothing.

15. After assessing old dialysate for cloudiness or sediment, discard.

Adapted from Walsh J, Persons CB, Wieck L: Manual of Home Health Care Nursing. Philadelphia, JB Lippincott, 1987

ACCESS TO CIRCULATION

In the use of hemodialysis, it is necessary to locate a method for accessing the circulation. There are two methods commonly chosen: arteriovenous (AV) shunt and fistula.

With an AV shunt, one cannula is placed into an artery and the other into a vein. The radial artery and cephalic vein are frequently selected as the site for cannulation. A shunt is an external device and thus may present some safety problems, such as rapid blood loss if it becomes disconnected. In the immediate postoperative period, the client's activities are limited to provide for maximal safety. Once discharged to home, the major nursing interventions include keeping the area of the shunt clean and observing frequently for clotting. Assessment of the patency of the shunt is accomplished by listening for a bruit and feeling for a thrill over the device.

An arteriovenous fistula is a surgically created anastomosis between an artery and a vein. Therefore, the arterial blood flows into the venous system, causing a marked dilatation of the veins and allowing for easy puncture. Generally this technique circumvents the problems of infection, clotting, and hemorrhage associated with a cannula. The major advantages of the AV fistula are that they can be used for months or years, they require fewer physical limitations, and they avoid the dangers and complications of an external device. The major complications from the fistula include hemorrhage, thrombosis, failure of the prominent vein to develop, infection, and ischemia of the involved hand (Thompson, 1986). The home health nurse should be aware that blood and blood pressures should not be taken in the arm with an AV fistula.

NURSING DIAGNOSES

A multitude of nursing diagnoses are applicable in the care of the client with renal failure at home. Assessment, interventions, and outcomes will be discussed in relation to each nursing diagnosis.

ANXIETY RELATED TO DISEASE PROCESS AND TREATMENT

A client with renal failure who is undergoing dialysis at home may experience anxiety due to the unfamiliar technical aspects of the various dialysis procedures and the uncertainty of his condition (Stark 1985). The level of anxiety is often proportionate to the level of knowledge and degree of confidence the client has concerning his treatment at home.

Anxiety can also be caused by some of the psychological consequences of the uremia. The production of toxins leads to encephalopathy, making the client lethargic and less mentally alert. The client may also suffer from poor concentration, confusion, and depression.

Assessment

Assessment begins with a discussion of the client's emotional state at present and reaction to home dialysis and other aspects of therapy. The nurse should attempt to elicit information concerning the client's knowledge of disease, prognosis, equipment, and procedures. While assessing this knowledge, the nurse may also be able to identify the client's perception of the effects of the disease process and treatment on his life. Careful assessment requires therapeutic communication and effective listening skills in order to elicit the client's true response.

Interventions

One of the most effective interventions for anxiety is the establishment of a trusting relationship between the client and nurse. As the client becomes secure in the relationship, he is better able to discuss concerns, thereby becoming better equipped to solve problems. Verbalization of client's feelings may be therapeutic. By providing the client with adequate and understandable information about dialysis the nurse will dispel many of the inherent fears of facing the unknown.

Throughout the course of the nurse/client relationship, it is important for the nurse to provide reassurance and support as needed.

Outcomes

The above interventions are interwoven. Anxiety will be alleviated as the client becomes aware of his own feelings and becomes more confident that he has someone to trust. As the relationship develops, the client and family will exhibit fewer signs of anxiety and the nurse will continue to gain insight about means of assistance.

INEFFECTIVE INDIVIDUAL COPING

The ability to cope can be related to the amount of effective support and previous coping patterns.

Assessment

The nurse must ascertain the various support systems available to the client and their effectiveness. In addition, an assessment should be obtained of the client's coping history. "How have you dealt with problems in the past?" may yield helpful information indicative of the client's ability to deal with stress. Verbal and nonverbal clues will provide information about current coping ability.

Interventions

Each client has unique coping skills. There are many ways to deal effectively with major threats and it is necessary that the nurse assist the client to utilize those means that benefit him most. Positive support and reassurance should be offered as the client exhibits healthy coping mechanisms.

Outcomes

The outcome of nursing interventions will result in more effective means of coping. In addition, the client should have enhanced self-awareness that will prove increasingly beneficial as dialysis continues.

ALTERATION IN FAMILY PROCESS

There are many reasons why the client with renal failure may have a potential for alteration in family process. Dialysis in the home setting will affect both the client and family. A disruption of the normal family process occurs from the intrusion of technical equipment, procedures, and the presence of health care professionals within the home.

Assessment

The assessment should begin with the determination of the client's role in the family and the ability to function in that role. If, for example, the client is the head of the household, the family will be forced to undergo changes in order to adjust. A thorough assessment will include each family member, observing reactions, effect, and interactions within the system.

Interventions

The nurse should encourage verbalization from each individual regarding the loved one's condition. It is also important that the family be educated about home dialysis and encouraged to participate whenever possible in the procedure (Lowry 1984). Matters of practical importance may also require intervention. Assistance with health and disability insurance, income supplementation, transportation, child care, and legal concerns may be required. The home care nurse is a liaison between client/family and community resources.

Outcomes

The threats of dialysis will be lessened as the family members gain appropriate knowledge. As the family becomes more comfortable, there will be a subsequent decline in anxiety

and they will be better able to provide support for the client. The more open and flexible the patterns of communication, the more successful the home dialysis (Palmer 1982).

ALTERATION IN FLUID AND ELECTROLYTE BALANCE

Renal failure can lead to a number of abnormalities in both fluid and electrolyte balance. The potential for fluid volume deficit is related to an increased fluid loss caused by the inability of the renal tubules to reabsorb electrolytes and water (Porth 1986). Clients may also experience vomiting and diarrhea related to retention of waste products. On the other hand, the client may have a fluid volume excess caused by retention of sodium and water due to a decreased number of functioning nephrons. Electrolytes, particularly sodium, potassium, and calcium, may also be abnormal due to varying rates of renal excretion and reabsorption.

Assessment

Careful assessment of the client's weight, temperature, pulse, respirations, and blood pressure will offer important data concerning fluid volume. Level of hydration can be observed by measuring skin turgor and noting the presence of edema (especially in dependent extremities and parts). With renal failure, fluid volume can fluctuate quickly and the client can change from hypovolemia to hypervolemia with little warning. Assessment must be continual and ongoing. An example of the many aspects to assess in differentiating hypovolemia and hypervolemia can be found in Table 12-1.

Assessment for signs and symptoms of electrolyte imbalance is important. The major electrolytes to monitor include sodium, potassium, calcium, and phosphorus. Signs and symptoms for abnormalities of each electrolyte are listed in Table 12-2. Assessment for metabolic acidosis is also necessary.

TABLE 12.1 Assessment for Hypovolemia and Hypervolemia

	Hypovolemia	Hypervolemia
Skin and SQ Tissue	Dry, loss of elasticity	Warm, moist, pitting edema, wrinkled skin
Face	Sunken eyes	Periorbital edema
Tongue	Dry, coated	Moist
Saliva	Thick, scanty	Excessive, frothy
Thirst	Present	May not be significant
Temp	May be increased	May not be significant
Pulse	Rapid, weak, thready	Rapid
Resp.	Rapid, shallow	Rapid dyspnea, moist rales
B.P.	Low orthostatic hypotension	Normal to high
Weight	Decreased	Increased

TABLE 12.2 Signs and Symptoms of Electrolyte Abnormalities

Electrolyte	Signs and Symptoms	
	Hyper— Low Levels	Hypo—High Levels
Sodium	Confusion Weakness Nausea Vomiting Abdominal cramps Twitching Seizure	Restlessness Lethargy Weakness Increased DTR
Potassium	Irregular pulse Muscle weakness Cramping Paresthesias Nausea, vomiting Hypoactive bowel sounds Cardiac dysrhythmias	Slow pulse Paresthesias Weakness; flaccidity Diarrhea Hyperactive bowel sounds
Calcium	Cardiac dysrhythmias Positive Chvostek's and Trousseau's signs Numbness and tingling	Nausea Vomiting Anorexia Cardiac dysrhythmias

Interventions

Harmful levels of blood urea nitrogen, creatinine, sodium, or potassium can be rectified by the contents of the dialysate. If, for example, the client has a subtherapeutic potassium level, the physician will prescribe an increased level of potassium to be added to the dialysate, the process of diffusion will result in a shift of necessary potassium into the blood.

Clients may require assistance in adhering to proper fluid restriction (500 ml to 1000 ml/day). Although unpleasant, such restrictions minimize the potential stress of fluid overload upon the circulatory system.

Interventions to maintain electrolyte balance are numerous. Sodium levels can be best safeguarded by maintaining intake of fluid and dietary sodium. Any nausea, vomiting, or diarrhea must be treated promptly to prevent hyponatremia. To maintain potassium levels, the client should be encouraged to maintain a normal dietary intake. Potassium supplements can be given if hypokalemia is a problem. If hyperkalemia occurs, it may be necessary to treat with an exchange resin, such as Kayexalate.

Clients should be taught the various dietary sources of calcium. If necessary, calcium supplements can be added. If hypercalcemia is a problem, mithramycin can be given (USP–DI 1987). Other electrolytes, such as phosphorus and magnesium, are best maintained through normal dietary consumption. Since magnesium is already elevated, it is best to avoid the use of drugs containing large amounts of magnesium, such as milk of magnesia, magnesium sulfate, Gelusil, Maalox, and Mylanta. Other drugs, such as Phosphajel and Basaljel, are given in an effort to bind the phosphate and excrete. Drugs of this type are often thought to cause diarrhea. Although some nurses might want to stop these drugs if the client develops diarrhea, it is important that she *do not* do so, since the drug is needed to help maintain normal electrolytes.

Outcomes

The outcome of assisting the client to achieve an adequate fluid level is optimal functioning and a decreased threat to other essential body functions. In addition, the client will maintain safe levels of sodium, potassium, calcium, and phosphorus. The client should maintain normovolemia and a serum pH and bicarbonate within normal limits.

KNOWLEDGE DEFICIT RELATED TO DIALYSIS AT HOME

The dialysis procedures are unfamiliar to most clients. Improvement in the knowledge base of both client and family will help to ensure compliance with regimens and treatments.

Assessment

Assess the client's general level of knowledge concerning renal failure and all related treatments. In addition to the understanding of the general problems encountered, the home health nurse should assess the knowledge concerning social and financial aspects of the disease and its treatment.

Interventions

Once the level of knowledge regarding disease and procedures has been assessed, careful explanations of the purpose and process of dialysis are provided (Shurr 1980). Several areas must be included in teaching. Aseptic technique in the handling of the dialysis equipment is explained. The components of the dialysis system must also be explained, together with their preparation, operation, cleaning, and maintenance. Teaching should include the initiation, monitoring during, and discontinuation of dialysis.

Emergencies related to the machine and the client's condition must be discussed carefully. In addition, education must be provided about daily care: diet, fluid restrictions, complications, care of peritoneal or blood access routes, medications, and prevention of infections. Teaching includes daily observational skills: temperature, pulse, respirations, blood pressure, weight, intake and output, and accurate record keeping (Thompson et al 1986).

Outcomes

The desired outcome is an accurate understanding of the purpose and procedure of dialysis. The client also will describe correct use of dialysis equipment. Methods to achieve a good nutritional status, avoid infections, monitor vital signs, and keep accurate records will be verbalized by the client and family. An understanding of complications will be evidenced along with understanding of when to call for medical assistance. Both the client and family should be able to accurately describe plans for follow-up.

DISTURBANCE IN SELF-CONCEPT RELATED TO ALTERED BODY FUNCTION

Clients in renal failure may suffer a disturbance in self-concept related to several factors. Because of the seriousness of the disease process, the client is dependent upon others to meet self-care needs. Changes in life-style and role functioning may result. The chemical changes inherent in renal failure may also lead to physical changes in the appearance of the individual. These changes include pale, bronze cast skin color, thin, brittle nails, and subcutaneous nodules.

Assessment

The assessment of disturbance in body image involves obtaining the client's response to living with a chronic illness and, in particular, altered renal function. Most of the cues to the client's response will be verbal and nonverbal. The nurse requires strong observation skills in order to correctly interpret the signs demonstrated by the client.

Interventions

Nursing interventions include supporting the client's strengths and motivations to live with dialysis. The goal that the client works toward is a return to as normal a life as is possible. This means that the client is not exhibiting signs of depression or anxiety, nor is he excessively concerned with the loss of normal renal function. The client should not exhibit signs of deficiencies in self-care needs, lifestyle, or role function. The nurse can assist the client during periods of discouragement by offering the information that is needed and offering continuing emotional support.

The essence of nursing is caring. It is an essential element required as the client adjusts to the myriad of changes and disturbances in his life. Listening attentively to worries and fears is very important. Touching —a hand on the client's arm—signifies interest, care, and silent communication. The nurse understands that sometimes just "being there" is an appropriate and effective intervention. Problems with sexual functioning (Gonsalves 1985) or loss of libido may also impact on one's self-concept and will be explored later. The fact that many persons learn to cope effectively with dialysis at home may be reassuring and comforting to the client. Nursing interventions should be aimed at enhancing the client's self-concept and worth as a vital human being. The home care nurse is in the ideal position to become a mainstay of support, information, and reassurance.

Outcomes

Upon successful interventions, the client will demonstrate adaptation to changes in the appearance of the body. Changes in life-style, roles, and independence will be accepted.

ALTERATION IN SKIN INTEGRITY

Due to the various complications related to chronic renal disease or dialysis, the client is at great risk for sustaining an alteration in skin integrity. Increased levels of blood urea nitrogen lead to a decrease in oil gland activity and an atrophy of the sweat glands (Guyton 1986). Pruritus may then result. Constant dryness and itching may become unbearable for the client, yet scratching will lead to further complications.

Assessment

The home care nurse performs a careful assessment of the client's skin, noting color, turgor, hydration, all indicating overall skin integrity. The assessment should include not only a thorough visualization of the skin, especially at the shunt or fistula site, but also palpation to determine temperature and resiliency. The dialysis catheter insertion site, whether on the arm or abdomen, should be inspected for evidence of rash, redness, or excoriation.

The skin may be dry and itch, conditions related to the calcium and phosphorous metabolism. The nailbeds and mucous membranes may appear pale secondary to the anemia. The skin itself may have a yellow brown cast due to the anemia and placement of melanin. Finally, bruises and petechiae may also be present.

Interventions

Interventions include both excellent skin care and instruction to prevent future diffi-culties, such as breakdown and infection. The client should be bathed with a lanolin-based soap to prevent dryness, and there should be an application of generous amounts of non-perfumed body lotion, such as Keri Lotion. In extreme cases of pruritus, it may be necessary to obtain a prescription for a medicated cream to control itching. If proper skin care and lotion do not provide relief, an antihistamine oral medication such as Benadryl may be required. Clients should be encouraged *not* to scratch dry skin as this may cause breakdown and eventual infection if not treated promptly.

Special precautions should be taken to protect the fistula or shunt used for dialysis. The functioning of the fistula or shunt is critical for the client with renal failure; consequently, skin care must center upon such protection. The client should avoid constriction in the arm with the shunt or fistula. Therefore, that arm is not used to obtain blood pressure measurements or blood samples. Clients should also be encouraged to wear loose-fitting sleeves that will not impede circulation in the arm. Lifting of heavy objects as well as sudden and extreme temperature changes should all be avoided. The arm should be carefully protected. Proper skin care and teaching techniques will yield an improved skin integrity and the prevention of potentially dangerous skin conditions. Comfort will increase as the client experiences relief from pruritus and a greater knowledge of skin care. If these interventions are not effective in alleviating the pruritis, an antihistaminic drug may be ordered.

Outcomes

With adequate nursing interventions, the client should experience no complaints of itching. The skin should demonstrate good turgor and level of hydration. The client should remain intact.

ALTERATION IN NUTRITION: LESS THAN BODY REQUIREMENTS

There are several factors that may compromise the nutritional status of the client with renal failure. A renal diet necessitates a restriction of both protein and potassium intake. Careless dietary patterns can cause several problems for the client. Proper nutrients must be obtained from the diet in order to replenish what is lost via dialysis, yet not in excess of what is necessary for therapeutic blood levels.

Assessment

A dietary history must be obtained during the initial phase of a nutritional assessment. The client and family are interviewed to determine the types and amounts of foods ingested, the addition of condiments and spices, and the amount of fluids consumed during each day. A calorie count can be calculated for a three-day period in order to determine the average caloric nutritional stability including serum albumin, protein and hematocrit will be within normal limits.

Interventions

Diets must be low in potassium, sodium, and protein since all of these substances may be difficult to eliminate through dialysis (Schreiber 1985). Therefore, it is necessary for the renal client to choose foods that will not burden his homeostatic mechanisms by causing an overload of any of the above. Teaching should center upon instruction related to foods that are "free" and can be easily ingested and those that are "dangerous" and may cause harm. A simple explanation about the disastrous outcome of high potassium on cardiac function will assist in the client's comprehension. Education should always be done when the client is comfortable, physically and emotionally. The nurse at home may ask for cans and packages of food representative of those consumed by the client. Then, the nurse reviews them with both client and family so they can be taught how to obtain nutritional information from labels and all can become sensitive to dietary considerations. The dietary requirements and rationale for clients in renal failure are outlined in Table 12-3. A consultation with a

TABLE 12.3 Dietary Requirements for Clients in Renal Failure

Considerations	Rationale
Limit protein intake 60–80 g/day	Protein breaks down into nitrogen waste that is difficult to filter.
Limit sodium intake 2 g/day	Sodium causes the retention of water; therefore, hypertension.
Limit potassium 1.5 to 2 g/day Serum K = 3.5	Increased potassium affects myocardium.
Caloric adjustments 2500–3000	Too few calories result in weight loss while too many cause weight gain.
Fluid intake daily 500–1000 cc	Too much fluid may result in retention.

registered dietitian would be appropriate at this time.

Outcomes

With the above interventions, the client will maintain adequate nutritional status with a normal weight. Measures of nutritional stability including serum albumin, protein, and hematocrit will be within normal limits.

ALTERATION IN SAFETY RELATED TO INFECTION

Clients who undergo dialysis are at risk for infection. In fact, some suggest that infection is a leading cause of death in clients with renal failure. This is due to reduced phagocytic activity and the atrophy of lymphoid tissue. Diminished lymphoid tissue results in decreased lymphocytic production, especially of B and T cells. These factors not only increase the risk of infection, but they also cause wounds to heal very slowly. In addition, the client undergoing peritoneal dialysis has a permanent abdominal catheter for dialysate infusion. The possibility of contamination from outside sources and the risk of peritonitis are ever present. Due to the external location of the AV shunt there is an increased threat of exposure to infectious agents. Therefore, a generalized susceptibility to infection resulting from weakened immune response and potential contamination from external catheters and dialysate place the renal patient in potential danger.

Assessment

Nursing assessment must occur frequently and include observations for signs and symptoms of infection, especially peritonitis. Elevated temperature, complaints of general malaise, tachycardia, and feeling warm and flushed are signs of infection. Peritonitis causes abdominal pain and the abdominal examination results in rebound tenderness — a classic symptom. Rebound tenderness is demonstrated by the presence of sudden pain when the examiner suddenly withdraws fingertips after deep palpation. This is a symptom of peritoneal inflammation. Attention should be paid to the insertion sites of the shunt, fistula, or peritoneal catheter for redness, swelling, or abscess.

Interventions

Nursing interventions should be aimed primarily at preventing infection. Clients are educated about the signs and symptoms of infection and taught that they must seek help as soon as this complication is suspected. Meticulous attention must be paid to infection precaution. Exposure to persons known to have infection should be avoided. Once the client appreciates that he is highly susceptible to infection helps him to understand the rationale for avoiding the presence of those with colds, flu, or other infections. Appropriate nutritional intake may help to keep the client healthy, as will care taken to obtain moderate exercise and maintain regular sleep patterns. Erratic diets and excess fatigue place additional stress on the already depressed immune system.

Clients require instruction concerning aseptic technique. For example, the need to wear a mask (as should with the nurse) while connecting dialysate and tubing should be understood. The AV fistula is entered using sterile insertion technique and care should be taken to avoid the possibility of contamination with cannula connections. All connections should be securely anchored in place to avoid their separation and exposure to contaminating organisms. Sterile gloves provide an additional deterrent to infection and should always be worn during the connections of tubing.

If the peritoneal outflow is cloudy, has sediment, blood, or is malodorous, peritonitis should be suspected and a sample should be sent for culture and sensitivity.

Outcomes

Successful outcomes are twofold: The patient and his family will know how to prevent infection and should infection develop in spite of precautions the patient and family will recognize its presence at the earliest stage of development. The client would be expected to be afebrile.

ACTIVITY INTOLERANCE RELATED TO ANEMIA

Anemia is a common finding in the client with renal failure since the kidney's ability to produce the hormone erythropoietin is decreased. This hormone stimulates the production of erythrocytes in the bone marrow and the consequence of lowered levels is anemia. The resulting picture is that the red blood cells (RBCs) are normal in configuration and size, but are present in inadequate numbers. The anemia appears to be as severe as the uremia. For example, the home health nurse can anticipate that the worse the uremia, the worse the anemia. In addition to the decreased numbers of RBC's, they also have a shortened lifespan.

Assessment

Assessment findings include skin pallor, fatigue, and changes in the complete blood count (CBC). The client is monitored for response to activity. For example, a pulse rate increase of more than 20 beats/minute above resting rate with activity is an indication of the client's inability to tolerate the exercise.

During activity, it is also important to monitor the client for marked increases in systolic blood pressure, and the occurance of specific symptoms including chest pain, weakness, diaphoresis, dizziness, or syncope. The CBC is monitored for decreases in RBC, hemoglobin and hematocrit. Generally, clients with renal failure have a microcytic, normochromic anemia evidenced by a decrease in overall RBC count. Changes in the RBCs may also lead to capillary frigidity.

Interventions

Clients are encouraged to obtain adequate rest and sleep. Activities should be interspersed with periods of rest to prevent and deal with feelings of fatigue. Iron supplements and dietary intake of high iron foods may also help to alleviate this troublesome problem. Although it is important for clients to achieve and maintain as much independence as possible, it is at times necessary for them to receive assistance in bathing, ambulating, or even feeding when fatigue becomes too great a burden.

Outcomes

The outcome of successful management is the patient's heightened ability to judge activity tolerance, monitor physical exertion, ingest adequate nutrients, rest as appropriate, and lead as normal a life as is possible. An outcome of no bleeding should also be expected.

ALTERATION IN SEXUAL FUNCTION RELATED TO FATIGUE AND DECREASED LIBIDO

There exists a very real potential for sexual dysfunction to occur in the client with renal failure. Sexual activity is dependent upon both physiological responses and psychological preparedness. The underlying pathophysiology that led to renal dysfunction may well interfere with a male's ability to achieve sexual satisfaction. Sexual problems for clients with renal failure arise due to psychological considerations. Depression, anxiety, fatigue, loss of control, and changes in bodily function tend to create diminished libido or sexual drive. It may be impossible for the client to think of sexual activity during the initial days of adjusting to dialysis because of disruptions in life-style, unfamiliar procedures, and uncertain future.

Assessment

The home health nurse should assess the client and spouse response to any change in their sexual activity.

Interventions

Nurses should offer support in this area by suggesting mutually pleasing sexual activity that does not involve intercourse. The couple can be taught that petting, fondling, hugging, kissing, and caressing can assist in making the client feel desirable and loved.

Appropriate assistance is best offered by the nurse who is comfortable with her own sexuality. This process takes special effort for some people and involves examining one's own feelings about homosexuality, masturbation, birth control, sex practices, and personal gender. While people have various views on all of the above, the nurse recognizes each person's right to have his own opinion and to practice what he wishes in his private life. Thus, the nurse remains nonjudgmental during both assessment and intervention in order to best assist patients and their partners. Satisfactory sexual adjustment for patient and loved one is the anticipated outcome of support, information, and counseling. A further discussion of interventions appropriate for

sexual dysfunction can be found in Chapter 10 (Circulation).

Outcomes

With successful interventions, the client will perceive himself as sexually adequate and acceptable. The client should be able to verbalize feelings concerning sexual activity.

ALTERATION IN COMFORT RELATED TO PAIN

Renal failure causes poor calcium absorption and calcium loss from bone (Paradiso 1986). Eventually, bone or musculoskeletal pain may result. In addition, muscle cramps related to electrolyte imbalances and irritation of the nerves may occur. The higher the level of nitrogenous waste product, the more likely is irritation of the nerves. Peripheral neuropathies demonstrated by burning, numbness, and tingling may also be associated with electrolyte imbalance and high serum levels of waste products.

Renal osteodystrophy occurs in 50% of all clients with uremia (Price and Wilson 1986). Generally, these problems are diagnosed by x-ray only, but have many important aspects for home health nurses to consider. Osteomalachia is softening of the bones that occurs due to the failure of calcium salts to be deposited in new tissue. Osteitis fibrosis occurs due to reabsorption of calcium from bone and replacement of these salts by fibrous tissue. The third type of renal osteodystrophy is osteosclerosis, which is the abnormal hardening of the bone characterized by areas of increased bone density (Price and Wilson 1986).

Assessment

The nurse should assess several parameters when the patient complains of pain: location, duration, quality, quantity, frequency, onset, alleviation and precipitating factors. Pain may or may not be correlated with poor calcium absorption. It is appropriate once again to assess the patient's diet. A diet poor in calcium could be the contributing factor to calcium deficiency.

Interventions

Interventions include dietary instructions and the possible supplementation of both vitamins D and C. The client and family must be cautioned to use care in manipulating the client's extremities, since they may be weakened by the presence of the renal osteodystrophy. Other techniques that may be effective in alleviating pain are discussed in detail in Chapter 16.

Outcomes

Successful interventions will cause the client to experience a reduction in muscle cramping and symptoms of peripheral neuropathies. Dietary compliance and absence of bone or musculoskeletal pain can also be expected.

ALTERATION IN CARDIAC OUTPUT

The cardiovascular system is affected by renal failure and uremia. Hypertension occurs in 80% of the patients with chronic renal failure (Price and Wilson 1986). Although the exact mechanisms are not understood, it is surmised that a decrease in blood flow to the kidney stimulates the juxtaglomerular apparatus to release renin and angiotensin I and II. Angiotensin II stimulates the adrenal medulla to release aldosterone. In turn, the aldosterone leads to sodium and water retention. The end result is an increase in arterial blood pressure. These events are outlined in Figure 12-1.

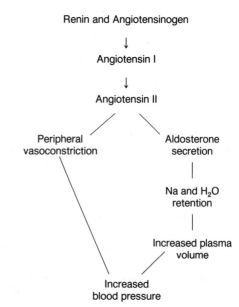

Figure 12-1. Mechanisms producing hypertension in renal failure.

Congestive heart failure may also occur with chronic renal failure. Generally, congestive heart failure is associated with hypertension, anemia, and sodium and water retention. Pulmonary edema can also occur secondary to hypertension and congestive heart failure (Porth 1986). This occurs secondary to volume overload, altered pulmonary capillary permeability, and a decrease in oncotic pressure secondary to protein. The pulmonary edema accumulates to a greater degree in the central portions of the lungs.

Pericarditis is a less often seen complication, but develops when the chemical control is poor. This is generally defined as when the BUN remains over 100 for a period of time. (Porth 1986).

Assessment

Cardiovascular status should be assessed in some of the traditional ways. Monitor the client's blood pressure with particular attention to diastolic pressure. Monitor pulmonary status, assessing the client for the presence of rales that would indicate congestive problems.

Periodic auscultation of heart sounds will assist in recognition of pericarditis. Auscultate for the presence of a friction rub, the sound of which is similar to that produced by rubbing pieces of hair together over the ear and is described as grating or scratchy. Press the diaphragm of the stethoscope firmly against the chest to hear the sound most accurately. Determine the exact location of the rub, usually best heard along the lower left sternal border. Pain may also accompany the pericarditis. The home health nurse must attempt to help the client describe the pain as accurately as possible to help differentiate the pain from other problems, such as myocardial infarctions, aortic aneurysms, and pulmonary emboli.

Interventions

The client's blood pressure should be carefully monitored. It may be necessary for the home health nurse to instruct both the client and family in the technique of taking blood pressure measurements. In renal disease, the blood pressure can change so quickly that it is necessary for the family to continue to monitor the pressure as often as possible. On each visit, the home health nurse's assessment should include not only the blood pressure, but also cardiac and pulmonary function.

Hypertension control in renal failure includes several interventions including sodium and water restriction, dietary control, and drug therapy. Daily weights may be of assistance in monitoring fluid control. A detailed description of management for hypertension can be found in Chapter 10.

Interventions for the potential of pericarditis are continual assessment and follow-up.

If the client describes pain, particularly discomfort on deep inspiration and change of position, pericarditis should be suspected and reported to the physician. The presence of a pericardial friction rub, as previously described, should also be reported to the physician.

Outcomes

Successful interventions will be identified as the client maintains a normal cardiac output and blood pressure. In addition, the client should be comfortable and pain free. The lungs should be clear to auscultation and percussion.

ALTERATION IN GASTROINTESTINAL STATUS

Deaths in clients with renal failure due to GI complications have been reported. There are three major types of problems including gastrointestinal bleeding, mouth sores, and GI symptoms.

Gastrointestinal bleeding may occur as the result of defective clotting mechanisms caused by the response of the blood marrow to the renal disease (Price and Wilson 1986). Specifically, platelet counts are decreased, which leads to the bleeding disorders. The increased amount of urea also leads to mucosal irritation that increases bleeding potential. A decrease in histamine stimulated gastric acid secretion that further increases the chances of GI bleeding. Finally, the vascular abnormalities that occur with renal disease also increase the probability of bleeds.

Mouth sores can occur not only because of the defective clotting mechanism, but also due to the high levels of urea produced as a waste product and eliminated through the mouth. The presence of the urea is irritating and causes tissue breakdown.

Assessment

Any vomitus or stool should be tested for blood. Hematocrit and hemoglobin counts should be done when possible. Observe the client for anorexia, nausea, and vomiting. Nonspecific complaints such as fatigue, malaise, and feeling cold may suggest blood loss.

Interventions

If any of the symptoms of GI distress occur, alter diet therapy if necessary. Antiemetic drugs, such as Tigan, may be needed. Frequent mouth care is provided to assist the client in the removal of the nasty taste in the mouth. Iron supplements should be taken with meals as ordered. The nurse continues to monitor the client for signs of GI blood loss and to recommend assessment of hemoglobin and hematocrit as needed.

Outcome

The expected outcome is normal GI function and the absence of nausea, vomiting, stomach ulcers, and bleeding.

ALTERED LEVEL OF CONSCIOUSNESS

With the electrolyte changes and build up of uric acid during renal failure, a metabolic encephalopathy can result. Uric acid has a depressant effect on the cerebrum and when present in large amounts, has an overall slowing effect. Abnormalities of any electrolyte affect cerebral activity; however, abnormalities of sodium and calcium are the most dangerous.

Assessment

On each visit, the home health nurse evaluates the client level of consciousness (LOC). Interviews with the family may provide additional information concerning the stability of or any changes in LOC. For example, a typical finding with metabolic encephalopathies is a variable LOC. Note, in particular, periods of agitation, depression, or excitement.

Interventions

Consistently orient the client. Instruct the family in appropriate techniques. Encourage the family to always reorient the client, never allowing the client to have his disoriented responses reinforced. Families sometimes grow tired of orienting the client, but it is important that they continue their efforts, no matter how often.

Techniques to maintain orientation abound. To support the verbal cues to reorient the client, clocks and calendars can be placed in areas where the client can readily review them. Keeping the client involved in his own care can also assist in preventing disorientation.

If the client suffers from metabolic encephalopathy, the interventions are mainly for prevention of additional loss of consciousness and worsening of condition. Additional safety concerns may arise and should be considered in the development of the plan of care.

Outcomes

In establishing the outcomes, the nurse should be careful to set realistic goals, dependent upon the extent of physiological compromise. With successful interventions, the client should be oriented to time, place, and person.

NURSING CARE DURING PERITONEAL DIALYSIS AND HEMODIALYSIS

In addition to the nursing diagnoses already discussed, there are specific types of nursing interventions that are required when the home health nurse supervises the delivery of care to the client undergoing peritoneal dialysis or hemodialysis. The specific potential problems are outlined in Table 12-4 for peritoneal dialysis and Table 12-5 for hemodialysis. These concepts are integrated in the abbreviated care plans at the end of the chapter.

PATHOPHYSIOLOGY OF URINARY OSTOMY

When bladder damage or disease results in urinary diversion, the bladder is bypassed and urine leaves the body via a stoma. Urostomy care requires expert nursing management in order to prevent skin problems and urine leaks. There is a variety of urostomy products available and the choice of which to use is determined by the shape and placement of the stoma, the condition of the skin, body weight, and financial resources.

NURSING DIAGNOSES

A variety of nursing diagnoses are appropriate for the patient with a urostomy. The following are examples that include nursing interventions and outcomes.

DISTURBANCE IN SELF-CONCEPT RELATED TO ALTERED BODY IMAGE

The presence of any ostomy represents a threat to the individual's body image. Ini-

TABLE 12.4 Peritoneal Dialysis: Potential Nursing Problems (Complications)

Problems	Nursing Actions
Inadequate preparation of client	Have client void before initiating dialysis. Place client in supine position with head of bed elevated to comfortable level.
Bleeding	Monitor for bloody drainage. Use pressure dressing if bleeding occurs.
Bowel perforation	Monitor for fecal contents in dialysate returns. Stool mixed with fluid.
Bladder perforation	Monitor for large urinary output.
Leakage of dialysate	Monitor for frequent need to change dressing. Weigh dressing and include in record of fluid loss. Protect skin at insertion site.
Insufficient dialysis return	Monitor for occlusion of catheter with fibrin or blood. Turn client side to side. Position client in semi-Flowler's. Prevent catheter malposition.
Obstruction, malposition, or kinks in catheter	Add heparin to dialysate if ordered. Maintain drip chamber of dialysate administration tubing 4 feet above patient. Anchor catheter to provide for adequate inflow and outflow.

TABLE 12.5 Hemodialysis: Potential Nursing Problems (Complications)

Problems	Nursing Actions
Excessive ultrafiltration rate	Ensure adequate operation of machinery prior to initiation of dialysis. Examine system for leaks or air. Change composition of dialysate as ordered. Alter regimen as ordered. Adjust flow rates Decrease positive pressure in blood chamber Decrease negative pressure in dialyzing solution

Poor blood flow	Use only mature arteriovenous fistula (*i.e.*, 2–4 weeks)
	Use smaller needles and slower blood flows in first runs.
	Monitor for signs of poor blood flow:
	    low flowmeter readings
	    collapsed tubing in arterial and/or venous side of dialysis tubing
	    abnormalities at vessel cannulation sites
	    discomfort associated with poor blood flow.

Air embolus	Avoid kinks in the tubing.
	Tape all connections.
	Monitor blood flow.
	Monitor for symptoms of air embolism:
	    chest pain
	    cyanosis
	    cough
	If air has been delivered to client, put in Trendelenburg position and turn on left side.
	Notify physician and prepare for transit to hospital.

Failure of shunt/fistula	Maintain flow rates. Apply sterile pressure dressing after dialysis. Continually monitor for patency of the shunt or fistula.
Needle dislodged	Clamp arterial and venous lines. Monitor vital signs. Apply pressure for 10 to 15 minutes. Both needles may be removed. Pressure dressing applied for 3 to 4 hours.
Improper needle position	Pull needle back slightly and retape. Place gauze square under nub of needle. (Decrease pump speed during this procedure.)

tially, the individual may be concerned with the physical aspects of his illness; that is, he is concerned with pure survival. However, once the threat of physical harm is overcome, the individual may then become concerned about his body image.

Assessment

Nursing assessment for the urostomy patient begins with an exploration of the meaning of the procedure for the patient, as well as its effect on body image. It is necessary to remember that body image is the perception both of how one sees oneself and how he feels others see him. The assault on self-concept resulting from urinary diversion surgery may be tremendous. A lifetime familiarity of body elimination is changed, elimination topics are considered off limits since they invade privacy and center on "unclean" body wastes, and sexual dysfunction in males is common. It is difficult to undergo such surgery without feeling that a major trauma has ensued.

Assessment should be done in private and at the patient's pace, to prevent feelings of further assault. The nurse can move from low emotionally charged areas such as the stoma, skin, and pouch to areas of higher intensity such as feelings of worth, attractiveness, and sexuality. The client should be encouraged to vent his feelings and discuss his concrete problems. He must also be allowed to discuss how he thinks his partner feels about the ostomy. The home health nurse will want to assess whether the client's perception matches those of the partner.

Interventions

Intervention in this area involves providing accurate information, correcting misconceptions, and offering a great deal of support and encouragement. Because the procedure and its complications are overladen with anxiety, the nurse may find the client initially unwilling to discuss the ostomy at length. By placing the topic open for exploration, the nurse gives the patient permission to talk about the ostomy now or later, according to his desire. The client will sense that nothing about the ostomy is off limits and that an interested, caring person will provide accurate and helpful information as the client becomes ready to receive it.

Outcomes

The expected outcome of nursing intervention is that the client will begin to adjust to the urinary diversion and a return to a normal way of life. The client and spouse should be able to discuss the ostomy freely and the client should be able to feel good about himself and the ostomy.

ALTERATION IN SKIN INTEGRITY

The presence of urine and various appliance adhesives and solvents on the skin have the potential to promote rashes or breakdown. Urine is very damaging to skin and can cause severe problems in breakdown.

Assessment

The peristomal area should be assessed during each pouch change, and the presence of redness, rash, blisters, or infection should be noted, as should specific areas surrounding the ostomy that are affected with breakdown.

Interventions

Skin should be carefully cleansed and patted dry to prevent skin abrasion. Properly fitting appliances may also be helpful in keeping the skin dry and intact. If preventive measures are unsuccessful, alternative approaches must be taken.

Karaya powder is very helpful in the promotion of skin healing and a small amount should be sprinkled on reddened skin or a rash before the skin barrier is applied. If the area looks infected, an anti-yeast powder (Mycostatin) should be applied or Neosporin, if a bacterial infection is present. A more detailed discussion of skin care techniques can be found in Chapter 17.

Outcome

A successful outcome is the maintenance of skin integrity. The skin around the stoma will be intact and without signs of irritation or infection.

KNOWLEDGE DEFICIT RELATED TO MANAGING THE UROSTOMY

Changing the bag and providing skin care may not be overly difficult, but keeping the appliance from leaking may provide a real challenge. The home health nurse will have several areas to consider while arriving at the nursing diagnosis of knowledge deficit.

Assessment

The patient at home is carefully assessed to ascertain knowledge about the ostomy, appliances, and their replacement. In some instances, the client may have been discharged from the hospital with minimal or no ostomy teaching provided. The home care nurse must determine what the patient has been taught and his level of comprehension. It may be necessary to describe the rationale for the ostomy before the client can be expected to learn the fundamentals of changing the appliance.

Interventions

The appliance change should be explained, the equipment gathered, and the old bag removed. Step-by-step, the bag is replaced. The procedure is outlined in the box below. The client should be encouraged to do this procedure as soon as he is mentally prepared. The client should also be taught to observe and manage the peristomal area. It can be very

---

Procedure to Change a Disposable Pouch

1. Prepare skin barrier by tracing correctly sized hole on paper cover of barrier wafer and cutting it. Remove the old bag and skin barrier.

2. Cleanse the peristomal area with warm water. Dry area. Place gauze or tampon in stoma to collect urine. Wipe with skin prep. Apply prepared skin barrier with properly sized hole. Mold into abdominal folds.

3. Remove paper back from faceplate on pouch. Remove gauze or tampon from stoma.

4. Place pouch on skin barrier. Hold in place. If belt is used, fasten ends to faceplate.

The procedure is the same for the reuseable pouch with the exception of cleansing procedures:

1. Empty pouch.

2. Rinse with warm water.

3. Instill white vinegar and allow to soak for 15–20 minutes.

4. Rinse with cool water. Allow to dry thoroughly, then powder inside to prevent adherence of bag on inside.

---

discouraging to both client and nurse if the appliance leaks shortly after being changed. Urine leaks will prevent the patient from a return to a normal life-style (Rolstad 1983). The fear of a urine leak will fill the patient with anxiety about being with others or leaving home. Patience and perseverance are necessary to deal with this problem.

Ensure that the skin is absolutely dry before applying the skin prep and, likewise, that it is dry before putting the skin barrier in place. Make sure that the hole in the skin barrier is not too large and that the opening in the face plate is the correct size. If the patient is obese, it is necessary to dry abdominal skin adequately between the folds and powder with karaya to counteract any moisture or oil in the skin. Skin folds should be smoothed before applying the skin barrier and it should be carefully manipulated into place as it warms and softens.

Continual problems with leakage necessitate beginning anew with different appliance products and asking for the assistance of another home care nurse or stomal expert at a medical supply company. Eventually, the proper combination will be found. It is imperative that the nurse continue to encourage the patient, letting him know that a proper solution will be developed.

Occasionally, the client may be physically or emotionally incapable of learning to change the appliance. In this case, a family member would need to be instructed in the required care. A consultation with an enterostomal therapist may be needed.

Outcomes

A successful outcome is the presence of a nonleaking appliance on the patient for at least 48 hours prior to the necessity of a bag change. The client and family will verbalize an understanding of the function and care of the ostomy.

ALTERED BOWEL ELIMINATION

NORMAL BOWEL FUNCTION

The patient who experiences an alteration in the elimination patterns of the large or small bowel is likely to undergo a tremendous amount of change, both physically and emotionally. Even the slightest disturbance to the gastrointestinal system may yield a barrage of complications that can have a deleterious effect on a patient's life-style. Unfortunately, gastrointestinal disorders are the number one cause for hospitalization for Americans (Thompson et al 1986). Many of these disorders result in long-term problems that cannot be resolved, leading to chronic alterations of normal elimination. Consequently, patients may be discharged from the hospital with permanent changes that require a great deal of adaptation for their success. Colostomies, for example, are becoming a more common procedure, requiring education and support for the client. The client may rely heavily upon the home care nurse to reinforce much of the information previously taught in the hospital.

PATHOPHYSIOLOGY

The digestive process is responsible for the chemical and mechanical breakdown of glucose, amino acids, and fatty acids. In conjunction with digestion, the intestines are the vehicle for absorption of the body's essential nutrients into the bloodstream. The small intestine is between 21 and 23 feet in length and usually two centimeters in diameter.

The first portion is called the *duodenum*, shaped like a "C," and followed by the *jejunum* and the *ileum*. The three sections of the small intestine work together to facilitate digestion and absorption, and to mix and propel food toward the large intestine and eventual elimination of the food.

The large intestine, on the other hand, is primarily responsible for only minimal absorption, and functions to control the transportation and storage of waste. It is made up of the *colon* and the *rectum*. The terminal ileum meets the colon at what is known as the *ileocecal valve*. It is at this point that the intestines are divided into large and small and where the elimination mechanisms change their function. Elimination is controlled by internal and external sphincters that allow the end waste products to be evacuated via the rectum.

Normal digestion, absorption, and elimination can be affected by disorders such as infection, disease, or obstruction, all of which alter the normal functioning of the body. Without access to necessary nutrients, or the ability to excrete harmful wastes, the body will not survive.

Diverticulitis is a common inflammatory disease of the bowel, which is the result of inflammation and obstruction following perforation of diverticula, herniated pockets of mucosa of the large colon. The inflammation generally is worsened by spreading to the surrounding intestinal walls. In extreme cases, perforation may cause leakage of intestinal contents and subsequent peritonitis. Diverticulitis most commonly afflicts those over 40 years of age. It is manifested by tenderness in the lower left abdominal quadrant, constipation and distention, a decrease in audible bowel sounds, and an increase in temperature and white blood cells. In some cases, the colon can actually be palpated upon physical examination, and blood may accompany bowel movements (Thompson 1980).

Another chronic bowel complication may be the result of obstruction, or the failure of intestinal contents to be propelled for expulsion. Obstruction can be mechanical or functional in its etiology. A mechanical obstruction results from impaction of stool, the presence of a tumor or hernia, adhesions in the bowel, or unresolvable inflammation. It may be simple and treated medically (medications, cathartics, etc.) or may become strangulated and require surgical intervention (Price and Wilson 1986). A functional obstruction, however, is also known as an *ileus* or the *loss of propulsion*. Most commonly, an ileus follows manipulation of the bowel during a surgical procedure. Gastric motility decreases considerably and may halt completely after surgical trauma to the bowel or long-term administration of narcotics. An obstruction is generally evidenced by abdominal cramping, chronic constipation, localized tenderness, vomiting, and dehydration, along with tachycardia, decreased urinary output, loss of skin turgor, and moisture to mucous membranes.

Surgery may be required to remove the obstruction. The degree of surgical complexity is related to the duration of the obstruction and the condition of the intestine surrounding it. If possible, the obstruction will be removed and an anastomosis performed at the site. In the case of a tumor, however, the obstruction must be relieved prior to the removal of the tumor. The large intestine is most frequently affected by cancer; therefore, a loop colostomy can be performed for bowel elimination and the return of homeostasis. The tumor can then be removed and if not malignant, the colostomy may be reversed.

Loss of bowel function may also be related to spinal cord injury. If the level of injury is such that it affects the bowel, a patient will no longer have control over elimination. The sensory, motor, autonomic, and reflex mechanisms are all at risk of damage below the level of spinal cord injury.

Regardless of the precipitating factors leading to elimination problems, the patient will require a great deal of support both in the hospital, and even more so when he returns home to live and cope with his change of life-style.

NURSING DIAGNOSES

A number of diagnoses are appropriate for individuals with alterations in elimination.

ALTERATION IN ELIMINATION: CONSTIPATION

Constipation can accompany any bowel disorder. Although often ignored as a minor annoyance, it can be the symptom of a more serious problem and should alert the home care nurse to carry out a thorough assessment.

Assessment

The client should be asked to describe his normal bowel patterns (number and frequency of bowel movements), and the duration of the current episode of constipation. A recent diet history may provide insight as to possible causes of constipation. The patient should also be questioned about abdominal pain, if present, including location, intensity, fluctuation, and duration. It should likewise be noted whether or not pain is caused as a result of palpation during a physical examination. The presence or absence of bowel sounds, in addition, will aid in the assessment of the patient's overall gastrointestinal system. With constipation, there will be an increased discomfort with palpation in the left lower quadrant. Bowel sounds may also be decreased.

Interventions

Assuming that the patient does not have an obstruction (visible via a barium swallow or enema), the interventions to counteract constipation center upon increasing gastric mo-

tility. The client should be encouraged to exercise as much as possible. If bedridden, range of motion exercises (either passive or self-initiated) will aid in increasing peristaltic activity. It should be explained that regular exercise, no matter how little, will help to prevent future problems with constipation.

The diet should be high in roughage such as raw fruits, vegetables, and bran and water content, both of which help to move waste products and lubricate the intestinal tract. If indicated, the patient may require the administration of peristaltic stimulants or laxatives or enemas to provide relief. The patient with a colostomy may require irrigation to relieve constipation. Appropriate orders for irrigating should be obtained.

Work with the client to establish a routine time for elimination. Once that time has been established, the client can drink warm fluids to help initiate the process. It is important that the nurse not treat constipation lightly, as it may be the manifestation of an underlying disorder, such as an intestinal obstruction.

Outcomes

The expected outcome from these interventions is that the client will experience normal bowel function. In addition, the client will be comfortable and without complaints of pain or bloating.

ALTERATION IN ELIMINATION: DIARRHEA

Diarrhea, especially of long duration, is an alteration in normal bowel activities. Like constipation it may accompany another disorder and should receive prompt attention. Diarrhea poses a significant threat to the client. Not only does it cause the client to be weak and lethargic, it may also lead to dehydration and electrolyte imbalance, both of which are extremely stressful for an already compromised system.

Assessment

When a client complains of diarrhea the nurse should note several important things. The amount, color, and consistency of the output and the frequency of episodes should be recorded. The client's energy level, especially complaints of sudden lethargy or malaise, should be evaluated. In order to rule out food poisoning or contact with a virus, the patient should be watched for 24 hours for an alleviation of symptoms. If the symptoms do not abate, the client should be monitored for signs of dehydration. The nurse should check urinary output, concentration, and specific gravity, the skin's turgor, and the visible moisture content in the mucous membranes. A blood sample may also be obtained in order to determine the status of the patient's electrolytes. Likewise, a stool sample may be sent to the laboratory for examination.

Interventions

Interventions center upon the cessation of the diarrhea and the replacement of lost fluids and electrolytes. If possible, fluids can be replaced orally via the ingestion of fluids and electrolyte supplements (potassium, sodium, etc.). If the patient is unable to drink to the degree necessary for replacement, intravenous (IV) routing may be necessary. The intravenous rate and electrolyte content will be determined by the preliminary and subsequent blood laboratory results. The client's hydration is further monitored by records of intake and output.

Meticulous care is essential for the prevention of skin breakdown, especially if the patient is bedridden. The skin should be kept clean and dry, using a mild, nonirritating soap. A and D Ointment may be applied to protect the skin from moisture and sitz baths may be necessary to alleviate the burning associated with diarrhea. If prescribed, Lomotil may be given after each episode of diarrhea (not to exceed the amount indicated per 24 hours) to slow or stop diarrhea. A low residue diet, including such foods as bananas, peanut butter without nuts, and applesauce, aids in alleviating diarrhea episodes.

Diarrhea is not only uncomfortable, but frequent episodes interfere greatly with a client's normal activities. The above assessment and interventions are aimed at the eventual outcome of relief for the patient with diarrhea. Relief will come most likely in a decrease in the number of episodes of diarrhea, followed by passage of formed stool.

Outcomes

If nursing interventions are successful, the client will not experience diarrhea. Should the diarrhea not be controlled, the client should not suffer any discomfort or skin breakdown.

KNOWLEDGE DEFICIT REGARDING OSTOMY CARE

As is true in the previous discussion of urinary ostomies, the client with a colostomy or ileostomy must possess a thorough knowledge of disease process, the ostomy itself, and all of its related care.

Assessment

Assess the client's and family's understanding of the disease process leading to the establishment of the ostomy. In addition to the knowledge of the disease, the client must understand the many aspects of care of the ostomy. Assess for knowledge concerning changing the ostomy bag, proper diet, skin care, and symptoms concerning complications.

Interventions

There are many new products developed and marketed each year, providing the ostomate with a variety of materials to help care for the ostomy. However, the client will never be adequately equipped until he possesses the vital knowledge necessary to accompany the technology. Therefore, the nurse in home care must keep abreast of the latest equipment and be attuned to the patient's true understanding of ostomy care. It should never be assumed that the client's knowledge is complete until the ability to demonstrate an appliance change, skin care, and dietary considerations has been documented. Depending on the client, this process may take quite a while.

The new ostomate may be very fearful about changing the bag, leakage, odor, flatulence, and having the appliance show under clothing. The greatest fear may be related to the inability to manage a bag change. Nursing interventions are aimed at assisting the client in managing his care. The client can be shown an appliance change and as soon as comfortable can assist in the procedure. It may be helpful to gather the equipment and use it as a visual aid while describing the procedures. The pieces of equipment can become familiar to the client before he attempts to change his own bag. The procedure for changing a disposable colostomy bag is outlined in the boxed material opposite.

Some pouches have built in skin barriers, gaskets, and outlet clips. Client preference and finances dictate equipment used. Alter procedure to accommodate special appliances. The procedure for changing the appliance is illustrated in Figure 12-2.

Outcomes

The eventual outcome of the instruction and encouragement provided will be a confident patient independent in the care of his ostomy. The client and significant others should express understanding of the care of the ostomy and knowledge of how to find assistance when needed.

Procedure for Changing a Disposable Colostomy Bag With a Skin Barrier

1. Remove old bag. Cleanse skin with warm water. Dry.

2. Measure size of stoma, cut skin barrier wafer to fit stoma.

3. Apply skin prep. Allow to dry.

4. Apply wafer to skin.

5. Attach appliance.

6. Fasten belt, if used.

POTENTIAL FOR STOMAL/PERISTOMAL COMPLICATIONS

The client who has undergone an ostomy procedure requires proper functioning of the stoma. It is important, therefore, to educate the client concerning stoma care and the signs of any pending disorders.

Assessment

The stoma should be checked often for color and blood supply. It is normal, especially immediately after surgery, for the stoma to bleed. Blood may appear on the cloth used to cleanse the stoma; the client should be instructed that this is normal, and a good sign of a proficient blood supply as evidenced by the many functioning capillaries. If the stoma appears dark purple, or dusky in color, it may be a sign that it is not receiving enough blood and is at risk for necrosis if not promptly treated by the physician. If the stoma "dies," a new procedure will be necessary in the attempt to yield a healthy ostomy.

The stoma should also be assessed for the presence of pain or discomfort, neither of which should remain after postoperative re-

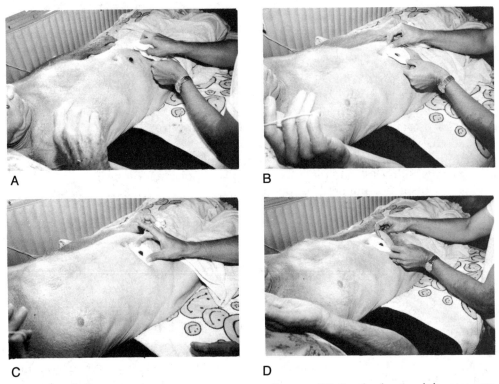

Figure 12-2. Procedure for changing ostomy appliances. *(A)* Gently clean and dry areas surrounding the ostomy. *(B)* Apply the shield, making sure its hole fits onto the ostomy. *(C)* Press the shield gently to remove all wrinkles. *(D)* Apply the pouch. (From Walsh J, Persons CB, Wieck L: Manual of Home Health Care Nursing, p 108. Philadelphia, JB Lippincott, 1987)

covery. The stoma should not be loose enough to allow for the passage of stool and should remain moist and supple. Check the surrounding skin for evidence of breakdown due usually to either feces or chafing from the ostomy equipment.

Interventions

Should breakdown occur, keep skin free from excess moisture or contact with the contents of the bag (empty frequently and rinse with warm water). Skin prep can be used to protect the skin from moisture and irritation by

the appliance. Redness, rash, or blistering may be due to adhesive or feces and should be treated with karaya powder. Skin should be bathed with water only and air dried. Allow the skin to remain exposed to air for 20 minutes.

Outcomes

The desired outcome for the above care is the maintenance of a healthy and viable stoma, and the skin that surrounds it. This will allow a patient to establish an uninterrupted pattern of ostomy care.

INEFFECTIVE INDIVIDUAL COPING RELATED TO ALTERED ELIMINATION PATTERN

The individual faced with a major life change, such as a colostomy, is likely to have difficulty coping at various stages of the illness. A nurse who can identify these difficulties is in an excellent position to offer help and advice as appropriate.

Assessment

The initial step is an assessment of the client's coping patterns, both past and present. Discussions of past difficulties and the client's manner of coping with them is less threatening initially than asking direct questions about coping with his colostomy. The way in which he responds to the question, verbally and nonverbally, will provide insight that can be used to help him in the future. It is necessary, of course, to establish a trusting relationship with the patient before asking questions that will require an exposure of his personal feelings. The home care nurse has the advantage of seeing the client in his own environment, making such trust easier, and providing clues about coping that would not otherwise be evident in the hospital.

In addition to questions about the past, the nurse might explore fictitious scenarios with the client to elicit information about coping in hypothetical situations. If, for example, the patient were asked, "What would you do if. . . ?", his responses could be used to clarify for himself and the nurse the ways in which he copes with stress. If it becomes obvious that the patient is exhibiting maladaptive coping mechanisms, it will become necessary to intervene.

Interventions

The most effective primary intervention begins with informing the client as to the results of the assessment. The nurse must take care not to appear condescending while sharing this information. A client is likely to feel extremely vulnerable while being offered details about himself. Once again, trust is a prerequisite for such intervention. The client must first admit to an inability to cope effectively with his colostomy before he will be open to receiving help. This assistance will come from the nurse in the form of gentle discussion about coming to terms with the illness, what it means to the individual, and how he can help himself by accepting the circumstances. Acceptance leads to growth, and if unable to grow, the client is at risk of emotional regression. Therefore, the nurse must attempt to develop a therapeutic relationship with the client, one which will serve as a catalyst for such growth. The outcome of these efforts will be the reward of seeing positive changes for the patient.

Outcomes

Successful nursing interventions will result in a client who is able to verbalize acceptance of the ostomy. Finally, the client should accept the care and responsibility for the colostomy and integrate it with other activities of his life. The client will exhibit signs of use of healthy coping mechanisms.

HOME CARE ASSESSMENT

As part of the overall nursing process, the home health nurse must also assess the home care environment. In this section, techniques for assessment of the home environment as it relates to problems with elimination will be discussed.

Careful assessment of the home environment includes both home and neighborhood. Important neighborhood considerations are socioeconomic status, safety, distances between homes, and access to the area. The nurse is able to formulate a care plan reflecting goals that are realistic and achievable when environmental assessment is performed (Bohnet 1980).

The client's residence should be examined for accessibility inside and out, considering location, stairs, obstacles, and room placement and size. Stairs are often an impediment for an easily fatigued client and consideration may be given to rearranging the living quarters to better accommodate a weakened physical condition. Basic utilities should be checked to determine not only if they are available in the home but if they are currently operational. Even in the wealthiest country in the world there are homes that lack running water, electricity, and heat. These are major concerns for someone who will be cared for at home with a new colostomy or who will undergo dialysis under less than optimal home conditions. The home may have utility hookups but ones that are not functional due to lack of payment. It may be possible to obtain assistance for needy persons by contacting the appropriate utility provider. All such avenues should be explored by the nurse and social worker.

It should be remembered that crowded home conditions create stress in family members. The addition of supplies, machinery, and equipment may add further insult to an already difficult and stressful situation. This, in turn, may create problems for a client who feels that his physical problem is creating problems for his family.

The family may feel pressured and resentful. Certainly the nurse will provide better care when these areas are explored, problems identified, and care delivered that is supportive, realistic, and goal-oriented. Careful assessment is the foundation of such care.

ABBREVIATED CARE PLAN: ALTERATION IN ELIMINATION: PERITONEAL DIALYSIS

Nursing Diagnosis	Assessment	Interventions	Outcomes
Alteration in Gas Exchange	Lung sounds, level of consciousness, cough	Place client in semi-Fowler position during dialysis. Provide oxygen therapy as needed. Provide quiet, restful environment.	Lungs remain clear Client experiences no respiratory distress.
Alteration in Cardiac Output	Weight (every 6 to 10 runs), blood pressure, urine output, pulse	Closely monitor adjustment of cardiac drugs. Continually evaluate for fluid overload. If arrhythmias occur, notify physician.	

ABBREVIATED CARE PLAN: ALTERATION IN ELIMINATION: PERITONEAL DIALYSIS (*continued*)

Nursing Diagnosis	Assessment	Interventions	Outcomes
		Alter runs of 1.5% and 4.25% of dialysate as needed to maintain volume.	

ABBREVIATED CARE PLAN: ALTERATION IN ELIMINATION: HEMODIALYSIS

Nursing Diagnosis	Assessment	Interventions	Outcomes
Alteration in Cardiac Output	Blood pressure, pulse rate, weight	Carefully prime machine as ordered.	Client will maintain a normal cardiac output.
		Administer saline, albumin, or blood products if hypotension occurs.	
		Ensure that all connections on machinery are tight.	
Alteration in Cardiac Output: Potential for Hemorrhage		Carefully secure needle in place.	
		Position extremity to prevent dislodgement of needle.	
		Closely monitor blood pressure during dialysis.	
		Monitor for potential complications: angina, arrhythmias, or electrolyte imbalance.	

References

Bohnet N: Total nursing assessment of the home care patient. Home Health Review I1I: 13, 1980

Chaffee E, Greisheimer E: Basic Physiology. Philadelphia, JB Lippincott, 1974

Chambers J: Assessing the dialysis patient at home. Am J Nurse 81:750, 1981

Gonsalves EL: Psychological aspects of home care for the patient with end-stage renal disease. Cleve-Clin-Q: Fall 52:299, 1985

Guyton A: Textbook of Medical Physiology, Philadelphia, WB Saunders, 1986

Johnson R: Home dialysis: The competition between CAPD and hemodialysis. JAMA 245:1511, 1981

Kirkby M, Fax M: Support systems as a factor in hemodialysis. Nephrol Nurse 4:19, 1982

Lowry M, Atcherson E: Spouse-assistants, adjustments to home, hemodialysis J Chronic Dis 37:293, 1984

Palmer S et al: Helping families respond effectively to chronic illness: Home dialysis as a case example. Social Work in Health Care 8:1, 1982

Paradiso C: The dialysis patient, the family, and the home health nurse. Home Healthcare Nurse 4:26, 1986

Porth CM: Pathophysiology. Philadelphia, JB Lippincott, 1986

Price SA, Wilson LM: Pathophysiology. New York City, McGraw-Hill, 1986

Rolstad B et al: Sexual concern in the patient with an ileostomy. Diseases at the Colon and Rectum 26:170, 1983

Schreiber MJ, Vidt DG, Cunningham RJ: Home therapy for kidney disease: Continuous ambulatory peritoneal dialysis and continuous cyclic peritoneal dialysis. Cleve-Clin-Q 52:291–297, 1985

Shurr M, Roy C: Components of a successful home dialysis program. Nephrol Nurse 2:5, 1980

Stansfield G: Coping with CAPD. Nursing Mirror 161(14):28–29, 1985

Stark CR: Home and in center hemodialysis patients—A descriptive study (survey). Nephrol Nurs 2(2):77–79, 1985

Thompson J, McFarland G, Hirsch J, Tucker, S et al: Clinical Nursing. St. Louis, CV Mosby, 1986

Wilson D, Conley SB, Brewer ED: Adaptation to home dialysis: The use of CAPD and CCPD in infants and small children. AA NNT J 10:49, 1983

USP-DI: United States Pharmacopia, Drug Information, 1987

ALTERATIONS IN SENSATION AND PERCEPTION

13

Mary Gokey
Charmaine Cummings

The nervous system transforms environmental energy into electrical energy and transmits this electrical energy from one part of the body to another (Goldstein 1983). The working unit for the transmission of this energy is the neuron.

The first neuron in the sensory system has a receptor, which is specialized to respond to certain environmental stimuli. The stimulus is received by the receptor and passes up the sensory fiber (a peripheral nerve), synapses at various levels in the spinal cord, travels through the thalamus and to the area of the brain's cortex that specializes in receiving input from the sense that was stimulated. Figure 13-1 illustrates the areas of the brain that comprise the sensory cortex.

Perception is the conscious recognition and interpretation of sensory stimuli through unconscious associations, especially memory, that serve as a basis for understanding, learning, and knowing, or for the motivation of a particular action or reaction (Hamilton 1983). Perception is thought to result from electrical impulses in the sensory cortex of the parietal lobe. Alterations of perception can lead to inaccurate views of oneself and the environment.

The sensory system does not work independently of the rest of the nervous system. For example, if we are to react to touch, the parietal cortex receives a message of pressure on the skin. The parietal area perceives this pressure. It, in turn, sends an electrical signal to the motor cortex in the frontal lobe, which relays a message to the muscles, and causes the body to move.

Disorders such as Guillain–Barré syndrome or stroke cause injury to the neurons so that the electrical impulses are impeded. In this chapter, some of the conditions that alter sensation and perception will be discussed, including cerebral vascular accident, Guillain–Barré, seizure disorders, and unconsciousness. These conditions are by no means limited to sensory–perceptual problems only, but they do interfere significantly with the client's ability to sense and perceive his environment.

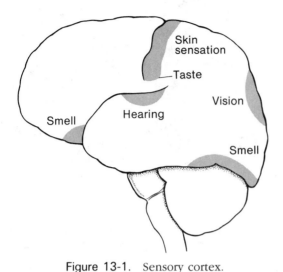

Figure 13-1. Sensory cortex.

CEREBRAL VASCULAR ACCIDENT

Cerebral vascular accident (CVA) or stroke is the third leading cause of death in the United States, behind heart disease and cancer. It claims 180,000 lives annually, and leaves thousands requiring some type of long-term assistance (Sahs 1976). Of every 100 persons who survive the acute phase of stroke, 10 may return to work without noticeable impairment, 40 will have mild impairment, 40 will be disabled enough to require special services, and 10 will need to be institutionalized (Sahs 1976).

Despite these dramatic statistics, the death rate from cerebral vascular disease has fallen 5% per year since 1969 (Barnett 1986). Presumably this is due in part to better control of hypertension and increased public awareness of the importance of lifetime treatment. The changes in attitude toward healthy diets, exercise, and the diminished consumption of cigarettes may also contribute to the decline in mortality. Another reason is thought to be

more effective treatment of stroke in its acute stages, with more clients surviving into the long-term phase. Death during this phase is usually attributed to other causes, such as cancer or cardiovascular disease (although stroke is certainly a part of the larger problem of cardiovascular disease). With shortened lengths of hospital stays the rule, the home health nurse can anticipate adding clients with CVAs to her case load.

PATHOPHYSIOLOGY

A cerebrovascular accident is the clinical expression of a pathological process involving the cerebral vasculature, either directly or indirectly, and resulting in a secondary abnormality in the brain (Kaplan 1986). Pathophysiological mechanisms of stroke are many. Generally a stroke occurs as a result of hemorrhage or occlusion. Pathogenesis of occlusive disease usually occurs as a result of thrombosis, embolism, or compression.

Types of Cerebral Vascular Syndromes

Transient ischemic attack (TIA) is a localized ischemic event producing a focal neurological deficit that lasts 24 hours or less, and does not leave a permanent deficit. Most TIAs occur abruptly, last usually 2 to 30 minutes, and recede quickly. TIAs occur in a particular vascular distribution, which frequently aids the physician in the diagnosis due to the clinical syndromes. The TIA is often viewed as a warning sign of the permanent neurological deficit that will follow if stroke occurs. According to Sutin (Kaplan 1986), 25% to 40% of clients experiencing more than one TIA will infarct within the next 5 years, 51% during the first year of the onset of TIA.

Some clinicians describe another type of localized ischemia, termed a reversible ischemic neurologic deficit (RIND). This ischemic event may last up to 3 weeks, but usually resolves in 24 to 72 hours. Other clinicians believe RIND is actually submaximal infarction, which is sometimes demonstrable on CT scan. Ultimately, the possibility of recurrence of symptoms with more devastating results should stress the importance of community education and treatment to prevent this from happening.

TIA syndromes are classified as either carotid or vertebrobasilar. Typically, the client may not recognize that symptoms suggest anything important. For example, the client may report that he "fainted." On further questioning, the fainting spell may be found to be one of many episodes. An astute home health nurse will recognize the pattern as a TIA. Generally, carotid TIAs affect the cerebral hemispheres and the deep nuclei of the brain. Vertebrobasilar TIAs occur due to ischemia of the brain stem, cerebellum, portions of the occipital and temporal lobes, thalamus and inner ear. The patterns of neurological deficits that occur during TIA depend on a variety of factors including the patency and structure of the arterial systems.

TIAs occurring in the carotid distribution tend to be hemispheric and include such symptoms as transient monocular blindness (*amaurosis fugax*), contralateral paralysis, weakness or clumsiness of one or both extremities, paresthesias, usually of the hand, dysphasia with involvement of the dominant hemisphere, dysarthria, and homonymous hemianopsia.

Vertebrobasilar insufficiency tends to affect both sides of the body. Combinations from weakness of the extremities to quadriplegia can occur. Attacks can occur without warning, without any disturbance in consciousness. Sensory components of vertebrobasilar TIAs include vision loss (cortical blindness), visual hallucinations, perioral tingling, numbness and paresthesias of the entire face or combinations of the extremities and, rarely, sudden and permanent deafness.

Vertigo, diplopia, dysarthria, dysphagia, clumsiness, and ataxia are other common complaints.

The most common cause of stroke is atherosclerotic thrombosis. Thrombotic strokes tend to evolve slowly and are frequently preceded by TIAs. Most clients have a history of hypertension and atherosclerotic disease of the cardiovascular or peripheral vascular systems. The risk factors linked to coronary heart disease, such as smoking, obesity, sedentary life-style and stress may be similar for thromboembolic stroke. Certain diseases, such as diabetes mellitus, which compromise circulation, sickle cell anemia and polycythemia, which tend to increase the viscosity of blood, are risk factors for thrombotic stroke. Reduced levels of high density lipoproteins, which are believed to carry excess tissue cholesterol to the liver, are other risk factors.

Various syndromes occur as a result of occlusion of specific cerebral arteries. Middle cerebral artery syndrome is usually secondary to occlusion of the internal carotid artery or embolism. Symptoms include contralateral hemiparesis and cortical sensory loss greater in the face and arm than leg, aphasia, and homonymous hemianopsia. Anterior cerebral artery syndrome is characterized by incontinence, paralysis, and cortical sensory loss in the contralateral leg, and slowness in mentation with perseveration. Occlusion of the internal carotid artery resembles the middle cerebral syndrome and may include the anterior cerebral distribution. This type of stroke can be quite devastating due to the potentially large amount of infarcted tissue. Posterior cerebral artery syndrome produces little or no paralysis, but may result in severe sensory losses to both pain and light touch. Homonymous hemianopsia is a frequent finding. Vertebrobasilar artery thrombosis gives rise to a number of syndromes, depending upon the arterial branch affected. The client may develop ataxia, facial pain or numbness, vertigo, nausea, vomiting, dysphagia, and dysarthria. With complete basilar artery occlusion the client may be paralyzed in all four extremities and in coma.

Embolic stroke usually occurs rapidly and without warning. The deficit at onset is usually severe but the chances of eventual recovery to near normal are good due to the breakdown and dispersion of the embolus. Frequently, embolic stroke occurs during the waking hours. Emboli are usually cholesterol plaques or mural thrombi fragments that travel from one part of a vessel and lodge further along the vessel. Secondary hemorrhage and edema can occur as blood seeps through the damaged vessel wall where the embolus originated. Emboli that originate in the heart can travel to the brain following cardioversion, cardiac dysrhythmias, valvular disease, or myocardial infarction. Seizures sometimes accompany embolism or stenosis.

Intracranial hemorrhage can be classified as either intracerebral or subarachnoid. Intracerebral hemorrhage is bleeding into the brain substance, or "parenchyma." Subarachnoid hemorrhage is bleeding into the subarachnoid space. Hypertension is widely accepted as the most significant risk factor for intracerebral hemorrhage, accounting for nearly 60% to 70% of intracerebral bleeding. Ruptured aneurysms and arteriovenous malformations (AVM) are the cause for most of the remainder. Ruptured aneurysms and AVMs are responsible for the majority of subarachnoid hemorrhages.

Intracerebral hemorrhagic stroke occurs without warning, when the client is usually up and active. It may evolve in minutes or days, depending on the rate of bleeding. As the expanding lesion exerts mass effect on surrounding tissue, the client may complain of headache, nausea, vomiting, followed by deterioration in level of consciousness and coma. Vital signs are unstable with acutely elevated blood pressure. Blood in the parenchyma follows the path of least resistance, frequently finding its way to the ventricles. Mortality rate for intracerebral hemorrhage is the greatest with 70% to 75% dying during the first 30 days (Kaplan 1986).

Unless an aneurysm is close enough to a structure to exhibit symptoms of compression, it will frequently go undetected before rupturing. Subarachnoid hemorrhage most often occurs during activity and presents with a very severe headache, nuchal rigidity, photophobia, and vomiting. Coma may ensue, depending on the extent of the hemorrhage. Complications of subarachnoid hemorrhage can be cerebral edema, communicating hydrocephalus, rebleeding, aseptic meningitis, and cerebral ischemia or infarction (Kaplan 1986). Rebleeding occurs most often during the period between 10 days and 14 days after the initial rupture. Vasospasm is another potential problem that occurs usually between the third and the eighth day, and can cause further ischemia and infarction to an already compromised brain. A summary of the various types of stroke can be found in Table 13-1.

NURSING DIAGNOSES

Clients who recover from the acute phase of stroke are frequently left with numerous deficits and are candidates for many more potential problems. The following nursing diagnoses are among the most common when caring for the stroke client. Each diagnosis includes the indications for the diagnosis, assessment methods, suggestions for nursing interventions, and the desired outcome.

ALTERATION IN COMMUNICATION

Infarction of the dominant side of the brain, most frequently due to an occlusion of the left middle cerebral artery or one of its

TABLE 13.1 Characteristic Features of Stroke*

	Embolus	Intracerebral Hemorrhage	Large Vessel Thrombosis	Lacune	Subarachnoid Hemorrhage
Location	Peripheral (cortical)	Deep (basal ganglia, thalamus, cerebellum)	Variable (depends on vessel)	Pons, internal capsule	Vessels at junction of the Circle of Willis
Onset	Sudden (maximum deficit at onset)	Sudden (deficit develops over minutes to hours)	Sudden, Gradual, Stepwise, or Stuttering	Sudden, Gradual, Stepwise, or Stuttering	Sudden; usually few or no focal signs
When	Awake	Awake and active	Asleep or inactive	Asleep or inactive	Awake and active
Warning (TIA)	None	None	Usually	Variable; TIA's may occur	None
Headache	Sometimes	Usually	Sometimes	No	Always (stiff neck)

*These characteristics are generally accepted principles regarding stroke; however, they are not hard rules, and stroke can present atypically. (From Weiner HL: Neurology for the House Officer. Baltimore, Williams & Wilkins, 1983)

branches, leaves the client with various communication deficits. Language is defined as the "symbolic formulation, vocal or graphic, of ideas according to semantic and grammatical rules for communication of thoughts and feelings" (Kaplan 1986). Speaking, writing, gesturing, hearing, and reading are all ways of communicating. Therefore, the client who has right-sided hemiplegia, loss of a properly functioning speech center, and visual impairments most likely has difficulty communicating.

According to Halper and Mogil, aphasia is an acquired language disorder resulting from neurological impairment that affects all language modalities including auditory and reading comprehension, oral and written expression, and gestures (Kaplan 1986). Many types of aphasia have been described, depending upon which part or parts of the brain have been infarcted. Three of the most common types of aphasia are global, Broca's, and Wernicke's aphasia.

Clients suffering from global aphasia tend to understand facial expressions, inflections in the voice and gestures, but cannot comprehend written or spoken language well, nor express themselves orally. Broca's aphasics speak slowly and laboriously. Difficulties with word finding (anomia), reading comprehension, and writing ability are present. Auditory comprehension is intact if the person is spoken to in slow, less complex sentences. Wernicke's aphasia is characterized by hyperfluent, meaningless speech and impaired auditory comprehension. Unlike the Broca's aphasic who is aware of his communication deficits, the Wernicke's aphasic is not aware of his, frequently seeming euphoric.

Assessment

The speech pathologist conducts an extensive evaluation of the aphasic client to diagnose the type of aphasia, identify the client's strengths and weaknesses, and prescribe and conduct therapy. The client should continue to see the speech therapist by outpatient or home visits. Recommendations for communication made by the speech pathologist are most helpful for the client, family, and the nurse.

The nursing assessment of the aphasic client begins with a thorough neurologic assessment for deficits such as hemiparesis, visual problems, and swallowing difficulties. Cranial nerves V, VII, IX, X, and XII should be evaluated carefully because they are important for articulating and phonating as well as for swallowing. For example, if food tends to pocket on one side of the mouth, involvement of cranial nerve VII can be suspected. Evaluate the client's hearing ability. The nurse may experience some difficulty evaluating the cranial nerves due to the client's aphasia. Understand the client's frustration and allow plenty of time for him to respond during the assessment.

On the initial visit, the questions the nurse asks will help to determine the extent of the client's communication skills. To determine whether the client comprehends the spoken word, ask him to perform simple commands, such as closing his eyes or grasping your hand. Be sure the commands are something the client is able to do physically. To test the client's ability to understand the written word, have him read some simple words. Do not start with complete sentences as the ability to process a whole sentence is lost in some aphasics. Establish whether the client can correctly answer simple "yes" and "no" questions. Also, establish whether the client can recognize simple pictures or objects. Ask the client to say what an object is. Does he say the right word, or does he say something unrelated to the object? A communication board can be a useful tool when communicating with some aphasics. This board has pictures that represent specific needs. The client simply points to the appropriate picture and the family is able to understand. Observe the client when he communicates with you or the family. Does he say what he wants, or does he gesture or point to the object he wants. Many aphasics have a selective retention of certain language modalities that should be identified and used to improve communication.

Interventions

One of the major responsibilities of the home health nurse will be to assist the family as it lives with the client's problems in communication. Help the family to maintain a calm, quiet, unhurried environment in the home, which will support the client's efforts at communicating. On each visit, encourage the client to speak, and praise all attempts. Encourage the family to understand the client's frustration when unable to communicate needs correctly. Request the family to encourage the client in all efforts to verbalize. Teach the family to keep the client involved in activities of the household. Isolation of the client will worsen the communication problems. Encourage the family to help the client participate in conversations throughout the day.

Problems with communication require expenditure of energy by the client. Efforts at communication are frequently more productive when the client is rested. Therefore, when possible, the home health nurse should attempt to schedule visits with the client during his most rested periods. Information can be gathered from the family which would indicate the client's fluctuation in communication abilities throughout the course of a normal day.

For a client with global aphasia, teach the family to capitalize on the client's ability to comprehend nonverbal cues, such as inflections in the voice or gestures. Point to objects in the house when speaking to stimulate the visual abilities of the client. Instruct the family to speak slowly, simply, and distinctly, and to supplement their speech with facial expressions. Help the global aphasic to learn gestures to communicate with the family and nursing staff. Sometimes a communication board is useful with these clients, although its use may be hampered by difficulty in pointing.

Because clients with Broca's aphasia usually have intact word comprehension, the home health nurse should teach the family to use "yes" and "no" situations and questions. The client can nod or point to "yes"/"no" on a board. Since the client with Broca's aphasia can usually comprehend the written word, use of "yes" and "no" questions can be an effective means of communication. These clients are usually aware of their communication deficit, which can lead to severe depression and withdrawal.

Lack of auditory abilities and awareness of his speech problems are the biggest problems for the client with Wernicke's aphasia. Reading comprehension and writing abilities are also severely impaired. Teach the family to reinforce single words with gestures. They should be cautioned not to constantly point out errors, but to repeat the desired word. Use nonverbal stimuli such as gestures and vocal inflections.

Outcome

The client will be able to communicate needs and desires effectively.

ALTERATION IN SENSORY – PERCEPTUAL PATTERNS

Sensory deficits of pain, temperature, proprioception, vibration, touch, graphesthesia, stereognosis and/or two-point discrimination are involved in most stroke syndromes. Visual dysfunctions such as homonymous hemianopsia are also common due to an infarct behind the optic chiasm.

Perceptual deficits may occur as a result of stroke, making rehabilitation much more difficult. Various types of apraxias and agnosias may be present as a result of stroke. Infarcts of the nondominant brain, usually the right side, cause interference with spatial ability, recognition of faces, perception of smells, sounds, and awareness of one's own body. This damage diminishes the client's ability to respond appropriately to life events that are occurring in the client's environment. There is a lack of stability in the perceptual world (Goldstein 1983). According to Goldstein, the right hemisphere readily becomes bewildered by the complexities of navigating in space and thereby dealing effectively with regard to activities of daily life. Clients with right-sided brain damage can also appear euphoric and unconcerned, or can deny or neglect their deficits. Clients who experienced a right-sided stroke usually do not function as well as those with left (dominant) hemispheric stroke. There are two possible explanations for this fact; the extent of the right-sided lesions and the inability of medical science to treat right damage as well as it can treat language-related functions (Goldstein 1983).

Assessment

Assessment of the sensory – perceptual altered client should include evaluation of the primary sensory modalities, such as touch, pain, vibration, two-point discrimination, position sense, and stereognosis. Visual fields should be tested for homonymous hemianopsia. Visual acuity and cranial nerves III, IV, and VII should be assessed for oculomotor function. Assess the client for unilateral inattention, or hemineglect. For example, the client may shave just one side of his face, or draw only half of a picture you ask him to copy.

Interventions

When the client has a sensory–perceptual alteration, the family will be vital in protecting him from injury. Clients with hemineglect may injure the affected side. Work with the family to assure that the client includes the neglected side during activities of daily living (ADLs). The family can monitor the bath and encourage the client to wash both sides of the body. This exercise will assist the client to establish the midline of the body and the presence of all extremities.

Too much auditory stimulation can produce sensory overload for the stroke client with auditory–perceptual problems. This can cause him to become confused or disoriented. Encourage the family to keep background noise to a minimum if the client shows signs of this disorder. The apraxic client can be taught to perform his own ADLs, such as dressing. In supervising this activity, the family should be taught to allow the client adequate time to complete the task.

According to Lieberman (Kaplan 1986), prognosis for sensory perceptual recovery has not been studied as much as motor recovery, although some studies show less than 50% recovery rate for pain sensation and two-point discrimination. The goal of the nurse should be to encourage the client to be as involved in family activities and activities of daily living as possible to stimulate the sensory–perceptually altered client.

Outcomes

The client will demonstrate beginning adaptation to visual and spatial perceptual defects.

The client will participate in more activities and will be free from injury related to the sensory–perceptual alteration.

POTENTIAL VISUAL DEFICIT

Homonymous hemianopsia is a frequent occurrence in stroke clients and results from infarction of brain tissue past the optic chiasm, in the optic tract, or optic radiations. The client experiences a field cut in half of the visual field. For example, the client may be able to see only half of a dinner plate, half of a person standing directly in front, or half of a newspaper. The client may not be aware of a person entering the room from the affected side. This visual deficit can be devastating to the client, causing fear and confusion.

Assessment

On an initial visit, the home health nurse will observe the client to assess whether he neglects part of the environment. This can be an initial evaluation through assessment of visual acuity and visual fields.

Interventions

Prior to the discharge of the client with homonymous hemianopsia from the hospital to home, the home health nurse can work with the family to set up the client's room to allow the client to observe the door where people enter. Furniture within the home should be strategically placed to reduce the chance of client injury. Instruct the family to place all meals within the client's visual field.

Another important intervention is to assist the client to learn how to cope with the impairment. On each visit, the home health nurse can reinforce the client's awareness of his environment. For example, the client can be taught to turn his head consciously to see objects on the neglected side. Involvement with ADLs will help to stimulate the client's perception and reduce neglect of self and surroundings. Specific approaches for the client are outlined in Table 13-2.

Outcome

The client will be able to adapt to the visual deficit.

IMPAIRED SKIN INTEGRITY

Alterations in skin integrity may occur due to diminished sensation and perception of pain, altered level of consciousness, and immobility of the affected extremities. Dehydration, overhydration, nutritional deficits, and breaks in skin integrity can also predispose the client to skin breakdown. Areas of the body that are particularly prone to decubitus ulcers are those lying over prominent bony areas, such as heels, ankles, sacrum, or shoulders. Skin that is rubbed by splints and braces, nasogastric tubes, and tight-fitting clothing is also susceptible to tissue breakdown and infection. Skin cells die due to compression of the blood supply, causing a sloughing and open necrotic area.

Assessment

On each visit, the home health nurse should assess the client's skin, especially over the bony prominences, and where pressure is evident and where skin touches skin (for example, under breasts). Inspect for cleanliness and any open areas caused by irritation or injury. Red areas are clues to compromised circulation. Nutrition and hydration status must also be evaluated since they are necessary ingredients for good skin repair. Peripheral vascular status should be assessed by palpating peripheral pulses to determine adequacy of circulation. Edema in extremities compromises blood flow to skin, thus predisposing it to ulceration. Assess for any pain or discomfort over susceptible skin, an early sign of skin breakdown.

Interventions

Prevention of decubitus ulcers is an important nursing responsibility when caring for a client following a cerebrovascular accident. If the client is wheelchair-bound, instruct the family to maintain the wheelchair cushion well padded and without wrinkles or lumps. If possible, teach the client to do wheelchair push-ups to relieve pressure on the sacrum and buttocks. Encourage the family to keep bed linens clean, dry, and wrinkle-free.

The family plays a vital role in maintenance of skin integrity. Assist them to develop a schedule for frequent changing of the client's position. Sheepskin, an air mattress, a draw sheet to decrease friction when turning the client, and heel or elbow pads can be beneficial preventive measures. Work with the family to institute a nighttime turning schedule if the client is immobile to such a degree that he requires assistance.

Ensure that the client receives adequate vitamins, protein, and hydration in the diet (see detailed discussion in Chapter 11). Selection of appropriate clothing for the client is important. Well-fitting clothes with bulky seams help the skin "breathe" and are generally most comfortable for the client. Teach the client to avoid extreme hot or cold temperatures and the use of heat lamps, heating pads, or hot water bottles. The client should also be cautioned not to carry hot beverages in his lap because of the risk of spillage. Water in the tub or shower should be tested by the family. The client can also learn to test water on the unaffected side with intact sensation. Instruct the client to wear shoes when sitting in a wheelchair because hot footplates can burn his feet. Protect all skin from the sun.

In the event that skin breakdown occurs, the home health nurse will institute a thera-

TABLE 13.2 Approaches for the Client With Perceptual Deficits

Deficit	Explanation	Approach
One-sided neglect	Failure to recognize objects or people from the affected side. May neglect affected side or propel wheelchair into the wall. May not dress, bathe, or use affected limbs.	Allow for increased stimulation to the affected side. Use that side as an assist when performing activities of daily living. Approach clients from the affected side. Encourage scanning of the visual field and actual manipulation of the affected limb.
Right–left disorientation	Inability to distinguish right from left.	Use terms like weak or strong and the blue door or the door next to the windows instead of right arm, left leg, door on the left or door on the right.
Body parts disorientation	Inability to discriminate body parts: may be unable to identify body parts when asked, may attempt to put trousers on upper extremities.	Give simple verbal instructions. Avoid use of gestures, but guide hand through hair or place spoon into mouth.
Apraxia	Inability to perform a learned task.	Encourage client participation in activities of daily living but with cueing and supervision to assist client through the routine.
Agnosia	Inability to recognize information through sensory input. May not recognize objects, pictures, symbols, people, room, etc. May be unable to recognize sounds. May have difficulty correcting posture.	When providing care, use a multisensory approach. Incorporate the use of other senses to recognize objects that once were recognized easily by sight or sound. Mark client's room with a symbol, sign, or other method that can be identified by the client. Simplify the environment. Place one item of food at a time in front of the client. Consult phone company for visual replacement of phone bells.

From Geibel CA, Kubalanza–Sipp: Nursing therapy and stroke rehabilitation. In Kaplan PE, Cerullo LJ (eds): Stroke Rehabilitation. Stoneham, MA, Butterworths, 1986

peutic regimen to begin to heal the area. A more detailed discussion of this therapy can be found in Chapter 16.

Outcome

The client will maintain intact skin. Specifically, there will be no areas of redness, irritation or skin breakdown.

SELF-CARE DEFICIT

Decreased muscle strength or paralysis, apraxia, and fatigue are among the many factors that hinder the client's ability to move about purposefully. With a decrease in mobility, compounded with possible depression, the stroke client is often unable to perform self-care functions.

Assessment

On an initial visit to the client, the home health nurse can assess for the presence of self-care deficits. The client's inability to carry out the activities of daily living indicates a self-care deficit. During this assessment, evaluate the client's sitting tolerance, balance, transferring, and ambulating capabilities and endurance. While the client performs some of these maneuvers, monitoring blood pressure, pulse and respirations will help indicate the level of activity tolerance. Assess the range of motion of all extremities. Muscle strength, and presence of flaccidity, spasticity, or contractures must also be evaluated.

Interventions

After this initial assessment, a realistic plan of care should be developed that considers the client's present abilities. Short-term, achievable goals should be set so the client will not become discouraged. Encourage independence with activities the client can perform.

Instruct the family in the most appropriate methods for meeting the remaining client needs.

In establishing a complete plan of care, it may be necessary to consult with other members of the health-care team. The occupational therapist works with the client to achieve independence or near independence in activities of daily living. A consultation with the occupational therapist can be helpful as the client attempts to learn to work within his limitations.

Several important areas should be included in the plan of care. The family and client should be taught how to incorporate active and passive range of motion exercises into daily activities. While the client is performing passive range of motion, instruct the family to provide good support under joints and not to pass the point of pain.

The family can help to guide the client in pacing the activities of the day. If the client has a decreased activity tolerance level, instruct the family to encourage the client to avoid activity immediately after meals since available energy will be utilized by the digestive system.

Along with activity, the client requires consistent periods of rest. An appropriate rest time is following meals. Remind the family that a good time to perform muscle strengthening or range of motion exercises is after these periods of rest. The best schedule is to space activity throughout the day and provide time to rest.

Outcome

The client will perform self-care activities within physical limitations.

ALTERATION IN NUTRITION: LESS THAN BODY REQUIREMENTS

Ensuring proper nutritional and fluid balance in the stroke client can be a difficult task.

Difficulties in maintaining nutritional status begin with the client's inability to self-feed due to a decreased level of consciousness, apraxia, hemiparesis, or hemiplegia. Immobility causes catabolism, a loss in the body's much needed nitrogen. Damage to cranial nerves V, VII, IX, X, and XII impede swallowing ability. Loss of self-esteem and depression can cause anorexia. Homonymous hemianopsia can cause the client to overlook half of a meal on a plate. Fluids are frequently difficult to swallow due to facial paralysis. The client's inability to communicate likes and dislikes can cause further depression and withdrawal.

Assessment

Begin with an assessment of the client's general nutritional status. Inquire about the client's premorbid weight and eating habits. Obtain a baseline weight, and ask the family to weigh the client at least weekly. Assess skin turgor, intake and output, and buccal mucosa for hydration status. Assess the mouth for dentition, status of dentures, whether the client can salivate or overproduces saliva. Assess the function of cranial nerves V, VII, IX, X, and XII. Observe the client's sitting posture and the ability to feed self. Evaluate the client's muscle strength and coordination and whether assistive devices are needed or are adequate.

Interventions

The client should be as well rested and alert as possible for meals. A quiet, relaxed environment will support the client's ability to concentrate on feeding and swallowing. Mouth care before meals may help improve the appetite. Instruct the family to remain with the client during meals because of the great potential of aspirating food. Suction equipment should be available for the dysphagic client.

The home health nurse must teach the family several techniques to assure the safety of the client during meals. Assist the client to a full high Fowler's position if in bed, or to a chair. Position the client slightly forward with a slight forward tilt of the head to aid in swallowing the food bolus. Set up the meal so it is within reach and can be seen if the client has a visual deficit.

Instruct the client and family in the techniques of safe eating when dysphagia is present. Small amounts of food should be placed toward the back and on the unaffected side of the client's mouth. Often clients will have diminished sensation and taste in the mouth. Food may collect in the affected side of the mouth, making chewing and swallowing more difficult. Teach the client to be cognizant that food is in the mouth and to use the tongue to catch the food and move it to the back of the mouth. Sometimes a mirror is helpful by letting the client see where the tongue is in relation to the rest of the mouth and to see where food has pocketed. Clients who have problems with overproduction of saliva can be helped by teaching them to use their tongue in the same manner to catch saliva and move it back to swallow.

Semi-solid foods that are moist and form a bolus easily are the easiest for the dysphagic client to swallow. Commercially prepared baby foods and pureed solids are nutritious and easily swallowed. Liquids are more difficult to control and tend to run out of the corners of the mouth. If the client has difficulty swallowing fluids, a fluid-filled straw placed in the mouth will allow him to swallow small, controlled amounts of liquid.

Speech therapists and occupational therapists are usually consulted in the hospital before the client comes home. Speech therapy assists the dysphagic client with muscle strengthening exercises and teaches him how to swallow. Assistive devices such as mugs or plate guards are prescribed for the hemiparetic client by the occupational therapist. Once in the home, it may be necessary for the home health nurse to continue consultation with speech and occupational therapists. Generally, a program of two to three visits per week for 1 to 2 months is ordered.

When oral feedings cannot be taken safely, nasogastric feedings, or a gastrostomy for long-term gastric feedings may be necessary. Commercially prepared feedings or blenderized food may be given. A detailed discussion of nasogastric feedings can be found in Chapter 11.

Outcomes

The client will not aspirate or choke, will maintain body weight, and will demonstrate the ability to swallow oral secretions, food, and fluid.

ALTERATION IN URINARY ELIMINATION

Alterations in urinary function are frequently experienced by clients with stroke. Urinary incontinence is a continuing problem for 20% of clients after 6 months following stroke, and 50% of clients in the nursing home 1 year following stroke (Rottkamp 1985). Factors found to be significant when urinary incontinence was present are age 65 years and older; presence of an acute illness besides stroke; hemiplegia; lethargy or somnolence; speech dysfunction; inability to follow directions; dependence in bathing and feeding; inability to walk with or without assistance (Adams and associates 1966). Rottkamp (1985) also suggests that psychological factors such as depression, anxiety, comfort/discomfort; urological factors such as 24-hour pattern of urination; urinary tract infection; fluid intake; bladder/sphincter dysfunction; urine constituents; and anticholinergic drugs; and environmental factors such as the urination control methods employed are signifi-

cant factors associated with urinary dysfunction.

Assessment

Assessment of the incontinent client's urinary pattern begins with discussing voiding habits prior to the CVA, including frequency, hesitancy of starting a stream, nocturia, dribbling, and previous urinary tract infections. Assess the client's current voiding pattern, including the same parameters. The factors described in the previous paragraph should also be included in the assessment. Evaluate the client's and family's reaction to urinary incontinence.

Interventions

Establish a toileting regimen based on the client's level of alertness, fluid intake, and bladder capacity. A flow sheet can be helpful in determining a pattern by monitoring fluid intake, times and amount voided, any incontinence, and an estimate of the amount. The family will be able to provide the home health nurse with this information.

Techniques to stimulate the voiding reflex may be necessary (see Chapter 14). Encourage the family to restrict the client's fluids after the evening meal to prevent nighttime incontinence. Drug therapy may be necessary at times to decrease involuntary bladder emptying. Incontinence briefs and male incontinence systems may be beneficial to promote self-confidence.

Outcome

The client will experience a normal pattern of elimination without incontinence.

ALTERATION IN PATTERN OF BOWEL ELIMINATION

Constipation and incontinence are problems frequently encountered by the client. Factors that influence these two problems include immobility, loss of muscle strength leading to retention, inability to respond to the urge to defecate, inability to communicate the need to defecate, and changes in routine and nutritional habits.

Assessment

Discussing previous bowel habits with the client will help the nurse determine what was normal for the client. Specifically, the nurse should assess whether the client used different aids for defecation and the frequency of bowel evacuation.

Since a cerebrovascular accident can interfere with a client's ability to perceive the need to evacuate the colon, this is an area the nurse will assess. Assess the client's ability to move and manipulate his clothing. Eating habits such as amount of fluids and roughage ingested and swallowing ability are evaluated. Assess whether the presence of aphasia impedes the client's ability to communicate the need to toilet.

Auscultate bowel sounds on each visit. Infrequent, low-pitched sounds may indicate constipation. Palpate the abdomen to detect any hard-formed stool indicating impaction. A mass in the lower left quadrant and frequent loose stools may mean impaction. Question the family about the consistency of the stool.

The family and client can be instructed to keep accurate stool records. This type of information will form the basis of the interventions.

Interventions

The stool regimen is based on the client's previous toileting habits since changes in routine can interfere with an established bowel schedule. The client's diet may need revision to include additional roughage and

fluids to stimulate colonic movement and prevent drying and slowing of feces. A warm drink such as coffee or prune juice in the morning stimulates the gastrocolic reflex. Activity during the day will also be beneficial. Glycerine suppositories or stool softeners are sometimes needed to maintain a regular stooling routine. Additional interventions can be found in Chapter 14.

Outcome

The client will maintain the usual pattern of bowel elimination.

POTENTIAL FOR INJURY

Limited mobility due to hemiplegia or hemiparesis, or sensory–perceptual alterations such as homonymous hemianopsia, loss of sense of pain and temperature, hemineglect, agnosia and apraxia can predispose the client to injury.

Assessment

There are two areas of concern for the home health nurse to assess: the client and the living environment. Both visual and sensory activity are important for safety. Visual acuity and visual fields are tested for deficits. The primary sensory examination should include testing pain, light touch, and position sense. Assess for hemineglect and agnosia. Evaluate the client's muscle strength and endurance, observe for involuntary movements.

On each visit, the home health nurse will want to assess the home environment for potential dangers. Assess the client's environment, especially the bedroom, bathroom, kitchen, stairways and doorways. Observe for placement of furniture, locks on doors, storage of medications, handgrips in the tub or shower or next to the commode, skidproof shower, rugs that will not slip, and obstacles such as toys or stools. Shower chairs and commodes should be equipped with brakes.

Interventions

Encourage the family to keep the environment as litter-free as possible. Remove excess furniture, and place objects within sight if the client is visually impaired. Teach the client how to compensate for defects in the visual fields. Encourage the family never to leave the client alone in the shower or bathtub, and always test the water temperature before the client enters the tub or shower. Also teach the client the importance of using a part of the body with intact sensation to test the temperature of the water. Stress the importance of never leaving the client unattended in a chair or commode if the client is unable to sit correctly, because of hemiplegia or paresis. If the client with a perceptual deficit is ambulatory, precautions may be needed to ensure that he does not wander away. Keeping the screens shut, doors locked, and outside gate (if applicable) locked will help prevent this from happening. Conduct client and family education about potential hazards and safety precautions.

Outcome

The client will not experience any falls or trauma.

ALTERATION IN FAMILY PROCESSES

The impact of stroke on the family can be overwhelming. Changes occur in family roles and in family members' ability to function. Sometimes families are unable to communicate effectively or express feelings with one another. Physical and emotional needs may not be met by the client or any other member. Overprotection or overcommitment may also interfere with family processes.

Assessment

Assess the family dynamics, coping strategies, knowledge of stroke and their attitudes toward each other. Chapter 3 offers more detail on assessment of family.

Interventions

Create a supportive environment for the family. Family counseling may support its efforts to cope. Educate the family about the sick role, stroke, deficits the client may have, and how to care for the client. Include family members in the care of the client, and teach them to let the client be as self-sufficient as possible. Encourage the family to divide duties at home so that one member does not provide all of the care. Prepare the family for periods of depression and overdependence by the client. Stroke clubs can provide support for both the family and the client. Publications written in lay terminology should be made available. Examples of these publications are listed at the end of this chapter.

Outcome

The family demonstrates the ability to function as a cohesive group.

POTENTIAL SEXUAL DYSFUNCTION

Sexual dysfunction encountered during rehabilitation is frequently a result of sensory–perceptual changes. Loss of self-esteem, changes in perception of the relationship between partners, sensory loss, visual deficits, and impaired ability to communicate can impair sexual functioning. Neurological deficits such as hemiparesis, hemiplegia, and urinary incontinence can also inhibit sexual relations.

Assessment

Sexuality is often a difficult subject for both client and partner to discuss, especially if a sexual problem is present. The nurse may need to anticipate this, and over time present the topic for discussion. This will allow the couple the opportunity to discuss any difficulties in a nonthreatening, clinical manner.

Interventions

Alternate methods of sexual play can be suggested by the nurse. Educate the partner as to where the client has intact sensation and to approach him from the side he can see if visually impaired. Aphasia interferes with communication between partners. They should establish other ways to communicate by both verbal or nonverbal cues. Muscle weakness and fatigability can impede sexual sharing. Experimenting with side-lying and supine positions will help the couple find a comfortable way to lie during coitus. If urinary incontinence is a problem, suggest that the client empty his bladder beforehand, or lie on top of a towel or disposable diaper.

If the couple is unable to establish a mutually satisfying sexual relationship, a referral to a specially trained counselor or urologist may be needed.

Outcome

Client and partner will experience a satisfying sexual relationship.

INEFFECTIVE INDIVIDUAL COPING

Fear of another stroke and depression about the status of physical condition contribute to the client's emotional reaction to a cerebral vascular accident. The interaction between brain pathology and emotional reaction is dependent upon premorbid personality; the direct consequences of the lesion itself; the manner in which the individual reacts to illness; and deficits (Goldstein and Ruthaven 1983). After damage to the brain occurs, many people develop exaggerated forms of their previous personality. Persons with an external locus of control may experience a high degree of helplessness and powerlessness as a result of their stroke. Certain types of lesions in certain parts of the brain also have implications for the individual's affective life (Goldstein and Ruthaven 1983). Some drugs may also produce depression, such as drugs to treat hypertension.

Assessment

Assess the effectiveness of the client's past coping skills. Observe his current behavior, noting strengths and weaknesses in reference to coping. Assess for the signs and symptoms of ineffective coping such as sleep disturbances, fatigue, difficulty in concentrating, and communication of feelings of inability to cope.

Interventions

Interventions such as letting the client make choices and allowing the client extended exposure to his successes help him overcome feelings of powerlessness and hopelessness and enhance self-esteem. Set goals with the client and encourage him along the way. Praise him when a goal is attained. The nurse should also be available to the client to listen and support him, keeping communication open at all times. The outcome of acceptance of the reality of the stroke and willingness to work to improve deficits are among the goals that can be mutually set.

Sometimes poststroke depression is so intense that it requires the attention of highly skilled mental health personnel. Referrals should be made without reservation.

Outcome

The client will demonstrate effective use of coping skills.

GUILLAIN–BARRÉ SYNDROME

Guillain–Barré syndrome is an acute, rapidly developing ascending or descending polyneuropathy of the peripheral nervous system. It is a relatively uncommon disease resulting in inflammation and demyelinization of the peripheral nerves.

The disease was first reported by Landry in 1859, as an acute, ascending, predominantly motor paralysis with respiratory failure and death. The syndrome is referred to by other names including postinfectious polyneuritis, acute polyradiculitis, inflammatory polyradiculoneuropathy and Landry–Guillain–Barré–Strohl syndrome. The etiology of the disease is unknown but has been linked to cell-mediated autoimmune origin. A theory of viral causation is also under investigation. Approximately 60% of the patients with the disease have reported mild afebrile respiratory or gastrointestinal symptoms 1 to 3 weeks prior to the onset of the syndrome. Other events that may precede Guillain–Barré include surgical procedures, influenza vaccination, or Hodgkins disease.

The Guillain–Barré syndrome affects 1.4 to 1.9 per 100,000 population (Kenner 1985). Both males and females are affected with a slightly higher percentage of men recognized. All races and ages are affected but onset is usually in the young to middle adult years. Seasonal clustering in the fall was reported by Dowling (1977), but it also appears that winter is a high incidence time. Guillain–Barré syndrome is reversible with 75% to 85% of patients experiencing complete functional recovery. The remaining individuals have some degree of permanent deficit. Expert nursing care during the acute and rehabilitative stages of the disease will decrease the possibility of permanent disability.

ANATOMY AND PHYSIOLOGY OF PERIPHERAL NERVES

The peripheral nervous system is one subsystem of the central nervous system. Peripheral nerves can be sensory, motor, or mixed with the majority being the latter. Since peripheral nerves branch repeatedly and travel to all parts of the body and organs, they are most vulnerable to attack in Guillain–Barré syndrome. A peripheral nerve consists of an axon, its perineural sheath, and the myelin sheath. The nerves covered by a myelin sheath have a white lipid coating produced by Schwann cells. Indentations occurring at 1 millimeter intervals are called *nodes of Ranvier*. The myelin and nodes allow rapid transmission of the impulse to occur, resulting in a "jump" from gap to gap; rather than a continuous transmission along the axon. Those smaller axons that do not have myelin sheaths or a thin coating conduct impulses more slowly than those with myelin sheaths (Figure 13-2).

A cross section of the spinal cord with its motor neuron and sensory neuron originating from the ventral horn and dorsal horn respectively illustrates the reflex arc of the cord. A signal is transmitted from the receptor site (skin) to the cord and out to the muscles for action (Figure 13-3*A*).

PATHOPHYSIOLOGY

The main pathologic event in Guillain–Barré syndrome is a diffuse inflammatory response occurring in the long peripheral nerves. This inflammatory response may be triggered after incubation of 5 to 21 days following a mild viral infection or other idiopathic event.

During the inflammatory response, lymphocytes and macrophages begin to phagocytize the myelin sheath at the nodes of Ranvier. Slowly the nodes widen, with edema

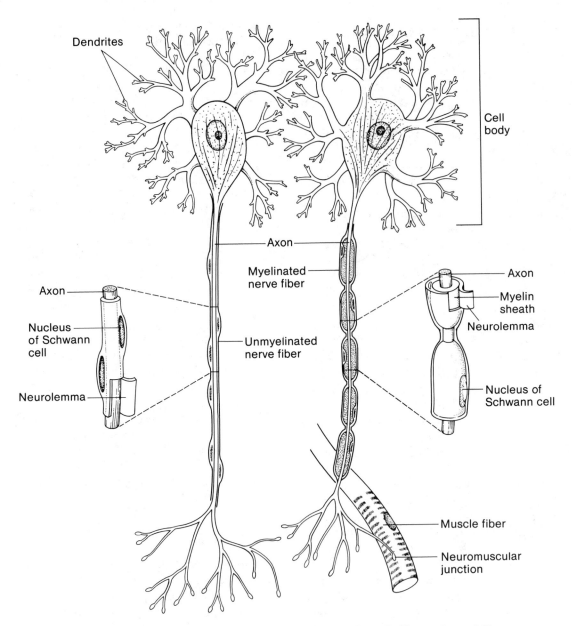

Figure 13-2. Typical efferent neurons: unmyelinated fiber (left), myelinated fiber (right). (From Chaffee EE, Lytle M: Basic Physiology and Anatomy. Philadelphia, JB Lippincott, 1980)

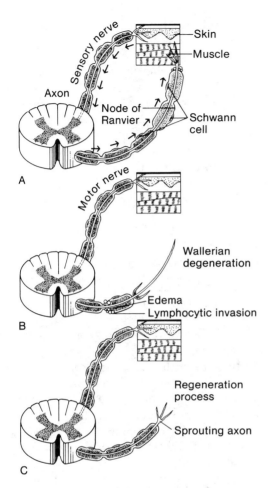

A

B

C

Figure 13-3. Pathophysiological changes in Guillain–Barré syndrome. Cross-section of reflex arc. (*A*) Normal anatomy and physiology of a motor nerve and sensory neuron. (*B*) Wallerian degeneration—injury to myelin sheath. (*C*) Regeneration process of axon. (From Kenner CV, Guzzetta CE, Dossey BM: Critical Care Nursing: Body, Mind, and Spirit, p. 730. Boston, Little, Brown & Co, 1985.

forming at the site of injury. As the inflammatory response progresses, degeneration of the axon occurs (Wallerian degeneration, Figure 13-3*B*). The degenerative process continues, affecting the heavily myelinated peripheral

motor nerves. The more thinly myelinated sensory nerves for pain, touch, and temperature are affected later by this same process. As the disease progresses, inflammation and consequential destruction of the more heavily myelinated cranial nerves such as the oculomotor, facial, glossopharyngeal, vagus, sensory accessory, and hypoglossal nerves has been reported. Finally, inflammation in the anterior horn cells of the spinal cord can develop.

Regeneration of the myelin sheath and repair of the peripheral nerve is a slow process in recovery from Guillain–Barré syndrome (Figure 13-3*C*). In some cases, secondary injury to the axon causes damage, leaving the patient with permanent neurological deficit. This deficit, occurring in 25% of the cases, presents itself with residual weakness, generally in the distal muscles of the lower extremities.

Clinical Progression

Major clinical manifestations of the disease vary and may be mild to severe. Characteristically, the initial neurologic symptoms are paresthesia (numbness and tingling) and muscle weakness of the lower extremities, which progresses to upper extremities, trunk, and facial area. Often these symptoms appear in "stocking and glove" fashion and, initially, rest may relieve the symptoms. The onset of symptoms follows approximately 12 to 14 days after a mild viral infection.

The symptoms progress rapidly (1 to 7 days) bilaterally into flaccid paralysis of lower motor neurons with no atrophy of muscles. Although ascending paralysis is usual, descending progression beginning with the cranial nerves has been noted. (Mills 1980). Sensory loss occurs less frequently and is less severe than motor loss. Sensory disturbances affecting the perception of cutaneous stimuli, vibration sense, and joint position are common. Pain is often experienced by the patient in varying degrees but often described as "pins and needles" progressing to cramping and frank pain in arms, legs, and buttocks.

As the paralysis ascends, respiratory involvement occurs when the intercostal muscles become weakened. Twenty percent of patients have respiratory involvement that has proved to be the indicator of severity of the illness. Death from respiratory insufficiency can result.

Cranial nerve involvement is characteristic of 75% of clients with Guillain–Barré syndrome. The facial nerve (VII) is the most affected, resulting in facial paralysis, such as inability to smile, frown, and drink through a straw, as well as loss of taste and sensation from the anterior two thirds of the tongue. Other cranial nerves less often affected are the glossopharyngeal (IX), vagus (X), spinal accessory (XI), and the hypoglossal (XII). Dysphagia and laryngeal paralysis will occur if nerves IX and X are affected. Involvement of the vagus (X) nerve is thought to cause autonomic dysfunction characterized by hypotension, hypertension, and sinus tachycardia. Hyper- and hypotensive crisis has been reported in the acute phase with dysrhythmias leading to cardiac arrest. Urinary retention and constipation can result during the first few days of the disease but long-term catheterization is often not required.

Diagnosis is usually based on the clinical manifestations and the course of the illness. Stages of the illness follow a distinct pattern with some variations. Stages are

1. Acute onset (Hours to 10 days) with a rapid development of weakness and paralysis
2. Involvement of both proximal and distal limbs and absent muscle atrophy
3. Static phase (days to several months) characterized by no further progression of paralysis and diminishing pain and sensory loss

4. Rehabilitative phase characterized by reappearance of muscle strength

Laboratory findings include albuminocytologic dissociation characterized by increases in cerebrospinal fluid (CSF) protein without an increase in cell count; moderate leukocytosis in the peripheral blood early in the illness; and a decrease in nerve conduction velocities and myopathy as demonstrated with nerve conduction velocity (NCV) studies and electromyelogram (EMG) wave patterns, respectively.

NURSING DIAGNOSES

The essence of nursing care centers on supportive measures. During the acute phase the patient will be hospitalized. As the patient stabilizes, weeks to months of meticulous nursing care based on multiple diagnoses will prevent further compromise and ensure full recovery from Guillain–Barré. Most of what has been written about this syndrome reflects the care needed in the acute care setting or in the rehabilitation setting. However, the static phase requires as much attention and concern.

INEFFECTIVE BREATHING PATTERNS

During the acute phase (1 to 4 days after onset) respiratory involvement may appear. The intercostal muscles and the phrenic nerves are affected by demyelinization. Shallow and irregular respirations leading to inadequate gas exchange are common. The vagus nerve involvement cause the bronchi to lose the ability to dilate and constrict alternately. Spasm occurs, allowing constant dilatation with loss of the protective mechanism of constriction in the presence of a foreign body. The patient's decreased mobility also contributes to the respiratory insufficiency. Pulmonary support with respiratory ventilation and elective tracheostomy may be indicated if the vital capacity falls below 50% of normal.

Once discharged home, it is possible that the client will continue to require support from mechanical ventilation. For a complete discussion of the nursing care involved in this therapy, see Chapter 9.

More likely, however, the client will be discharged to home without mechanical ventilation. Should this be the case, the home health nurse's top priority will be to work with the family to maintain constant monitoring of the respiratory status.

Assessment

There are two important aspects to assess in the homebound client with Guillain–Barré syndrome. One aspect involves the need for assessment of the family and the other aspect involves the home health nurse's assessment of the individual client.

Since the family will be with the client daily, they will need to be taught the various components of a respiratory assessment. Because of the weakness of respiratory muscles caused by the disease process, the family should be taught to monitor the client for signs of increasing respiratory muscle weakness. For example, signs such as a weakened cough, increased respiratory rate, increased pulse, and any change in client's color can be considered as possible signs of respiratory distress. The family should be taught to notify the home health nurse and/or physician immediately if these signs are noted.

On each visit to the home, the home health nurse should perform a detailed assessment of the respiratory system. Parameters to include are respiratory rate, presence of gag, cough and swallow reflexes, breath sounds, skin color, nailbeds. The nurse will want to ask the family for an evaluation of the client's respiratory status, including specific aspects such as certain times of the day when the client seems more fatigued and times

when the client experiences difficulty in respiratory control.

Interventions

The family is the major provider of care for the client. In addition to monitoring the client's respiratory status, the family will need instruction concerning the possible mechanisms for maintaining a patent airway.

Supplemental oxygen may be needed. The presence of this equipment in the home setting is a safety hazard. Consequently, the family will require directions and support in the care of this equipment.

If feasible, teach the family to help the client cough and deep breathe every 2 hours. It may also be necessary to gently remove secretions through suctioning. Positioning changes should be accomplished on this time schedule as well, to prevent atelectasis. If the client has difficulty in mobilizing secretions, it may be necessary to perform chest physical therapy and postural drainage. These techniques are described in Chapter 9.

Outcomes

The client will maintain a patent airway, and an adequate breathing pattern.

SENSORY–PERCEPTUAL ALTERATION

Peripheral sensory nerves are affected by Guillain–Barré syndrome to varying degrees. Vibration, position sense, and deep pain sensation are usually affected. Frequently, clients experience a burning sensation of the skin. Cranial nerve involvement may decrease the sense of taste and present swallowing difficulty.

Assessment

The home health nurse will periodically want to assess the deep tendon, plantar, and abdominal reflexes. Generally, as the client is recovering, this assessment will reveal diminished deep tendon reflexes with absence of plantar and abdominal reflexes. Periodic assessment of sensation and position sense will reveal progression or remittance of sensory symptoms. The family can assist in the assessment by monitoring the client's ability to swallow. The family can also offer information concerning the client's perception of pain.

Interventions

Teach the family to handle the client's extremities gently since grabbing may cause extreme pain. Inform family members that the client's muscles are so sensitive that even the pressure of linen on them is extremely painful. Reinforce the need to turn the client frequently, since the ability to sense pressure on an area of skin is diminished. Always teach client and family the dangers of placing hot objects near denervated areas of the body, since injury can result. Many clients experience a burning sensation of the skin due to the perceptual changes. This can be relieved by a fan or by placing a cool, refrigerated cloth on the extremity. The client will probably also want to wear the smallest amount of clothing possible. For example, a very light cotton shirt may be the most clothing he is able to tolerate. Finally, assist the family to monitor the client for aspiration of foods and fluids that may occur due to cranial nerve involvement.

Outcome

The client will not experience complications from the alterations in sensory–perceptual function.

ANXIETY

The rapid onset of grave symptoms with total dependence on the care-giver initiates high levels of anxiety and stress in the client with Guillain–Barré syndrome. Anxiety is related to helplessness, decreased ability to communicate, and hopelessness of the totally dependent state. Many patients fear permanent paralysis with fear of financial crisis due to lost occupation.

The transfer from hospital to home can cause tremendous anxiety on the part of the client and family. While hospitalized, the client has most likely been cared for in an intensive care unit, where he received one-on-one attention and care. Once transferred out of the critical care unit, the client was still monitored very closely. With that amount of supervision while hospitalized, the thought of returning home without constant supervision from health care professionals may provoke some anxiety.

Family members may also experience anxiety as they consider the amount of responsibility they have in caring for the client at home. They may also feel overwhelmed by the amount of information given to them.

Assessment

Assessment for stress and anxiety reactions should include talking to the client/family to determine the level of their anxiety and fear; observing body language, such as facial expressions; analyzing acting out behavior; and determining the level of denial.

During the initial visit to the home, the nurse will want to evaluate the client's and the family's understanding of the disease, the care required, and their responsibilities. Many home health nurses may find it helpful to visit with the client and family prior to discharge from the hospital. In this way, a relationship can be established and perhaps some of the inevitable anxiety will be diminished.

Interventions

Interventions can help the client reduce anxiety and stress while gaining more independence. The nurse should develop a rapport with the client and family that fosters open verbalization of feelings. The client/family need knowledge of the normal progression of the disease.

When the client goes home, anxiety about procedures can be reduced through instruction and skill practice. After the home health nurse has identified the specific reasons for anxiety, it is important to deal with each of the issues. For example, if family members are anxious because they are afraid of what may happen during an emergency, make sure that they have all of the information needed and availability of needed resources. In the initial stages after discharge, the home health nurse may need to visit the client and family several times a week. Once several weeks have passed, they should begin to feel in control to a greater degree. If the feelings of anxiety continue, teach relaxation exercises to the client and family.

Outcomes

Client's and family's behavior demonstrate decreased anxiety. They are able to effectively communicate their feelings.

ALTERATION IN COMFORT: PAIN

Sensations of pain ranging from tingling and burning to deep muscle pain described by clients as "cramping" and "throbbing" have been reported in Guillain–Barré syndrome. This pain results from degenerating sensory nerves and irritated nerve endings at the myoneural junction.

Assessment

The nurse should periodically question the client about the location, duration, and quality of the pain sensation. Body language such as frequent repositioning and tensed facial expression are often exhibited during pain.

Change in mood may also indicate change in pain quality.

Interventions

Frequent change in position or use of pillows to support body parts may relieve cramping. Range of motion exercise can change the character of pain sensation. Providing the client with distractions such as radio and television or hobbies can help to decrease awareness of pain.

Analgesic therapy may be needed to relieve pain, particularly during the acute and static phases. Generally, non-narcotic analgesics are effective.

Outcomes

The client will maintain a comfort level and experience minimal pain.

ALTERATION IN TISSUE PERFUSION

Alteration in tissue perfusion in the client with Gullain–Barré syndrome occurs because of degeneration of the vagus nerve. This degeneration causes vasomotor instability, including cardiac dysrhythmias, and hypertensive crises. Another common vasomotor change is hypotension, due to interruption of the reflex arcs that control circulation.

Assessment

Frequent assessment of vital signs is essential. The family can assess vital signs particularly when the client's position is changed. Instruct the family to monitor for hypotension, hypertension, tachycardia or bradycardia, and diaphoresis. On each visit, the home health nurse may wish to assess the client's response to position change in a similar way.

Interventions

Interventions will be directed toward maintaining safety for the client. Reinforce with the family the importance of the client wearing Ace bandages or antithromboembolic stockings that are beneficial in alleviating hypotension. Instruct the family to change the client's position slowly to decrease the possibility of hypotension. The family should also be encouraged to monitor the client for pulse, blood pressure, facial flushing, and diaphoresis as indications of autonomic dysfunction. The family can be instructed to check the blood pressure with a regular cuff.

Outcome

The client will experience no complications from the alterations in tissue perfusion or vasomotor instability.

IMPAIRED PHYSICAL MOBILITY

The Guillain–Barré syndrome causes muscle weakness leading to paralysis and sensory deficits. Once discharged to home, the client will continue to experience these changes in physical mobility.

The impaired physical mobility will be accompanied by other complications, including potential skin breakdown and the presence or urinary calculi. Skin breakdown is discussed separately. Urinary calculi may be formed, due to the breakdown of bone and the resulting release of calcium.

Assessment

On each visit, the home health nurse will assess muscle tone and strength as described in Chapter 14. Frequent observation of joints for deformity such as footdrop or wrist drop is essential.

The nurse will also want to ask the family if they have noted any change in the client's urine, specifically the presence of sedimentation. If a calculus has formed, the client may experience pain, urinary frequency, urgency, and, possibly, a fever.

Interventions

Prevention of complications of immobility can be accomplished by adherence to a strict plan of intervention. If the client is bedridden, turning every 2 hours is necessary. As soon as possible, the family should be taught to assist the client into a chair.

Contractures can be prevented by use of passive and active range of motion exercises. Active range of motion is performed on all areas that the client can mobilize. This will strengthen muscles and provide the feeling of accomplishment of a task. Proper alignment of limbs is accomplished with the use of trocanter rolls and foot boards.

Interventions to prevent formation of renal calculi will include forcing fluids such as cranberry juice up to 2000 cc/day providing the patient has an intact swallowing reflex; observing the urine for color, amount, and consistency; and instructing the patient and or family to report signs of flank pain. Mobilization of joints through active and passive range of motion will lessen likelihood of bone breakdown with release of calcium that could form renal calculi.

Outcome

The client will be free from the complications of alteration in physical mobility.

SELF-CARE DEFICIT

Clients with Guillain–Barré syndrome will be unable to perform activities of daily living, particularly in the acute and static phases of their condition. Many of these activities will be completed by the family. The client may not have the muscle control needed to accomplish these normal activities. Cranial nerve involvement may lead to difficulty in swallowing and chewing.

Assessment

On a periodic basis, the home health nurse will want to assess for the factors needed to complete activities of daily living. These include motor strength and cranial nerve involvement. The family will be able to offer information concerning the client's ability to complete normal activities of daily living.

The nurse will also want to assess the cough and gag reflex periodically. As cranial nerve function returns, these reflexes will improve.

Interventions

Until the client regains motor strength, the family's assistance will be needed for completion of self-care activities. The nurse must instruct the family and client in skills needed to enhance self-care in all areas such as feeding, bathing, and toileting.

Since the client's swallowing reflex may be impaired, foods that can be easily swallowed should be provided. Small, frequent meals will decrease fatigue. Emergency procedures for choking should be taught to all family members. Assistive feeding devices can be obtained, such as utensils with built-up handles for easier grasp.

The family will need instruction on bathing the client. Instruct the family that during the bath, skin integrity should be assessed and special attention paid to reddened areas. Since sensation of heat or cold is decreased, assessed and special attention paid to reddened areas. Since sensation of heat or cold is decreased, bath water temperature should be warm, not hot, to prevent burns. The family

should encourage the client to participate as much as possible.

During the acute phase, urinary retention may occur, necessitating the use of a Foley catheter, but rarely is this for more than a few days. Urinary sphincter control is usually present during most stages. Fluid intake should be increased to promote urination and prevent infection.

Bowel elimination is also of importance in proper digestive functioning and may be compromised by immobility and loss of self-care. If problems occur, stool softeners may be prescribed. Sphincter control remains intact. Incorporating fibrous foods in the diet and liquids when the swallowing reflex returns will help to prevent bowel complications.

Maintaining as much self-care as possible in the Guillain–Barré patient will increase positive self-regard and enhance rehabilitation.

Outcome

The client will be able to participate in self-care activities within the physical limitations imposed by the Guillain–Barré syndrome.

INEFFECTIVE FAMILY COPING

Often, the onset of Guillain–Barré syndrome is rapid and symptoms are of a considerable magnitude. The client and family experience fear and anxiety from a lack of knowledge of the disease, its progression, and prognosis. Although the client is alert, with vision and hearing intact, the ability to communicate verbally is often impaired. Consequently, the ability to cope with the situation is compromised.

Assessment

The clients and family coping style can be assessed by determination of previous problem-solving techniques. A major part of the assessment will be to determine the client's and family's expectations for recovery.

Interventions

On each visit, encourage expression of feelings and anger by both the client and family. While at home, encourage the family to include the client in social activities and meals whenever possible. Routine visits by the home health nurse and social worker can support family coping style.

Outcomes

The client and family will articulate their feelings and concern. They will also demonstrate utilization of successful coping styles.

ALTERATION IN SKIN INTEGRITY

During the static and rehabilitation stages of the syndrome, the client will continue to be confined to the bed, wheelchair, or chair. For that reason, there is a continued concern with maintenance of skin integrity.

Assessment

On each visit, the home health nurse should assess the skin for areas of redness or breakdown. Areas of skin over the bony prominences should be carefully evaluated. Adequate nutrition is also important in preserving skin integrity. An assessment of nutrition status is needed. A more detailed discussion can be found in Chapter 16.

Interventions

The major interventions include turning, careful positioning, and maintenance of nutritional status. See Chapter 16.

Outcome

The client will maintain skin integrity.

KNOWLEDGE DEFICIT

Guillain–Barré syndrome is a long-term problem and, as such, presents the client and family with many challenges. The home health nurse provides invaluable support to them as they live through the many stages of the disease. One of the major responsibilities of the nurse is to provide the family and client with the information needed to make appropriate decisions.

Assessment

On each visit, assess the family and client for changing needs for information. For example, on one visit, they may only need information concerning the care and the next visit, want information about the future and prognosis for the client.

Interventions

Teach the family and client aspects of the care already described. Make certain the family is aware of the many safety concerns in the care of the client. Assist the family in its understanding of the therapies and their implementation. The family and client should have a good understanding of any drugs used in the care of the client.

Outcome

The client and family should verbalize an understanding of the disease, its treatment, and prognosis.

SEIZURES

The word "epilepsy" is of Greek origin meaning *to be seized by a force from without.* It has been called *falling sickness, fit, convulsion* and *seizure.* Epilepsy is a chronic syndrome denoting a tendency to recurrent seizures. A seizure is a sudden, violent involuntary contraction of a group of muscles that may be paroxysmal and episodic. A seizure represents a symptom of a transitory disturbance in brain function.

This cerebral dysfunction was first described by John Hughlings Jackson (1835–1911) as occasional sudden, excessive, rapid, and focal discharges of gray matter in the brain (Barry 1983). Epilepsy, seizure disorder, convulsion, and seizure will be used interchangeably in this chapter. Seizure disorder has become a more common term since the word "epilepsy" has negative connotations in today's society.

Approximately 1% of the population (2–4 million) in the United States suffer from seizure disorders, many of whom are children. Of all persons with seizures, 25% have recurrent seizures while on medications, 10% are institutionalized, and 5% are home-bound invalids. The annual cost of the problem in the United States is $3 billion.

The etiology of the seizure disorder is usually a physical or chemical stressor creating a lower neuronal threshold for diffuse brain activity. Any untoward group of stimuli can cause seizure activity in most normal people.

Seizure disorders can either be acquired or idiopathic. Acquired seizures are often caused by cerebral trauma, lesions, or biochemical means. Cerebral lesions account for a large category of seizures. Included in this group are neoplasms of the brain; infectious diseases such as meningitis; cerebral circulatory disturbances such as stroke, hypertension, and vasospasm; and trauma as related to head injury, contusion, or birth injury (anoxia). Biochemical inducement of seizures is caused by alcohol, electrolyte imbalance, drug overdose, vitamin deficiency, and metabolic disorders such as diabetes mellitus. Post-traumatic epilepsy can follow head injury at any time but onset is most common between 6 months and 2 years post-trauma.

The above conditions and diseases are not inclusive of all etiologies of seizure disorders. Any condition that causes cerebral irritation through injury or chemical means can precipitate neuronal discharge (Hickey 1985).

CLASSIFICATION OF SEIZURES

An older classification of seizures included grand mal, petit mal, psychomotor (temporal), and focal motor (Jacksonian). In 1981, the International Commission on Classification reclassified seizures and, due to advanced diagnostic technology, new categories listed in Table 13-3 are now in common use.

The two major categories in this classification are partial and generalized seizures. Partial seizures are broken down into two groups and generalized seizures subdivided into four subgroups.

Partial seizures originate from a localized activation of neurons and involve only a partial area of the brain. Hence, consciousness and memory are not severely impaired. Subcategories include simple partial seizures (Jacksonian–focal) and complex partial seizures (psychomotor). Simple partial seizures generally originate from the motor cortex of the frontal lobe and the irritated site in the brain is opposite the side of the body movement. Complex partial seizures originate in the temporal lobe and are often associated with loss of consciousness. Many sensory experiences precede the seizure, such as illusions, olfactory and gustatory sensations, and dizziness.

Generalized seizures originate from diffuse neurons firing bilaterally. During grand mal seizures, there is a sudden loss of consciousness with tonic convulsions alternating with clonic convulsions. Following the sei-

TABLE 13.3 Characteristics of Seizures

Type of Seizure	Etiology	Characteristics	Clinical Signs	Aura	Postictal Period
Generalized Seizures					
Tonic–clonic (grand mal)	Most common	Generalized (characterized by loss of consciousness for several minutes)	Aura Cry Loss of consciousness The fall Tonic–clonic movements Incontinence	Yes Flashing lights Smells Spots before eyes Dizziness	Yes Need for sleep 1 to 2 hours Headache common
Absence (petit mal)	Usually occur during childhood and adolescence Frequency decreases as child gets older	Sudden impairment in or loss of consciousness with little or no tonic–clonic movement Occur without warning Have tendency to appear a few hours after arising or when person is quiet	Sudden vacant facial expression with eyes focused straight ahead All motor activity ceases except perhaps for slight symmetric twitching about eyelids Possible loss of muscle tone Consciousness returns	No	No
Myoclonic General Tonic–clonic	May antedate by months or years	May be very mild or may have rapid, forceful movements	Sudden involuntary contraction of muscle group, usually in extremities or trunk No loss of consciousness	No	No

Partial Seizures	Atonic	Not common	Peculiar generalized tonelessness	Person falls in flaccid state Unconscious for minute or two	Rarely	No
	Simple partial (Jacksonian-focal)	Occur almost entirely in patients with structural brain disease	Dependent on site of focus May or may not be progressive	Commonly begin in hand, foot, or face	Yes Numbness Tingling Crawling feeling Nausea	Yes
	Complex partial (psychomotor)	Occur at any age	Sudden change in awareness associated with complex distortion of feeling and thinking and partially coordinated motor activity Longer than absence Automatisms	Behaves as if partially conscious Often appears intoxicated May do antisocial things such as exposing self or carrying out violent acts Autonomic complaints may occur Chest pain Respiratory distress Tachycardia Gastrointestinal distress Urinary incontinence	Yes Complex hallucinations or illusions	Yes Confusion Amnesia Need for sleep

Adapted from Phipps WJ et al: Essentials of Medical-Surgical Nursing, 3rd ed, p 809. St Louis, CV Mosby, 1985

zure the patient awakens slowly, is confused, and disoriented. Grand mal seizures usually occur as a single event, but if the patient experiences a second before fully conscious, the term *status epilepticus* applies. This is a medical emergency to be treated with immediate medical management. Absence seizures (petit mal) is the second type of generalized seizure characterized by an abrupt cessation of activity with loss of consciousness lasting no longer than 30 seconds. Children over 4 years of age but not yet adolescent frequently have this type of seizure disorder.

PATHOPHYSIOLOGY

The basic unit of the nervous system is the neuron. Through polarization and depolarization, neurons have the ability to generate an electrical "action potential." This discharge is then passed on to other neurons in the central nervous system or to innervate muscles at the myoneural junction. In the brain the normal neuron fires approximately 200 times per second.

Seizures result from a few abnormally hyperactive and hypersensitive neurons that form a focus. These eliptogenic neurons become excited, causing rapid repetitive depolarization that is often diffuse in nature. This hyperactive stimulus excites other neurons, causing a seizure. During seizures, a neuronal discharge may reach a rate of 1000 firings a second. When the cells in the focus stop firing, the other neurons follow slowly, normal activity returns, and the seizure is over. The tonic phase of the generalized seizure commences when the increased excitation of the neurons spreads to the subcortical, thalamic, and upper brainstem. At this time, consciousness ceases and autonomic system activity occurs, such as salivation, tachycardia, and increased blood pressure.

The clonic phase commences as inhibitory neurons of the anterior thalamus, cortex, and basal ganglia begin to fire, changing the burst of electrical firing to an intermittent quality becoming less and less frequent. The neurons are then "exhausted" (Adams and Victor 1981).

The postictal period is characterized by deep sleep followed by confusion and lethargy. Headache has been reported and temporary aphasia and paresis may occur. Early muscle rigidity is followed by flaccidity.

During the seizure, electroencephalogram (EEG) picks up amplified electrical activity from the neurons. In the normal adult, alpha and beta waves are present with their own characteristic patterns. Abnormal EEG waves seen with seizure disorders include delta and theta waves. EEG tracings are helpful in diagnosis of seizure disorder but not conclusive since 10% of the population who have never experienced a seizure have abnormal waves. Consequently, EEGs must be combined with other information, such as history, to confirm seizure disorder.

Treatment for seizure disorders falls into three categories: removal of precipitating factors, drug therapy, and surgical intervention. If the causative or precipitating factor can be identified, it should be corrected. For example, if a tumor is causing focal seizures, surgery to extract the lesion can be performed. Drug therapy will be discussed under nursing diagnoses. Surgical intervention is indicated in 5% of clients with seizure disorders. Often patients who have not responded to medical management can have enhanced quality of life with surgery. Patients with unilateral focus that will not cause major neurological deficit if extracted are good risks for this treatment.

NURSING DIAGNOSES

The goal of nursing management for clients in the home setting with a seizure disorder will include protecting the client from injury during a seizure, promoting social contact, and providing information. It is unlikely that the home health nurse will see a client only because of a seizure disorder. Generally, the client will be referred because of another medical diagnosis. The major nursing diagnoses for the client with a seizure disorder will be discussed in the following pages.

POTENTIAL FOR INJURY RELATED TO SEIZURE ACTIVITY

A client is at high risk for physical injury during a seizure. The home health nurse plays a vital role in assuring that the client and family understand the potential risks and are equipped to minimize them.

With generalized seizures, when the client loses consciousness, becomes disoriented, and/or suffers decreased sensory–perceptual ability, injury potential is high. Head injury from falling, burns, drowning, and automobile collision are a few examples of possible injury in this population. Often patients have no warning of the seizure; consequently, safety measures cannot be instituted by them, but if the seizure occurs in an environment where family or other trained individuals are present, injury can be averted.

Assessment

Assessment of risk factors including environmental hazards in the home/work setting can be evaluated. Gather information about the client's ability to realize that a seizure is eminent and the ability to institute safety precautions to prevent injury. Life-style and activities of daily function must be assessed for their safety if a seizure occurs. Finally, assess the client's and family's understanding of the necessity for safety measures before and during a seizure.

Interventions

Instruction should be provided to the client concerning safety precautions such as taking showers instead of tub baths, avoiding swimming alone, and similar information. The family members must be instructed in safety precautions to be utilized during a seizure. The family should also be taught the parameters to assess during the seizure. Finally, interventions to reorient the client in the postictal stage are essential. The boxed material below and on page 378 provides pertinent information.

Outcome

The client will be free from injury during and after a seizure.

Procedure: Safety Precautions for Clients With Seizure Disorders

1. Avoid dangerous situations.

- Do not operate dangerous machinery.
- Do not swim alone.
- Do not climb to high or dangerous places.
- Do not drive a car. Many states have restrictions for patients with seizure disorders.

2. Take care of yourself when seizures occur.

- If you have a warning, lie down in a safe place.
- Wear an emergency medical identification band to alert others who are trying to help you.
- Teach others what to do if you have a seizure.

Procedure: Protection of Client During a Seizure

1. Remain calm. This will reassure the client if he has not lost consciousness.

2. Stay with the client to ensure his safety.

3. If client is out of bed, help him to the floor to prevent falling. If in bed, put side rails up or place chairs next to bed so client will not roll out. Pad sides with blanket.

4. If client hasn't clenched teeth, place a soft object or rolled handkerchief between his teeth. Dentures should be removed if possible. Don't force anything between clenched teeth.

5. Remove or loosen client's tight clothing such as scarf, tie, or belt.

6. Turn the client on his side with head back and face slightly downward.

7. Place a pillow or other soft material under the client's head or hold his head in your lap.

8. Don't restrain the client during the seizure. Hands can be gently held to prevent injury from banging. If client is wandering just protect from floor.

9. Keep crowds or spectators away from the client.

10. Reassure and reorient the client if seizure has left him frightened or disoriented.

11. If another attack begins before regaining consciousness, it may signal the onset of status epilepticus. Call a physician or rescue squad. Stay with the client, maintain client airway.

12. If ordered by a physician, give oxygen after the seizure.

Gathering Seizure Information

When you witness—and cope with—a client's seizure, observe him carefully to collect the information needed by the physician. Ask yourself the following questions, and do your best to remember what you saw.

- Exactly what time did the seizure occur?
- What was the client doing just before the seizure, or what were you doing to him?
- How did the seizure develop? Gradually or suddenly? Did he complain of premonitory sensations? What part of his body started moving first? How did the convulsion spread?
- If your client has been taking anticonvulsant drugs, when was his last dose?
- Did your client change his position during the seizure?
- Did he chew, froth at the mouth, or roll his eyes?
- Were his eyes open throughout the seizure? If they were, what did his pupils look like? Did they dilate or constrict? Together or unilaterally?
- What were the client's respirations like?
- What was the color and temperature of his skin?
- Was he incontinent?
- When did he regain consciousness? And how did he act then? Was he alert? Active? Or sleepy? Did he remember anything about the seizure or what preceded it? Did he have any injuries?

Document everything you remember in your nurse's notes. Notify the physician of your findings.

SENSORY – PERCEPTUAL ALTERATION

Clients experiencing seizures may have a sensory–perceptual alteration immediately prior to, during, and following the event. Prior to the seizure, many patients experience an aura that has a sensory sensation such as a ringing in the ears, or smelling an unpleasant odor. This aura is part of the seizure and is postulated to arise from the area of the "discharging" focus. During the seizure, the patient may (depending on type) experience sensory sensations such as olfactory, gustatory, or auditory experiences. Vague visceral sensations and autonomic sensations have been reported. For example, patients have experienced profuse diaphoresis, tachycardia, and "gooseflesh." Postictally, the patient may be stuporous, aphasic, and experience paresis.

Assessment

Presence of an aura should be documented and may lead to a fuller understanding of the seizure event. Instruct the family to observe the client's consciousness level following the seizure. When the client is able, he should be asked to describe sensory sensations.

Interventions

Teach the family other interventions following the seizure, such as reorienting the client to the environment and observing for signs of aphasia, paresis, or paralysis of an extremity. The family should be encouraged to maintain verbal, touch, and eye contact with the client following the seizure to reduce anxiety. Once the seizure has ceased, the family should be encouraged to provide a quiet atmosphere so the client can rest.

Outcome

The client will experience only limited alterations in sensory–perception following the seizure.

SOCIAL ISOLATION

Problems of a social, psychological, and behavioral nature frequently accompany a seizure disorder. Often clients are viewed by others as having a "handicap." Epilepsy imposes feelings of fear, alienation, and depression. The client fears the seizure and the embarrassment following the event. Consequently, many individuals with epilepsy avoid social contact.

Assessment

The home health nurse must assess the client's social situation. On an initial visit, the nurse can pose questions concerning the client's activities and community involvement. Realistic evaluation of the client's ability to carry out social functions is also assessed at this time.

Interventions

Nursing interventions can encourage the client to seek social contact. Often the establishment of a trusting relationship with the home health nurse will provide the basis for further outside contact. Discuss feelings of loneliness and fear of embarrassment with the client, helping him to identify possible social outlets and develop solutions to embarrassing circumstances. Finally, help the client identify support groups such as the Epilepsy Foundation.

Outcome

The client will seek interactions with individuals outside of his home.

POTENTIAL FOR INJURY RELATED TO DRUG THERAPY

Drug therapy can control or reduce seizure activity in many clients with a seizure disorder. Certain drugs are more effective for particular types of seizures. One drug can be utilized, followed by an addition of another if seizure activity continues. Therapeutic levels of drugs must be maintained and monitored. Drug toxicity can occur with many of the medications, as well as side-effects. (See the list displayed below.

Drugs Commonly Used to Treat Seizures

BARBITURATES
Phenobarbital (Luminal)
Mephobarbital (Mebaral)
Metharbital (Gemonil)
Primidone (Mysoline)

HYDANTOINS
Phenytoin; formerly call diphenylhydantoin (Dilantin)
Mephenytoin (Mesantoin)
Ethotoin (Peganone)
Phenacemide (Phenurone)

OXAZOLIDINEDIONES
Trimethadione (Tridione)
Paramethadione (Paradione)

SUCCINIMIDES
Phensuximide (Milontin)
Methusuximide (Celontin)
Ethosuximide (Zarontin)

OTHER
Carbamazepine (Tegretol)
Valproic acid (Depakene)
Diazepam (Valium)
Clonazepam (Clonopin)
Paraldehyde

Assessment

The home health nurse will periodically assess the client for signs of drug toxicity. The major common side-effect from anticonvulsant drugs is blood dyscrasias. The home health nurse should, therefore, assess the client for signs of bone marrow depression such as fever, sores, and bruising.

Other signs of toxicity are cerebellar symptoms including ataxia and tremors. Periodically the home health nurse should perform point-to-point testing and other measures of cerebellar activity. These techniques are described in Chapter 14 under Multiple Sclerosis.

Interventions

The client and family should be taught all of the needed information concerning the drugs. They must understand the goals of therapy, expected effects, and side-effects. They must appreciate the importance of taking the drugs as prescribed. Any side-effects should be reported to the nurse. The home health nurse must then decide whether the physician should be notified for a possible change in regimen.

Outcome

The client will maintain drug regimen and will experience minimal toxic or side-effects.

NONCOMPLIANCE TO DRUG REGIMEN

Noncompliance is defined as *the extent to which a person's behavior deviates from a prescribed health regimen.* Often clients with epilepsy may be noncompliant concerning their medications. In the vast majority of epileptic clients, seizures are controlled by drug therapy. Often the client may not experience a seizure for long periods of time. Consequently, clients feel they no longer need the medication and withdraw from the regimen.

Another factor contributing to noncompliance relates to the side-effects that are a consequence of long-term drug therapy. Side-effects causing undue distress encourage discontinuation of the medication. Unfortunately, discontinuation of medications may also precipitate seizures.

Assessment

The home health nurse must assess the client's and family's knowledge of medication therapy and their ability to adjust to the new health regimen. Follow-up to assess the client's adherence to therapy is essential.

Interventions

Interventions to promote compliance to the individual treatment plan include several factors. The client and family must be taught about the drugs, toxic symptoms, and need for routine evaluation. The home health nurse should allow the client to express any feelings about the diagnosis and medication plan. After the client has been stabilized, it may be useful to refer the client to a support group. The home health nurse can also assist the client to understand the consequences of noncompliance.

Outcome

The client will be compliant with the drug regimen.

THE UNCONSCIOUS CLIENT

"Consciousness is the state of awareness of the self and the environment and coma is its opposite, *i.e.*, the total absence of awareness of self and environment even when the subject is externally stimulated" (Plum and Posner 1982). Conscious behavior requires arousal, or wakefulness, and awareness, or content of cognition and affect. The reticular activating system of the upper brain stem controls arousal. It receives input from somatic and special sensory pathways and serves to activate the cortex. Awareness is a function of the higher level cerebral cortex in addition to the reticular activating system.

Various states of altered consciousness exist between consciousness and coma. Terms such as obtundation, stupor, semicoma and coma are used to describe various levels of consciousness. Definitions of these and other terms used by health care workers to classify altered states of consciousness frequently vary from person to person.

PATHOPHYSIOLOGY

Impairment of consciousness is a symptom of conditions that destroy or widely depress functions of both cerebral hemispheres, the brain stem activating systems, or both. Lesions such as hemorrhage, infarction, neoplasm, abscess, and head injury encroach on vital structures in the brain stem or deep diencephalon. Extrinsic disorders and metabolic dysfunction caused by anoxia or ischemia, hypoglycemia, hepatic encephalopathy, uremia, drugs, and acid–base disruptions can cause alterations in consciousness. Encephalitis, subarachnoid hemorrhage, concussion, and postictal states are examples of intrinsic diffuse dysfunction that can widely depress function of brain structures. The availability of 24-hour nursing care will be needed.

NURSING DIAGNOSES

INEFFECTIVE AIRWAY CLEARANCE

Maintaining a clear airway is of paramount importance when caring for an unconscious client. Airway blockage may occur as a result of many reasons. The client's inability consciously to clear his upper airway is lost, so accumulated mucous secretions or vomitus may be aspirated. Injury and edema of mucous membranes or poor positioning of the client's neck can contribute to an ineffective airway clearance and poor gas exchange. Immobility causes pooling of secretions in the gas exchange airways, thus impeding respiration.

Assessment

Assessment of respiratory function should include observing the client for the ability to breathe, noting chest expansion, muscles used for breathing, changes in respiratory rate and depth, coughing ability and characteristics of sputum. Tachypnea and tachycardia may indicate respiratory distress. Stridor is indicative of upper airway compromise, and may be so loud it is heard without a stethoscope. Cyanosis may be present in the lips, earlobes, nose, and knees and is evidence of inadequate oxygen saturation. Auscultation of all lung fields must be done at least every 8 hours, or more frequently as indicated. Rhonchi or wheezes usually indicate partial obstruction of airway passages by secretions or mucosal swelling. Crackles (rales) are frequently heard with congestive heart failure, pneumonia, and bronchitis.

Interventions

The home health nurse must protect the client from aspiration by assuring proper positioning, preferably with the head elevated, the neck straight, and the client side-lying to facilitate drainage of secretions. Never place the unconscious client on his back, as the tongue may fall back and occlude the pharynx. To promote gas exchange, the client must be turned and repositioned frequently.

Oropharyngeal and tracheal suctioning is used to keep the airway clear of secretions. Preoxygenation with 100% oxygen using a manual resuscitation bag, or the "sigh" control on a ventilator for 1 minute prior to suctioning, and limiting catheter passage to 10 seconds is recommended to prevent hypoxemia and hypercapnia. To facilitate passing the suction catheter in the client without an artificial airway, place the client in the Fowler's position and hyperextend his neck. Gently insert the catheter during inspiration. Before beginning the procedure, explain to the client the purpose of suctioning and what he will feel.

Artificial airways are sometimes indicated in the unconscious client. An oropharyngeal airway may be useful to help protect the airway and facilitate ventilation and suctioning, although complications such as alceration of the hard palate and cleft tongue can occur. A tracheostomy is necessary for the unconscious client requiring prolonged mechanical ventilation. Meticulous care of the tracheostomy will help prevent infection and minimize tracheal damage. Artificial humidification and adequate systemic hydration will be needed to maintain moist mucous membranes. These procedures are discussed in detail in Chapter 9.

Outcomes

Nursing interventions should assist the client in protecting his airway and keeping it clear of mucus and blood. The goal is to maintain adequate aeration of the lungs for gas exchange.

INEFFECTIVE BREATHING PATTERNS

The unconscious client may require supportive oxygen therapy if breathing patterns are inadequate. Conditions that alter the function of the respiratory centers in the brain stem, such as hemorrhage, tumor, or increased intracranial pressure, or injury to the phrenic nerves controlling the diaphragm will cause insufficient respiratory function and a resulting impaired gas exchange.

Assessment

Assessment of the client's respiratory status is performed as described under the heading "Ineffective Airway Clearance."

Interventions

The client diagnosed as having an ineffective breathing pattern will require oxygen by mask or nasal cannula, or may require long-term mechanical ventilation. Care of the mechanically ventilated client is discussed in detail in Chapter 8. Again, positioning and turning the client are done to prevent stasis of secretions, and meticulous care of an artificial airway is recommended to prevent infection and tracheal breakdown.

Outcome

The client will be oxygenated and exhibit an effective breathing pattern.

SENSORY – PERCEPTUAL ALTERATION

Loss of intact integration between the reticular activating system and the cerebral cortex results in the functional loss of arousability and content of consciousness. Consequently, the unconscious client has a very limited ability to respond to environmental stimuli since he is unable to process incoming stimuli.

Assessment

Sensory–perceptual assessment of the unconscious client begins with establishing the level of consciousness (LOC). Arousability is assessed immediately upon entering the client's room. If the client is not awake, call out his name (verbal stimuli). Progress to light touch, light pain, and then more noxious stimuli if the client remains unresponsive. The Glasgow Coma Scale (Table 13-4) is most useful in measuring and grading the neurological responses of the unconscious client. Coma is considered to be a total score of seven or less.

Discretion must be used when applying deep painful stimuli. Pressure on the manubrium rather than rubbing the sternum with knuckles will cause less bruising and produce a noxious stimulus to which the client may localize. Pressure on the nailbed or the Achilles tendon is acceptable for assessing movement and strength, but the client will not be able to localize this stimulus easily. Care must be taken to prevent gouging the client, so the examiner's fingernails must be short. The Glasgow Coma Scale also scores the motor responses to stimulation.

Content of consciousness can be tested only if the client is arousable. Establish orientation by asking questions pertaining to person, place, and time. The client who was unconscious and waking up may not be able to answer these questions. He should be given the appropriate information for future assessments. Assess the client's ability to follow simple commands by directing him to "blink your eyes." "Squeeze my hand." "Let go of my hand," and so forth. The primitive grasp reflex can give false hope to the family. If the client is able to let go upon command, he is more likely following commands.

Verbal response is also assessed to determine level of consciousness. The Glascow Coma Scale is also used to measure the verbal response of clients. Speech requires an intact cerebral hemisphere and cranial nerves V, VII, IX, X, and XII. Speech is assessed as being clear, appropriate, inappropriate, aphasic, incomprehensible sounds, or no response.

TABLE 13.4 Glasgow Coma Scale

Response	Stimulus	Score
Best Eye Opening Response	Opens eyes spontaneously	4
	Opens eyes to speech	3
	Opens eyes to pain	2
	Does not open eyes	1
Best Motor Response	Motor response with verbal command	6
	Responds to localized pain	5
	Moves from examiner in response to localized pain	4
	Decorticate Posturing	3
	Decerebrate Posturing	2
	No Response	1
Best Verbal Response	Carries on conversation	5
	Conversant but confused	4
	Inappropriate words	3
	Incomprehensible sounds	2
	No response	1

From Teasdale G, Jennett B: Assessment of coma and impaired consciousness: A practical scale. Lancet 2: 81–84, 1974

Assessing the sensory cranial nerves in the unconscious client is difficult. Cranial nerve I is not generally assessed. Visual acuity cannot be tested, but the client's reaction to the bright light may be noted. Cranial nerve V, whose sensory component consists of sensation of the face, may be assessed by testing the corneal reflex, although it is not a good idea to test this indiscriminately due to the potential for corneal abrasion. The acoustic nerve (cranial nerve VIII), with hearing and vestibular functions, is assessed by talking to the client and testing Doll's eyes and caloric responses. The unconscious client may not appear to respond to the nurse's voice or to the voice of a family member, due to the depth of coma. Nevertheless, the nurse must encourage the family to continue to speak with the client as a means of providing stimulation for the client. Cranial nerves IX and X are assessed by testing gag and swallow reflexes.

Interventions

Nursing interventions for the sensory–perceptually altered client include stimulating each of the sensory modalities. Stimulation is necessary to prevent sensory deprivation and to elicit the responses the client is capable of making. Stimulation should also be frequent, consistent, brief, and meaningful. Responses to the stimulation are noted, such as turning of the head toward auditory stimuli, or following a moving object with the eyes.

Auditory stimulation should consist of talking with the client, identifying who the care-giver is, what is being done for him, orienting him, encouraging family members to talk to him, reading to him, and playing music he enjoys. Somatosensory stimulation includes baths or showers, washing the face, rubbing the client with lotion or soft cloths, light or deep touch, and brushing the hair. Visually stimulate the client by moving him to different rooms if possible, or elevate the head of the bed to give a different perspective. Show brightly colored pictures or pictures of familiar faces, pull up the shades, and encourage visual tracking with bright objects or lights. Kinesthetic stimulation would include elevating the head of the bed, transferring the client to a chair if tolerated, range of motion exercises, and turning the client. Orally stimulate the client with different tastes, temperatures, and mouth care. Finally, pleasant odors may be used to stimulate olfaction.

Outcomes

Through proper stimulation, the client will be given the opportunity to respond within his limitations. Progression in responses may be monitored, and stimulation exercises may then progress.

ALTERATION IN MOBILITY

Immobility causes problems for all body systems. The respiratory system is affected by decreased chest expansion, decreased respiratory rate, diminished cough and vital capacity, which lead to pneumonia and atelectasis. The heart is required to work harder. Blood pools in extremities, predisposing the client to venous thrombosis. Immobility causes osteoporosis, joint fibrosis, muscle shortening, contractures, and peripheral nerve damage by improper positioning. Negative nitrogen balance contributes to muscular atrophy and skin breakdown. Elimination is affected, resulting in constipation and renal calculi.

The following nursing diagnoses in part reflect the diagnosis of alterations in mobility. The author has chosen to discuss them separately under each respective diagnosis.

ALTERATION IN TISSUE PERFUSION

Immobility causes an increased work load on the heart. Loss of neurovascular tone and voluntary muscle movement result in sluggish blood flow especially through the extremities, causing a pooling effect of the blood. Orthostatic hypotension may result.

Assessment

Check the client's vital signs periodically. The home health nurse will also want to assess other parameters of perfusion, including pulses and skin temperature.

Interventions

To stimulate the neurovascular reflexes, slowly elevate the head of the bed, or sit the client in a chair, if possible. Monitor the client's vital signs, particularly the blood pressure before and while his head is elevated. Turning the client, passive range of motion exercises, and use of thigh-high elastic stockings or bandages will help to minimize the pooling of blood in the extremities.

Outcome

The client will remain normotensive.

POTENTIAL FOR VENOUS THROMBOSIS

The unconscious client is at risk for deep vein thrombosis. Venous stasis occurs when the normally vertical position of the body is recumbent. Venous blood flow depends upon the movement of muscles and the competency of one-way valves. Platelets and red blood cells may collect in pockets next to the valve cusps, interfering with blood flow. The decreased blood flow causes an imbalance between precoagulants and anticoagulants, causing the formation of venous thrombi. Immobility also causes the loss of calcium from bones, causing more formed elements in the blood stream. Dehydration may also be present, compounding the increased hemoconcentration. If a thrombus is large enough, it can impede arterial flow, eventually causing the loss of the limb, or can detach from the vein wall and cause pulmonary embolism or stroke.

Assessment

Assess peripheral pulses frequently, and remove antiembolic stockings at least every 8 hours to assess color, temperature, and tenderness.

Interventions

Nursing interventions are directed at improving circulation and minimizing the risk of deep vein thrombosis. To improve venous flow, elevate the legs 15°, as much as possible, perform passive range of motion exercises, and avoid pressure on the popliteal spaces. Avoid massaging the legs, which could dislodge fragments of a clot. Prevent dehydration of the client.

Outcome

The client will not develop venous thrombosis.

IMPAIRED SKIN INTEGRITY

Skin breakdown is a potential problem when caring for the unconscious client, as it is for any immobilized or sensory–perceptually altered client. Refer to the same diagnosis under the heading "Cerebral Vascular Accident."

POTENTIAL FOR INJURY: CORNEA AND CONJUNCTIVA

The unconscious client is frequently unable to close his eyelids completely. Incomplete eyelid closure places the client at risk for corneal and scleral irritation and infection from lack of tearing, inability to blink or sense a foreign object in his eye.

Assessment

Assess the eyes for dryness and irritants. The cornea should be transparent, smooth, glossy, and moist; the palpebral conjunctiva should be pink, and the bulbar conjunctiva should be clear.

Interventions

Any irritant should be removed manually with a moist sterile Q-tip or piece of gauze, or with a saline flush. Administer artificial tears or lubricating ointments as needed. Artificial tears must be instilled at frequent intervals. Lubricating ointments protect the cornea, but ointment already in the eye should be removed before reapplying because of the possibility of foreign irritants being lodged in the ointment. Humidifiers will help to keep the cornea moist. Remember that clients who are waking up from coma will be more disoriented if unable to see clearly through ointment. Antibiotic drops such as neomycin may be needed to control eye infections.

Eye patching or taping may be necessary to keep eyelids closed. Eye shields may be useful in protecting the eye. Be certain that the eyelid is completely closed before applying the patch or shield.

Outcome

The client will not experience an injury to the cornea.

ALTERATION IN URINARY ELIMINATION: INCONTINENCE

The loss of voluntary inhibitory function over sphincter control results in urinary incontinence. Spontaneous micturation occurs with normal sphincter responses when a particular bladder volume is reached. Since the bladder generally empties well, urinary tract infection does not occur unless other predisposing factors are present, such as an indwelling catheter.

Assessment

Assess the client for residual urine periodically.

Interventions

A closed system indwelling catheter is usually necessary for the female. Males may use the external condom catheter, or placement of a urinal.

Urinary track infection is a potential problem with indwelling catheter use. The need for strict cleanliness when caring for an indwelling catheter can not be overemphasized. Typically, meatal care with soap and water is done twice daily, although the literature differs concerning the success of this method in controlling urinary tract infections. A study published by the Department of Urology, St. Paul–Ramsey Medical Center (Cass and Ireland 1985) states that the combination of antibacterial lotions used during perineal washings in conjunction with oral antibacterials were useful in preventing recurrent urinary tract infection in 32 women. Infection rate was reported at 0.5 per patient year.

Cranberry juice has also proved to be useful in reducing bacterial adherence to the bladder wall (Sobota 1984). Keeping the client well hydrated and the catheter unkinked and secured also contribute to keeping the client infection-free. Monitor the client for signs and symptoms of infection, such as fever or sediment in the urine. Some physicians will order intermittent irrigations with an antibacterial solution to prevent infection, although this technique has also not proved effective in preventing infection. Avoid irrigating the system, but if it is necessary to disconnect the closed drainage system, disinfect the connecting junctions with 70% isopropyl alcohol, and irrigate the pinched catheter with the same solution before reconnecting.

Outcomes

The drainage system should remain unobstructed and the client free of infection.

ALTERATION IN STOOL ELIMINATION: CONSTIPATION

Constipation is a frequent problem associated with immobility. Dehydration and changes in nutritional intake, whether total parenteral or enteral feedings, contribute to hard feces and impaction.

Assessment

Auscultating and palpating all four abdominal quadrants for bowel sounds and masses is an important first step. Nursing interventions are intended to maintain a regular bowel program and to prevent constipation.

Interventions

Monitor and record frequency of stool evacuation, consistency, and presence of occult blood. Prevent dehydration, since clients with increased intracranial pressure are frequently fluid restricted. Stool softeners and laxatives may be a necessary part of a bowel program. Enemas may be given if not contraindicated by increased intracranial pressure.

Outcome

The client will maintain normal bowel elimination.

ALTERATION IN NUTRITION: LESS THAN BODY REQUIREMENTS

The unconscious client is unable to take in sustenance by mouth, and is therefore at risk of alteration in nutrition, less than body requirements. Negative nitrogen and calcium balance also result from immobility. A head injured client is especially at risk for severe malnutrition, because of a high catabolic rate.

Assessment

Nutritional assessment should include evaluation of the client's general nutritional status. Observe the client's general musculoskeletal appearance. Skin should be inspected for turgor and dryness. Mucous membranes are assessed for hydration or injury, and the tongue is inspected for swelling or trauma. Obtain the client's weight and weigh him on a twice weekly basis at least, if possible. Monitor intake and output.

Interventions

Alternate methods of providing nutritional support for the unconscious client include tube feedings and total parenteral nutrition. The unconscious client will most likely require a high calorie, high protein content in his diet. High protein feedings produce an osmotic diuresis, so the nurse must ensure that the client is well hydrated. Various enteral feedings are available, and will be specified by the physician. Enteral feedings may be given through a nasogastric tube, or a gastrostomy or jejunostomy may be in place to minimize potential aspiration.

Administration of tube feeding may be done continuously or intermittently. Whichever method is used, it is important to assess placement of the tube before beginning feedings, or every 4 hours during continuous feedings. Monitor residual gastric contents and hold the feeding for 1 hour if greater than 100 milliliters. Let tube feedings warm up to room temperature before feeding. Maintain the head of the bed elevated at 30° to 45° during and for at least 1 hour after feeding if intermittent, or at all times if continuous. Keep the cuffed tracheostomy inflated to prevent aspiration. Assess the client for signs of aspiration such as respiratory distress, coughing, increased secretions, and cyanosis. It is beneficial to add food coloring to tube feedings to assist the nurse in determining aspiration. Have suction available at all times.

Central parenteral nutrition may be indicated for clients who require additional nutrition or are unable to tolerate tube feedings. Solutions provide protein or amino acids, dextrose, vitamins, minerals, trace elements, electrolytes, and water. A central silastic catheter in the superior vena cava is needed to accommodate the high amount of dextrose. Meticulous care of the catheter and insertion site is needed to prevent occlusion and infection. A complete discussion of parenteral nutrition can be found in Chapter 11.

Outcomes

The client's body weight and nutritional status will remain stable.

POTENTIAL FOR JOINT CONTRACTURES

Immobility causes loss of muscle mass and joint contractures. Joints become fibrotic and less pliable. Muscle fibers shorten, and contractures develop.

Assessment

Assessment of joint movement is performed during range of motion exercises. Motion should be smooth and within normal range of movement.

Interventions

Perform range of motion exercises every 2 hours for every joint, moving the joint through complete range at least two times. Proper physiologic alignment should be maintained when positioning the client. Trochanter rolls should be used to prevent external rotation of the hip. A pillow is placed under the superior leg while the client is side-lying to prevent hip displacement and direct pressure on the lower leg. Special splints or even rolled up washcloths can be used to splint the hand. Sometimes rigid clients can injure themselves with their fingernails by gouging their hands. Splinting can help prevent this from happening. To prevent footdrop, use a footboard, or special supportive boots to stabilize the foot in a normal position. Elevate dependent extremities to prevent edema. A firm mattress provides support to the musculoskeletal system.

Abnormal posturing, such as rigid flexion or extension, or abnormal muscle movements make positioning more difficult. These clients should be repositioned more often than every 2 hours as their rigidity increases metabolic activity and their risk for skin breakdown.

Outcome

Joint motion will remain within normal limits.

INABILITY TO PERFORM SELF-CARE

The unconscious client depends completely upon the care-giver for hygiene needs, nutritional needs, and toileting. Nutrition, elimination, skin and eye care have been discussed previously. Bathing, mouth care, grooming, and dressing are additional activities of daily living that are performed routinely by the nurse and/or family.

Interventions

Bathing the client, in addition to other skin care measures, is important not only for reasons of hygiene, but also to stimulate the sensory–perceptually altered client. Daily baths may not be necessary unless the client is diaphoretic or incontinent. A superfatted soap is useful for the client with dry skin. Lotions may also be used, and are useful in washing the client who is incontinent of stool.

Mouth care is done at least every 2 to 4 hours to keep the mucous membranes moist and intact, and to prevent tooth and gum disease. Use a toothbrush for brushing the teeth, and suction simultaneously. Massage the gums and parotid glands to stimulate circulation and prevent blockage of the glands. Keep the lips moist by applying lotion and Vaseline regularly. A humidifier is helpful in keeping skin, mucous membranes, and eyes moist.

Keep the hair clean, combed, and out of the client's face. Braiding long hair keeps it out of the way. Nails should also be kept short to prevent the client from injuring himself.

Outcome

The client will be maintained in a clean, comfortable state.

POTENTIAL FOR INJURY: SEIZURES

Depending upon the cause of the client's coma, seizures are a potential problem. Refer to the section on seizures in this chapter for the appropriate nursing care plan.

ALTERATIONS IN FAMILY PROCESSES

Caring for an unconscious family member in the home is a very stressful situation that can affect the family's ability to function cohesively. The goal is that the family support each other, form a cohesive group, and adapt to the situation.

Assessment

To reduce alteration in the family process, the nurse assesses the family structure, coping strategies, and knowledge of the client's condition.

Interventions

Create a supportive environment for the family. Listen attentively and encourage family members to express their feelings. Educate the family if a knowledge deficit is present, and include them in the care of the client. The nurse must remember that the family's wishes must be respected. The nurse will play a vital role in supporting the family as it copes with a difficult situation.

Outcome

The family will exhibit effective coping skills.

ASSESSING THE HOME ENVIRONMENT

Refer to discussions in Chapters 9 and 10 under this heading.

ABBREVIATED CARE PLAN: THE UNCONSCIOUS CLIENT

Nursing Diagnosis	Assessment	Interventions	Outcomes
Ineffective Airway Clearance	Chest expansion Accessory muscles Coughing Rate and depth of respiration Sputum	Monitor for signs and symptoms of ineffective airway clearance. Correctly position the client to prevent aspiration and to promote drainage of secretions. Turn and reposition every 2 hours. Never place client on his back.	The client will maintain clear airways for adequate aeration of all lung fields and optimal gas exchange.

ABBREVIATED CARE PLAN: THE UNCONSCIOUS CLIENT (*continued*)

Nursing Diagnosis	Assessment	Interventions	Outcomes
		Suction as needed.	
		Provide oxygen therapy and humidification.	
		Prevent infection and dehydration.	
Ineffective Breathing Pattern	Chest expansion Accessory muscles Coughing Rate and depth of respiration Sputum	Constantly monitor respiratory status. Provide oxygen therapy. Provide for potential mechanical ventilatory assistance. Turn and reposition at least every 2 hours. Prevent infection and tracheal injury from artificial airways.	The client will maintain adequate oxygenation and promote effective breathing patterns.
Sensory–Perceptual Alterations	Level of consciousness Response to touch Glasgow Coma Scale Cranial nerves	Use stimulation techniques for all the senses: olfactory, visual, somatosensory, auditory, and kinesthetic.	The client will respond to the best of his ability, will not be sensory deprived, and may progress to prefunctional skills.
Alterations in Mobility		Support all body systems as outlined in following diagnoses.	The client will maintain well-functioning body systems.
Alterations in Tissue Perfusion	Blood pressure Pulse Skin temperature	Stimulate the neurovascular reflexes by placing client in as upright a position as tolerated. Monitor client for orthostatic hypotension. Turn and reposition the client every 2 hours.	The client will remain normotensive.

(continued)

ABBREVIATED CARE PLAN: THE UNCONSCIOUS CLIENT (*continued*)

Nursing Diagnosis	Assessment	Interventions	Outcomes
		Perform range of motion exercises every 2 to 4 hours.	
		Use thigh-high antiembolic stockings or Ace wraps.	
Potential for Venous Thrombosis	Peripheral edema Temperature Color Tenderness Assess peripheral pulses	Promote venous flow by elevating the legs 15°, passive range of motion exercises. Avoid pressure on popliteal spaces. Avoid massaging calves. Prevent dehydration.	The client will not develop deep vein thrombosis.
Potential for Impaired Skin Integrity	Skin redness Areas of breakdown Nutritional status Pain or discomfort	Prevent decubitus ulcers. Teach client to mobilize as much as possible. Keep wheelchair pads and bed linens clean, dry, and wrinkle-free. Ensure adequate hydration and nutrition. Teach safety factors.	The client will maintain intact skin.
Potential for Injury: Cornea and Conjunctiva	Dryness Irritation	Remove foreign materials by using a sterile, moist Q-tip or gauze. Administer artificial tears or lubrication ointment. Administer antibiotics as ordered to prevent infection.	The client will maintain a healthy cornea and sclera.

ABBREVIATED CARE PLAN: THE UNCONSCIOUS CLIENT (*continued*)

Nursing Diagnosis	Assessment	Interventions	Outcomes
		Patch or tape eyes as necessary.	
Alteration in Urinary Elimination: Incontinence	Residual urine Incontinence	Control incontinence; an indwelling catheter or external condom catheter may be required. Maintain a clean, closed system. Cranberry juice will interfere with adherance of bacteria to bladder wall. Prevent dehydration. Monitor intake and output. Irrigate with antibacterials as ordered.	The client will be kept dry of urine, have a clean and unobstructed drainage system, and be free of urinary tract infection.
Alteration in Stool Elimination: Constipation	Bowel sounds Tenderness	Monitor and record frequency, character, consistency of stool. Monitor for occult blood. Prevent dehydration. Administer stool softeners and laxatives as ordered. Give enema as last resort.	The client will evacuate stool on routine basis.
Alteration in Nutrition: Less than Body Requirements	Skin turgor Mucous membranes Weight Intake and output	Conduct thorough nutritional assessment. Weigh biweekly. Monitor intake and output. Administer enteral feedings as prescribed. Have suction available at all times.	The client's body weight and nutritional status will remain stable.

(*continued*)

ABBREVIATED CARE PLAN: THE UNCONSCIOUS CLIENT (*continued*)

Nursing Diagnosis	Assessment	Interventions	Outcomes
		Monitor for signs and symptoms of aspiration.	
		Add food coloring to enteral feedings to assist in detecting aspiration.	
		Take meticulous care of central line if receiving TPN.	
Potential for Contractures	Range of motion	Do range of motion exercises every two hours.	Joint motion will remain within normal limits.
		Maintain client in proper alignment, using rolls, pillows, splints, and special supportive boots.	
		Prevent footdrop and peripheral edema.	
Inability to Perform Self-Care	Motor abilities Sensory abilities	Perform hygiene measures, mouth care, skin care, eye care, grooming, and dressing for the client.	The client will be maintained at a high level of cleanliness as he is totally dependent upon others for ADLs.

References

Adams M, Baron M, Caston MA: Urinary incontinence in acute phase of cerebral vascular accident. A descriptive study of hospitalized patients. Nurs Res 17(1): 37–44, 1966

Adams R, Victor M: Principles of Neurology. New York, McGraw-Hill, 1981

Barnett H, Stein B, Mohr J, Yatsu F: Stroke: Pathophysiology, Diagnosis, and Management. Vols I and II. Edinburgh, Churchill Livingstone, 1986

Barry K, Texeira S: The role of the nurse in the diagnostic classification and management of epileptic seizures. Neurosurg Nurs, 15(4): 243–249, 1983

Cass AS, Ireland GW: Antibacterial perineal washing for prevention of recurrent urinary tract infections. Urolology 25(5): 492–495, 1985

Dowling PC: Guillain–Barré syndrome in greater New York–New Jersey. JAMA (238): 317, 1977

Goldstein G, Ruthaven L: Rehabilitation of the Brain Damaged Adult. New York, Plenum, 1983

Hamilton HK: Definitions: The Nurses' Reference Library. Springhouse, PA, Intermed Communications, 1983

Hickey J: The Clinical Practice of Neurological and Neurosurgical Nursing. Philadelphia, JB Lippincott, 1985

Kaplan PE: Stroke Rehabilitation. Stoneham, MA, Butterworths, 1986

Kenner CV, Guzzetta CE, Dossey BM: Critical Care Nursing: Body, Mind and Spirit. Boston, Little, Brown & Co, 1985

Mills N, Plasterer H: Guillain–Barré syndrome: A framework for nursing care. Nurs Clin North Am 15(2): 257–263, 1980

National Institutes of Health: Epilepsy: Hope through Research. NIH Publication 81-156. Bethesda, MD, National Institutes of Health, 1981

Plum F, Posner J: The Diagnosis of Stupor and Coma. Philadelphia: FA Davis, 1982

Rottkamp BC: A holistic approach to identifying factors associated with an altered pattern of urinary elimination in stroke patients. J Neurosurg Nurs 17(1): 37–44, 1985

Sobota AE: Inhibition of bacterial adherence by cranberry juice: Potential use for the treatment of urinary tract infections. J Urol (131): May, 1984

Sahs AL, Hartman EC, Aronson SM: Guidelines for Stroke Care. Bethesda, MD, Public Health Service, 1976

Suggested Readings

Abels L: Critical Care Nursing: A Physiologic Approach. St. Louis, CV Mosby, 1986

Ballenger M: Seizures. Emergency 17(4): 46–52, 1985

Bedbrook G: Lifetime Care of the Paraplegic Patient. Edinburgh, Churchill Livingstone, 1985

Behrends E, Coronado M, Bryant C: Nutrition in neuroscience. J Neurosurg Nurs 14(1): 44–46 1982

Brunner LS: Suddarth DS: Textbook of Medical–Surgical Nursing. Philadelphia, JB Lippincott, 1984

Carpenito LJ: Nursing Diagnosis: Application to Clinical Practice. Philadelphia, JB Lippincott, 1983

Carroll P: Caring for ventilator patients. Nursing '86 16(4): 34–39, 1986

Colbert A, Schoch N: Respirator use in progressive neuromuscular diseases. Arch Phys Med Rehabil 66(11): 760, 1985

Eisenson J: Adult Aphasia, 2nd ed. Englewood Cliffs, NJ, Prentice-Hall, 1984

Griswold K, McKenna M, Ropper A: An approach to the care of patients with Guillain–Barré syndrome. Clin Rev Crit Care, 13(1): 66–72, 1984

Hughes M: Seizure disorders. Heart Lung 9(3): 154, 1983

Kinney AB, Blount M, Dowell M: Urethral catheterization; pros and cons of an invasive but sometimes essential procedure. Geriatr Nurs November/December: 258–263, 1980

Mahoney EH: Nutritional care of the brain damaged patient. ARN November/December: 17–19, 1975

McConnell J: Preventing urinary tract infections. Geriatr Nurs November/December, 1984

Nikas DL: Neurologic assessment of altered states of consciousness, Parts I, II, and III. Focus Crit Care: 10(5): 10–14 (1983); 10(6): 10–13 (1983); 11(1): 54–58 (1984)

Porter RJ: Epilepsy. Philadelphia, WB Saunders, 1985

Rich J: Generalized motor seizures. Nursing '86 16(4): 33, 1986

Samonas R: Guillain–Barré syndrome. Nursing '80 10(8): 35–41, 1980

Snyder M: Stressor inventory for persons with epilepsy. J Neurosci Nurs 18(2): 71–73, 1986

Swift, N: Helping patients live with seizures. Nursing 1978 June: 24–30, 1978

Thompson J et al: Clinical Nursing. St. Louis, CV Mosby, 1986

Tikkanen P: Landry–Guillain–Barré–Strohl syndrome. J Neurosurg Nurs 14(2): 74–81, 1982

Tucker C: Safety assessment for the postictal confusional phase following complex partial seizure. J Neurosurg Nurs 17(3): 201–209, 1985

Publications About Stroke for the Lay Person and Health Care Worker

Aphasia and the Family: American Heart Association, 1969

Facts About Strokes: American Heart Association, 1968

Facts About Women

Fundamentals of Stroke Care

How You Can Help Your Doctor Treat Your High Blood Pressure: American Heart Association, 1983

Nutrition Counseling for Cardiovascular Health; A Consumer Guide: American Heart Association.

Recipes for Fat-Controlled Low Cholesterol Meals: American Heart Association, 1975

Seven Hopeful Facts About Stroke: American Heart Association, 1980

Strokes, A Guide For the Family: American Heart Association, 1981

Stroke: Why Do They Behave That Way? American Heart Association: 1981

The 1984 Report

The Physician's Guide. How To Help Your Hypertensive Patients Stop Smoking: U.S. Department of Health and Human Services, Public Health Service, National Institutes of Health, 1984

What You Should Know About Stroke And Stroke Prevention. U.S. Department of Health and Human Services, Public Health Service, National Institutes of Health, 1981

The 1984 Report Of The Joint National Committee on Detection, Evaluation, and Treatment of High Blood Pressure. U.S. Department of Health and Human Services, Public Health Service, National Institutes of Health, 1984

Facts About . . . Women: Heart Disease and Stroke. U.S. Department of Health and Human Services, Public Health Service, National Institutes of Health,

Fundamentals of Stroke Care. U.S. Department of Health and Human Services, Public Health Service, National Institute of Neurological and Communicative Disorders and Stroke, 1976

14

ALTERATIONS IN LOCOMOTION

Jeanette Hartshorn

Successful attempts at locomotion require integration of both neural and musculoskeletal systems. In this chapter, some of the conditions that alter locomotion will be described; nursing care of individuals with these problems in the home setting is its focus. Specific conditions of spinal cord injury and multiple sclerosis will be discussed. Although each of these problems has a chronic component, the goal of this chapter is to describe the acute aspects of care of these individuals.

SPINAL CORD INJURY

Spinal cord injury is one of the most devastating injuries an individual can sustain. Data indicate that 60% of spinal cord injuries are sustained by persons between the ages of 15 and 30 with males comprising the majority of the group (Collins 1984). Despite the many advances in medical care of these individuals, the prognosis for complete recovery remains poor. Therefore, the individual is left with the need for long-term care, with expert nursing care as its cornerstone.

PATHOPHYSIOLOGY

The spinal cord is located in a relatively small space, making it prone to injury from a number of different forces. Damage to the cord occurs through a variety of mechanisms, including hyperextension, hyperflexion, and vertical compression (Fig. 14-1).

Following injury, a hemorrhagic lesion forms primarily involving the central gray matter. Chromatolysis, vacuolation, and alterations in cytoplasmic density and stainability are also observed (de la Torre 1981). Minimal edematous changes in white matter, more marked in internal than in external layers, have also been identified. The mechanical distortion of spinal cord tissue after compression trauma promotes not only intrinsic biochemical changes within the injured cells but also related changes involving extraneural tissues, particularly the blood vessels supplying the cord tissue (Collins 1984). Thus, the infiltration by platelets and red cells into the perivascular spaces will serve to worsen the intraneural damage normally accompanying the tissue distortion.

Following extravasation of the blood ele-

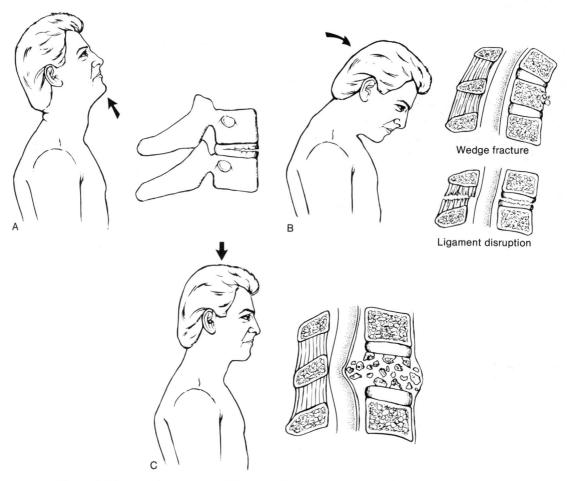

Figure 14-1. Hyperextension (*A*), hyperflexion (*B*), and vertical compression (*C*) are common mechanisms of spinal cord injury.

ments, polymorphonuclear leukocytes leak into the cord tissue, heralding various degrees of cellular necrosis. Moderately severe impact lesions of this type also involve interactions with the myelin sheath, leading to neuronal degeneration in the central gray matter. Within 24 to 48 hours following this type of injury, fibrocytic cells increase substantially (de la Torre 1981). Moderate to severe cavitation of the central gray matter occurs following stabilization of the injury.

Distal to the site of trauma, wallerian degeneration or demyelinization of the axon sheath occurs. This change is characterized by swelling of the myelinated axon, which then breaks into fragments and finally disappears from the tissue. When the axon regrows, in limited circumstances, the glial processes retract, and if synaptic contact is restored between cells, sensory–motor function may return to a degree. The way in which the healing of the injury proceeds is directly influenced by the severity and site of the injury, and by the time elapsed between trauma and the observed physiopathologic changes (De LaTorre 1981).

FUNCTIONAL LOSS

The degree of functional loss in the client is related to the level of injury. Figure 14-2 outlines the loss of function related to the level of injury.

There are eight cervical vertebrae. When damage occurs to the first two cervical vertebrae, the individual will suffer total quadriplegia and respiratory paralysis. The third, fourth, and fifth cervical vertebrae innervate the diaphragm with the peripheral phrenic nerve. Therefore, C3, C4, and C5 offer functional control over diaphragmatic excursion (Adelstein and Watson 1983). Damage to C3 and C4 causes total quadriplegia, a weak diaphragm, and absent intercostal movement. In addition to the diaphragm, C5 also innervates the trapezius muscle along with the spinal accessory nerve (CNXI). Thus, C5 regulates the individual's ability to perform a shoulder shrug.

The fifth and sixth cervical segments innervate the deltoid, biceps brachii, brachioradialis, and triceps muscles. This innervation includes the axillary, musculocutaneous, and radial nerves that allow arm elevation, supinated forearm, and neutral forearm flexion (Adelstein and Watson 1983). Damage to the fifth and sixth cervical region causes quadriplegia with gross arm movements. The diaphragm may be impaired initially, but function may return with time. The sixth cervical segment, in conjunction with the seventh and eighth, control forearm and wrist extension. Specifically, the extension carpi radialis and carpi ulnaris muscles are innervated. C7 and C8 also control wrist flexion (Guyton 1986). Damage to the sixth and seventh cervical segment causes quadri-

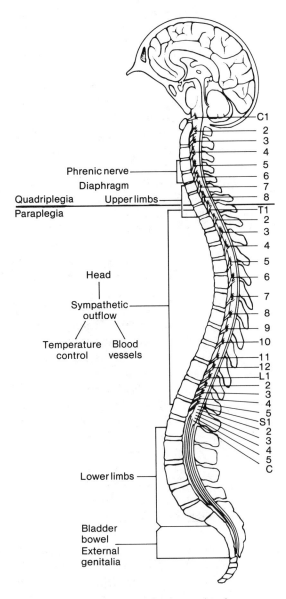

Figure 14-2. Diagram of relationship between level of lesion and degree of functional loss.

plegia with biceps and deltoid function, but no triceps function. Damage to the seventh and eighth segments causes quadriplegia with triceps function but no intrinsic hand function.

Grip and finger spreading are controlled by the eighth cervical and first thoracic segments. The first through the twelfth thoracic segments innervate the intercostal, rectus abdominis, and oblique muscles (Guyton 1986). These segments involve thoracic and lumbocervical peripheral branches and also influence respiration through intercostal muscles. In addition, the segments influence the muscles of the trunk.

Damage to the first through fifth thoracic segments produces paraplegia with diaphragmatic breathing, loss of leg, bladder, and bowel function. Arm function is intact and sensation is present to the nipple line. When there is damage to the sixth through twelfth thoracic segments, the individual is paraplegic with no abdominal reflexes at T6, and all abdominal reflexes at T12 (Guyton 1986). Generally, with this level of injury, there is spastic paralysis of the lower limbs. Damage to T12 is generally accompanied by sensation present to the groin area.

The first three lumbar segments control hip flexion through innervation of the iliopsoas muscle and the peripheral femoral nerve. Knee extension is controlled through L2, L3, and L4. These segments innervate the quadriceps femoris muscles involving the peripheral femoral nerve. The fourth lumbar through the second sacral segment control foot dorsiflexion and knee flexion.

This control originates through innervation of the extensor halluces, digitorum, biceps femoris, and hamstring muscles. The peripheral deep peroneal and sciatic nerves are included (Guyton 1986). Hip flexion, through the gluteus maximus muscle, and plantar flexion, through the gastrocnemius muscle, are also controlled through L5–S2.

When damage occurs to a segment below the level of L2, the individual may have mixed sensory–motor loss and bladder, bowel, and sexual loss depending on the nerve roots damaged. Should the conus medullaris be damaged, there will be bowel and bladder sphincter dysfunction, lower leg weakness, sacral dermatome hypesthesia or anesthesia and back pain. If the cauda equina is involved, there will be asymmetric, atrophic, and areflexic paralysis indicating involvement of the lower motor neurons (Adelstein and Watson 1983). Sensory root loss causing decreased sensation in the outer aspect of the legs, ankles, posterior lower limbs, and saddle area will occur. Damage to the cauda equina also causes sphincter dysfunction.

Sacral segments innervate the sphincter muscles through the pudendal peripheral nerves. Damage to sacral segments 1–5 causes loss of bladder, bowel, and sexual function. Some foot displacement may be present. Loss of sensation caused by this type of injury involves the saddle area, scrotum, perineum, penis, anal area, and upper third of the posterior aspect of the thigh.

NURSING DIAGNOSES

There are multiple nursing diagnoses for the client with a spinal cord injury. For each of the following diagnoses, appropriate assessment, planning, interventions, and outcomes will be described.

INEFFECTIVE BREATHING PATTERNS

Changes in innervation due to the injury and problems specifically caused by immobility make the client with a spinal cord injury a likely candidate for ineffective breathing patterns. Whether or not a client with a spinal cord injury will develop respiratory complications is also dependent upon the level of injury.

With immobility from any cause, there is an increase in the work of breathing, an increase in intraesophageal pressure, and a slight decrease in tidal volume. The end result is that more effort is required to expand the lungs and exchange gas. Immobility can be complicated by decreased strength of the muscles of respiration, which will lead to decreased chest expansion. The pressure of the bed against the chest also decreases expansion, predisposing the person to shallow breathing. Lack of activity decreases the normal stimulus to deep breathing (Guyton 1986). All of these factors lead to stasis of the normal secretions of the lung. If these mucous secretions become static, they form a good medium for bacterial growth. In addition, when a person is supine, the effects of gravity tend to draw the mucus in a bronchiole toward the bottom, leaving dry upper epithelium. This epithelium is more vulnerable to bacterial invasion, which in turn can lead to pneumonia. Atelectasis may occur if static secretions become thick and block a bronchiole. If a person is unable to cough, for example, if he is too weak, unconscious, or in pain, pneumonia is possible.

Clients with high-level cervical cord injury have reduced lung volume and capacity and poor oxygen exchange with CO_2 retention (Adelstein and Watson 1983). Each client demonstrates a variable cough, a progressive decrease in thoracic compliance, and elastic recoil of lungs because of decreased volume. These same individuals require total respiratory support, at least for a prescribed period of time. The cough reflex is significantly impaired by paralysis of the intercostal and abdominal muscles.

Assessment

Initial assessment of the respiratory function of the client with a spinal cord injury should include respiratory rate and respiratory excursion. Lung sounds are assessed for the degree of movement of air and the presence of adventitious sounds. Specific respiratory parameters, such as tidal volume and vital capacity, are measured. When warranted, arterial blood gases can be assessed for levels of oxygen, carbon dioxide, and pH in the blood.

Interventions

A number of interventions can be used to promote effective breathing patterns in the client with a spinal cord injury. Clients should be positioned in a way that promotes gravitational movement of the diaphragm. Special beds, such as the Roto-Rest bed have been designed for this purpose. Other techniques that may help are turning the client at least every 2 hours, assisting with deep breathing exercises, and the use of incentive spirometry. Throughout the utilization of these various therapies to improve breathing patterns, it is important for the nurse to continue to monitor the client's response. The family's assistance will be needed to implement these interventions successfully.

Outcomes

An expected outcome for the client with an ineffective breathing pattern is the client's attainment of a normal breathing pattern. Specific parameters demonstrating achievement of this outcome include a normal rate and rhythm of respiration and normal arterial blood gases.

INEFFECTIVE AIRWAY CLEARANCE

The client with a spinal cord injury may also experience ineffective airway clearance. For these clients, there are several reasons for their condition, including stasis of secretions, poor or nonexistent cough effort, and immobility.

Assessment

To assess for ineffective airway clearance, monitor for adventitious breath sounds, rapid, shallow respirations, dyspnea, and cyanosis. An increased heart rate may also be present. Should the ineffective clearance worsen, gas exchange may become impaired. In this situation, the client may become irritable, restless, and confused. Adequate nursing interventions should prevent the client from developing this serious consequence.

Interventions

Several interventions may help to support effective airway clearance. Fluid intake should be maintained at around 2500 cc/day. There may be some clients (*i.e.*, those with decreased heart function or renal disease) who may not be able to tolerate a fluid level of that magnitude. By increasing the daily fluid intake, it is possible to liquefy secretions, thereby improving the client's ability to cough and expectorate the secretions. The use of humidified air through an artificial or natural airway can be another method for decreasing the thickness of secretions and improving the individual's ability to expectorate (Ulrich, Canale, and Wendell 1986).

Nursing care techniques such as turning the client and encouraging him to cough and breath deeply can aide in the removal of secretions. Clients can be taught respiratory exercises to increase movement of secretions.

Outcomes

Successful interventions should result in the client's ability to maintain a clear airway. Normal, clear breath sounds, normal respiratory rate, and absence of signs of respiratory distress can be used as indicators of the effectiveness of the interventions.

ALTERATION IN NUTRITION

Clients at any stage of recovery from a spinal cord injury are at risk for an alteration in nutrition. The immobility caused by the cord injury leads to a slowed metabolic rate. The immobile client may also suffer from an inability to feed himself. Thus, the injured client can experience an alteration in nutrition of less than body requirements. A multitude of nutritional problems, including negative nitrogen balance, negative calcium balance, and paralytic ileus, may also occur.

Negative nitrogen balance may develop as a result of immobility. Normally, anabolism (protein synthesis) is in balance with catabolism (protein breakdown). During immobilization, a marked increase in urinary nitrogen (byproduct of protein metabolism) excretion occurs. The marked urinary excretion of nitrogen results in a negative nitrogen balance, representing a depletion of stores for protein synthesis necessary in tissue healing after trauma or surgery.

Negative calcium balance also occurs as a result of immobility (Maynard 1986). Calcium is mobilized from the bone in the process of bone reabsorption and is excreted in excess of dietary intake. Calcium is normally present in the urine and is dissolved if the urinary volume, *p*H, and citric acid concentration are normal. With immobility, calcium output changes while citric acid concentration remains the same, thus altering the important ratio between calcium and citric acid. Urinary *p*H rises slightly, rather than falling, as would be necessary to retain an acid urine. The volume rises slightly, but not in proportion to the calcium increase. These factors combine to make precipitation of calcium and formation of stones quite likely.

Paralytic ileus may also occur with immobility. During the acute stage following injury, many clients experience loss of bowel sounds and abdominal distention from the loss of peristaltic movements in the intestines. Peristaltic activities are mediated by the parasympathetic nervous system, and the exact cause of paralytic ileus in these clients is generally attributed to the sudden paralysis and interruption of impulse pathways. Severe gastric dilation from a paralytic ileus can interfere with diaphragmatic functioning. Vomiting can also occur, placing the client at risk for aspiration.

Assessment

Several parameters should be assessed by the nurse in evaluating the nutritional status of the client with a spinal cord injury. The home health nurse should assess the client for signs of malnutrition. Weight, and serum levels of blood urea nitrogen, albumin, protein, and hematocrit and hemoglobin are indicators of nutritional status. Electrolyte levels, particularly calcium, will provide important information concerning nutritional status. Additional information concerning nutritional assessment can be found in Chapter 11.

Interventions

Once the spinal cord injured client is returned to a home setting, it is likely that the individual will be taking oral feedings. Certain assistive devices may be required to supplement returning muscle and nervous function. Generally, clients are fitted with these devices before they are discharged from the hospital. Should their needs for assistive devices change, a consultation with an occupational therapist would be required. When possible, the client should be in a high Fowler's position while eating. Actual positioning, however, is dependent upon the stability of the spine. While feeding, the family should be instructed in safety techniques to prevent aspiration.

On occasion, it may be necessary to supplement feedings for the spinal cord injured client. These supplements may range from periodic administration of cans of feedings (such as Magnacal or Ensure) to continuous enteral tube feedings. Refer to Chapter 11 for a discussion of nutritional products and their use in the home.

Outcomes

The goal of these interventions is to help the client maintain adequate nutritional status. Specific parameters that indicate normal nutritional status include normal weight, normal laboratory values such as BUN, albumin calcium, and protein, and tolerance for activity.

ALTERATION IN BOWEL ELIMINATION

Clients with spinal cord injury can experience alterations in elimination for a number of reasons. One of the most common forms of this alteration is constipation. Several anatomical and physiological principles explain why constipation is a common problem.

The large bowel musculature has its own neural center within the intestinal wall that responds to distention caused by fecal contents. This type of innervation is usually not greatly affected by cord injury. However, the client may suffer from loss of the sensation of fullness in the lower bowel, loss of awareness of bowel evacuation, loss of ability to control the rectal sphincter, and loss of the ability to contract the abdominal muscles and to expel the stool (Ulrich, Canale, and Wendell 1986).

Other causes may also promote the development of constipation in the spinal cord-injured client. Those on restricted diets may not receive adequate amounts of roughage and fluids. With immobility, the muscle begins to lose strength and the individual may not have enough muscle strength to pass stool. The perineal and abdominal muscles used in defecating are weakened by bed rest and may be affected by the level of injury. The client should be assessed for fecal impaction. One of the early signs of impaction is constant leakage of stool from the rectum.

Fecal impaction is a serious problem and requires specific and prompt treatment. The usual treatment includes oral stool softeners, increased fluid intake, oil retention enema, digital removal and breaking up of impaction, and a cleansing enema.

Assessment

Assessment of the client for potential alterations in elimination is important. Bowel sounds should be auscultated routinely. High-pitched sounds may indicate the presence of diarrhea or the beginning of closure of a paralytic ileus. On the other hand, distant and muffled bowel sounds generally indicate constipation. While palpating the abdomen, hardness in the left lower quadrant may indicate constipation, leading to impaction. Clients will also be aware of a feeling of fullness and abdominal discomfort.

Interventions

Prevention is one of the most effective interventions for constipation. Unless contraindicated, clients should maintain fluid intake at 2500 cc in 24 hours. Foods high in fiber and substances that stimulate peristalsis, such as warm liquids or prune juice should be encouraged.

Several techniques may be needed to help facilitate emptying of the rectum for the spinal cord-injured client. A routine time for defecation should be established. The gastrocolic reflex will stimulate emptying of the colon 20 to 30 minutes after a meal. Placing the client in a high Fowler's position will assist in defecation. However, this type of positioning will be acceptable only when the spine has been stabilized.

Pharmacological agents may be needed to assist in the process of bowel evacuation. Several different groups are used, such as stool softeners and laxatives. Stool softeners can be used as an integral part of any bowel management program. Drugs such as Colace are given to assist in the management of the bowel program, but have no direct laxative effect. Stool softeners are frequently given daily, while laxatives can be given on a more sporadic basis. It is preferable that a bowel management program be established without the addition of drugs.

Outcome

A successful bowel management program will result in a client with a normal bowel evacuation routine. The client should experience no sign of bowel abnormalities.

ALTERATION IN URINARY ELIMINATION

Clients with spinal cord injury may experience problems due to flaccidity and areflexia.

Clients may have experienced problems in urinary control due to the presence of spinal shock. Spinal shock occurs as early as 30 to 60 minutes following cord injury and involves the complete or nearly complete suppression of all reflex activity below the level of the injury. Tendon reflexes diminish or disappear, temperature control and vasomotor tone are lost. Bladder and bowel paralysis resulting in urinary retention, ileus, and fecal retention may also occur. Spinal shock occurs because of the sudden loss of impulses from the descending pathways, which normally maintain the cord neurons in a ready state of excitability. This transient inability of the cord to respond is referred to as *spinal shock.* Occasionally in a client with complete cord transection, sacral reflexes may be present immediately after transection (Grundy and Russell 1985). These reflexes show a diminished response and commonly reflex activity returns following recovery from spinal shock and, without the modulating influence of the central cortex, reflexes are hyperactive.

There is wide variation in the duration of spinal shock for some instances resolving in several days while others require several months. No specific medical treatment has been identified for spinal shock (Rudy 1984).

Although spinal shock generally occurs soon after the time of injury, the effects may last for several months. While it is not common for the client at home to experience such a problem, it remains a possibility.

Assessment

Assessment of the client includes monitoring intake and output, and assessing for signs of either urinary retention or incontinence. Signs of urinary retention include frequent voiding of small amounts of urine, and complaints of urgency. The client may experience bladder fullness associated with discomfort in the suprapubic region.

Interventions

Once discharged to home, clients may continue to experience retention or incontinence. Several measures can be implemented to promote complete bladder emptying. Stimulate trigger zones of the reflex sacral arc (*e.g.*, tap suprapubic area, stroke inner thigh, perform anal sphincter stretching). Repeat stimulus as necessary to empty bladder (the goal is to have residual urine of less than 100 cc). If stimulation of the trigger zones is not effective, continue to provide the stimulation periodically. It may take up to 9 months for strong reflex sacral arc activity to return. Always place the client in a normal position for voiding unless contraindicated.

If signs of urinary retention persist, it may be necessary to implement intermittent catheterization. Both client and family should be instructed in this technique if it is to be routinely used.

If incontinence is a problem, maintain consistent fluid intake to prevent over-distention of the bladder. The client should avoid drinking caffeinated beverages, since caffeine increases urine production and can cause bladder spasm. Limiting oral intake of fluids prior to bedtime will help to decrease the risk of nighttime incontinence.

Outcomes

Success of nursing interventions will be achieved when the client does not experience urinary retention or incontinence.

IMPAIRED PHYSICAL MOBILITY

The major characteristic of the immobile individual is an inability to purposefully move within the physical environment, including transfer, ambulation, and locomotion. For the client with a spinal cord injury, the degree of impairment of physical mobility is related to the level of injury.

After a spinal cord injury, impaired physical mobility leads to several additional problems. One of the most obvious changes attributed to impaired physical mobility is a loss of muscle strength and mass. Muscle strength and endurance for exercise decrease (Mitchell and Loustau 1981).

Through fibrosis, muscle and joint mobility is decreased or lost when these structures are not used. Normal mobility is dependent upon the free movements of the joints and their muscular attachments. When the joints and muscles are not used, the normal metabolic activity within joints and muscles is altered, leading to a loss of mobility (Mitchell and Loustau 1981).

Connective tissue fibers are continually being laid down in the subcutaneous tissues, muscles, and joint capsules. The normal range of motion of joints and muscles keeps this fibrous network loose and helps it to stretch to accommodate the maximum range of movement of any one joint. When motion is limited, the normal stretching forces are absent and the collagen meshwork becomes less pliable. A dense collagen network may form in as few as 5 days of immobilization (Mitchell and Loustau 1981).

Fibrosis within a muscle leads to progressive shortening of the muscle in a contracted shape. If the fibrosis is sufficiently severe, contractures may become permanent deformities. Poor alignment of body parts during prolonged bed rest may lead to deformed posture through atrophy of muscles, fibrosis, and contractures.

Assessment

In assessing the client with impaired physical mobility, it is necessary to check frequently the range of motion of all extremities. Muscle strength and tone can similarly be assessed on a routine basis. To test muscle tone, the nurse notes whether ridigity (increased resistance throughout range of motion of the joint), spasticity (increased muscular resistance to brisk movement of the joint), and clonus (oscillation between flexion and extension of the foot when brisk pressure is applied to the sole) are elicited by passive motion. Muscles are also palpated for tenderness or spasm.

Muscle strength is tested in the following ways. To test the shoulder girdle, press down on the client's arms after he abducts them to shoulder height. Upper extremities are tested by evaluating biceps, triceps, wrist dorsiflexion, hand grasps, and strength of finger abduction and extension. Lower extremities are tested through the hip flexors, abductors and adductors, knee flexors and extensors, foot dorsiflexors, invertors and evertors. Muscle strength is graded as normal, minimal, moderate, severe weakness, or paralysis (Bates 1987).

Interventions

A major goal in caring for the immobile client is to prevent complications such as contractures. Both active and passive range of motion exercises are needed on a frequent basis. As the client is maintained on bed rest, proper positioning is essential. Support for extremities should be used at all times. Frequent turning of the client and repositioning may also help in maintaining proper alignment. When possible, the nurse may also assist the client in performing muscle conditioning exercises. Muscle-setting exercises, in which the muscle is contracted as hard as possible for 10 seconds and then released, are a type of isometric exercise that may be helpful. Resistive exercises, those in which the muscle contracts in pushing or pulling against a stationary object, can be used to help maintain strength. The family should be carefully instructed in the proper technique for these exercises (Ulrich, Canale, and Wendell 1986).

Equipment may also interfere with the client's mobility. Halo braces are devices to stabilize cervical injuries (Fig. 14-3). The traction and stability of the halo is achieved through screws attached to the skull and to struts of a metal frame that are encased in a rigid plastic vest. This metal framework and head halo permit no flexion, extension, or rotational movements of the neck, thus completely immobilizing the site of injury or fusion, allowing callus formation (Rudy 1984).

Nursing interventions can be implemented to assist the client in dealing with the halo device. The client can be reminded of the need for the brace and taught about its function. Gentle massage to the client's shoulders and utilization of a turn sheet when moving the client may help in decreasing any possible discomfort caused by the device. Family members should be taught safety procedures to be used in the event of an emergency for

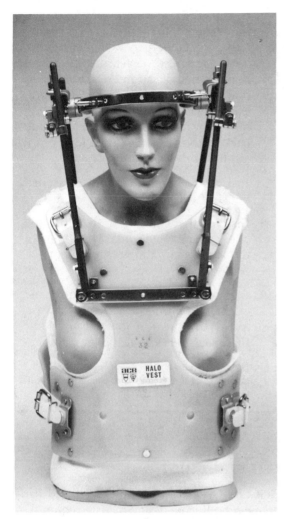

Figure 14-3. Halo-vest traction.

the client. Specific procedures for the care of the client in a halo brace can be found in the boxed material in the opposite column.

Outcome

Successful nursing interventions will result in the client maintaining the maximal possible mobility within the limitations caused by the injury.

Halo-vest Traction

INTRODUCTION: Halo-vest traction immobilizes the head and neck after trauma to the cervical vertebrae. The procedure can be performed in the emergency room. The halo-vest allows the client some mobility, while keeping the cervical vertebrae in alignment.

EQUIPMENT:
Hydrogen peroxide
Sterile water or normal saline
Cotton-tipped applicators
Povidone-iodine ointment
Sterile gauze
Two wrenches

PROCEDURE

1. Examine the halo-vest unit to ensure that all parts are securely fastened and that the head is centered within the halo. Check the edges of the halo-vest by inserting a finger to determine if it is too tight. Check the pins to ensure proper tightness.

2. The client's chest and back should be washed daily. This is accomplished by loosening the bottom velcro straps. By reaching under the vest, the chest and back can be cleansed.

3. Check skin daily for areas of potential breakdown.

4. Utilize a hair dryer to dry the sheepskin, which lines the brace, if it becomes moist with perspiration.

5. Cornstarch or dusting powder can be used to prevent itching.

6. Keep two conventional wrenches taped to the front of the vest at all times in order to remove the vest during an emergency.

(continued)

7. Assess the client for the need for mild analgesics to control headache, spasm of the neck muscles, and discomfort at pin sites.

PIN CARE

1. Remove the dressing from each pin site (if applicable).

2. Inspect the pin sites for evidence of bleeding, CSF leak, swelling, redness, or purulent drainage.

3. Remove hair from around the pin site as necessary.

4. Cleanse the pin sites with cotton-tipped applicators dipped in hydrogen peroxide solution.

5. Rinse the sites with sterile water or sterile normal saline to remove the hydrogen peroxide.

6. Cleanse pin sites with povidone-iodine ointment

7. Replace sterile dressing.

SPECIAL HOME HEALTH IMPLICATIONS

1. On each visit, assess cranial nerves VI, IX, and XII, which may be damaged by pin placement.

2. Assess the client for motor, sensory, and pulmonary function on each visit.

3. Instruct the family in signs and symptoms of motor, sensory, and pulmonary complications.

4. Instruct client and family to avoid contamination of pin sites.

5. Instruct the family in the use of the halo-vest. They should feel comfortable providing for client's daily hygiene and for potential emergencies while halo-vest is being used.

6. Instruct the family in the proper procedure for removal of the halo-vest in the event of an emergency. In the event of a cardiac arrest, detach the wrenches, remove the distal anterior bolts, and pull the two upright bars outward. Then unfasten the velcro straps and remove the front of the vest. Use the back of the vest as a board for cardiopulmonary resuscitation (CPR).

7. Instruct the family in the jaw-thrust maneuver for CPR.

8. Instruct the family not to allow the client to ambulate alone. The weight of the vest may throw the client off balance.

9. Instruct the family never to move the client by pulling on the bars or vest. Avoid any pressure on the apparatus that may affect cervical alignment.

(Adapted from Walsh J, Persons CB, Wieck L: Manual of Home Health Care Nursing. Philadelphia, JB Lippincott, 1987)

SELF-CARE DEFICIT

Self-care tasks are activities performed daily to meet bodily needs and that are required so that the client may participate in society. Therefore, dependence in this area may impede one's participation in activities with friends and family. Most self-care activities require a significant amount of upper extremity function, which poses obvious problems for clients with cervical cord injury.

Assessment

The spinal cord-injured client can suffer from varying levels of self-care deficit. While assessing the client, the presence of an inability to move in the bed and transfer from bed to chair, difficulty in grasp and grip, and difficulties in utilizing tools and utensils indicate the presence of self-care deficits. Once noting these difficulties, the nurse plans care to minimize the deficit to the greatest extent possible. The client should be involved with his own care, maintaining independence whenever possible.

Interventions

Consultation with other health-care professionals, such as physical and occupational therapists, may be needed. In particular, occupational therapists can be consulted for assistance in developing new types of utensils that can be used by a client with a weakened grasp. Occupational therapists can also teach the client methods of dressing despite the restrictions imposed by the injury.

Another strategy that may be effective in helping the client become independent is to schedule care for times when the client is most likely to participate to the fullest extent. The client will be most able to do this when he is rested and comfortable. For example, scheduling activities when analgesics are at peak action or after rest periods may be helpful in encouraging client participation. Some research indicates that ability to participate in care may also be related to the individual's circadian rhythm (Hall 1979). Assessment of the client's "best" time may help in the development of the nursing care plan.

As the nurse continues to promote independence in the individual client, the family must be taught about the client's current abilities and future potential. The family can be used to help encourage the client's independence.

Outcomes

Successful outcomes of these strategies will be documented by the client's ability to par-ticipate in his care to the maximal extent possible.

IMPAIRED SKIN INTEGRITY

Maintenance of skin integrity is a major problem for the client with a spinal cord injury. Pressure sores or decubitus ulcers are commonly seen. The lack of muscle tone, voluntary movement, and perception of pain are factors in the development of pressure sores. However, the most important factor is the lowered tissue resistance to pressure caused by interruption of the vasomotor pathways.

Pressure sores involve cutaneous and subcutaneous tissue and occur in areas of the body subjected to unrelieved pressure, such as the back of the head, the sacrum, heels of the feet, and trochanters. Skin and subcutaneous tissue die, slough away, and leave areas of ulceration (Sugarman 1985). Cells in these tissues die because sufficient nutrients cannot diffuse from the capillaries to the cells, and their waste products cannot be carried away. This lack of diffusion to and from the capillaries occurs because pressure on the tissues is greater than the hydrostatic pressure in the capillary. This pressure difference effectively opposes diffusion from the capillaries, leading to tissue ischemia. Prolonged tissue ischemia leads to the development of pressure sores (Ulrich, Canale, and Wendell 1986).

Assessment

Since prevention of pressure sores is a top priority in caring for the client with a spinal cord injury, skin assessment is performed on each visit. Generally, one of the first signs of skin breakdown is the presence of reddened areas. Assessment of the skin should include all areas of the body, with particular attention to the elbows, ear lobes, sacrum, and heels of the feet.

Other parameters to assess include the nutritional status of the individual and other medical problems present at the same time. Wound healing is slowed in those with poor nutritional status. These individuals, therefore, are more likely to suffer from pressure sores. Medical problems, such as diabetes mellitus, may also lead to potential problems in skin breakdown.

While assessing these parameters, the nurse assesses the client's risk for development of pressure sores. Other factors that contribute to the development of ulcers include debilitated conditions, edema, anemia, and trophic skin changes.

Interventions

The family is a crucial element in the skin care program for the client with a spinal cord injury. The nurse can instruct the family to reposition the client at least every 2 hours to relieve pressure on body parts. Skin should be kept clean and dry, particularly in areas prone to the development of pressure sores. When the nurse notes reddened areas, an early sign of skin breakdown, threatened areas of the skin should be protected immediately. Enterostomal therapists with a knowledge of comprehensive skin care should be consulted for decubitus care.

Specific treatment of pressure sores varies. The use of an occlusive plastic film (Op-Site) has gained some popularity over the last few years. This film covers the area, keeps bacteria out, and allows granulation tissue to develop. A number of antibacterial creams have also been recommended for various types of pressure sores. Periodic application of heat is useful in the treatment of existing areas of skin breakdown. Most severe pressure sores may require surgical debridement and plastic surgery. A more complete discussion of skin care can be found in Chapter 17.

Outcome

If the interventions are successful, the client should not experience any areas of redness or breakdown.

ALTERATION IN TISSUE PERFUSION

Alteration in tissue perfusion in the spinal cord-injured client can occur secondary to hypotension or hypertension. The most common reason for a hypertensive response is autonomic dysreflexia.

AUTONOMIC DYSREFLEXIA

Autonomic dysreflexia is a response generally initiated by stimulation of sensory receptors from a distended bladder or bowel that send impulses to the lower spinal cord. Normally, stimuli from the muscle cause impulses to travel via the pelvic and presacral nerves to the spinal cord and via the lateral spinothalamic tracts, posterior columns, and other ascending pathways to the brain. Below the level of spinal cord injury, these impulses activate a massive sympathetic reflex with arteriolar spasms in the vasculature of the skin and splanchnic vascular bed resulting in an elevation of blood pressure and symptoms of sympathetic outflow. Normally, this increased blood pressure stimulates the baroreceptors in the carotid sinus and aorta, sending signals via the glossopharyngeal and vagus nerves to the basomotor center in the brain. The efferent impulses are then sent to the heart, resulting in bradycardia via the vagus vasculature via decreased sympathetic flow through the spinal cord (Rudy 1984).

If injury to the cord occurs above the level of visceral outflow, the response of the vasomotor center is bradycardia, which is mediated via the vagus nerve. But the vasomotor center cannot send impulses past the site of lesion in the spinal cord to counteract hypertension by vasodilation. Thus, severe hypertension persists. Vasodilation will occur in segments above the lesion possessing normal sympathetic supply (Rudy 1984).

Hypotension, specifically orthostatic hypotension, may also occur. One major reason for hypotension involves peripheral pooling of blood resulting from the loss of sympathetic control over peripheral vessels. In addition, the loss of muscle tone in the extremities resulting from paralysis and decreased mobility can also cause orthostatic changes.

Assessment

The family can assist in assessment of tissue perfusion by monitoring the blood pressure. They can be warned that if the client suffers from orthostatic hypotension, the decrease in blood pressure may be accompanied by light-headedness and possibly, syncope.

The symptoms associated with autonomic dysreflexia are multiple. With autonomic dysreflexia, the marked systemic hypertension associated with the sudden rise in intracranial pressure is experienced by the client as a pounding headache and nasal congestion. Sweating of the face and neck, flushing, and enlarged pupils may also occur.

Interventions

Several nursing interventions will assist in the prevention of orthostatic hypotension. Passive range of motion exercised at least every 2 hours will increase circulation throughout the masculature. Thigh-high elastic wraps or hose will also improve circulation. The client and family should be taught appropriate ways of positioning to prevent pooling of blood in the extremities. Clients should change position slowly when moving. Finally, an abdominal binder may be required to assist in maintenance of blood pressure. The abdominal binder increases pressure on the aorta and limits the amount of blood that will be able to flow to and pool in the extremities. Therefore, the abdominal binder should be applied before the client is assisted to a sitting position (Ulrich, Canale, and Wendell 1986).

The major treatment of autonomic dysreflexia is to identify and treat the cause. Generally, checking the bladder and rectum will reveal the cause. During this time, the blood pressure should be carefully monitored. If the blood pressure does not decrease with the removal of the cause, it may be necessary to administer antihypertensive drugs such as Apresoline. Autonomic dysreflexia should be viewed as a medical emergency and treatment instituted immediately.

Outcomes

Successful interventions will result in a client who is normotensive, particularly during position changes, and free from symptoms of decreased blood pressure. Finally, the client should not experience autonomic dysreflexia.

SEXUAL DYSFUNCTION

Clients with spinal cord injury may suffer from sexual dysfunction related to the level of cord injury. Decreased libido from loss of sensory and motor function below the level of spinal cord injury may be experienced. Impotence can occur for many reasons including the presence of a urinary catheter, fear of urinary or fecal incontinence, and fear of rejection from the partner. Many men also suffer from impotence related to a decreased ability to maintain an erection.

Assessment

Assessment for potential sexual dysfunction is best completed over a period of time. The nurse listens for any verbalization of sexual concerns from the client. As the home health nurse establishes a long term relationship with the client and family, subtle indicators of difficulty in maintaining sexual relationships may be evident.

Interventions

Once the assessment is complete, the home health nurse communicates concern and interest in assisting the family to work through the problems. An important responsibility for the nurse at this time is to provide adequate information to the family. Questions must be answered as completely and honestly as possible.

Several specific interventions may help. The nurse can discuss alternate ways of expressing sexuality, such as massage or cuddling. Inform the male client and his partner of techniques for eliciting and maintaining reflexogenic erection. A penile prothesis may also be advised. Always include the partner in all discussions related to sexuality. Possibly, the problems related to sexuality will require counseling from someone with specific training in this area.

Outcome

Successful interventions will result in the client being able to demonstrate a beginning acceptance of changes in sexual functioning.

INEFFECTIVE INDIVIDUAL COPING

Spinal cord injury causes the client to confront multiple problems. Emotional reactions that can be expected include denial, anger, and depression. Each nurse works with the client to help in developing methods for dealing with all of the feelings relative to the injury.

Assessment

Psychological support of this client should begin at the time of injury. Once the client is transferred from the acute care institution to the home, additional emotional responses can be expected. As the individual becomes more physically stable, the client may experience some denial of the extent of his injury and eventually some depression. When an understanding develops about the extent of injury and what it means in terms of overall functioning, anger may result. Feelings of inferiority, inadequacy, powerlessness, lack of self-worth, and despair may also occur.

Interventions

As the client progresses through each of these stages, the nurse can best assist by encouraging expression of feelings. The nurse learns about the client's perception of his condition and his expectations. Education may be needed at this time to help the client maintain a realistic view of the future. Goals are mutually set by the nurse and client, so that the client can experience the satisfaction of goal attainment. Nurses can do much by repeatedly expressing confidence in the client's ability to perform successfully, always emphasizing the positive. Working towards maintaining communication that is open and honest, and being sensitive to the client's need for acceptance are interventions that are frequently successful in working with these individuals. The home health nurse can also assist the client to identify all support systems. These may include the family, friends, neighbors, and community groups (Ulrich, Canale, and Wendell 1986).

There are times, however, when the nurse is not the best person to help the client work through these problems. In this situation, the nurse should consider asking for consultation with a clinical nurse specialist in psychiatric nursing who can establish a relationship with the client and offer the needed support.

Outcomes

A successful outcome is demonstrated when the client utilizes effective coping skills. Demonstration of these outcomes includes verbalization by the client concerning the injury, identification of methods to deal with individual stressors, and recognition of support systems.

POTENTIAL FOR FAMILY CRISIS

As the client works through various stages of anger, depression, and denial, so does the family. There are a multitude of factors that combine to help form the attitudes of the family toward the situation. For example, the family may suffer from guilt, thinking that it may have been able to do something that would have prevented the injury. The length of time required for hospitalization of the client may produce an additional strain on the family. Members may disagree as to the best decisions to be made on behalf of their family member.

Assessment

In assessing the family relationship, it is important to accept the family as they are. The approach to the family should be one of determining how they are coping, trying not to impose any personal beliefs on the group. Assess the family dynamics, coping strategies, knowledge of disease process, and attitudes.

Interventions

Interventions for the family parallel those for the individual. Initially, it is important to give the family members the opportunity to express their feelings. Support groups for families may assist in their process of adjustment.

Support groups, composed of friends and family of the person who suffered the physical loss, are organized to increase the members' knowledge and participation in the grieving process, and in rehabilitation plans. In addition, group members can benefit from the instillation of hope, recognition of the universality of tragedy, close relationships with others, and the expression of strong emotions. A support group may enable the family to work through its own grief by identifying with others and by learning how to provide its injured family member with the best support within the family's capabilities.

As with the individual, additional counseling may be required for the family. While working with the family, the nurse may assess pathological responses among family members and note that the family group is suffering from inadequate coping mechanisms. At this time, a consultation with a psychiatric clinical nurse specialist or other mental health clinician may be of particular value.

Outcomes

Successful interventions for the family will result in evidence of improved relationships between client and family members. Evidence of family tension should be minimal.

ANXIETY

The home-bound client with a spinal cord injury frequently suffers from anxiety related to several factors. One of the major causes of anxiety in this client is the potential effect of the injury on the client's life-style. Early in the course of therapy, the client may experience anxiety related to transfer from the hospital setting to home. Immobilized clients may feel a loss of control once they are discharged from the hospital. In the hospital, personnel are always available to assist if the client experiences any ill effects from the injury. However, once transferred home, the client may be concerned that family members are inadequately prepared to deal with potential problems. For this reason, family members should be actively involved in teaching prior to the client's discharge from the hospital.

Assessment and Interventions

The home health nurse can assess the client by noting both physical and psychological signs of anxiety. For example, irritability, restlessness, tachycardia, and verbalization of fears and concerns may all indicate potential anxiety. Nursing interventions to help control the anxiety will be related to the actual causes of anxiety. Offering emotional support by expressing interest in the feelings of the individual and by demonstrating sensitivity to changes in the client's mood can help to decrease anxiety. Once a relationship is established with the client, counseling from the home health nurse can assist the individual to develop good coping skills useful in reducing the anxiety.

Outcomes

The effectiveness of these interventions will be demonstrated by a reduction in the apparent signs and symptoms of anxiety. Another expected outcome is that the client will verbalize a decrease in anxiety.

ALTERATION IN SENSORY–PERCEPTUAL PATTERNS

Clients with spinal cord injury may suffer from sensory perceptual alterations related to a decreased ability to move the head. Sensory information may be lost due to loss of integrity of the ascending spinal pathways.

Assessment

Assessment of the client should include visual field testing and tactile stimulation. Visual field testing allows the nurse to determine the individual's peripheral vision. Response to tactile stimulation should be assessed over the client's body.

Interventions

Several techniques may be useful in assisting the client with decreased visual fields. Prism glasses can be used when the client is supine to allow for reading. Mirrors can be positioned in such a way to permit the client to see more of the surrounding area. Family members can be taught always to approach the client within the confines of his existing visual field. Once areas of good response have been located, touch the client in these areas to increase the amount of tactile information. Encourage the family to assist in this intervention. Occupational therapists can be consulted for additional techniques in increasing response to tactile stimulation (Ulrich, Canale, and Wendell 1986).

Outcome

These techniques should assist the client to establish normal sensory–perceptual patterns.

KNOWLEDGE DEFICIT

Throughout the course of recovery, the family and client will require information. The major areas of concern include prevention of complications, knowledge of procedures and protocols, and adequate information concerning community resources and emergency care facilities.

Assessment

Assess the client's and family's knowledge concerning the disease process and treatment.

Interventions

The home health nurse must teach the client about the many potential complications for the home-bound client with spinal cord injury. Major complications, including contractures, thrombophlebitis, orthostatic hypotension, skin breakdown, autonomic dysreflexia, and injury have been discussed while the nurse assesses the client and intervenes to prevent these complications. Teaching of both client and family can be accomplished. The family should be able to verbalize the symptoms of any complications. For example, any signs of infection (cloudy, foul-smelling urine, fever, chills), unsuccessful bowel or bladder programs, skin breakdown, or decreased range of motion should be reported.

While implementing specific procedures, such as suctioning, skin care, transfer and range of motion exercises, the nurse can also instruct the client and family during a home visit. The nurse can then ask for demonstrations of these techniques in order to assess periodically the family's need for further teaching (Ulrich, Canale, and Wendell 1986).

The home health nurse must also teach the family about appropriate referrals. Since the client is still considered to be acutely ill, the family must be able to access emergency assistance if necessary. The importance of keeping follow-up appointments with the physician and clinic should be emphasized. The family should be able to reach a health-care professional at any time assistance is needed.

Outcomes

Successful interventions will be demonstrated by the client being able to verbalize an understanding of the plan of care. The family and client should be able to discuss the signs and symptoms of complications and should know how to reach help outside of the home when necessary.

An abbreviated plan of care for the client with a spinal cord injury is shown below.

ABBREVIATED CARE PLAN: SPINAL CORD INJURY

Nursing Diagnosis	Assessment	Interventions	Outcomes
Ineffective Breathing Pattern	Respiratory rate Excursion (lung sounds) Tidal volume	Instruct client to deep breathe and cough every 2 hours. Position in semi- to high Fowler's. Increase activity as tolerated.	Client will maintain an effective breathing pattern.

(continued)

ABBREVIATED CARE PLAN: SPINAL CORD INJURY (*continued*)

Nursing Diagnosis	Assessment	Interventions	Outcomes
Ineffective Airway Clearance	Lung sounds Dyspnea Irritability Confusion	Maintain adequate fluid intake. Suction as needed. Utilize chest physical therapy and postural drainage.	Client will maintain clear, open airways.
Alteration in Nutrition	Weight BUN Albumin Calcium	Utilize safety precautions while feeding client. Provide assistive device as needed. Offer supplemental feedings.	Client will maintain an adequate nutritional status.
Alteration in Bowel Elimination	Bowel sounds Palpate abdomen Fullness or discomfort	Maintain fluid intake. Implement measures to assist in evacuation of rectum at regular intervals. Administer stool softeners or laxatives as needed.	Client will evacuate stool according to a usual routine.
Alteration in Urinary Elimination	Intake and output Frequent voiding Urgency Discomfort Incontinence	Utilize mechanical methods to promote complete emptying of bladder. Place client in a position conducive to normal voiding. Perform catheterization as needed. Monitor oral intake.	Client will not experience urinary retention or incontinence.
Impaired Physical Mobility	Range of motion Muscle tone Muscle strength Mobility	Perform range of motion exercises. Utilize assistive devices. Encourage mobility.	The client will achieve maximum physical mobility.

ABBREVIATED CARE PLAN: SPINAL CORD INJURY (*continued*)

Nursing Diagnosis	Assessment	Interventions	Outcomes
Self-Care Deficit	Ability to move in bed Transfer Grasp and grip	Utilize assistive devices. Encourage client and family participation in care.	Client will participate in daily care.
Impaired Skin Integrity	Redness Nutritional status Diabetes Risk factors	Prevent skin irritation. Keep skin clean and dry. Change position frequently.	Client will maintain skin integrity and not experience any areas of redness or breakdown.
Alteration in Tissue Perfusion	Blood pressure Headache Nasal congestion Flushing	Monitor for signs of autonomic dysreflexia and orthostatic hypotension. Identify measures to decrease the pooling of blood in the extremities. Encourage client to change position slowly.	Client will be normotensive and not experience autonomic dysreflexia.
Ineffective Individual Coping	Depression Feelings of inadequacy	Assist client to identify methods to assist in coping. Encourage development and utilization of support systems. Provide referral for counseling as needed.	Client will utilize effective coping skills.
Potential for Family Crisis	Family dynamics Coping strategies Attitudes Knowledge	Establish relationship with family. Provide support groups. Refer for counseling as necessary.	Family will demonstrate evidence of good relationships.
Potential for Anxiety	Irritability	Implement measures to decrease anxiety.	Client will experience a decrease in anxiety.

(continued)

ABBREVIATED CARE PLAN: SPINAL CORD INJURY (*continued*)

Nursing Diagnosis	Assessment	Interventions	Outcomes
Sexual Dysfunction	Restlessness Tachycardia Attitudes Past behaviors	Explain all procedures. Communicate interest and support for client and family. Provide information for client. Initiate referral to additional counseling if necessary.	Client will demonstrate beginning acceptance of sexual dysfunction.
Potential Knowledge Deficit	Knowledge of disease process Treatment	Instruct in methods to prevent and treat complications; spinal cord injury. Instruct in procedures and techniques. Reinforce protocols of therapy. Instruct family in emergency procedures.	Client will demonstrate requisite knowledge concerning spinal cord injury.
Alteration in Sensory-Perceptual Patterns	Visual fields Response to tactile stimulation	Use prism glasses as needed. Increase tactile stimulation.	Client will demonstrate normal sensory—perceptual patterns.

MULTIPLE SCLEROSIS

Multiple sclerosis (MS) is a chronic disease characterized by the presence of numerous areas of demyelinization in the central nervous system. It is a disease of young adults with the highest incidence in those 20 to 40 years of age. The incidence of the disease appears to be higher in the northern Atlantic states, the Great Lakes, and the Pacific Northwest.

Normal conduction occurs through transmission of impulses in myelinated fibers. With multiple sclerosis, normal conduction through the nerve fiber is destroyed.

PATHOPHYSIOLOGY

Multiple sclerosis represents a disseminated demyelinization of individual neurons. The involved areas become edematous, inflamed, and pink. Quickly, macrophages are mobilized to remove the degenerating myelin. The end result of the action of the macrophages is the production of a shrunken area of demyelinization, called a *plaque*. Neither the axon cylinders or cell bodies are destroyed, but the scar disrupts the nerve fiber conduction. Thus, the normal saltatory conduction will be impaired and slowed.

Remission in multiple sclerosis occurs due to healing of the demyelinated areas by sclerotic tissue. Eventually, the symptoms become permanent due to nerve fiber degeneration.

THEORIES OF CAUSATION

The cause of multiple sclerosis remains unknown although there are three major theories that have been proposed to explain this process. One theory involves a virus. One explanation of the virus theory is that of migration: if adults move from high-risk areas to low-risk areas, they retain a high risk for developing multiple sclerosis. However, if migration occurs before age 15, there is a decreased incidence of the disease. This theory is consistent with a possible viral etiology that has a long latent period between initial exposure and clinical onset of the disease (Price and Wilson 1986). It has been proposed that the mechanism of action for these changes may be an autoimmune reaction attacking the myelins.

Several viruses have been identified as possible causative agents in multiple sclerosis. Rubella viruses have been suspected by several investigators. If this virus is involved, it is probably contracted early in life, lies dormant for several years, and then stimulates an autoimmune response.

Genetic factors have also been implicated in multiple sclerosis. Genetic factors render some persons more susceptible to central nervous system invasion by "slow" viruses. The slow viruses have a long incubation period and may develop in conjunction with abnormal immune status.

Finally, histocompatibility antigens, more common in multiple sclerosis than controls, may be related to deficient immunologic defense against viral infection. As with myasthenia, the probable cause of MS is a combination of all of these.

Recent evidence suggests that an immune system response may be involved in multiple sclerosis. Immunoglobulins have been implicated in this immune response. Immunoglobulins are proteins that have either demonstrable antibody activity or chemical and antigenic structures closely related to antibodies or their fragments. All of the immunoglobulins (IgG, IgA, IgM, IgD, and IgE) are widely distributed in body fluids and secretions. It appears that immunoglobulin G (IgG) may be involved in the process of multiple sclerosis (Price and Wilson 1986).

DIAGNOSTIC STUDIES

Several studies assist in the diagnosis of multiple sclerosis, including cerebrospinal fluid analysis, evoked potentials studies, and neuroradiologic studies.

Cerebrospinal fluid analysis reveals elevated total protein (45–75 mg/100ml) and elevated gamma globulin. When the gamma globulins are exposed to electrophoresis, oligoclonal bands are produced in about 95% of patients with MS. Finally, a myelin basic protein assay, an index of active demyelinization, can be measured (Holland et al 1981).

Evoked potential studies indicate a delay in the transmission of neural signals. Although these results are not specific to a particular disease process, they may add necessary data that assist in the diagnosis of MS. Visual evoked potentials, which measure transmission through the optic nerve, have been shown to be abnormal even in patients without visual symptoms (Farlow et al 1986). Thus evoked potential studies may offer an early indication of the presence of MS.

Several neuroradiologic studies may also add valuable information. Electroencephalograms (EEGs) demonstrate abnormalities in about one third of the patients with MS if studies during an acute exacerbation. The abnormalities are identified as slow waves, which appear to be a nonspecific reaction of the brain to an acute local pathological process. Computerized tomography (CT) scans demonstrate a nonspecific ventricular enlargement and cortical atrophy in less than half of the patients with MS (Price and Wilson 1986).

CLINICAL SYMPTOMS

Symptoms and their severity vary considerably in multiple sclerosis. As the disease progresses, symptoms reflect lesions at more than one location within the central nervous system (CNS). In addition, symptoms are referable to several anatomic foci. Symptoms may appear, remit, then reoccur, and worsen.

Although there is wide variance in the symptoms, there are several that are found most commonly. Optic atrophy, Charcot's triad (nystagmus, scanning speech, and intention tremor), signs of pyramidal tract disease (intention tremor, atomic gait, and loss of vibratory sensation), absent abdominal reflexes, and bilateral Babinski's reflex are common. Other symptoms will be discussed under the appropriate nursing diagnoses.

CLINICAL COURSE

Multiple sclerosis is a chronic, progressive disease. Although the onset is usually slow, in rarer cases it can be rapid and abrupt. Gener-

ally, the clinical course is identified by symptoms that occur at separated time intervals.

Specifically, patients with MS may follow several clinical courses. The benign form is characterized by mild or completely remitting attacks with long symptom-free periods. The most common type, exacerbation-remitting, is characterized by periodic acute onset of symptoms followed by partial or complete recovery, with plateaus of stable disability.

The less common forms are slowly progressive and rapidly progressive. The slowly progressive form shows no clear exacerbation and remissions. There is a slow, but steady, deterioration in function. The rapidly progressive form is a continuous functional deterioration over several months or years with high susceptibility to further disabling or life-threatening complications (Price and Wilson 1986). The home health nurse may be working with patients from any one of these categories.

NURSING DIAGNOSES

There are many nursing diagnoses that are appropriate for the patient with MS. In the following pages, the major diagnoses will be described.

POTENTIAL FOR INEFFECTIVE AIRWAY CLEARANCE

Not all clients with MS will experience ineffective airway clearance. However, those with progressive disease and particularly those who are bedridden are at risk for problems in airway clearance due to weakness of the involved muscles. In addition to problems in mobilizing secretions, the client is at risk for aspiration pneumonia.

Assessment

The family will be able to monitor the client for problems in airway clearance. They should be taught to monitor the client carefully while he is eating or drinking. They should evaluate the client's cough for its strength and ability to produce secretions.

On each visit the home health nurse should assess the same parameters. Lung sounds should be assessed for the presence of adventitious sounds, including rales, rhonchi, and wheezes. As a test for the client's ability to cough, the home health nurse can periodically assess vital capacity.

Interventions

The home health nurse will work with the client and family to assure that the client participates in breathing exercises as often as possible. Should the client experience respiratory muscle weakness, incentive spirometry can be used to improve muscle activity.

Several additional techniques can be used to facilitate removal of secretions. These include increasing fluid intake to 2500 cc/day unless contraindicated. Inspired air can be humidified and mucolytic agents used as needed. Physical techniques of percussion, vibration, and postural drainage can also be effective in mobilizing secretions. Once the secretions have been mobilized, it may be necessary to assist the family in an understanding of suctioning techniques.

Outcomes

The client will be expected to have normal respiratory patterns and maintenance of clear, open airways. He will not exhibit any signs of difficulty in airway clearance.

ALTERATION IN MOBILITY

Clients with multiple sclerosis experience alterations in mobility for several reasons including spasticity, muscle weakness, and cerebellar involvement.

Unilateral or asymmetrically distributed spastic weakness occurs in all four limbs. Profound spasticity leading to muscle spasm is not uncommon. The spasticity can cause spontaneous leg jumps. These commonly occur while in bed and during the night and may then awaken the client.

The client may complain of fatigue and heaviness in one leg and may noticeably drag or have poor control over the leg. These changes generally will interfere with the client's ability to walk.

Cerebellar involvement may occur as the disease progresses. With involvement of the cerebellum and corticospinal tracts, uncoordinated voluntary movements may be seen. The client will complain of loss of balance and coordination.

Assessment

Assessment for alterations in mobility are multiple. The best assessment techniques to be used for spasticity are to evaluate deep tendon responses. When spasticity occurs, the tendon reflexes are hyperactive. The home health nurse can also anticipate a Babinski reflex in the lower extremities experiencing the spasticity.

Muscle strength is assessed by watching the client ambulate. If the client experiences muscle weakness, the gait will be unsteady. The nurse also assesses for the more obvious signs of dragging a leg or complaints of pain and stiffness in the extremities.

Cerebellar assessment will help the home health nurse to evaluate the client's coordination. To test for ataxia, the nurse may assess the Romberg sign. For this test, ask the client to stand with his feet together, arms at his side, and close his eyes. The normal individual will sway slightly. However, the client with cerebellar involvement will sway to the extent that he may lose his balance. Instructing the client to open his eyes will usually prevent him from falling. The home health nurse must recognize that safety is a concern in using this test technique. Therefore, the nurse should safeguard the client, preventing him from falling during the test.

Coordination can also be assessed through rapid alternating movements. With this technique, the client is asked to supinate and pronate his hands rapidly on his lap. He is asked to complete this as quickly as possible. A client with cerebellar disease will not be able to complete this test quickly.

Asking the client to walk "heel to toe" is another test for cerebral function. Clients with cerebellar involvement will be unable to walk by placing a heel directly in front of the toes of the other foot. In other words, the client will be unable to walk a straight line. If the home health nurse discovers this finding, it is likely that the client will also experience ataxia.

A final component of cerebellar assessment is to monitor for involuntary movements. These include tremors (both resting and intention), fasciculations, and spasms.

Interventions

Several nursing interventions may be useful in combating spasticity. Daily stretching exercises along with passive or active range of motion exercises help to maintain muscle tone and action. Warm tub baths also can help. However, the nurse must be certain the bath water is *warm* only, since hot water will increase metabolic demands, and will increase weakness. Other interventions that may help to alleviate the spasticity include massage of spastic areas and application of traction, braces, or splints (requiring a physician's order).

Safety issues become a concern when the client experiences cerebellar symptoms. The presence of intention tremors and ataxia present obvious safety problems. Exercises with weights and stabilization devices may help to diminish the effects of intention tremors. Instruct the client and family that excessive physical exertion will increase the tremors. The family should be instructed in ways to assist the client while he is undergoing activities that increase the risk of safety problems. For the client with intention tremors, such activities include eating, particularly hot beverages.

Cerebellar involvement may produce ataxia. A consultation with a physical therapist may be needed to improve the client's gait. The home health nurse can reinforce the gait training and encourage the family to do the same. Supportive equipment such as walkers may be helpful to the ataxic client. The client should be encouraged to ambulate as much as possible, but to avoid excessive fatigue. As with intention tremors, excessive fatigue will also increase ataxia.

Outcomes

The client will be expected to achieve maximum physical mobility and will not experience any of the complications associated with immobility.

ALTERATION IN NUTRITION

Nutritional status can be altered due to several factors including anorexia, dysphagia, and tremors. Some clients with multiple sclerosis experience anorexia due to their decreased activity, anxiety, and sometimes depression. Others may experience the reverse; due to their boredom they may begin to overeat. When cerebellar involvement occurs, the client may develop dysphagia. If the client has tremors and spasticity, he may experience difficulty in feeding himself.

Assessment

Several parameters should be assessed for evaluation of the nutritional status of the client with multiple sclerosis. Parameters such as weight, and triceps skinfold measures can be completed on each visit from the home health nurse. A 72-hour nutritional history or calorie count may be beneficial in determining actual dietary intake. If necessary, the physician can be contacted to order specific tests such as BUN, serum albumin, protein, hemoglobin, hematocrit, cholesterol, and transferrin levels. A more complete discussion of nutritional assessment is found in Chapter 11.

Interventions

One of the home health nurse's top priorities is to assure adequate nutritional intake. Nursing interventions such as feeding the patient and the use of hand braces may be required as aids in providing adequate intake of nutrients. For the client with a small appetite or who is anorexic, the diet should be high in calories and high in protein. If nutritional intake is limited, multiple vitamins may be added to the diet.

For clients who may become depressed or who are immobilized, obesity may become a problem. Once the client begins to gain weight, with the lack of mobility and possible boredom, it may become very difficult to lose weight. Therefore, the patient's weight should be carefully monitored, at lease several times a week.

If spasticity and tremors are present, it may be necessary to prepare the family to feed the patient. The use of hand braces may be required to begin to assure adequate intake of nutrients. If the client experiences dysphagia, the family should be taught not only to assist the client with meals, but also to utilize safety procedures to prevent aspiration during mealtimes. The family should be warned that aspiration can occur anytime the client is eating or drinking.

Outcomes

The client will be expected to maintain normal nutritional status. The family will be able to intervene for problems related to tremors and dysphagia.

LOSS OF SENSATION

Several sensory changes occur in the client with multiple sclerosis. Paresthesia is one of the most common problems. These symptoms are most likely to result from degeneration of the white matter, particularly within the spinal cord.

Assessment

To begin a sensory assessment, the home health nurse will want to ask a series of questions on each visit. The client may complain of numbness, tingling, and the experience of pins and needles in the extremities, which is one of the early signs of sensory changes. Further proprioceptive disorders may also cause a decreased response to temperature and vibration. Some clients may also experience pain. Fifth cranial nerve root involvement may also result in impairment of facial sensations and loss of corneal reflex. In fact, this may be an early indication of multiple sclerosis. Clients may also experience transient, electriclike shocks upon neck flexion (Lhermitte's sign). This finding coincides with destruction in the posterior columns of the spinal cord.

A second aspect of the assessment will be to perform a sensory assessment. Periodically, the home health nurse will want to test all of the primary sensory functions, including tactile sense (light touch), superficial pain, deep pain, vibratory sense, position sense, and temperature. The assessment is completed with the client's eyes closed and proceeds with testing of corresponding body parts on each side of the body. The client will be asked to compare sensations on one side to the same sensations on the opposite side. The client should be able to do the following things during the assessment; interpret sensations correctly (sharp versus dull, hot versus cold); discriminate which side of the body is being stimulated; locate the point on the body where the stimulus is being applied, and if this is proximal or distal to the previous stimulus (Rudy 1984).

Interventions

Once an alteration in sensation is identified, the nursing interventions will be directed towards maximizing safety for the client. Teach both family and client the importance of avoiding extremes of heat and cold since the client with a sensory disorder may not be able to distinguish between these variables. Clients should not be allowed to use heating pads unless they are under direct supervision of a family member. Instruct the client to use visual cues to interpret data usually interpreted in other ways. For example, the client should assess his extremities for lesions or cuts, since he may not be able to feel them. Teach the client to avoid skin trauma.

Outcomes

Clients would be expected to experience minimal complications from existing sensory deficits. The skin should remain intact.

POTENTIAL FOR INJURY RELATED TO VISUAL DEFECTS

Visual changes often represent the initial symptoms of multiple sclerosis. Blurred vision, abnormal visual fields with blind spots (scotoma), diplopia, and vision lost (from several hours to days) are common symptoms referred to as *optic neuritis.* Diplopia result-

ing from brain stem lesions affecting the nuclei or fiber tracts of the extraocular muscles may occur in isolation from other symptoms. Similarly, nystagmus, representing cerebellar involvement may also occur.

Assessment

Assessment of visual abilities is completed through several techniques including visual field testing and visual acuity.

The home health nurse must also assess the potential safety risks presented by changes in visual abilities. Talk with the family and client and attempt to learn how the visual changes interfere with the client's ability to perform his activities of daily living.

Interventions

Objects should be placed within easy reach of the client to prevent injury. Keep the client oriented to the environment and help him to learn methods to compensate for his loss. The use of eye patches may be useful for the patient with diplopia and blurred vision. The home health nurse may need to recommend the use of eye patches to the physician.

Once the visual impairment is identified, it may be possible to assist the client in taking advantage of books with an enlarged type face that he may be able to read. There are also a number of companies who provide books and magazines that have been placed on audiotapes.

Any visual impairment in the client with multiple sclerosis may produce feelings of inadequacy and helplessness. The home health nurse should encourage the client to verbalize his feelings about these changes. Although there are so many different symptoms of multiple sclerosis, often the visual changes are the most dramatic and cause the most change in the individual's life-style.

Outcomes

Clients will experience satisfactory visual functioning. The compensatory measures used will assist the client in his daily activities.

ALTERATION IN PATTERN OF URINARY ELIMINATION

Alterations in patterns of urinary elimination such as incontinence and retention may occur for a variety of reasons. Lesions of the efferent pathways of the corticospinal tract lead to disorders of sphincter control with resulting incontinence. Reduced bladder capacity associated with spastic bladder can also cause incontinence.

Urinary retention, related to hypotonic bladder, associated with interruption of afferent pathways from the bladder, can occur. As a result of the retention, urinary tract infections may also occur.

Assessment

The home health nurse will begin the assessment with an evaluation of possible symptoms of incontinence. The family and client can offer a report of any problems with incontinence. Comments from the client concerning an inability to respond to physical clues to empty the bladder should be carefully evaluated.

If urinary retention is a concern, the client may experience several symptoms including frequent voiding of small amounts of urine, complaints of urgency, bladder fullness, and suprapubic discomfort. Information concerning intake and output will also be helpful; retention should be suspected if the fluid intake exceeds output. If retention is a problem, the home health nurse will want to palpate the client for bladder distention on each visit.

In the client with urinary retention, the presence of a urinary tract infection should be suspected. Symptoms such as frequent voiding of small amounts of urine, complaints of urgency, bladder fullness, suprapubic discomfort and fever are consistent with an infection.

Interventions

There are many nursing interventions that may assist the client and family in coping with alterations in urinary elimination.

Measures should be instituted that help the client to the bathroom every 2 to 3 hours. Oral fluid intake in the evening can be limited to decrease the possibility of nighttime incontinence. Clients can also be taught perineal exercises in order to improve sphincter tone, which will assist in maintenance of continence. These exercises include stopping and starting stream during voiding, pressing the buttocks together, and then relaxing the muscles.

One of the goals for the home health nurse is to assist the patient and family in the implementation of measures to prevent urinary retention. These include performing actions that will help to facilitate voiding, such as running water, pouring warm water over the perineum, or placing the client's hands in warm water. The client can also be instructed to perform the Credé's technique to facilitate emptying of the bladder.

In extreme cases it may be necessary to utilize either intermittent catheterization or an indwelling Foley catheter. If an indwelling catheter is used, it must be changed every month. With intermittent catheterization, the home health nurse will teach the client and/ or family to perform the technique.

If a urinary tract infection occurs, the client should be encouraged to increase his fluid intake to 2000 cc per day. Vitamin C and cranberry juice have been helpful in decreasing the incidence of the infections (Ulrich, Canale, and Wendell 1986).

Outcomes

The client will experience urinary continence and no urinary retention. The client will also be free from urinary infections.

SEXUAL DYSFUNCTION

With a decrease in genital sensation and a decrease in urinary sphincter control, sexual dysfunction can occur. Impotence has been reported in male patients with MS and is thought to be related to lesions of the spinal cord (Szasz et al 1984). A decreased libido related to weakness, fear of urinary incontinence, and spasms of the hips and legs have also been described (Szasz et al 1984).

Assessment

Refer to discussion under Spinal Cord Injury.

Interventions

Some interventions that may help include discussing alternative methods of sexual gratification and identification of other erotic areas. A more complete discussion can be found under the same nursing diagnosis in the section on Spinal Cord Injury.

Outcome

The client will demonstrate a beginning acceptance of changes in sexual function.

IMPAIRED COMMUNICATION

Dysarthria and scanning speech (words broken into syllables with pauses between the syllables) produce a profound speech impairment for the individual with MS. Communication can be further impaired because of ataxia of the vocal mechanisms associated with cerebellar lesions.

Assessment

On each visit, the home health nurse will assess for difficulties in verbal communication. The specific patterns of speech should be noted. Look specifically for problems in articulation and slowed speech.

Interventions

The nurse must establish a means of communication and listen carefully when the client talks. Speech therapists can be contacted to teach the patient exercises to strengthen the muscles of phonation. Communication can be facilitated by helping the family to anticipate the client's needs, thereby decreasing the burden on the client to communicate. Teach the family to ask question that can be answered with short phrases or words. Above all, the patient and family should work to maintain a calm approach and allow ample time for the client to communicate.

Outcome

The client will effectively communicate needs and desires.

ALTERATION IN THOUGHT PROCESSES

As the multiple sclerosis progresses, the individual may experience euphoria. This unrealistic feeling of well-being is due to involvement of the white matter of the frontal lobes. This symptom does not occur in all patients with MS. Other thought processes such as memory, problem solving abilities and general emotional responses may also be affected.

Assessment

There are many methods that can be used for assessment of memory. Remote memory is tested by asking questions such as "when and where were you born?"; "How old are you now?" "How old were you when you were married?" Responses to these questions can be checked with the family. Intermediate memory can be tested by referring to personal and general events of the last 5 years. Recent memory can be tested by questions concerning recent events, such as "When were you released from the hospital?"

A problem-solving ability can be tested by asking the client to respond to questions that would require some judgment and problem-solving skills before answering. For example, questions could be used such as "what would you do if you locked your keys in your car?"; "What would you do if the smoke alarm went off in your home?" However, the home health nurse must, take into account the client's life experiences and his mode of living. The questions should be structured in such a way that the client is able to perceive the circumstances of the situation described.

On each visit, the home health nurse will evaluate the emotional stability of the client. Listening to the client and watching his facial expressions and general movements constitute ways of evaluating general mood and emotional response. The client should be assessed for outward displays of anger, hostility, or euphoria. During this assessment, the input of the family will be invaluable. For example, outwardly, the client may appear calm and relaxed to the nurse, but the family may have experienced a very different side of the client. The nurse will also want to develop an impression of how labile the client's responses may be.

Interventions

Nursing interventions to assist the client in coping with alterations in thought processes are numerous. Inherent in the use of any nursing interventions is an understanding of the degree of involvement of the client and whether the problem identified is of organic or psychological basis. For example, euphoria in the patient is consistent with damage in the white matter of the frontal lobe. Therefore this symptom has a physiological base and cannot be changed with interventions. Rather, interventions will be directed towards helping the client and family cope with the changes.

Several interventions can assist the client with impaired memory. These include encouraging the client to write down questions or concerns. The home health nurse can also provide written or taped instructions/information whenever possible for the client.

If the client suffers from problems with reasoning, the nurse can intervene by trying to keep environmental stimuli to a minimum. The family will be instrumental in maintaining an environment that will support the client. Allow adequate time for teaching sessions. The home health nurse can also teach the family to encourage the client to validate all decisions with them. Both the family and nurse can be instrumental in assisting the client to problem-solve.

A major role for the home health nurse is to help the family and client develop realistic expectations of the client's ability to learn, understand, and remember information. The family plays a critical role in helping maintain the client's safety.

Outcome

The client will be able to utilize compensatory mechanisms for the alterations in memory, problem solving, and emotional responses.

DISTURBANCE IN SELF-CONCEPT

Clients with multiple sclerosis undergo a number of physical and mental changes that necessitate changes in their life-style and roles. The goal of nursing interventions for this problem is to assist the client in formulating an improved self-concept.

Assessment

Nursing assessment for this diagnosis will help to determine the meaning of all of the changes in the individual client caused by the disease. The changes in appearance, dependency, change in life-style and roles and their effect on the individual must be assessed. Encourage the client to verbalize his feelings concerning the changes. Unfortunately, there are no specific ways to evaluate the client's self-concept. Rather, through expert critical analysis of the client's responses, the nurse must begin to understand the overall effect of the changes.

Interventions

There are several specific nursing interventions that may be of some assistance as the nurse works to help the client develop an improved self-concept. Assist the client to identify strengths and qualities that have a positive effect on his self-concept. The nurse can also assist the client to identify various coping techniques that have been used successfully in the past. Although the client may have several coping techniques that are used frequently, he may not be able to identify them as techniques. Through discussion and analysis, the home health nurse may be able to assist the client in proper identification of these techniques.

The family and significant others will play a vital role in assisting the client to develop an improved self-concept. Assist the family to develop the skills to listen attentively to the client. Help the family to identify others who may be able to spend time with the patient and to offer support. Provide information about and encourage utilization of community agencies or support groups.

If the client continues to experience a disturbance in self-concept, the home health nurse may need to consult with the physician for the purpose of recommending psychological counseling. That type of support may be beneficial for short-term or long-term therapy.

Outcome

The client will demonstrate adaptation to the changes imposed by the disease process. The client and family will be able to verbalize their feelings to the home health nurse.

KNOWLEDGE DEFICIT

The pathophysiology, treatment, and prognosis of multiple sclerosis are quite detailed and intricate. Clients tend to progress more rapidly and experience less complications when they have a good understanding of all of the necessary information. As the stages of the disease change, the client and family will require additional information.

Assessment

With every change in therapy, the home health nurse can assess the client's and family's understanding of the processes they are experiencing. Simple questions such as "How have things been since my last visit?" will help to uncover many things and may be instrumental in identifying where the knowledge gaps can be found.

Interventions

The client and family should understand the potential for possible exacerbation and return or progression of the disease. Thus the client should avoid infections, extreme fatigue, and emotional stress, all of which can precipitate an exacerbation. Teach all of the signs and symptoms of exacerbation, so that the family and client will be able to access appropriately the health care system.

Offer extensive information on the disease process, treatment, drug therapy, and follow-up. Keep the family and client informed about community referrals and knowing when and where to call for help. From time to time, fads in the treatment of multiple sclerosis surface and clients may be tempted to utilize unusual methods for treatment. Make sure that the clients have the necessary information to make informed decisions relative to these treatments.

Work with the client and family to prevent premature disability due to despair and resignation to the disease. Allow the client time to grieve. Once he is ready, help him to explore future goals and assist him in making realistic plans. Help the client avoid activities that would serve to hurt his self-concept.

Offer assistance by referrals to vocational counselors and possible financial counselors. Be alert to the need for additional help within the home for normal family responsibilities.

Outcomes

The client and family will be able to identify methods to maintain independence. They will also be able to identify ways to decrease the risk of disease exacerbation. Client and family will verbalize an understanding of the identified plan of care.

IMPAIRED SKIN INTEGRITY

When the client with multiple sclerosis has remained immobile for a period of time, the potential exists for a breakdown in skin. Prolonged or uneven pressure on the tissues,

the use of splints and braces, and the presence of urinary incontinence can worsen the problem.

Assessment

The family can be instructed to inspect the client's skin on a daily basis. In particular, they should check areas such as bony prominences, dependent areas, skin under the braces, and the perineal area for redness and breakdown. On each visit, the home health nurse should assess the same areas. A detailed account of skin assessment can be found in Chapter 17.

Interventions

An extensive discussion on interventions to decrease the potential for alteration in skin integrity can be found in Chapter 17.

Outcome

The client would be expected to maintain skin integrity. No reddened areas would be noted.

SELF-CARE DEFICIT

With the physical limitations imposed by the progression of multiple sclerosis, the client will most likely experience a self-care deficit. He will experience difficulty, therefore, in completing the normal activities of daily living.

Assessment

See the discussion under Spinal Cord Injury.

Interventions

All interventions that help to increase the client's ability to perform self-care activities are beneficial (see discussion under Spinal Cord Injury). In addition, if the client experiences intention tremors, the use of weighted eating utensils may help. Clients who experience impairments in visual function will require assistance from the family in identifying the location of various self-care objects.

Outcome

The client will perform self-care activities within his physical limitations.

ALTERATION IN BOWEL ELIMINATION

The decreased activity associated with multiple sclerosis may cause constipation. Improper diet, particularly one low in fluids and fiber, may serve to worsen the situation.

Assessment

The assessment of a client for constipation is discussed in detail under Spinal Cord Injury.

Interventions

The interventions are discussed under Spinal Cord Injury.

Outcome

The client will maintain a normal pattern of bowel elimination.

POTENTIAL FOR INJURY RELATED TO DRUG THERAPY

In the recent past, ACTH and immunosuppressive therapy have been used to decrease the severity of an exacerbation of MS. Although this therapy has taken place in the hospital, it can be expected that it will soon take place in the home.

Assessment

ACTH is an anterior pituitary hormone that stimulates the adrenal cortex to produce and secrete adrenal cortical hormones. This effect is meant to assist the individual positively in coping with the stress of an illness. ACTH produces two major types of effects; glucocorticoid (metabolism of fats, proteins, and carbohydrates) and mineralocorticoids (sodium and water balance).

Thus, use of the drug can cause several effects on the patient. There may be sodium and water retention leading to hypertension and congestive heart failure. Hypokalemia can occur resulting in alkalosis, weakness, and an irregular pulse. ACTH will increase insulin requirements and may produce symptoms of diabetes in latent diabetics. Since ACTH causes protein catabolism, negative nitrogen balance can result, leading to weight loss, anemia, anorexia, fragile and thin skin, and poor wound healing. With ACTH, there may be a sympathetic response to stress that can produce stomach ulcers.

Interventions

The general dosage of ACTH is 40 to 50 units twice a day for 7 to 10 days. Intravenous infusion is 500 cc of D5W with 80 units of ACTH for 3 days, followed by 40 units IM every 12 hours for 7 days. During this therapy the patient must be observed for the above symptoms and the usual steroid precautions instituted.

The family will be instrumental in helping the home health nurse follow the client's response to these potentially dangerous drugs. The family should be taught the name, dosage, action, and expected effects of the drugs. They should always be given an emergency number to call in the event of an untoward drug reaction.

Outcome

The client will experience minimal side-effects from the drugs.

ASSESSING THE HOME ENVIRONMENT

Prior to the transfer of the client with a spinal cord injury from the hospital to home, several aspects of the home environment must be evaluated. Factors such as the location of the bathroom, electrical capabilities, and availability of equipment must be evaluated.

The home must also be carefully evaluated for the safety needs of the client with multiple sclerosis. Adequate electrical outlets must be available to support needed equipment. Methods for communication must be established so that the client will be able to have his needs met in a timely manner.

References

Adelstein W, Watson P: Cervical spine injuries. J Neurosurg Nurs 15(2): 65–71, 1983

Bates B: A Guide to Physical Examination and History Taking. Philadelphia, JB Lippincott, 1983

Collins WF: A review of treatment of spinal cord injury. J Surg 71(12): 974–975, 1984

de la Torre JC: Spinal cord injury. Spine 6(4): 315–335, 1981

Farlow MR, Markand ON, Edwards MK, et al: Multiple sclerosis: Magnetic resonance imaging, evoked responses, and spinal fluid electrophoresis. Neurology 36(6): 828–831, 1986

Grundy D, Russell J: ABC of spinal cord injury. Later management and complications. II. Br Med J (Clin Res) 292(6522): 743–745, 1985

Guyton AC: Textbook of Medical Physiology. Philadelphia, WB Saunders, 1986

Hall LH: Circadian rhythms, implications for geriatric rehabilitation. Nurs Clin North Am 11(4): 631–638, 1976

Holland NJ et al: Overview of multiple sclerosis and nursing care of the MS patient. J Neurosurg Nurs 13(1): 28–33, 1981

Maynard FM: Immobilization hypercalcemia following spinal cord injury. Arch Phys Med Rehabil 67(1): 41–44, 1986

Mitchell PH, Loustau A: Concepts Basic to Nursing. New York, McGraw-Hill, 1981

Price SA, Wilson LM: Pathophysiology. New York, McGraw-Hill, 1986

Rudy EB: Advanced Neurological and Neurosurgical Nursing. St. Louis, CV Mosby, 1984

Sugarman B: Medical complications of spinal cord injury. Quart J Med 54(213): 3–18, 1985

Szasz G, Paty D, Maurice WL: Sexual dysfunctions in multiple sclerosis. Ann NY Acad Sci 436: 443–452, 1984

Ulrich SP, Canale SW, Wendell SA: Nursing Care Planning Guides. Philadelphia, WB Saunders, 1986

Suggested Reading

Albion JH: Multiple sclerosis: A chronic care focus. Nurs Pract (5): 29–35, 1983

Aranson B: Multiple sclerosis: Current concepts and management. Hosp Pract 17: 81–89, 1982

Bamford E, Grundy D, Russell J: ABC of spinal cord injury. Social needs of the patient and his family. Br Med J (Clin Res). 292(6519): 546–548, 1986

Brackett TO, Condon N, Kindelan KM, Bassett L: The emotional care of a person with a spinal cord injury. JAMA 252(6): 793–795, 1984

Braughler JM, Hall ED: Current application of "high-dose" steroid therapy for CNS injury. A pharmacological perspective. J Neurosurg 62(6): 806–810, 1985

Clifford DB, Trotter JL: Pain in multiple sclerosis. Arch Neurol 41(12): 1270–1272, 1984

Cotman CW, Nieto–Sampedro M: Progress in facilitating the recovery of function after central nervous system trauma. Ann NY Acad Sci 457: 83–104, 1985

Coyle PK, Sibony PA: Tear analysis in multiple sclerosis. Neurology 36(4): 547–550, 1986

Davies GM: The problems of nursing patients with advanced multiple sclerosis at home. J Adv Nurs 4: 635–635, 1979

DeJong G, Branch LG, Corcoran PJ: Independent living outcomes in spinal cord injury: Multivariate analyses. Arch Phys Med Rehabil 65(2): 66–73, 1984

DeVivo JJ, Fine PR: Spinal cord injury: Its short-term impact on marital status. Arch Phys Med Rehabil 66(8): 501–504, 1985

Dudas ST, Stevens KA: Central cord injury: Implications for Nursing. J Nurosurg Nurs 16(2): 84–88, 1984

Egerton J, Grundy D, Russell J: ABC of spinal cord injury. Nursing. Br Med J (Clin Res) 292(6516): 325–329, 1986

Frankel D: Long-term care issues in multiple sclerosis. Rehabil Lit 45(9–10): 282–285, 1984

Friedman–Campbell M, Hart CA: Theoretical strategies and nursing interventions to promote psychosocial adaptation to spinal cord injuries and disability. J Neurosurg Nurs 16(6): 335–342, 1984

Giesser B: Multiple sclerosis. Current concepts in management. Drugs 29(1): 88–95, 1985

Grundy D, Russell J: ABC of spinal cord injury. Later management and complications. I. Br Med J (Clin Res) 292(6521): 677–680, 1986

Green BC, Pratt CC, Grigsby TE: Self-concept among persons with long-term spinal cord injury. Arch Phys Med Rehabil 65(12): 751–754, 1984

Hall ED, Braughler JM: Glucocorticoid mechanisms in acute spinal cord injury: A review and therapeutic rationale. Surg Neurol 18(5): 320–327, 1982

Hart LK: Fatigue in the patient with multiple sclerosis. Res Nurs Health 1(4): 147–157, 1978

Howard M, Corbo–Pelaia SA: Psychological after-effects of halo traction. Am J Nurs 82(12): 1839–1843, 1982

Kinnersly D, Grundy D, Russell J: ABC of spinal cord injury. Transfer of care from hospital to community. Br Med J (Clin Res) 292(6520): 607–609, 1986

Kurtzke JF, Beebe GW, Norman JE, Jr: Epidemiology of multiple sclerosis in US veterans: III. Migration and the risk of MS. Neurology 35(5): 672–678, 1985

LaRocca NG: Psychosocial factors in multiple sclerosis and the role of stress. Ann NY Acad Sci 436: 435–442, 1984

Levine AM: Management of multiple sclerosis. How to improve the quality of life. Postgrad Med 77(5): 121–123, 126–127, 1985

Limid S, Chia JK, Kohli A, Cid E: Chronic pain in spinal cord injury: Comparison between inpatients and outpatients. Arch Phys Med Rehabil 66(11): 777–778, 1985

Luce JM: Medical management of spinal cord injury. Crit Care Med 13(2): 126–131, 1985

Lugger L: Spinal cord injury: Nutritional management. J Neuosurg Nurs 15(5): 310–312, 1983

Meyers AR, Feltin M, Master RJ et al: Rehospitalization and spinal cord injury: Cross-sectional survey of adults living independently. Arch Phys Med Rehabil 66(10): 704–708, 1985

Mickey MR, Ellison GW, Myers LW: An illness severity score for multiple sclerosis. Neurology 34(10): 1343–1347, 1984

Myllynen P, Kammonen M, Rokkanen P et al: Deep venous thrombosis and pulmonary embolism in patients with acute spinal cord injury: A comparison with nonparalyzed patients immobilized due to spinal fractures. J Trauma 25(6): 541–543, 1985

Richards JS: Psychologic adjustment to spinal cord injury during first postdischarge year. Arch Phys Med Rehabil 67(6): 362–365, 1986

Sanders EA, Rewlen JP, Van der Velde EA et al: The diagnosis of multiple sclerosis. Contribution of nonclinical tests. J Neurol Sci 72(2–3): 273–285, 1986

Sargant C, Braun MA: Occupational therapy management of the acute spinal cord-injured patient. Am J Occup Ther 40(5): 333–337, 1986

Schapiro RT, van den Noort S, Scheinberg L: The current management of multiple sclerosis. Ann NY Acad Sci 436: 425–434, 1984

Scheinberg LC, Van den Noort S: Editorial. Multiple sclerosis treatments. Neurology 36(5): 703–704, 1986

Stanton GM: A needs assessment of significant others following the patient's spinal cord injury. J Neurosurg Nurs 16(5): 253–256, 1984

Sterman AB, Coyle PK, Panasci DJ et al: Disseminated abnormalities of cardiovascular autonomic functions in multiple sclerosis. Neurology 35(11): 1665–1168, 1985

Sypert GW: Early management of spinal injuries. Am Fam Physician 29(5): 113–122, 1984

Toth LL: Spasticity management in spinal cord injury. Rehab Neurosurg (1): 14–17, 1983

Wise G: Learning to live with multiple sclerosis. Nurs Times 81(15): 37–40, 1985

Wood J, Stell R, Unsworth I et al: A double-blind trial of hyperbaric oxygen in the treatment of multiple sclerosis. Med J Aust 143(6): 238–240, 1985

Woolsey RM: Rehabilitation outcome following spinal cord injury. Arch Neurol 42(2): 116–119, 1985

ALTERATIONS IN NEUROENDOCRINE CONTROL

15

Angela P. Clark

Many disorders fall under the neuroendocrine category. These include thyroid, pituitary, and metabolic disorders. Of these, metabolic disorders, specifically diabetes mellitus, are seen more commonly.

Although diabetes is a common phenomenon, it is also one that may progress into an emergency. In this chapter, the general phenomenon of diabetes will be discussed. The acute manifestations of the disease including diabetic ketoacidosis and hyperosmolar coma will be presented, and the role of the home health nurse in the care of the client with diabetes will be emphasized throughout.

DIABETES MELLITUS

Diabetes mellitus is a chronic, hereditary disease characterized by high blood glucose and the urinary excretion of glucose. All or part of the ability to use carbohydrates has been lost because of a deficiency in insulin or an inability of the body to use any available insulin.

PATHOPHYSIOLOGY

There are two main types of diabetes mellitus. Type I diabetes is insulin-dependent (IDDM) and Type II diabetes (NIDDM) is noninsulin dependent. The two types both fit the above definition of inability to use carbohydrates and hyperglycemia, but the causes are quite different.

In Type I diabetes, there is an insulin deficit due to islet cell (pancreas) loss. It is thought to be associated with a genetic predisposition to respond to a particular virus or some autoimmune phenomenon resulting in islet cell antibodies. Type I often has an abrupt onset with acute symptoms, such as diabetic ketoacidosis. The genetic predisposition is seen in a specific human leukocyte antigen (HLA) (Clark 1985). The onset of Type I diabetes seems to peak around puberty, with females diagnosed at a slightly earlier age than males. It is one and a half times more common in whites than in blacks. There will be about 13,000 new cases this year of this type of diabetes. Type I comprises 5% to 10% of all cases of diabetes (Coughlin and Kahn 1986).

434

Type II diabetes has a very different origin. It is associated with a deficiency in the quantity and quality of insulin receptors that normally facilitate the movement of glucose into the cell. Thus, if glucose molecules cannot enter the cell, hyperglycemia will result. When insulin levels are measured in the typical overweight patient with Type II diabetes, normal or increased amounts of insulin are present. However, the insulin cannot be used by the cells because a structural part of the cell is abnormal—the receptor site.

A recent study (Haffner et al 1986) demonstrated that the distribution of body fat influences insulin resistance. It has long been known that obesity was linked to insulin resistance. This study found a more centralized distribution of body fat in Mexican Americans, who have three to five times the prevalence of NIDDM, or type II diabetes as the normal population. This is the most common type of diabetes and occurs in about 90% of all cases. Typically, clients are overweight, older at the time of diagnosis, and have a family history of diabetes. These individuals may require insulin periodically for hyperglycemia during stress, but do not have the basic lack of insulin production seen in Type I diabetes (American Diabetes Association 1981). An estimated one in 25 persons over age of 20 has Type II diabetes (Coughlin and Kahn 1986).

Insulin is normally produced by the beta cells in the islets of Langerhans. About 50 units of insulin are produced daily and a larger amount is usually stored in the pancreas. The stored insulin awaits the stimulus of glucose for its release. When the glucose level rises, as after food intake, the pancreas immediately begins to produce and secrete insulin. The insulin then facilitates the movement of glucose into the cell to be used in energy production. A few select tissues do not require insulin to facilitate glucose entry, such as the brain and liver. Insulin also increases glycogen storage into the tissues, which can later be converted back to glucose, if needed.

NURSING DIAGNOSES

Because of the complexity of the nature of diabetes and its many complications, almost all of the nursing diagnoses might be seen in the population of clients with diabetes mellitus. However, this chapter will describe the primary ones seen most commonly in the care of diabetic clients. Assessment data, selected interventions, and outcomes for evaluation will be discussed.

ALTERATION IN TISSUE PERFUSION: PERIPHERAL SYSTEM

One of the leading complications of diabetes is microvascular disease, or large vessel disease. It can be manifested in several ways; however accelerated peripheral vascular disease is a major and much feared complication. The amputation rate is 17 times greater for a person with diabetes than a nondiabetic. The prevention of diabetic foot disease and good foot care are major goals for these clients.

While microvascular disease is *most* commonly seen in persons with Type II diabetes, clients who have Type I diabetes may also be at risk because of their predisposition to neuropathy, which can be a part of the disease process. The disease process is similar to the atherosclerosis seen in the normal population but occurs at an earlier age and advances more rapidly.

There has been some disagreement as to the exact pathology in diabetic foot disease. Some clinicians believe it to be a function of small-vessel disease (microaniopathy) but physiologic research has not supported this theory. Actually, the same amount of small vessel disease has been seen in diabetics and nondiabetics in vessels as small as 10 mm (LoGerfo and Coffman 1984).

Diabetic peripheral vascular disease is associated with involvement of the arterioles and the larger arteries. These arteries control peripheral vascular resistance and regulate capillary blood flow; thus they play a critical role in tissue perfusion (Levin and O'Neal, 1983). There may also be some functional changes in the capillaries in the diabetic circulation. A major cause of foot disease may be diabetic neuropathy, particularly in the presence of a normal arterial system.

Assessment

The home health nurse will want to evaluate the client for the multiple risk factors that appear to be related to the development of peripheral vascular disease. These include hypertriglyceridemia, hypertension, and cigarette smoking. Obviously, each of these risk factors can be controlled to some degree and should be evaluated with the client. It appears that a combination of these risk factors is particularly harmful (Levin and O'Neal 1983).

The client should also be assessed for signs of peripheral vascular disease including cool extremities, changes in skin color, diminished arterial pulsations, gangrene, claudication, blood pressure changes in extremities, and slow healing of lesions.

Nursing assessment of the client should begin with data about the history of any foot and leg problems, such as years of "coldness" or leg aches. The client may be unaware of decreased circulation. Next, the home health nurse should proceed with a thorough examination of the feet and legs, to determine the presence (or absence) of pedal and popliteal pulses, color, skin temperature, shiny skin, and loss of hair on foot or toes. If the feet or legs are cool, pulses diminished, or there is a loss of hair a venous or arterial insufficiency should be suspected. Determine how the client cares for his feet. Lastly, assess for the presence of the associated risk factors of hypertension, elevated lipids, or cigarette smoking.

Intervention

There are several nursing interventions for this diagnosis. Teach the client to do a systematic inspection of his feet *daily* to check for any red or bruised areas, blisters, fungal infections, calluses. If the client's vision is impaired, teach a family member to do this. Stress the importance of good footwear that is well fitting, wearing new shoes only a few hours a day until they are stretched and more resilient. The feet should be washed daily and a thin layer of vaseline or lanolin applied to seal in normal moisture (see Nursing Diagnosis: Impaired Tissue Integrity). To avoid injury and other potential problems, the need for keeping the toenails clipped should be stressed. If the family is unable to assist the client in clipping of the toenails, it may be necessary to refer the client to a podiatrist.

Cigarette smoking must be avoided by these clients. In addition to being associated with an increase in foot disease, smoking leads to a high incidence of amputations (LoGervo and Coffman 1984). A single cigarette may narrow arteries and reduce blood flow for as long as 1 hour (Levin and O'Neal 1983). Smoking may cause intimal narrowing or may be related to platelet aggregation.

The client should be told to seek further evaluation of any new lesion or ulcer. In the early stages, chances of successful treatment are much greater. The physician may use vascular laboratory studies to detect peripheral vascular disease areas, such as studies using a Doppler.

Another nursing intervention involves helping the client to develop strategies for the reduction of hypertension and elevated lipids. One study has found that higher systolic blood pressures were associated with "poorest" levels of glucose control (Klein, Klein, and Moss 1984). Dietary control is the most important intervention to decrease lipids. The use of drug therapy may also be indicated. A further discussion of these interventions can be found in Chapter 10.

If a lack of sensation in the feet is present (peripheral insensitivity), teach the client about the dangers of this symptom and plan (with him) ways to avoid complications. For example, a lack of pain from new shoes is no indication that it is alright to wear them all day. Stress that pain is a *reminder,* so the absence of pain takes on special significance. Brand (1983) discusses several diagnostic and therapeutic areas related to shoes, shoe inserts, and walking management. The reader is referred to this source if needed. Another safety measure is to teach the client to test his bath water with his hands rather than with his feet. Encourage him to fill the tub with cold water first, then add hot water. This should protect the client from a burn.

Several other nursing interventions may assist the client in living with the day-to-day changes caused by diabetes. Instruct the client to change positions slowly in order to allow time for normal mechanisms to adjust to position changes. Encourage the family to maintain a room temperature that is comfortable for the client. Often, the client feels "cold" and may require a higher environmental temperature for comfort than does the family.

Active leg and foot exercises can assist in the promotion of circulation. Counsel the client to avoid the use of constrictive hosiery. If the physician orders peripheral vasodilator drugs, assist the client and family in monitoring for potential effects.

Outcome

An expected goal for this nursing diagnosis is that the client will be able to assess circulation in his feet and legs and take appropriate action. Effective individualized nursing interventions can help the client reach this goal.

ALTERATION IN TISSUE PERFUSION: CARDIAC SYSTEM

Tissue perfusion is altered in the diabetic client by involvement of the cardiovascular system. Coronary artery disease is the most common cause of death in Type II diabetes, but it is also found in clients with Type I. Diabetes is a well-known risk factor for heart disease.

There are three layers in the artery walls — the intima, the media, and the adventia. The intima, the innermost layer, comes in direct contact with the blood. Fibrous thickening of the intima begins in infancy and progresses from that point. Atherosclerosis initially involves the intima but progresses until the media is involved. When this happens, elastic membranes are destroyed and the vessel wall can be stretched and dilated, predisposing the client to possible aneurysms. In addition, the intima can undergo necrosis as a result of plaque formation (Levin and O'Neal 1983).

None of the conventional heart disease risk factors completely explain the excess occurrence of heart disease in diabetic patients. Much remains to be known about the relationship of diabetes and heart disease. It is possible that some less traditional risk factors may be found to be related, such as the increased platelet adhesiveness seen in diabetics or the increased fibrinogen concentrations (Barrett-Conner and Orchard 1985).

One very important aspect of diabetic heart disease is the incidence of painless or asymptomatic myocardial ischemia. It may be explained partially by diabetic neuropathy involving cardiac afferent nerves (Hume et al 1986). This finding is well established in the literature but not well understood. In clients with known diabetes, blood glucose control after myocardial infarction is often poor and may contribute to increased mortality. Myocardial infarction induces several metabolic changes, including excess catecholamine secretion and suppression of endogenous insulin secretion (Husband et al 1985).

Another factor involving diabetes and heart disease is the influence of myocardial infarction on glucose intolerance. Many nurses have noted the hyperglycemia seen postinfarction for many days. In one study, 65% of patients without known diabetes had fasting hyperglycemia that lasted over 10 days. After 1 month, it decreased to 20% (Fein and Scheuer 1983).

Assessment

Key signs of alteration in tissue perfusion that the home health nurse should note include chest pain and complaints of fatigue. Other areas to assess include history of any chest pain, shortness of breath, fatigue, palpitations, or blood pressure changes. The nurse should evaluate which of the cardiac risk factors are present in the client, such as elevated lipids, obesity, sedentary life-style, birth control pills, hypertension, and cigarette smoking. Find out what medications the client is taking that may affect cardiovascular status. Assess dietary habits and other life-style factors.

Check major pulses and auscultate the precordial area, listening for an S_3 (pre- or early congestive heart failure) or an S_4 (hypertension). Note the rate and rhythm of the heart, as hypoxia of the heart can predispose the client to arrhythmias.

Interventions

After a data base is developed, the home health nurse can plan needed nursing inter-

ventions. The client may need education about medications—type, timing, side-effects—to ensure protection of the heart function. Educate him about high risk factors that may influence his future health, such as cigarette smoking.

If the client ever experiences chest pain, discuss the importance of reporting this to his physician if there is any change in its pattern. The nurse may teach the client to check his blood pressure at home to evaluate any blood pressure change.

Outcome

The client should be able to detect any physical changes related to cardiac function and seek consultation when needed.

IMPAIRED THOUGHT PROCESSES

An alteration or impairment in thought processes may be seen in the person with diabetes for one of several reasons, including impaired cerebral perfusion and hypoglycemia.

Cerebral metabolism is dependent on circulating serum glucose in the brain. There is little or no glucose storage in the brain, so the circulating glucose is fuel for energy needs. When serum glucose levels are low, this energy source is compromised, and significant adaptation time is needed to switch to the use of fatty acids as a secondary source. Both hypoglycemia and hyperglycemia have been shown to alter normal electrocardiograph activity.

Hypoglycemia is a continuous threat for the person who is insulin-dependent. A recent study (Casparie and Elving 1985) determined that clients need to be taught to respond more adequately to changing circumstances during daily living and to be more alert to warning signs that may reduce the incidence of hypoglycemia. In this study, the subjects experienced hypoglycemia due to administration of more insulin than needed by the client, improper combinations of short-, intermediate-, and long-acting insulins, and client errors in administration of the drug.

The effect of serum glucose changes on selected verbal skills was evaluated by Holmes et al (1984). Results showed significantly disrupted naming or labeling skills during hypoglycemia. Accuracy was not always impaired but the rate of response was very slow. During hyperglycemia, subjects did not have significant impaired skills in verbal fluency, but a trend toward poorer performance was seen.

Hyperglycemia results when there is too much glucose and not enough insulin present. The deficiency of insulin may be relative or absolute. There are several possible causes for hyperglycemia including too little insulin, improper eating habits, and decreased exercise.

Hyperglycemia may also result from emotional stress. When an individual is upset, epinephrine from the adrenal medulla is released into the blood, increasing the rate of glycogenolysis and hence the discharge of glucose from the liver. Also, the adrenocorticotrophic hormone (ACTH) causes a release of glucocorticoids from the adrenal cortex, promoting gluconeogenesis.

Infection and fever also increase blood glucose levels by activating the adrenal medulla and cortex, which produce epinephrine and cortisol respectively.

Assessment

Symptoms that may indicate an impaired thought process include impaired attention span, impaired recall abilities, impaired perception, impaired decision making, or inappropriate behavior. Nurses who have seen clients during an insulin reaction recognize that many of these are present.

Other signs that may be present include nervousness, irritability, numbness in lips or tongue, tachycardia, nausea, headache, blurred vision, or a sleepy feeling. If hypoglycemia is suspected, a blood glucose level below 50 mg/dl can be expected. The signs and symptoms of hypoglycemia and hyperglycemia are shown in the boxed material below.

Interventions

The client and his family should be taught key data about hypoglycemia and hyperglycemia: What it is. How to recognize it. How to treat it, and dangers associated with it. The

---

Signs and Symptoms of Hyperglycemia and Hypoglycemia

HYPERGLYCEMIA

Glycosuria
Polyuria
Polydipsia
Polyphagia
Acetone breath
Serum glucose 140 mg/dL

HYPOGLYCEMIA

MILD:
  Cool
  Irritable
  Tired, weak
  Headache
  Hunger
  Personality changes
MODERATE:
  Nausea
  Sleepiness
  Disorientation
  Fainting
  Decreased level of consciousness
SEVERE:
  Coma
  Convulsions

nurse in the home environment is in a good position to evaluate unique features of the client's life-style and anticipate factors that may influence hypoglycemia: fluctuations in activity levels, changing mealtimes, or inconsistent morning awakening times.

Encourage the client to monitor blood glucose levels regularly and when hypoglycemia or hyperglycemia is suspected. A study by Cox and Gonder-Frederick (1986) found that the majority of 79 subjects did *not* confirm low blood glucose before taking action to raise the glucose levels. The authors believe the study showed clients used perceived cues of hypoglycemia alone, rather than also checking blood glucose. Certainly, clients need to know their own body cues, but teach them it is also possible to misinterpret symptoms. When possible, validate symptoms with blood glucose levels. The techniques for monitoring glucose are described later in this chapter.

Initial treatment for hypoglycemia in the home setting (or job) is 10 to 15 grams of a simple carbohydrate. This can be met with 2 or 3 glucose tablets, Glutose, or Reactose (or related product) according to package instruction, 6 to 8 Lifesavers, 4 ounces of a regular soft drink or orange juice (with no added sugar!), or 2½ teaspoons of granulated sugar. If that is not effective, repeat in 5 to 10 minutes. If the client is confused or drowsy, someone else should give him sugar in a concentrated form, rubbing it into the inside of the cheek or under the tongue. Products such as Instant Glucose, Reactose Paste, or cake icing in a tube can be used. In addition, Glucagon can be injected by a family member. If the client has passed out, he should be taken to the hospital for intravenous glucose. This response also represents a medical emergency. Call Emergency Medical Services (EMS) immediately for transport to the hospital.

The site of insulin injections can influence hypoglycemia. Faster absorption of insulin occurs in the abdomen than in arms or legs. The arms are the next fastest site, the legs being the slowest. Thus, if a client moves injection sites daily from one part of the body to another, he may experience altered absorption times (Koivisto and Felig 1980). The nurse should teach the client to stay in the same injection area for as long as possible (*i.e.,* arms or legs or abdomen).

Be certain the client knows the major characteristics of any insulin he takes: type, onset time, duration, peak time, and number of units. If possible, help the client to evaluate his own body's response to the insulin, as there is some inherent variability of insulin absorption rates in various persons. According to Haycock (1986), it may approach 50% variation between clients. A summary of insulin types, onset of action, and other important parameters can be found in Table 15-1.

Suggest that the client educate neighbors and coworkers to recognize signs of hypoglycemia. They need to know when to call for medical help and what not to do if the client becomes unconscious.

Interventions for the client with hyperglycemia are similar. The client and family must understand the possible symptoms, confirm the problem through determination of blood glucose, and notify the home health nurse and/or physician. A physician's order will be needed to adjust insulin dosages.

Outcome

A realistic goal for this client is to learn to detect and treat early signs of hypoglycemia. Avoiding numerous insults to the brain's metabolism will probably aid in maintaining the best possible physiologic status in the future.

IMPAIRED TISSUE INTEGRITY

This nursing diagnosis highlights one of the areas of necessary vigilance in diabetes care.

TABLE 15.1   Insulin Types and Administration

Action	Preparation	Onset	Peak	Duration
Short	Regular Insulin	½–1	1–4	6–8
	NPH	1–2	6–8	12–24
Intermediate				
	Lente	1–2	6–12	14–24
	Protamine Zinc	4–6	18+	36–72
Long				
	Ultralente	4–6	8–24	36

(Time shown is in hours)
Adapted from United States Pharmacopeia—Drug Information, 1988

There are several possible etiologies for the tissue damage that may occur. Among these are alterations in circulation secondary to both microvascular or macrovascular disease, impaired physical mobility, lack of sensation from diabetic neuropathy, or knowledge deficits about good skin and foot care.

Impaired tissue integrity is commonly seen in the person with Type II diabetes, but clients with Type I diabetes may also have some impairments. Microvascular disease, or large vessel disease, is most commonly seen in Type II diabetes. Large vessels, such as those found in the lower extremities, may be affected.

Assessment

The nurse who is assessing the client for impaired tissue integrity should utilize every opportunity to teach the client during the assessment period. This will facilitate self-care at home for years to come.

During the assessment, the nurse should evaluate the client's skin for color, temperature, intactness, and pulses. Question the client about factors that could cause or relate to impairments in various tissue: cigarette use, presence of hypertension, how new shoes are adapted into daily routines, usual routines for wound care, visual patterns for inspection and care, and his knowledge of injury hazards to the skin found in the home environment.

Interventions

Interventions for this diagnosis are numerous. Primary ones include teaching the client to perform a complete skin assessment, with emphasis on the feet; educating the client about the rationale for the decreased circulation seen in diabetes; alerting the client to the dangers of wound infection and circulatory impairment, such as gangrene, but doing this in a sensitive manner, not emphasizing additional fear and anxiety; and supplying the client with literature on foot care. Many pamphlets are available listing numerous points for safety (example: never walk barefooted; do not do "bathroom surgery" on corns or callouses, etc) that will supplement the client's learning.

If a client reports having difficulty with

wound healing, check the blood glucose level. Hyperglycemia can interfere with healing. A blood test evaluating glycosolated hemoglobin (AI_c) may help to evaluate long-term control as it reflects a mean blood glucose of the previous 4 to 6 weeks. This test is fairly inexpensive ($10–$15) and can be done at most laboratories.

Once a wound is present, an area of concern to many clinicians is how to care for it to reduce the chance of infection. A recent article (Levin and Spratt 1986) cautioned caregivers about recommending soaking the feet. As a preventive method, it is inappropriate since it increases dryness and does not increase moisture pliability of the skin. Instead, they suggest washing the feet once or twice a day, followed by immediate drying. This still leaves a little moisture on the skin that should then be sealed with a lubricant, such as hand cream or plain white petrolatum in small amounts.

Heavy coatings should be avoided since it is not the lubricant that increases pliability and moisture of the skin—it simply seals in moisture after the bathing. Diabetic neuropathy contributes to a decrease in sweating that causes some of the dryness. Slight, constant perspiring makes normal skin pliable.

Good oral hygiene should be stressed. The prevention of dental caries and peridontal disease is best achieved by careful home care and regular professional supervision (Villeneuve, Treitel, and D'Eramo 1985). Elevated salivary glucose levels and higher *Candida albicans* counts may contribute to caries in the patient with diabetes. Oral home care should include regular brushing and flossing, and irrigating if gum recession or surgery has occurred. Proper nutrition with a diet rich in minerals and vitamins is suggested. Studies have shown that small daily vitamin C supplements may reduce gum inflammation and increase healing potential.

Outcome

An expected outcome for this problem is that the client will be able to detect any early skin breakdown and practice preventive care. The client should also be able to describe possible hazards in the home environment and to outline planned alterations needed to avoid injuries to the skin.

POTENTIAL FOR INFECTION

Nowhere is the potential for infection more apparent than in the client with diabetes mellitus. There are several factors that support this situation. The decrease in blood supply (from macroangiopathy and microangiopathy) may be associated with an increase in infections. Some changes in phagocytic function have been detected in hyperglycemia, including defects in phagocyte engulfment and intracellular killing of bacteria. Conflicting research results have been seen regarding deficits in antibody production in diabetes, although some researchers have documented decreased antibodies to *Staphylococcus aureus,* and *Escherichia coli* and *Corynebacterium diphtheriae* (Casey 1983).

The home health care nurse may find several conflicting opinions in the literature about infectious processes in diabetes. While the common allegation is that all infections are more common and more severe in diabetes, close scrutiny of the literature reveals this is true for only certain infections, but not all.

A recent study (Bryan, Reynolds, and Metzger 1985) noted several infections appearing to be unique to persons with diabetes. These include malignant otitis media due to *Pseudomonas* aeruginosa, polymicrobial osteomyelitis of the small bones of the feet, candidiasis of the skin and mucous membranes, urinary tract infections, and skin infections from nonclostridial gas gangrene.

Assessment

The nurse should both assess the client for this nursing diagnosis and teach him how to care for it on an ongoing basis. Nursing assessment should include careful inspection of the skin for the presence of clinical signs of infection. Assessment should also include an evaluation of the client's knowledge of the major clinical signs of infection (Can the client read a thermometer accurately?), his knowledge of the most common sites for infections, and usual practices related to the skin and insulin injections. Therefore, the nurse is not only concerned about existing infections, but also about the client's ability to recognize future infections.

Interventions

Interventions for this nursing diagnosis follow from the assessment areas. The nurse should stress regular and systematic assessment of the skin and soft tissue. Increased skin and nasal carriage of *S. aureus* has been found in diabetics and may be twice as common as in the nondiabetic client. Local tenderness, warmth, and redness may be present in areas of skin infections.

The nurse should teach the client the major signs of infection. The above data regarding skin infections should be mentioned, as should the importance of the presence of fever, and how to check for it. One study (Clark 1986b) found most subjects were unable to discriminate local skin infections from allergy signs and symptoms.

In addition, signs of urinary tract infections should be discussed. The majority of controlled studies have found a two to fourfold higher incidence of bacteriuria in diabetic women. Some of the reasons for this include urinary stasis caused by neuropathy, underlying renal disease, and impaired host defenses (Casey 1983).

Teach the client the most common sites for infections, including the skin, urinary tract, pneumonia in the lung, periodontal disease, ear infections, and gallbladder (Casey 1983). The risk of vaginal infection is also high. Assist the female client to perform careful and consistent perineal care in order to prevent this complication.

Some studies have found bacteremia to be significantly increased in diabetes. Teaching the client to monitor for a systemic infection may be more difficult because of the lack of local signs, but nevertheless it is possible for the client to monitor for such a condition. Encourage the client to check for fever and to monitor blood glucose levels and urinary ketones, both of which will be elevated in major infections.

Teach the client to seek medical consultation when he recognizes or even suspects an infectious process. The professional caregiver can then add other information to the data base, such as the presence of leukocytosis, the differential white blood cell count (WBC), and relevant cultures. Assist the client and family in monitoring for the effects of antibacterial or antiviral therapy.

Finally, practices related to the skin and insulin injections are undergoing close scrutiny and evaluation. The research literature is abundant with reports of diabetics who are reusing disposable syringes, and not using alcohol skin preps (Aziz 1984; Hodge et al 1980; Collins et al 1983; Clark 1986a). These studies and others have shown no deleterious effects of syringe reuse. Some subjects have used the same syringe up to 7 days or longer with no deleterious effects. Clark (1986a) described 43% of subjects averaged 5.9 times per syringe.

Several factors may be related to the lack of infections from these techniques. Schade and Eaton (1982) reported the bactericidal properties of commercial insulin. They concluded that insulin contaminated with 5×10^5 bacteria found on the skin will self sterilize within 24 hours. It is hypothesized that the additives in the insulin account for this effect. In addition, it may be likely that a person can become infected (versus colonized) from his own skin flora.

This research can cause conflict for the home health nurse who wants to protect the client from any possible harm from these practices. It is suggested that nurses continue to monitor related recommendations from research findings and insulin manufacturers. The legal standard of care may now be in the process of being redefined (Clark 1985). Some nurses are choosing not to recommend reuse of syringes at this time, others tell clients of the two alternatives, while others clearly recommend the reuse. Before recommending a particular practice to a client, the physician should be consulted. Since the research does not present an unquestionable protocol, many physicians continue to have strong preferences for one technique or the other.

Outcome

A possible outcome for the client related to the potential for infection is that he will be diligent in monitoring his body for signs of infections. The nurse can help him learn content needed to better accomplish this goal.

ALTERATION IN BOWEL ELIMINATION: DIARRHEA

"Diabetic diarrhea" is an increasingly recognized complication in clients with longstanding diabetes. This nursing diagnosis can guide the home health care nurse to be alert to this condition and watch for cues that the client may be experiencing it. Some clinicians believe patients do not associate diarrhea with diabetes and therefore may fail to mention it to a care-giver.

The syndrome of "diabetic diarrhea" was first described in 1936 and since that time has remained a challenge to both the client and clinician. The most consistent and characteristic feature is the intermittency of diarrheal attacks, with spontaneous remissions and exacerbations of varying length. During the acute phase, the client may have 20 to 30 loose stools. The diarrhea often occurs at night or late evening. Steatorrhea (fat in stool) is often present (Ellenberg 1983).

There are several physiologic factors that have been identified as causative mechanisms. Normal exocrine pancreatic secretion is usually present. On examination, biopsy of small intestine mucosa is normal, though one or more components of autonomic nervous system pathology is usually present (Ellenberg 1983). The pathogenesis of diabetic diarrhea is not completely clear. Autonomic neuropathy plays a fundamental role but is poorly understood (Barkin and Skyler 1983).

A related but somewhat different condition that may be seen is fecal incontinence. It has been described in the client with long-standing diabetes and may be due to decreased rectal sensation, or impaired function of the external sphincter, or both. An interesting study by Wald and Tunuguntla (1984) showed that biofeedback training may improve external sphincter function and thus fecal soiling.

Assessment

Nursing assessment for this diagnosis should begin with data collection and attentiveness to cues from the client. Persons with chronic diarrhea may be reluctant to broach the subject, so the nurse needs to take the initiative (Funnell and McNitt 1986). If it appears to be present in the client, inquire about patterns of its occurrence. Diarrhea will most often be seen in young adults, is more common in females, and will usually occur in clients with other neuropathies or retinopathy (Barkin and Skyler 1983). Specific parameters to assess include increased frequency of stools, a sense of urgency, loose liquid stools, and cramping.

Interventions

The client should be taught to recognize diarrhea as a treatable complication of diabetes that many other persons also experience. Early medical intervention is indicated. The nurse may suggest Metamucil, a dietary fiber, to increase stool bulk (Barkin and Skyler 1983; Funnell and McNitt 1986). Antibiotics appear to help the process, usually ampicillin or tetracycline with dose and duration individualized, based on results (Barkin and Skyler 1983). Lomotil is beneficial for most clients. In addition, good glycemic control (low blood glucoses) appears helpful. Additional fluid therapy may be necessary since dehydration may occur.

The home health nurse can also suggest measures that will assist in allowing the bowel to rest. For example, the client should be instructed to avoid certain foods such as spicy foods or those high in fat content. Certain foods that may produce gas (*i.e.*, cabbage, onions, prunes, baked beans) should be avoided. Small frequent meals, avoiding extremely hot and cold foods, will also be of assistance in lessening the diarrhea.

Outcome

The client will seek early treatment for the condition. In addition, the client will not experience any dehydration or electrolyte imbalance related to the diarrhea.

ALTERATION IN URINARY ELIMINATION: RETENTION

Urinary bladder problems are often a common clue to the presence of autonomic neu-

ropathy. They affect men and women equally and the incidence may rise with age and duration of diabetes (Funnell and McNitt 1986).

The most outstanding feature is an insidious and progressive urinary retention, with the interval between voidings once or twice per day. While the volume may be very large (1000 cc), the client does not generally recognize the need to empty the bladder. In fact, some falsely believe that fewer voidings may represent improvement of the polyuria associated with hyperglycemia.

When a loss of efferent impulses from the bladder occurs, the need to void is not recognized and the bladder will distend and become hypotonic. This hypotonia then leads to difficulty initiating micturition.

Assessment

The home health nurse should assess the client for bladder distention, dribbling of urine, and the absence of urine output. Another sign for the nurse to evaluate is the presence of urinary tract infections from the stasis and retained urine. Query the client about the length and type of symptoms. Other diagnostic data may be obtained from cystometric (bladder) studies done by a qualified urologist.

Interventions

The nursing interventions for this diagnosis are very important in helping the client avoid further complications. The home health nurse can help the client to develop a schedule to try to empty the bladder every 3 to 4 hours, which will keep the urine volume less than 300 cc with each voiding. The Crede's maneuver (manual pressure), along with tightening of the abdominal muscles, may help empty the bladder completely (Funnell and McNitt 1986). Some drugs may help, such as cholinergic or parasympathetic agents.

Teach the client to recognize early signs of a urinary tract infection and to seek early treatment. Ascending pyelonephritis can follow neurogenic incompetency. In the early stages of a neurogenic bladder, there may be no signs of pyuria or bacteriuria. However, in advanced stages of the diabetic neurogenic bladder, gross infection is usually apparent (Ellenberg 1983).

Encourage the client not to rely on urine glucose evaluation since the retention will cause unreliable amounts of glucose. Blood glucose should always be checked, particularly when an infection is present.

As a last resort, surgery may be recommended. A transurethral resection of the bladder is indicated to weaken the vesical neck sufficiently to allow the incompetent detrusor muscle to expel bladder contents. Results have been good; however, side-effects such as retrograde ejaculation have been seen (Ellenberg 1983).

Outcome

A goal for the client with bladder retention is to be able to successfully manage a bladder control program of timed voidings.

ACTIVITY INTOLERANCE

Activity intolerance may occur in a client with Type I or Type II diabetes. However, it is probably most commonly seen in the person with Type II. It is this client who is most apt to be overweight and sedentary. Obesity and inactivity both contribute to the development of glucose intolerance.

Assessment

Several features are included in an assessment of this client, including a history of previous exercise intolerance, a deconditioned status, verbal reports of fatigue or weakness, and an abnormal heart rate or blood pressure

in response to physical activity. All of these are things that the home health nurse could elicit in a skilled interview with the client.

In addition, the home health nurse should query *all* clients with diabetes about their activity and exercise patterns. Try to elicit factual and accurate information before planning activity changes. In addition, assessment of cardiovascular parameters (blood pressure and heart rate) at rest and after some physical activity will assist in planning an exercise prescription.

Determine how much medication the client is taking and the type of insulin taken so that insulin peaks and durations can be considered. Lastly, determine daily calorie intake and meal spacing so the timing of exercise will be most beneficial. The nurse may wish to recommend a medical evaluation by a physician before initiating or suggesting any strenuous exercise.

Interventions

The home health nurse must encourage the client to participate in an exercise program. The benefits of exercise and activity are numerous for the person with diabetes. An improvement in insulin sensitivity and some possible improvement in glucose tolerance has been seen. Exercise may lessen the effects of cardiovascular risk factors. Consistently, increased work capacity may reduce the overall insulin or oral hypoglycemic dose requirements (Rifkin 1984).

One of the primary cardiovascular risk factors amenable to exercise is circulating levels of lipoproteins. A reduction to very low density lipoprotein (VLDL), low density lipoprotein (LDL), cholesterol and triglycerides may follow regular physical training. Exercise is also associated with an increase in high density lipoprotein, which may offer some protection against cardiovascular disease (Rifkin 1984).

Assist the client to determine what activities he most enjoys — such as walking, golfing, or jogging. Suggest three to four exercise sessions per week, beginning with very low workloads with gradual increases.

Each exercise session should include warm-up and cool-down periods, with some combination of stretching exercises and strength building. Consider referral or dialog with a physical therapist or fitness specialist.

A very important intervention is to teach the client that prolonged and vigorous exercise can lead to significant *hypoglycemia*. The client should be alert for signs and symptoms of hypoglycemia during exercise and for the next several hours. He should always carry or wear identification of self and his diabetic condition. The client should *always* have a source of carbohydrate available to treat hypoglycemia.

Another intervention is to teach the client to monitor his cardiovascular status. Have him locate and calculate his pulse rate for 1 minute before, during, and after the exercise period. One formula currently used by some is to determine the maximal heart rate (MHR) by subtracting the age from 220. A poorly conditioned individual should aim for a target heart rate of 60% of MHR, whereas a better conditioned individual might aim for 80% of MHR (Aschenbrener, Clark et al 1986).

An evaluation of any physical problems should precede the actual exercise program. The selection of appropriate footwear and/or evaluation of the feet is suggested before running or jogging. Clients with hypertension should avoid anything that might raise blood pressure significantly, such as intense exercise involving the arms and upper body, Valsalva's maneuvers, or weight lifting (Rifkin 1984).

There are some other precautions to consider. The client with Type II diabetes should be supervised or cautious during exercise if he has poorly controlled, labile blood glucose, or is at significant risk for developing complications due to proliferative retinopathy, neuropathy, or significant atherosclerosis. The client with Type I diabetes should be supervised or cautious during exercise if he is unable to prevent hypoglycemia during prolonged exercise, or if it is poorly controlled (blood glucose > 300 mg/dl). Many persons who have initiated exercise with a high glucose level (over 250–300 mg/dl) have a rise in blood glucose, rather than the expected decrease. Adjustment of insulin and diet are needed to make exercise a safe endeavor in these persons. One study (Schiffrin and Parikh 1985) found that the intake of 25 to 30 grams of glucose prevented hypoglycemia during an *unplanned* postprandial exercise, whereas a reduction of insulin dose was used for *planned* exercise periods.

Outcome

An expected outcome is that the client can develop and maintain an exercise program. Other outcomes may be considered, such as a reduction in blood pressures and heart rate after some time period. Beneficial changes in lipoprotein levels may be seen after some months.

SEXUAL DYSFUNCTION

This nursing diagnosis may be seen in male or female clients with diabetes, though more literature is available to describe it in males. An estimated 50% of the diabetic men may suffer from impotence.

While poor glucose control may affect penile erection ability, most of these men are impotent because of diabetic neuropathy with microscopic damage to nerve tissue. Usually, it is only the erection ability that is impaired, with normal libido, ejaculation, and orgasm (Funnell and McNitt 1986). The nerves that innervate the arteries of the penis are damaged and do not allow the normal dilatation of the arteries, thus preventing an erection.

It is important to consider other possible causes of impotence. These include psychogenic, or drug-induced, causes and testosterone deficiency. Psychological causes of impotence probably account for over 90% of impotence in the general population (Ellenberg 1983). One distinguishing factor is that libido is decreased in psychogenic impotence, but is normal in neuropathy.

Retrograde ejaculation is another manifestation of diabetic neuropathy in males. In this condition, orgasm occurs but there is no accompanying ejaculate. Catheterization of the bladder at this time reveals urine swarming with live, active sperm, thus establishing the diagnosis (Ellenberg 1983).

There is little documented evidence concerning sexual dysfunction in diabetic females. One recent study showed no difference in sex interest and orgasmic reaction between diabetic women with and without neuropathy. A startling finding was the lack of effect of diabetes on sexual performance as compared with nondiabetic women (Ellenberg 1983). In contrast, other studies have shown decreased orgasmic response in women with diabetes (Funnull and McNitt 1986).

Assessment

Assessment data for the nurse to obtain should be comprehensive. What is the present level of glucose control? Obtain a description of what client symptoms are and how long they have been present. Impotence caused by psychogenic causes tends to have a sudden onset, whereas that caused by diabetes will have a gradual (over months or years) onset. Inquire about nocturnal and morning erections — these are absent in neu-

ropathy and present in psychological impotence (Rifkin 1984).

An inexpensive way to screen for organic or neuropathic impotence is the "stamp test." A strip of postage stamps is placed around the base of the penis before going to sleep. A nocturnal erection will tear the stamps apart. One caution is that this will only confirm an erection, but not adequate penile rigidity (Clements et al 1985).

Find out what medications the client is taking. Many of the antihypertensives can cause impotence, as can phenothiazines, antidepressants, and alcohol.

Interventions

Most clients will not readily volunteer information about sex. They must be queried tactfully. If the blood glucose is poorly controlled, help the client to see the relationship of blood glucose elevation to impotence. Identify possible causes of hyperglycemia and develop corrective strategies.

If the sexual dysfunction is permanent, there is no specific treatment modality at the present time. The nurse may suggest referral to a urologist who specializes in a mechanical device, such as a penile implant. The specialist can provide noninvasive studies of penile blood flow and proper evaluation.

The frequency of impotence is directly proportional to the frequency of the inquiry and the direct manner in which the client is asked. Many men are relieved to learn of an organic cause for impotence. Some may have been accused of infidelity (Ellenberg 1983).

Other nursing interventions for the male client include supportive counseling with both partners. An open discussion and presentation of the facts may alleviate some of the anxiety and may help in emotional adjustment. Referral to a qualified psychiatrist or family therapist may be needed.

Outcome

One possible outcome for this client is that he will seek professional help for any sexual dysfunction present. The nurse can assist the client and spouse to deal with this often-neglected area. The Sex Information and Education Council of the U.S., Inc. (SIECUS) advocates that education in sexual health concerns, needs, and therapies be integrated with professional education in all health care fields (Manley 1986).

SENSORY – PERCEPTUAL ALTERATION: VISUAL

Diabetes is the leading cause of new cases of blindness in the United States. The classic eye disease seen is diabetic retinopathy. Five years after diagnosis of diabetes, approximately 30% of diabetics show some detectable signs of retinopathy, although the overall vision is still good. Ten years after diagnosis, the figure rises to about 50%, and after 20 years, 85%. One recent study found retinopathy in 9% of children younger than 13 years (Klein et al 1985).

There are two main types of retinopathy, nonproliferative (also called *background*) and proliferative. In nonproliferative retinopathy (less severe), there are aneurysms, hemorrhages, edema, exudates, and new vessels in the eye. Over time in some persons, this progresses to proliferative retinopathy. Only about 10% of diabetics appear to develop the proliferative type (severe). In proliferative retinopathy, the hemorrhages are much more severe. There is glial cell proliferation and eventually retinal detachment and blindness may occur (L'Esperance and James 1983).

The precise cause is not known. Diabetic retinopathy appears to be a response to ischemia of the retina. In addition, high levels of sorbital accumulation inside the retina have been linked with hyperglycemia. In the retina, glucose is converted to sorbitol when the enzyme aldose reductase is present.

Inhibition of this enzyme may be part of future treatment. Other pathological factors that may be related include increased red cell aggregation, metabolic control, and growth hormone levels (L'Esperance and James 1983).

Assessment

Nursing assessment for this diagnosis begins with obtaining data from the client concerning changes in sensory acuity. The nurse should inquire about changing visual perceptions the client is experiencing and compare present vision to past vision acuity.

Many nurses are able to do a basic examination of the internal eye using an ophthalmoscope. It is highly recommended that clients with suspected and undiagnosed retinopathy be referred to an eye specialist immediately. The nurse is referred to a good physical examination textbook for specific methods of visualizing the fundus of the eye. Some nurses have found it helpful to spend time with an ophthalmologist looking into dilated eyes to learn eye landmarks and to gain proficiency and confidence in this skill. Access the fundus for indications for mild retinal vascular damage including increased light reflex, arteriolar tortuosity, narrowing and arteriovenous nicking. More severe damage would include retinal hemorrhage, exudates, and papilledema.

Other assessment data should include information about blood glucose measures. Determine what the recent levels have been and how often they are measured.

Interventions

There are several nursing interventions for this diagnosis. The home health nurse should be certain the client has a current evaluation of his vision and a determination about the presence of retinopathy. If no visual disturbances are seen, a baseline examination is still encouraged. If the client has some visual impairment but not blindness, help him to evaluate his life-style to determine what assistance and alterations are needed. For example, if he has both impaired vision and neuropathy, teach someone else to help him do a regular assessment of his feet. Does he need help in locating aids to draw up insulin? Can he see syringe unit markers?

The client who is legally blind needs help and support to maintain independence. It is often difficult for persons who are blind to find appropriate resources to maintain self-care. Hoover (1985), chairman of the National Task Force on Diabetes and Blindness, notes that many persons who have unsuccessful treatment not only are disappointed by the results but must cope with hearing the ophthalmologist say, "I'm sorry, but there is nothing more I can do for you." This is potentially devastating to the client. The nurse should be available to listen to the client express his frustrations, and to suggest small goals aimed at more independence. For example, there are numerous devices for purchase to assist the blind person with drawing up and administering insulin. (See Herget 1983). The nurse can suggest a nearby office of the American Diabetes Association as a resource to obtain samples and information about some materials.

If the client has difficulty seeing well enough to draw up insulin, the home health nurse may need to prepare prefilled syringes for a certain period of time. The use of magnifying devices may also help the client to maintain independence while drawing up insulin.

The client may need information about treatments for retinopathy. Fluorescein angiography may be used to evaluate eye vessels. It has been available since 1961 and is an invaluable assist to planning treatment. Photocoagulation, or laser therapy, is used to destroy neovascular complexes, to obliterate areas of microinfarctions, and to destroy leaking vessels. This treatment has been very successful for many persons with retinopathy, but in some few individuals does not effect much change. The other main treatment is the vitrectomy, a surgical procedure. In this surgery, a needlelike cutting and aspirating device is introduced into the central cavity of the vitreous area of the eye. Then blood membrane and fibrin are delicately removed and replaced with a clear Ringer's solution. Studies have shown that 50% – 70% of patients have good results (L'Esperance and James 1983).

Outcome

A reasonable goal for this client is to be able to make informed decisions about eye status evaluations and treatment. The home health nurse can provide needed support and information to meet this goal.

ANXIETY

Diabetes is a disease that requires many life-style changes and has potentially severe complications. Anxiety is a part of life for many clients with the disease. Possible etiologies of the anxiety can include threat to self-concept, threat of death, or threat to health status. Because of recent findings linking elevated glucose levels with some of the complications, pressure exists to maintain normoglycemia. It is difficult to balance insulin requirements, physical activity, and diet intake on a 24-hour basis.

Psychological stress is believed to increase blood glucose and insulin requirements. Stress activates the sympathetic nervous system and elevates several hormones, such as catecholamines and growth hormone. In addition, free fatty acids and, possibly, ketones may be elevated.

There are many examples in the literature concerning persons who have documented hyperglycemia in response to stress. However, few methodologically sound research studies have been done to study this problem. Kemmer and others (1986) subjected 27 patients to two acute psychological stresses: mental arithmetic and public speaking. All subjects had increased heart rate, elevated blood pressure, elevated plasma epinephrine, and norepinephrine levels. However, no stress-induced changes were seen in blood glucose, free fatty acids, glucagon, or growth hormones. The author concluded that short-lived psychological stimuli causing marked cardiovascular responses with marked elevation of catecholamines and cortisol are unlikely to disturb metabolic control in Type I diabetes. Other studies (Carter et al 1985) found variations in response to stress and concluded the effect of psychological stress on metabolism in Type I diabetes was quite idiosyncratic, but reliable within patients. It may result in hyperglycemia but apparently does not in every person. More controlled research is obviously needed.

An excellent comprehensive article (Holmes 1984) concerning the impact of diabetes on the psychosocial aspects of life may be helpful to the nurse. This resource discusses the first year of diabetes, the next succeeding period of relatively good health, on to the time the client has to cope with more symptoms and impaired functioning.

Parents of diabetic children report significant anxiety. The literature indicates that mothers typically bear the burden of diabetes care. Some have reported neurotic or other psychopathologic behaviors. Kovacs and others (1985) reported on a longitudinal study of 74 sets of parents with newly diagnosed school-aged children. They found no evidence of blatant neurotic behaviors but instead found initial mild depression, anxiety, and overall distress. Twenty-five percent had a mild grief reaction. Most appeared to be coping by the end of the first year with anxiety scale score reduction.

Assessment

The nurse needs to skillfully interview the client and observe for verbal and nonverbal cues for this nursing diagnosis. Subjective defining characteristics include increased tension, overexcited, jittery, worried feelings, and a sense of helplessness. Objective characteristics may include insomnia, signs of sympathetic stimulation, poor eye contact, focus on self, and facial tension.

Interventions

Nursing interventions for this diagnosis should follow the assessment. If the client can identify any specific concerns, help him to problem-solve and reach possible solutions. One strategy that some have found useful is to encourage the client to discuss his worst fears. This may help him to learn to separate what is real from what is imagined. Psychiatric consultation may be very helpful (Holmes 1984).

Give clear explanations using neutral language. For example "kidney insufficiency" may be less anxiety-producing than "kidney failure." Provide information for the client including reading material so that he can have factual information about good glucose control. Encourage and assist him to evaluate his own glucose response to emotional stress by checking blood glucose levels at home when there is aware of any special stress.

Outcome

A goal for this nursing diagnosis is that the client will be able to reduce his anxiety about diabetes. The home health care nurse can provide continuity of care to assist with this goal.

ALTERATION IN NUTRITION

Dietary control is one of the most important features of the care of diabetic clients. One of the major goals for the home health nurse is to assist the client as he develops mechanisms to assure compliance with the prescribed diet.

Assessment

A major component of assessment is to determine whether the client understands the various aspects of the prescribed diet. The second major area for assessment includes a nutritional assessment (See Chapter 11).

Interventions

Diabetic diets are prescribed with a twofold purpose: to discourage the ingestion of foods with high sugar and fat content and, secondly, to correct or avoid obesity. Insulin-dependent clients are generally on diets with no special caloric restrictions, although the amount of fat, carbohydrate, and protein is generally prescribed. Noninsulin-dependent clients will often be on a diet with calorie restrictions.

The balanced diabetic diet should contain calculated quantities of carbohydrate, protein and fat, and normal amounts of vitamins and minerals. One of the most common types of diets is the exchange-measured diet. This diet was developed with the belief that the foods containing the same food value can be exchanged with one another without altering the person's basic dietary prescription. Foods are divided into six basic categories, including milk, vegetables, fruit, bread, meat, and fat. The foods in each list contain the same number of calories and the same amounts of protein, fat, and carbohydrate. This system allows the client considerable flexibility. Diabetic diet exchange lists can be found in Table 15-2.

Outcome

The client and family should demonstrate knowledge and understanding of the diabetic diet regime.

POTENTIAL FOR INJURY: COMPLICATIONS OF DIABETES

Two major complications may threaten the diabetic client, diabetic ketoacidosis and hyperosmolar, nonketotic coma. Although any client experiencing one of these complications would require immediate hospitalization, it is the home health nurse who may be responsible for identifying the problems and assuring the client access to the appropriate health-care agency.

Diabetic ketoacidosis results from a severe insulin deficiency. As the deficiency continues, serum glucose increases until the renal threshold for resorption of glucose has been exceeded. Glucose then begins to spill into the urine. The severe hyperglycemia then causes an osmotic diuresis that draws fluid from the intracellular and interstitial spaces into the intravascular compartment.

The body quickly begins to search for energy from noncarbohydrate sources. Fat is broken down into glycerol and free fatty acids, which in turn increase the amount of ketoacids or ketone bodies. Large amounts of acetoacetic acid produce acetone.

Hyperosmolar coma is a comatose state that develops in individuals with adult-onset diabetes. This condition is identified by hyperglycemia, hyperosmolality, hypernatremia and dehydration. Adults over the age of 60 are most commonly affected by this condition. It is rare in younger individuals.

(Text continues on p 457)

TABLE 15.2 Diabetic Diet Exchange Lists

List 1. Milk Exchanges
Carbohydrate: 12 grams; protein: 8 grams; fat: trace: calories: 80

Nonfat Fortified Milk		*Low-Fat Fortified Milk*		*Whole Milk* (omit 2 fat exchanges)	
Skim or nonfat milk	1 cup	1% fat fortified milk (omit ½ fat exchange)	1 cup	Whole milk	1 cup
Powdered (nonfat dry, before adding liquid)	⅓ cup	2% fat fortified milk (omit 1 fat exchange)	1 cup	Canned, evaporated whole milk	½ cup
Canned, evaporated—skim milk	½ cup	Yogurt made from 2% fortified milk (plain, unflavored) (omit 1 fat exchange)	1 cup	Buttermilk made from whole milk	1 cup
Buttermilk made from skim milk	1 cup			Yogurt made from whole milk (plain, unflavored)	1 cup
Yogurt made from skim milk (plain, unflavored)	1 cup				

List 2. Vegetable Exchanges
Carbohydrate: 5 grams; protein: 2 grams; calories: 25

Cooked Vegetables (one exchange is ½ cup)

			Raw Vegetables (use as desired)
Asparagus	Eggplant	String beans (green or yellow)	Chicory
bean sprouts	Green pepper	Summer squash	Chinese cabbage
Beets	Greens	Tomatoes	Endive
Broccoli	Mushrooms	Tomato juice	Escarole
Brussels sprouts	Okra	Turnips	Lettuce
Cabbage	Onions	Vegetable juice cocktail	Parsley
Carrots	Rhubarb	Zucchini	Radishes
Cauliflower	Rutabaga		Watercress
Cucumbers	Sauerkraut		

Starchy Vegetables (listed under Bread Exchanges)

(*continued*)

TABLE 15.2 Diabetic Diet Exchange Lists (*continued*)

List 3. Fruit Exchanges
Carbohydrate: 10 grams; calories: 40

Apple	1 small	Mango	½ small
Apple juice	⅓ cup	Melon	
Applesauce (unsweetened)	½ cup	canteloupe	¼ small
		honeydew	⅛ medium
Apricots, fresh	2 medium	watermelon	1 cup
Apricots, dried	4 halves	Nectarine	1 small
Banana	1 small	Orange	1 small
Berries		Orange juice	½ cup
blackberries	½ cup	Papaya	¾ cup
blueberries	½ cup	Peach	1 medium
raspberries	½ cup	Pear	1 small
strawberries	¾ cup	Persimmon, native	1 medium
Cherries	10 large	Pineapple	½ cup
Cider	⅓ cup	Pineapple juice	⅓ cup
Dates	2	Plums	2 medium
Figs, fresh or dried	1	Prunes	2 medium
Grapefruit	½	Prune juice	¼ cup
Grapefruit juice	½ cup	Raisins	¼ cup
Grapes	12	Tangerine	1 medium
Grape juice	¼ cup		

Cranberries may be used as desired if no sugar is added.

List 4. Bread Exchanges
Carbohydrate: 15 grams; protein: 2 grams; calories: 70

Bread		Frankfurter roll	½
White (including French and Italian)	1 slice	Hamburger bun	½
		Dried bread crumbs	3 tablespoons
Whole wheat	1 slice	Tortilla, 6″	1
Rye or pumpernickel	1 slice		
Raisin	1 slice	*Cereal*	
Bagel, small	½	Bran flakes	½ cup
English muffin, small	½	Other ready-to-eat un-sweetened cereal	¾ cup
Plain roll, bread	1		

(*continued*)

TABLE 15.2 Diabetic Diet Exchange Lists (*continued*)

List 4. Bread Exchanges (*Continued*)

Puffed cereal (unfrosted)	1 cup		Lima beans	½ cup
Cereal (cooked)	½ cup		Parsnips	⅔ cup
Grits (cooked)	½ cup		Peas, green (canned or frozen)	½ cup
Rice or barley (cooked)	½ cup			
Pasta (cooked), spaghetti, noodles, macaroni	½ cup		Potato, white	1 small
			Potato, mashed	½ cup
Popcorn (popped, no fat added)	3 cups		Pumpkin	¾ cup
Cornmeal (dry)	2 tablespoons		Winter squash, acorn, or butternut	½ cup
Flour	2½ tablespoons		Yam or sweet potato	¼ cup
Wheat germ	¼ cup			

Crackers

Arrowroot	3
Graham, 2½″ square	2
Matzoth, 4″ × 6″	½
Oyster	20
Pretzels, 3⅛″ long × ⅛″ diameter	25
Rye wafers, 2″ × 3½″	3
Saltines	6
Soda, 2½″ square	4

Dried Beans, Peas, and Lentils

Beans, peas, lentils (dried and cooked)	½ cup
Baked beans, no pork (canned)	¼ cup

Starchy Vegetables

Corn	⅓ cup
Corn on the cob	1 small

Prepared Foods

Biscuit, 2″ diameter (omit 1 fat exchange)	1
Corn bread, 2″ × 2″ × 1″ (omit 1 fat exchange)	1
Corn muffin, 2″ diameter (omit 1 fat exchange)	1
Crrackers, round butter type (omit 1 fat exchange)	5
Muffin, plain, small (omit 1 fat exchange)	1
Potatoes, French fried, length 2″ to 3½″ (omit 1 fat exchange)	8
Potato or corn chips (omit 2 fat exchanges)	15
Pancake, 5 × ½″ (omit 1 fat exchange)	1
Waffle, 5″ × ½″ (omit 1 fat exchange)	1

(*continued*)

TABLE 15.2 Diabetic Diet Exchange Lists (*continued*)

List 5. Meat Exchanges: Lean Meat
Protein: 7 grams; fat: 3 grams; calories: 55

Beef: baby beef (very lean), chipped beef, chuck, flank steak, tenderloin, plate ribs, plate skirt steak, round (bottom, top), all cuts rump, spare ribs, tripe	1 ounce	Fish: any fresh or frozen	1 ounce
		canned salmon, tuna, mackerel, crab, or lobster	¼ cup
		clams, oysters, scallops, shrimp	5 or 1 ounce
		sardines, drained	3
Lamb: leg, rib, sirloin, loin (roast and chops), shank, shoulder	1 ounce	Cheese containing less than 5% butterfat	1 ounce
Port: leg (whole rump, center shank), ham, smoked (center slices)	1 ounce	Cottage cheese, dry or 2% butterfat	¼ cup
		Dried beans and peas (omit 1 bread exchange)	½ cup
Poultry: meat without skin of chicken, turkey, Cornish hen, guinea hen, pheasant	1 ounce		

Medium-Fat Meat

For each exchange of medium-fat meat omit ½ fat exchange

Beef: ground (15% fat), corned beef		Liver, heart, kidney and sweetbreads (these are high in cholesterol)	1 ounce
(canned), rib eye, round (ground commercial)	1 ounce	Cottage cheese, creamed	¼ cup
		Cheese: mozzarella, ricotta, farmer's cheese, Neufchatel, Parmesan	3 tablespoons
Pork: loin (all cuts tenderloin), shoulder arm (picnic), shoulder blade, Boston butt, canadian bacon, boiled ham	1 ounce	Egg (high in cholesterol)	1
		Peanut butter (omit 2 additional fat exchanges)	2 tablespoons

High-Fat Meat

For each exchange of high-fat meat omit 1 fat exchange

Beef: brisket, corned beef (brisket), ground beef (more than 20% fat), hamburger	1 ounce	(commercial), chuck (ground commercial) roasts (rib), steaks (club and rib)	

(*continued*)

TABLE 15.2 Diabetic Diet Exchange Lists (*continued*)

List 5. Meat Exchanges: High-Fat Meat (*Continued*)			
Lamb: breast	1 ounce	Poultry: capon, duck (domestic), goose	1 ounce
Pork: spare ribs, loin (back ribs), pork (ground), country style ham, deviled ham	1 ounce	Cheese: Cheddar types	1 ounce
		Cold cuts 4½″ × ⅛″ slice	1
Veal: breast	1 ounce	Frankfurter	1 small

List 6. Fat Exchanges *Fat: 5 grams; calories: 45*			
Margarine, soft, tub, or stock (made with corn, cottonseed, safflower, soy, or sunflower oil only)	1 teaspoon	Nuts, other*	6 small
		Margarine, regular stick	1 teaspoon
		Butter	1 teaspoon
		Bacon fat	1 teaspoon
Avocado (4″ in diameter)*	⅛	Bacon, crisp	1 strip
		Cream, light	2 tablespoons
Oil, corn, cottonseed, safflower, soy, sunflower	1 teaspoon	Cream, sour	2 tablespoons
		Cream, heavy	1 tablespoon
Oil, olive*	1 teaspoon	Cream cheese	1 tablespoon
Oil, peanut*	1 teaspoon	French dressing†	1 tablespoon
Olives*	5 small	Italian dressing†	1 tablespoon
Almonds*	10 whole	Lard	1 teaspoon
Pecans*	2 whole	Mayonnaise†	1 teaspoon
Peanuts*		Salad dressing, mayonnaise type†	2 teaspoons
Spanish	20 whole	Salt pork	¾″ cube
Virginia	10 whole		
Walnuts	6 small		

From American Diabetes Association and The American Dietetic Association: Exchange Lists for Meal Planning, 1976.
*Fat content is primarily monosaturated.
†If made with corn, cottonseed, safflower, soy, or sunflower oil can be used on fat modified diet.

There are several conditions that increase the likelihood of hyperosmolar coma. These conditions include medical conditions (*i.e.*, severe burns, dehydration), medical procedures (*i.e.*, hyperalimentation), and drugs (*i.e.*, phenytoin, alcohol). These factors act as stressors that increase the body's need for insulin. There is inadequate insulin available, leading to increased levels of glucose in the blood. This is followed by a decrease in peripheral utilization of glucose by muscle and liver cells and because the liver increases its glucose production as a result of glycogenolysis and gluconeogenesis.

The serum glucose levels of hyperosmolar coma are much higher than in diabetic ketoacidosis. Because of hyperglycemia, the osmolality increases, stimulating the hypothalamus to release ADH and causing the distal and collecting tubules to become more permeable to water. Generally, there is no ketosis produced since sufficient amounts of insulin are produced to prevent or inhibit lipolysis.

Assessment

The clinical signs of diabetic ketoacidosis and hyperosmolar coma are outlined in Table 15-3. The home health nurse may first suspect the development of either complication if

TABLE 15.3 Clinical Signs of Ketoacidosis and Hyperosmolar Coma

Clinical Signs	Diabetic Ketoacidosis	Hyperosmolar Coma
Duration	Variable	Recent onset
Age	All ages	>50 Years
Events	Infection stress	Stress steroids
Mortality	5%	50%
Blood Sugar	400–800	>900
Dehydration	Variable	Severe
PH	Low	Normal
Breathing	Kussmaul	Normal
Serum Acetone	Present	Absent

there are mental changes. Glycosuria and hyperglycemia can also be expected.

Interventions

If the home health nurse suspects diabetic ketoacidosis or hyperosmolar coma, it is imperative that the client be transferred to the hospital immediately. Prior to that time, the home health nurse can be most influential by assuring that the client maintain other aspects of care to prevent the complications from occurring. Assure that the client and family understand the potential problems posed by mismanagement of diabetes.

Outcome

The client will not experience any complications of diabetes.

NONCOMPLIANCE

Inadequate patient compliance with prescribed treatment may be the most serious obstacle in effective diabetes management (Rosenstock 1985). There is no problem any more frustrating for the nurse than to deal with the diabetic client who is classified as noncompliant. Noncompliance is generally defined as an informed decision not to adhere to a therapeutic recommendation. The etiologies include patient value systems (health beliefs, spiritual values, cultural influences) and client–provider relationships.

Compliance may be measured by several other variables. Knowledge, frequently the only one addressed in patient teaching programs, is not a consistent predictor of compliance. Clients may know a good deal about the link between hyperglycemia and long-term complications, yet fail to adhere to diet and exercise prescriptions. Other variables used to measure compliance include the client's perception of disease severity and his personal susceptibility, perceived efficacy of treatment, and perceived barriers to action (Jenny 1983).

A recent study (Ary et al 1986) looked at the patient/client perspective for nonadherence. Both Type I (N=24) and Type II (N=184) groups were included and few differences were seen in the two groups. Subjects reported adhering least well to dietary and physical activity components of the regime. Comments from subjects regarding noncompliance included:

"Just this once." "A little won't hurt." "You only live once." (grant self-permission); "Just can't make myself walk." (poor self-control); "My fingers are too bruised to test today." "I am aging and don't feel up to exercise." (negative physical reasons).

The most common reasons given for dietary noncompliance were situational factors of eating out in restaurants and inappropriate food offers from others. Negative physical reactions were the most commonly reported reasons for nonadherence to exercise. Twenty-three percent of subjects reported forgetting to take oral hypoglycemics at times. One patient reported being too embarrassed to check blood glucose in front of family members. Consistent with previous adherence research, adherence to one aspect of the diabetes regimen was not strongly related to adherence in other areas.

Compliance with diabetic regimens may be even poorer than with regimens for other chronic diseases. This is not surprising when one considers the complex, life-long duration of the behavior changes needed in diabetes. From the client's point of view, noncompliance may have a quite rational basis. Most adults know that even perfect compliance will not take away the disease process or its symptoms (Rosenstock 1985).

An interesting study (House et al 1986) looks at difference in patient versus physician perceptions of nonadherence to diet. Physicians perceived dietary noncompliance as being largely under the patient's control, whereas patients maintained their noncompliance was out of their control. Patients rated environmental causes over motivational ones as the major reason for noncompliance, but physicians rated motivational factors as highest (80%).

Numerous other studies have clearly documented noncompliance in many other areas of diabetes care. Behaviors included lack of foot care, lack of urine testing or blood glucose testing, unacceptable insulin administration technique, and smoking cigarettes (Rosenstock 1985).

Assessment

There are several defining characteristics for this nursing diagnosis. These include: (1) behavior indicative of failure to adhere by direct observation, or statements by patient or significant others; (2) objective tests (physiologic markers, such as hemoglobin AI_c, which measures a mean blood glucose of the previous 4 to 6 weeks); (3) evidence of the development of complications; (4) evidence of exacerbation of symptoms; (5) failure to keep appointments; and (6) failure to progress. The nurse can use these to assess her client for compliance.

Interventions

Several nursing interventions can be suggested. The nurse should talk with the client in a nonjudgmental manner. She should do a thorough assessment of his knowledge and spot areas where he needs instruction. Get the client to discuss areas in which he needs help. Gather data about his life-style and make recommendations concerning how he might adjust his treatment to his personal needs and preferences. Assess finances for supplies and food as well as activity and rest patterns. Be sure you know current and usual blood glucose levels and client practices for measuring. Richardson (1982) suggests an assessment tool that assesses usual behaviors; treatment plan and suggested behavioral changes; and evidence of compliance.

Supply the client with both verbal and written information specific to his learning needs. Be aware of his reading level and make certain he can understand any written material. Several studies have documented a mismatch between reading and comprehension levels of the client with the level of oral instruction and printed materials. McNeal and others (1984) evaluated a diabetes education program and found that over half of the participants could not fully comprehend educational materials at fifth grade level, while nearly all written materials and oral instructions were presented at ninth grade level or above. Thus, one factor in noncompliance may be the inability to read and comprehend the treatment plan. This presents a challenge to the home health care nurse to be able to assess comprehension levels of clients with a variety of backgrounds. Educational level is certainly one factor to consider.

In preparing or adapting written materials, avoid three-syllable (or greater) words, substituting simpler words with the same meaning. For example, use sugar or glucose instead of glucose molecules. Streiff (1986) discusses several readability indices that can be applied to patient education literature. This study evaluated several types of materials including diabetes literature and found averages of 7.7 to 14.1 grade level reading comprehension. This study found that the client's last grade completed in school (mean = 3.1 grades) was significantly higher than their actual reading levels. The majority of study participants (54.7%) read at levels that did not allow them to comprehend any of the materials.

A written contract between the client and care-giver has often been used to aid the client to meet health improvement goals. Both agree on a treatment plan, time frame, and a specific goal or goals. When the client reaches the goal, a sense of self-efficacy is enhanced and he may be able to go on to a more difficult goal (Rosenstock 1985). Goals should be very specific: to lose 5 pounds in 2 months; to check and record blood glucose levels at least twice a day; to reduce daily cigarettes smoked from 26 per day to 15 per day.

Chief obstacles to maintaining new behaviors are high-risk relapse situations for which the client may lack coping skills. Among the high-risk situations that may cause relapse are negative emotional states; interpersonal conflicts (e.g., family arguments); social pressures (e.g., temptations at a party to eat, drink, smoke) (Rosenstock 1985). Help the client to anticipate some of these and not to use them as an excuse for not maintaining new behaviors.

For example, the use of alcohol in social situations can be a problem. If the client insists on drinking, teach him to do it wisely— use "dry" drinks, avoiding beer, cordials, sweet wine; calculate the alcohol in the diet and decrease fat intake; *never* drink instead of eating. Alcohol can cause a precipitous drop in blood glucose if inadequate food is ingested. It prevents the release of stored glucose and is metabolized like a fat (Campbell and Ruhlman 1985).

The home health nurse may face decisions about the safety shortcuts taken by clients and the need to offer a recommendation, for example, not aspirating the syringe before giving insulin or reusing the insulin syringe (see Potential for Infection). The nurse needs to keep up with current literature and support research in the exploration of these topics. The basis of expertise is the application of scientifically based interventions (Clark 1985).

Outcome

A reasonable goal for this client is to be able to set small behavioral goals to improve health status, and to meet these goals. The home health nurse can assist by providing appropriate interventions.

KNOWLEDGE DEFICIT

There are several etiologies for this diagnosis in the diabetic client including lack of exposure; lack of recall; information misinterpretation; cognitive limitation; lack of interest in learning; and unfamiliarity with information resources. Many research studies have helped to identify the cause of knowledge deficit in the client with diabetes.

Major deficits in knowledge have been reported by several investigators. The National Health Survey of 1965 (cited in Etzwiler 1983) showed that only 10% of those persons studied had sufficient knowledge to choose the proper foods. Lawrence and Cheely (1980) reported that knowledge and management errors were widespread even among persons who had previously demonstrated correct skills. Two-thirds of the patients in the study made at least one error, and one-third had multiple errors. This study did not find a progressive deterioration of performance to be related to years since diagnosis or interval between knowledge assessment.

One of the most valuable studies to help health professionals recognize the occurrence of lack of content recall was done by Page and colleagues (1981). In this study, patients only recalled an average of two recommendations out of seven presented. Most surprising, 40% of the content recalled by patients was not given by any of the professionals! These studies suggest that there are a number of factors operating in the diabetic client's understanding and recall of important information.

Assessment

Assuring the knowledge of the client and family is one of the major priorities for the home health nurse. For the first several visits, it may be necessary to continue the assessment and to validate problems as they are identified. A possible approach for this assessment is shown in Table 15-4.

An assessment should include an evaluation of basic essential content areas. For the person with Type I diabetes mellitus, evaluate knowledge of prescribed injection care and technique, recognition and treatment of

TABLE 15.4 Assessment For Diabetic Client

General	Specific	Client's Knowledge
Diabetes	Pathophysiology	
	Causes	
	Signs and	
	Symptoms	
	Treatment	
	Hypoglycemia	
	and	
	Hyperglycemia	
Glucose Monitoring	Urine test for	
	sugar and acetone	
	How collect urine	
	Specific times	
	Recordkeeping	
	Blood glucose	
	testing	
Foot Care	Inspection	
	Safety	
	Nail Care	
	Signs and	
	Symptoms to	
	Report	
Diet	Restrictions	
	Exchange Lists	
Insulin	Type	
	Duration	
	Side-effects	
	Administration	

hypoglycemia, the understanding of diet restrictions, knowledge about complications and their prevention and detection, how to plan for exercise, the importance of self-glucose monitoring of blood versus urine-testing. In addition, determine what resources the client is aware of for his own continuing education.

Interventions

Nursing interventions for knowledge deficits are numerous. Assisting the client in making an education diagnosis may be very helpful. The nurse can assist the client in safely choosing priorities for knowledge acquisition. The major areas to include in the teaching are shown in the boxed material at right.

Suggestions for resource materials and organizations can be given. Many patients have gained valuable content information from their local chapter of the American Diabetes Association. In many large cities, diabetes teaching programs are available for outpatient as well as inpatient instruction. Community health clinics may offer content classes for the patient and his family.

Memory is an important area to consider when in the process of the patient teaching. As Figure 15-1 illustrates, the patient has to

---

Objective of Teaching Program For Diabetic Client

CLIENT UNDERSTANDS:

1. Reason for, correct methods, and times for urine/blood testing

2. Insulin sites, rotation pattern, insulin injection technique, and preparation of syringes

3. Uses, action, and administration of oral hypoglycemic agents, if appropriate

4. Exchange lists, diet calculations, free foods, foods to avoid, and snacks

5. Causes, symptoms, treatment, and prevention of hypoglycemia and hyperglycemia

6. Complications of diabetes

7. Foot care techniques

---

remember the content in order to apply it. Guyton (1986) describes a good deal of interesting information about the physiology of memory. For example, persons learn best when they can relate new information to pre-

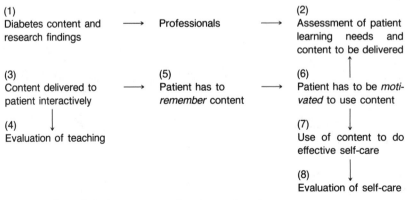

Figure 15-1. Conceptual model: the process of patient education

viously known areas of content. (The reader is referred to that text for more detail). In the diabetic client, remembering the content taught may be a major problem.

The home health nurse can use this diagram to assist in teaching. According to the model, the nurse must not only present the content to the client, but must also assist the client to develop and maintain the motivation needed to assure retention of content. The model also suggests that the client will recall content better if he is forced to apply that content. Thus, a good strategy would be to have the client demonstrate techniques (*i.e.*, insulin administration) or restate information to the home health nurse.

In addition to the general knowledge needs already described, the diabetic client also requires specific information concerning his individualized treatment plan. Specific information concerning insulin (boxed material, below), or the use of oral hypoglycemics (boxed material, at right) should be provided. All clients should be encouraged to carry a carbohydrate source with them at all times. The need for uniformity in diet, exercise, and hypoglycemic agents administration

---

Instructions For Administration of Oral Hypoglycemics

1. Take medication as prescribed.

2. Notify nurse or physician if unable to tolerate food or fluid.

3. Strictly adhere to diet.

4. Dosage may need adjustment if client experiences increased stress.

---

should be stressed. The client should be aware of change in insulin and glucose needs associated with illness or stress. Encourage all clients to wear medic-alert identification.

Considering the importance of teaching the diabetic client, many researchers have begun to look for ways to improve the existing system. Arbogast and Dodrill (1985) describe the use of computer-entered data to communicate between the patient at home and a primary care giver in a health facility. Their article shows how this can be accomplished using pushbutton telephones to enter data without expensive computer equipment in the home.

Outcome

An expected outcome for this client is to verbalize what his educational needs are and where he can find resources to meet them. Support by the nurse in the home setting can facilitate this process.

SELF-GLUCOSE MONITORING AT HOME

In the past decade, self-glucose monitoring has become an established part of diabetes care. By testing his own glucose levels, the client can gain a sense of control and confidence in managing his own disease. The role

---

Instructions For Administration of Insulin

1. Store bottle of insulin currently being used at room temperature ($\leq 75°$ C).

2. Store unopened bottle of insulin in refrigerator.

3. Check expiration date and discard outdated bottle of insulin.

4. Do not use insulin that has changed color.

5. Plan meals and snacks keeping onset, peak action, and length of action of insulin in mind.

of the home health nurse is to provide information, to assist in evaluation of various types of equipment, and to serve as a role model and educator in the interpretation of results.

Part of the impetus for self-monitoring glucose levels came as a result of research linking good glucose control (normal or near-normal glucose levels) with prevention or delay in some of the long-term complications. If the client knows his glucose level from day to day, some believe he will be more likely to work at reducing it if needed. It can eliminate the frustrating delays in obtaining readings only through the physician's office.

Urine glucose testing is no longer recommended for evaluation of current glucose levels. It does not provide information about glucose levels below the renal threshold and can be misleading and uninformative for many clients when the threshold is unknown. The lag time between blood glucose rise and urine spill can vary from 20 minutes to 2 hours, thus leading to misinterpretation of the actual glucose state at a given time (Valenta 1983). The client should still test urine for ketones as instructed. Presently there is no other way for this to be done at home.

There are numerous reasons to check blood glucose levels. (See the displayed material at right.)

There are several types of glucose meters available. Prices vary and new products are continually being introduced. Blood glucose reflectance meters are used to give a numerical reading. The client puts a drop of blood on a strip and inserts the strip into the meter to obtain a reading. The meter "reflects" color changes and converts it to a number.

The average meter cost is about $150.00. Most of them are lightweight (less than 1 pound), have built-in timers to guide the user and operate with power from a battery. Some of the newer models have a special feature of memory storage of glucose values. This could

---

Reasons For Home Monitoring of Glucose

1. To allow the client to work toward good (or "tight") diabetes control (blood glucose <150 mgl dl)

2. To make decisions about insulin doses

3. To validate cues the client is feeling, such as perceived hypoglycemia

4. To get immediate feedback when needed

5. To evaluate glucose levels during pregnancy to protect the fetus from dangerous levels

6. To evaluate irregular physical exercise

7. To diagnose hypoglycemia in the client who is unable to detect its symptoms

8. To provide data for insulin pump users, or those taking multiple daily injections

---

be very helpful for the client who is forgetful, too busy to record values, is blind, or has other visual problems. All meters have to be calibrated and procedures vary, depending on the brand. Some have control test strips, while others have control solutions that mimic blood at a set glucose level. Medicare and most insurance companies will pay for the meter if its use has been prescribed by the physician. An example of the monitor is shown in Figure 15-2.

In addition to the meter, test strips must be purchased and used. Many clients are surprised to find that this is the most expensive item for self-glucose monitoring. Some strips are made for meter use only, while others may also be used and read visually with a color chart giving ranges of glucose. Most

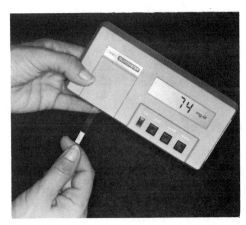

Figure 15-2. Using a glucose meter to measure capillary blood glucose. (From Walsh J, Persons CB, Wieck L: Manual of Home Health Care Nursing, p 284. Philadelphia, JB Lippincott, 1987)

strips can be blotted before reading, eliminating the rinsing step of earlier methods. The strips average about 50 cents each. Some strips may retain their color for several days according to their manufacturers claims, which may help the nurse evaluate findings a few days later.

Finger-sticking devices are available from several manufacturers. These range in price from about $9 to $28 for the basic device and about $5 per 100 for the lancets. Most of the devices use a hidden spring-operated method so the client does not feel he is sticking himself. There are some clients who may not want to purchase a meter but will still want to measure blood glucose levels at home. The nurse can suggest purchase of strips for visual reading. These come with color charts in various glucose increments, ranging from 20 mg/dl to 800 mg/dl, with about 9 increments in between. Some clients use this system before moving on to using a meter.

Some clients have tried to save money by splitting strips in half. This practice can compromise the precision of the strips although many persons are able to test successfully with a carefully split strip. Manufacturers obviously cannot vouch for the accuracy of their product unless used as directed. Only one meter presently on the market will accept split strips (Orzeck 1986).

The puncture site is cleansed with an alcohol swab and allowed to air dry before the puncture is made. A small needle (25 gauge, 5/8 inch needle, or small lancet) is used to make the puncture. The hand may then be dropped below the heart and the finger milked to obtain a large hanging drop (Peterson 1983). The drop is then placed on the strip. The nurse may suggest prewarming the hands if necessary to obtain a good drop of blood. Often individuals try to cover the strips too slowly and obtain false high test results (Tomky 1986). The client should be instructed about the easiest and least painful technique to obtain a drop of blood. Only a small drop of blood is necessary to do the test. The concentration of glucose is nearly the same in the extravascular fluid as in the blood, so a tiny finger puncture is sufficient (Peterson et al 1983). The client should be taught to rotate fingers used and to use the outer edges (or sides of the fingers) where there are fewer nerve endings.

Encourage the client to check expiration dates on strips and to store them in a moisture-free environment. Suggest that the client place the owner's manual for the meter in a safe place and refer to it frequently. It will provide instructions for use and care of the meter and strips.

If questions arise that you are unable to answer, contact the physician or other specialist in diabetes care. Most large cities have a diabetes education facility that teaches both inpatients and outpatients. The diabetes educator there may be available as a resource person if needed. Call the nearest chapter of the American Diabetes Association for information about resources.

The usual recommendations are that

clients test their blood 3 to 4 times a day, and as needed. The frequency may depend on what the treatment goals are — what it is the physician and client hope to accomplish. Some clinicians suggest that clients use glucose monitoring to test their individual responses to various types of foods and to exercise.

The physician may suggest the client alter his insulin dose based on blood glucose results. If this is done, be certain the client has written guidelines. For example, if the glucose level is over 150 mg/dl at 6 PM, add 2 units of regular insulin to the 6:30 PM injection. The client should record glucose values and insulin adjustments in a written form for discussion with the physician and other care-givers.

There are several related research studies that look at psychosocial aspects in clients using self-glucose monitoring. One study showed a decrease in anxiety, depression, and insomnia in subjects who were monitoring. Another found significant anxiety relief in parents with diabetic children (Peterson 1983).

Several researchers have questioned how accurate the glucose levels may be. Results indicate that clients testing glucose levels at home need to be regularly reminded of the importance of their evaluation of blood glucose. Carelessness is to be avoided! To test the accuracy of the technique, a venous blood sample can be drawn at the same time the client tests his glucose level. The two results can then be compared. Discrepencies between the two should be evaluated by the home health nurse.

The home health care nurse can assist the client with self-glucose monitoring in many ways. Providing information and resources can be an essential role. Helping the client develop routines and evaluating his techniques can help him reach maximal benefits. Clients with either Type I or Type II diabetes

can benefit from better glucose control and self-glucose monitoring. The procedure is outlined in the boxed material below.

Procedure For Blood Glucose Monitoring

EQUIPMENT

Lancets or prepared Autolet
Alcohol sponge (if soap and water not available)
Clean hand towel or paper towel
Reagent test strips
Cotton balls
Paper towel (if using glucose meter)
Wash bottle (if applicable)
Stopwatch or watch with second hand
Color chart or glucose meter and calibration equipment

PROCEDURE

1. Warm up and calibrate the glucose meter (if used).

2. Remove a reagent strip from the bottle and immediately replace the cap. Check the unreacted reagent strip with the O block on the color chart.

3. Discard reagent strips after 4 months.

4. Do not store strips in sunlight.

5. Clean the puncture area thoroughly with soap and warm water. Gently manipulate the puncture site.

6. Dry the puncture site with a clean towel or fresh paper towel.

7. Do a fingerstick using either a sterile, individually wrapped lancet or Autolet. Wait a few seconds to allow blood to begin to flow.

8. Facilitate flow by gently massaging the surrounding tissue toward the puncture site.

9. Use lancets only once to prevent infection.

10. Wipe away the first drop with a cotton ball. Collect a second drop. Apply a large drop of blood sufficient to cover the entire reagent area of the strip. Keep the strip level to avoid spilling the drop.

11. Stop blood flow by applying manual pressure over the wound with a cotton ball. Clean the puncture site with soap and water after the test is complete.

12. As the blood is placed on the strip, immediately begin timing for 60 seconds (Dextrostix or Chemstrip bG).

13. Prepare the strip for comparison with the color chart or interpretation with a glucose meter:

    For Dextrostix
    - Immediately wash the reagent area for 2 seconds with a sharp, constant stream of water using a wash bottle.
    - Immediately compare the color block with the color chart on the package.
    - If using a glucose meter, blot the strip on a clean paper towel and insert the strip into the prepared device.

    For Chemstrip bG
    - Wipe the blood off the reagent strip with a cotton ball.
    - Time for an additional 60 seconds.
    - Compare the color block with the color chart on the package.
    - Interpolate results that fall between two color blocks on the color chart.

Procedure For Insulin Pump

EQUIPMENT

Prescribed type and amount of insulin
A syringe that fits the pump, fitted with a butterfly needle and polyurethane tubing (size 25 needle)
Dressing ($1.5'' \times 2''$) of polyurethane or other see-through material to facilitate frequent monitoring of skin condition at the needle insertion site
Soap and water
Alcohol sponge or providone–iodine sponge
Prescribed supplies for measuring blood glucose levels
Chart to document patterns of blood glucose determinations

PROCEDURE

1. Develop a regular schedule of caring for the pump, to include charging and changing the batteries according to the manufacturer's specifications, and changing the syringe, tubing needle, and insertion site.

2. Fill the syringe each day with the prescribed amount of insulin to last one day.

CHANGING THE NEEDLE, TUBING, AND INSERTION SITE (EVERY 2 DAYS)

1. Prepare the site with soap and water, followed by applying providone–iodine or alcohol.

2. Apply a skin barrier to the insertion site.

3. Insert the needle at a 30° to 60° angle. Tape it in place by means of a see-through polyurethane patch. Secure the tube with hypoallergenic tape or polyurethane.

(continued)

OPERATION OF THE PUMP

1. Wear the pump on the belt or in a pocket.

2. Attach a syringe with the prescribed amount of insulin (usually rapid acting) daily.

3. Inject a bolus of insulin prior to meals.

Adapted from Walsh J, Persons CB, Wieck L: Manual of Home Health Care Nursing. Philadelphia, JB Lippincott, 1987

INSULIN PUMPS

Small portable pumps are used for the continuous administration of regular insulin. The pumps are worn externally and inject insulin subcutaneously into the abdomen through an indwelling needle site (Fig. 15-3). Insulin is infused through the pump at a low, set rate. However, larger amounts can be given as needed.

Insulin pump therapy is generally initiated while the client is hospitalized. Generally, the client undergoes intense education about

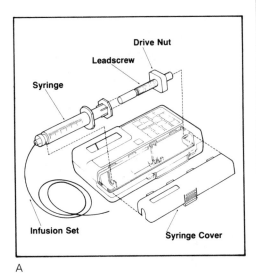

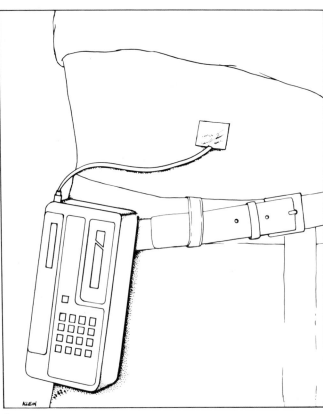

A   B

Figure 15-3. (*A*) Insulin infusion pump. (Courtesy of Cardiac Pacemakers, Inc., St. Paul, MN.) (*B*) Insulin pump in place. (From Walsh J, Persons CB, Wieck L: Manual of Home Health Care Nursing, p 383. Philadelphia, JB Lippincott, 1987)

Assessing The Home Environment

Kitchen	• Assess refrigerator, stove, sink, hotplate, etc. • Assess what foods client has in refrigerator and cupboards. • Does client understand and can he afford prescribed dietary alterations? Possible consultation with nutritionist to work with client and/or support persons to incorporate low-cost dietary modifications with family meals when applicable? • Explore possibility of Meals on Wheels. • Explore with client abundance of "sugar free" foods on the market.		person should pretest bath water. • Heating pads, heat lamps, hot water bottles, electric blankets, etc., should only be used under supervision. • Use of air mattresses, sheeps skin, etc., when appropriate. • Medicare/Medicaid and some insurance carriers will pay to have a podiatrist care for toenails. In many areas, home visits are available. • Shoes should always be worn to prevent injury.
		Decreased Visual Activity	
Poor Tissue Perfusion	• Assess client's ability to monitor feet and leg status. • Lower temperature of water heater to prevent accidental scalding. Reinforce that a family member/support		• Assess client's ability to benefit from sight-saving devices developed for insulin-dependent diabetics, *i.e.*, large numbered syringes; magnified set-up prefill syringes if patient cannot function independently (according to state and agency guidelines)

the operation of the pump prior to discharge. The home health nurse will be responsible for monitoring the client's ability to regulate use of the pump.

A complication to be expected from the insulin pump is infection at the site of injection. Hypoglycemia may also occur due to error in calculation of the insulin dosage. Diabetic ketoacidosis may also occur if insufficient amounts of insulin have been administered. The procedure for use of the insulin pump can be found in the boxed material on pages 467 and 468.

Procedures for the assessment of the diabetic client's home environment can be found in the displayed material on page 469.

ABBREVIATED CARE PLAN: DIABETES MELLITUS

Nursing Diagnosis	Assessment	Interventions	Outcomes
Alteration in Tissue Perfusion in Peripheral System	Risk factors Cool extremities Decreased pulsations Gangrene Claudication Hypertension	Assess status of foot and leg circulation, teaching client as you do so. Evaluate and educate for the presence of elevated lipids, hypertension, or cigarette smoking. Teach good basic foot care practices. Stress that any new lesion on the foot is significant. Refer client to physician for vascular studies if condition worsens.	Client will be able to assess circulation in his feet and legs and take appropriate action.
Alteration in Tissue Perfusion in the Cardiac System	Chest pain Shortness of breath Fatigue Heart sounds	Assess for key cardiac risk factors and educate the patient to alter life-style to reduce the risk. Note physical exam findings: cardiac rate and rhythm, S_3, S_4, pulses.	Client will be able to detect physical changes related to cardiac function and seek consultation when needed.

ABBREVIATED CARE PLAN: DIABETES MELLITUS (*continued*)

Nursing Diagnosis	Assessment	Interventions	Outcomes
		Educate the client about his medications.	
		Discuss the importance of monitoring for any changes in chest pain pattern.	
		Be sure the client knows that many diabetics do not experience chest pain.	
Impaired Thought Processes	Impaired attention span Nervousness Irritability Blurred vision	Teach key data re: hypoglycemia: what it is, how to recognize and treat.	Client will learn to detect and treat early signs of hypoglycemia.
		Identify factors that may predispose client to hypoglycemia.	
		Check blood glucose levels during suspected hypoglycemia to validate cues.	
		Treat home hypoglycemic reactions with 10–15 g of a simple carbohydrate.	
		Frequent area change (*i.e.,* from abdomen to arm or leg) can alter insulin absorption. Be certain the client understands differences.	

(*continued*)

ABBREVIATED CARE PLAN: DIABETES MELLITUS (*continued*)

Nursing Diagnosis	Assessment	Interventions	Outcomes
		Evaluate knowledge of insulin taken.	
		Have the client educate neighbors and coworkers about hypoglycemia.	
Impaired Tissue Integrity	Skin, for color, temperature Cigarette use Hypertension	Teach the client to do a complete skin assessment, with emphasis on feet.	Client will be able to detect any early skin breakdown and practice preventive care.
		Educate about the rationale for decreased circulation.	
		Alert the client about the dangers of wound infections and circulatory impairment but do not unduly increase his anxiety	
		Provide educational materials on foot care.	
		Suggest checking blood glucose levels when wounds do not heal.	
		Encourage foot washing (not soaking) once or twice a day followed by a thin layer of lubricant as a sealer.	
		Instruct client to brush and floss teeth regularly.	

ABBREVIATED CARE PLAN: DIABETES MELLITUS (*continued*)

Nursing Diagnosis	Assessment	Interventions	Outcomes
Potential for Infection	Skin Signs of infection	Assess knowledge of signs of infection, skin assessment procedures and practices. Teach the major clinical signs of infections. Educate client about the most common sites for infection. Suggest client seek medical consultation when infections are present or suspected. Be aware of the reported practices related to insulin syringe reuse and monitor research. Answer client's question truthfully and allow him to determine his own decision about syringe reuse.	The client will be diligent in monitoring for signs of infections.
Alteration in Bowel Elimination: Diarrhea	Frequency of stools Urgency Cramping Bowel sounds	Teach recognition of condition as a treatable complication of diabetes. Suggest Metamucil to increase dietary fiber. Suggest client see physician for other	Client will seek and obtain early treatment for diarrhea.

(continued)

ABBREVIATED CARE PLAN: DIABETES MELLITUS (*continued*)

Nursing Diagnosis	Assessment	Interventions	Outcomes
		medications: antibiotics, Lomotil. Encourage good glycemic control (low blood glucose).	
Urinary Retention	Bladder distention Dribbling Urinary tract infections	Evaluate history of absent or decreased urine output combined with large volumes of urine when voiding. Develop a schedule to have client empty bladder every 3–4 hours, aided by manual pressure. Teach the client to recognize early signs of a urinary tract infection and to seek early treatment. Encourage the use of blood glucose rather than urine glucose for reliable evaluation.	Client will be able to manage a program of timed voidings to decrease retention.
Sensory–Perceptual Alteration: Visual	Fundus of eye Glucose Acuity	Assist the client to obtain a current eye exam by an eye specialist to determine status of retinopathy and vision. Evaluate client's life-style to assist in making alterations when vision is impaired.	Client will be able to make informed decisions about eye status evaluations and treatments.

ABBREVIATED CARE PLAN: DIABETES MELLITUS (*continued*)

Nursing Diagnosis	Assessment	Interventions	Outcomes
		For the client with blindness, support and actively work to help client obtain help needed to maintain independence.	
		Provide information about treatment choices — vitrectomy, and laser photocoagulation.	
Anxiety	Tension Overexcited Eye contact	Encourage client to discuss perceptions of his health.	Client will be able to reduce anxiety about diabetes.
		Allow client to discuss his worst fears and assist him to problem solve solutions.	
		Give clear explanations using neutral language.	
		Refer client for psychiatric consultation if anxiety is incapacitating.	
		Anxiety and stress may elevate glucose levels in many persons. Be sure client is monitoring and knows his unique response to emotional stressors.	
Alteration in Nutrition	Knowledge of diet Nutritional assessment	Provide diabetic diet exchange lists.	Client and family demonstrate

(*continued*)

ABBREVIATED CARE PLAN: DIABETES MELLITUS (*continued*)

Nursing Diagnosis	Assessment	Interventions	Outcomes
		Monitor client understanding.	understanding of diabetic diet.
Potential for Injury	Glucose Respiratory pattern Level of consciousness	Teach client and family signs of complications. Transfer client to hospital as needed.	Client will not experience any complications of diabetes.
Noncompliance	Glucose Complications Exacerbation of symptoms	Use a nonjudgmental manner with client. Assess life-style and personal needs and preferences. Assess financial status. Help client to set goals and how he will meet them. Assess reading and comprehension level of client and provide oral and written instructions to match. Develop a written contract *with* the client, setting small achievable goals.	The client will be able to set small health improvement goals and to meet them.
Knowledge Deficit	Knowledge of injections Diet Exercise Blood glucose monitoring Urine testing	Assess for basic knowledge of essential content. (educational diagnosis) Assist client to set goals for increasing knowledge based on his individualized needs and priorities.	Client will continue to increase his knowledge base.

ABBREVIATED CARE PLAN: DIABETES MELLITUS (*continued*)

Nursing Diagnosis	Assessment	Interventions	Outcomes
		Help client to locate resources for his continuing education.	
		Teach client information in a manner that facilitates long-term memory storage.	
Activity Intolerance	Previous exercise tolerance Current patterns Current medications	Encourage participation in exercise.	Client will develop and maintain an exercise program.
		Assist in determination of appropriate exercises.	
		Teach to monitor cardiovascular status during exercise.	
Sexual Dysfunction	Glucose level Description of symptoms	Develop sensitive assessment.	Client will seek help as needed.
		Provide referrals as needed.	
		Offer supportive counseling.	

References

American Diabetes Association: Office guide to diagnosis and classification of diabetes mellitus and other categories of glucose intolerance. Diabetes Care 4: 335, 1981

Arbogast JG, Dodrill WH: Diabetes home monitoring by telephone data entry. Primary Care 12: 573–579, 1985

Ary DV, Toobert D, Wilson W et al: Patient perspective on factors contributing to nonadherence to diabetes regime. Diabetes Care 9: 168–172, 1986

Aschenbrener R, Clark A et al: Teaching Standards for Diabetes Mellitus, 4th ed. Austin, TX, American Diabetes Association, 1986

Aziz S: Recurrent use of disposable syringe–needle units in diabetic children. Diabetes Care 7: 118–120, 1984

Barkin J, Skyler J: Diabetes and the gastrointestinal system. In Ellenberg M, Rifkin H (eds): Diabetes Mellitus Theory and Practice, 3rd ed. New

Hyde Park, NY, Medical Examination Publishing, 1983

Barrett–Connor E, Orchard TJ: Insulin-dependent diabetes mellitus and ischemic heart disease. Diabetes Care (Suppl)1: 65–70, 1985

Brand P: The diabetic foot. In Ellenberg M, Rifkin H (eds): Diabetes Mellitus Theory and Practice, 3rd ed. New Hyde Park, NY, Medical Examination Publishing, 1983

Bryan CS, Reynolds KL, Metzger WT: Bacteremia in diabetic patients: Comparison of incidence and mortality with nondiabetic patients. Diabetic Care 8: 244–249, 1985

Campbell KS, Ruhlman G: Recreational drugs and diabetes: Alcohol, nicotine, and caffeine. Practical Diabetology 4: 16, 1985

Carter WR, Gonder–Frederick LA, Cox DJ et al: Effects of stress on blood glucose in IDDM. Diabetes Care 8: 411–412, 1985

Casey J: Host defenses and infections in diabetes mellitus. In Ellenberg M, Rifkin H (eds): Diabetes Mellitus Theory and Practice, 3rd ed. New Hyde Park, NY, Medical Examination Publishing, 1983

Casparie AF, Elving LD: Severe hypoglycemia in diabetic patients: Frequency, causes, and prevention. Diabetes Care 8: 141–145, 1985

Clark AP(a): Current reported practices related to insulin injections. Diabetes 35 (Suppl 156A), 1986

Clark AP(b): Diabetic ketoacidosis. In Guzzetta CE, Dossey BM (eds): Critical Care Nursing: Body, Mind, Spirit, 2nd ed. Boston, Little, Brown & Co., 1986

Clark AP: Legal implications of being an expert. Diabetes Educator 11 (Suppl)1: 52–56, 1985

Clements R, Bell D: Diabetic neuropathy: Part II. Diabetic complications 1: 3–5, 1985

Collins BJ, Richardson SG, Spence BK et al: Safety of reusing disposable plastic insulin syringes. Lancet 8324: 559–561, 1983

Coughlin SH, Kahn R: Diabetes in America: Where do you fit in? Diabetes Forecast 39(4): 27–31, 1986

Cox DJ, Carter WR, Gonder–Frederick L: Without warning. Diabetes Forecast 39(2): 40–43, 1986

Ellenberg M: Diabetic neuropathy. In Ellenberg M, Rifkin H (eds): Diabetes Mellitus Theory and Practice, 3rd ed. New Hyde Park, NY, Medical Examination Publishing, 1983

Etzwiler D: Patient education and management: A team approach. In Ellenberg M, Rifkin H (eds): Diabetes Mellitus Theory and Practice, 3rd ed. New Hyde Park, NY, Medical Examination Publishing, 1983

Fein F, Scheuer J: Heart disease in diabetes. In Ellenberg M, Rifkin H (eds): Diabetes Mellitus Theory and Practice, 3rd ed. New Hyde Park, NY, Medical Examination Publishing, 1983

Funnell MM, McNitt P: Autonomic neuropathy: Diabetics' hidden foe. Am J Nurs 85: 266–270, 1986

Guyton A: Textbook of Medical Physiology. Philadelphia, WB Saunders, 1986

Haffner SM, Stern MP, Hazuda HP et al: Hyperinsulinemia in a population at risk for noninsulin dependent diabetes mellitus. N Engl J Med 315: 220–224, 1986

Haycock P: Insulin absorption: Understanding the variables. Clinical Diabetes 4: 97–103, 118, 1986

Herget M: For visually impaired diabetics . . . devices that help the client administer insulin and monitor glucose. Am J Nurs 83: 1557–1560, 1983

Hodge RH Jr, Krongaard L, Sande MA et al: Multiple use of disposable insulin syringe–needle units. JAMA 244: 266–267, 1980

Holmes CS, Koepke KM, Thompson RG et al: Verbal fluency and naming performance in Type I diabetes at different blood glucose concentrations. Diabetes Care 7: 454–459, 1984

Hoover J: The national task force on diabetes and blindness. Diabetes Educator 10: 27, 1985

House WC, Pendleton L, Parker L: Patients' versus physicians' attributions of reasons for diabetic patients' noncompliance with diet. Diabetes Care 9: 434, 1986

Hume L, Oakley GB, Boulton AJ et al: Asymptomatic myocardial ischemia in diabetes and its relationship to diabetic neuropathy: An exercise electrocardiography study in middle-aged diabetic men. Diabetes Care 9: 384–388, 1986

Husband DJ, Alberti KG Julian DG: Methods for the control of diabetes after acute myocardial infarction. Diabetes Care 8: 261–267, 1985

Jenny J: A compliance model for diabetic instruction. Rehabil Lit 44: 258–263, 299, 1983

Kemmer FW, Bisping R, Steingruber HJ et al: Psychological stress and metabolic control in patients with Type I diabetes mellitus. N Engl J Med 314: 1978–1984, 1986

Klein BE, Klein R, Moss SE: Blood pressure in a population of diabetic persons diagnosed after 30 years of age. Am J Public Health 74: 336–339, 1984

Klein R, Klein BE, Moss SE et al: Retinopathy in young onset diabetic patients. Diabetic Care 8: 311–315, 1985

Koivisto VA, Felig P: Alterations in insulin absorption and in blood glucose control associated with varying insulin injection sites in diabetic patients. Ann Intern Med 92: 59–61, 1980

Kovacs M, Finkelstein R, Feinberg TL et al: Initial psychologic responses of parents to the diagnosis of insulin-dependent diabetes mellitus in their children. Diabetes Care 8: 568–575, 1985

Lawrence PA, Cheely J: Deterioration of diabetic patients' knowledge and management skills as determined during out-patient visits. Diabetes Care 3: 214–218, 1980

L'Esperance F, James W: The eye and diabetes mellitus. In Ellenberg M, Rifkin H (eds): Diabetes Mellitus Theory and Practice, 3rd ed. New Hyde Park, NY, Medical Examination Publishing, 1983

Levin M, O'Neal L: Peripheral vascular disease. In Ellenberg M, Rifkin H (eds): Diabetes Mellitus Theory and Practice, 3rd ed. New Hyde Park, NY, Medical Examination Publishing, 1983

LoGerfo FW, Coffman JD: Current concepts. Vascular and microvascular disease of the foot in diabetes. N Engl J Med 315: 1615–1619, 1984

Manley G: Diabetes and sexual health. Diabetes Educator 12: 66–69, 1986

McNeal B, Salisbury Z, Baumgardner P et al: Comprehension assessment of diabetes education program participants. Diabetes Care 7: 232–235, 1984

Orzeck EA: Self-testing. Blood glucose monitoring: Technology for taking control. Diabetes Forecast 39(3): 8–13, 1986

Page P, Verstraete DG, Robb JR et al: Patient recall of self care recommendations in diabetes. Diabetes Care 4: 96–98, 1981

Peterson C, Jovanovic L, Brownlee M: Home glucose monitoring. In Ellenberg M, Rifkin H (eds): Diabetes Mellitus Theory and Practice, 3rd ed. New Hyde Park, NY, Medical Examination Publishing, 1983

Richardson B: A tool for assessing the real world of diabetic noncompliance. Nursing 17: 68–73, 1982

Rifkin H (ed): The Physician's Guide to Type II Diabetes (NIDDM): Diagnosis and Treatment, New York, Diabetes Association, 1984

Rosenstock IM: Understanding and enhancing patient compliance with diabetic regimens. Diabetic Care 8: 610–616, 1985

Schade DS, Eaton RP: Bactericidal properties of commercial U.S.P. formulated insulin. Diabetes 31: 36–39, 1982

Schiffrin A, Parikh S: Accommodating planned exercise in Type I diabetic patients on intensive therapy. Diabetes Care 8: 337–343, 1985

Streiff LD: Can clients understand our instructions? Image 18: 48–52, 1986

Tomky D: Getting the most out of self blood glucose testing. Diabetes Forecast 39: 45–47, 1986

Valenta CL: Urine testing and home blood glucose monitoring. Nurs Clin North Am 18: 645–659, 1983

Villeneuve M, Treitel L, D'Eramo G: Dental care for the person with diabetes mellitus. Diabetes Educator 11: 44–47, 1985

Wald A, Tunuguntla K: Anorectal sensorimotor dysfunction in fetal incontinence and diabetes mellitus. Modification with biofeedback therapy. N Engl J Med 310: 1282–1285, 1984

ALTERATIONS IN REPRODUCTION

16

Karen S. Edmondson
Vicki Embiscuso
Corine Bonnet

Women experiencing a high-risk pregnancy and families with high-risk newborns and infants may require the interventions of the home health nurse. For example, the physician may request close monitoring of a pregnant patient in the home setting. For some, more frequent visits to the physician may be too stressful. The home health nurse may visit the patient as often as three to six times per week. Recently, some insurance companies have been recommending this procedure, rather than an extended prenatal hospitalization.

Similarly, the care of the high-risk infant requires supervision from the home health nurse. With this intense supervision, prolonged hospitalization for the infant may be avoided.

HIGH-RISK PREGNANCY

Most pregnancies have a favorable outcome; however those pregnancies at risk are open to more unfavorable results. A number of factors

and conditions may contribute to risk and have an adverse effect on the lives of both the pregnant woman and her unborn child. This chapter will be directed toward four of the more commonly occurring risks. These are pregnancy-induced hypertension, diabetes mellitus, threatened premature delivery, and placenta previa. These conditions are usually monitored by frequent visits to the physician's office or frequent hospitalizations. Typically, there is not a need for continuous nursing assessment and care in the home. However, the future may hold a place for care in the home of high-risk pregnancy. In this event, an important strategy in caring for those clients with a high-risk pregnancy is the development of a communication network with all care providers involved in the client's health management. These providers include the obstetrician or perinatal specialist, a physical therapist, nutritionist, obstetric nurses in both inpatient and outpatient settings, and a social worker. A key role for the home health nurse may be in coordination of communication among the network of providers.

PREGNANCY-INDUCED HYPERTENSION

Pregnancy-induced hypertension (PIH), previously known as *toxemia*, is a syndrome characterized by hypertension and proteinuria and often accompanied by edema. It is usually divided into conditions of preeclampsia and eclampsia. Preeclampsia describes the occurrence of hypertension, proteinuria, and edema after the 20th week of gestation, and eclampsia includes the symptoms of preeclampsia plus seizures. PIH frequently contributes to perinatal morbidity and mortality. While much is now known about this condition, the cause remains unclear.

Pathophysiology

Pregnancy is accompanied by a number of dramatic changes. The cardiac output increases in the first trimester and reaches a maximum of 30% to 40% above the nonpregnant level by the 24th week of gestation. In addition to the increase in cardiac output, the total blood volume increases by approximately 40% to 50%. The increase in plasma volume contributes to hemodilution and physiologic anemia of pregnancy. Since arterial blood pressure is the result of cardiac output and peripheral resistance, it is interesting to note that in pregnancy there is a reduction rather than an increase in arterial blood pressure. Vascular resistance also normally decreases during pregnancy; however, in PIH the vascular resistance increases (Burrow and Ferris 1982, p 1), particularly in the first pregnancy. Women pregnant with multiple fetuses, diabetes mellitus, and chronic hypertension are also predisposed to PIH. In addition, it is more common in lower socioeconomic circumstances and in women who receive limited or no prenatal care.

The two important signs of preeclampsia —hypertension and proteinuria—are abnormalities of which the pregnant woman is usu-

ally unaware. Hence, the importance of early and continuous prenatal care to facilitate detection cannot be stressed too strongly. Once the symptoms include headaches, visual disturbances, nausea or vomiting, oliguria, hyperreflexion or epigastric pain, the PIH is usually more severe (Pritchard et al 1985).

One of the first signs of PIH may be development of edema. The woman may notice her rings have become tight. When weight gain exceed 2 pounds in a given week or 6 pounds in a month, PIH must be suspected. Sudden and excessive gain is characteristic of abnormal retention of fluid. In more severe cases the nondependent edema may become visible; examples are puffiness of eyelids or fingers. Extreme cases may involve waterlogging with a weight gain of 10 pounds or more in a week (Pritchard et al 1985, p 541).

PIH is defined as a rise in blood pressure of 30 mm Hg in systolic pressure and 15 mm Hg in diastolic pressure over the first trimester baseline. This must occur on two occasions at least 6 hours apart. First trimester baseline evaluation is important for comparison since the blood pressure tends to drop during the second trimester from hypovolemia. Mild hypertension is also represented by a sustained blood pressure of 140/90. The rise in blood pressure indicates vasospasm, particularly of the arterioles, and is probably the most reliable prognostic sign. Therefore, any persisting diastolic pressure of 90 mm Hg should be closely monitored (Pritchard et al 1985, p 540).

Proteinuria usually occurs after the rise in blood pressure and edema and can be the most ominous sign. Proteinuria varies from case to case and also from hour to hour in the same woman. In early preeclampsia, proteinuria may be minimal or entirely lacking. Presence in concentrations greater than 300 mg/L in a 24-hour collection or 2+ or greater by dipstick method on two occasions 6 hours apart is usually significant (Knupple and

Drucker 1986, p 365). The degree of proteinuria is best correlated with the extent of glomerular lesion in the kidney (Burrow and Ferris 1982, p 11). However, any urine proteinuria should be reported and investigated. The investigation would include questions related to events of dysuria, vaginal itching, burning or foul odor, back pain, suprapubic pain, or fevers.

With mild cases of preeclampsia the woman may feel fine; however if the condition progresses toward eclampsia, she may experience symptoms of headache, nausea and/or vomiting, epigastric pain, oliguria, and visual disturbances. Headache is not common in milder cases of preeclampsia, but women who develop eclampsia frequently complain of severe headache prior to convulsion. It may be in the frontal or occipital region and ordinary relief measures such as rest, snacks, or analgesia are of no avail.

Visual disturbances range from a slight blurring of vision, or spots before the eyes, to blindness in eclampsia. Vasospasm of the cerebroarterial vasculature is thought to be responsible for visual disturbances and headaches in this condition (Whittaker, Hull, and Clochesy 1986, p 403).

Epigastric pain or pain in the right upper quadrant is a symptom of severe preeclampsia and is a warning of imminent convulsion. It is thought to be the result of the stretching of the liver, possible by edema and hemorrhage (Pritchard et al 1985, p 541).

Central nervous system irritability may be detected in the development of hyperreflexia. Normal reflexes are graded at 2+, while 3+ or 4+ are considered hyperactive. Clonus may not be present in 3+ hyperreflexia, but is present in 4+.

NURSING DIAGNOSES

There are multiple nursing diagnoses for the woman with PIH. Four diagnoses that address the greatest number of needs will be included, accompanied by appropriate assessment, goals, and expected outcomes.

ALTERATION IN TISSUE PERFUSION

Pregnancy is normally a time of change in hemodynamics. Preeclampsia (PIH) is a condition of vasospasm or increased constriction of the vasculature throughout the body. The vasospasm causes marked peripheral resistance and thus a rise in blood pressure. As these changes occur, generalized tissue perfusion become of greatest concern.

Assessment

A potentially serious consequence of vasospasm is a decrease in urinary output and a decrease in placental blood flow (Ouimette 1986, p 119). As vasospasm continues and renal blood is reduced, edema develops. This occurrence further compromises normal tissue perfusion.

Interventions

Interventions in PIH are directed toward prevention or minimizing progression of the disease. Bed rest with bathroom privileges is usually ordered by the physician. The left side-lying position is recommended to reduce the weight of the gravid uterus on the inferior vena cava and facilitate venous return (from extremities). This will promote reduction of blood pressure and edema. Trips outside the home should be restricted to visits to the physician's office.

Diet should be well balanced. Protein intake is recommended at 70 to 80 grams per day. A low sodium diet is no longer ordered unless known kidney damage exists. However, the client should be instructed to use no added salt and to decrease consumption of fried foods. Suggestions for baking, broiling, or poaching meats and fish can be given for food preparation. The diet should also include an adequate fluid intake of at least 8 to 10 glasses of water daily. Soda and caffeinated beverages should be used sparingly. The woman should be advised to expect an increase in urine output and that this is a good sign. Along with an increase in fluid, fiber should also be included in the diet to prevent constipation.

Outcome

A desired outcome for the pregnant woman with alteration in tissue perfusion is that she will deliver a healthy infant at term and that sequelae from the PIH will not develop in her own health.

KNOWLEDGE DEFICIT RELATED TO PIH

Since PIH is more common in the primipara, it is a condition that requires in-depth patient education and support. The woman must be encouraged to remember that PIH not only affects her body, but the development of her unborn child. It is crucial that the nurse investigate the emotional status of any pregnant woman on prolonged bed rest for a high-risk condition in pregnancy. A number of important facts may surface during conversations with these women that will affect our attempts at teaching. These will include guilt from "causing" the problem or from not planning or necessarily wanting the pregnancy; from inability to comply with the medical regimen for situational reasons such as other children in the house; from single parenthood; or from poverty.

Assessment

Initial assessment of knowledge deficit related to PIH will include eliciting information including level of education, previous health care practices, knowledge of desirable health care, and desire to give birth to a healthy child.

If the woman is able to read and will read, the knowledge deficit can be rectified much more easily. However, if the client is adolescent or from a low socioeconomic family, this becomes a greater challenge. In some instances adequate diet and bed rest cannot be achieved without hospitalization.

Interventions

Interventions are planned for the knowledge deficit diagnosis after a careful assessment of the woman's assets and values she holds for her pregnancy. Printed materials must be appropriate for the reading level of the client. The importance of compliance with the medical regimen must be tempered to meet the educational needs without engendering undue fear. Since PIH usually occurs after the woman has felt her baby move within her body, she may tend to worry too greatly if the printed materials contain advanced pathophysiology.

If the client with PIH reads little, the nurse may achieve more by developing a positive nurse–patient relationship. She may focus attention on the woman's postpartal plans. By this method the nurse may determine the patient's goals and then design interventions that will assist her to meet those expectations.

Outcome

The desired outcome of interventions planned for knowledge deficit is that the woman will gain necessary information to comply with the therapeutic regimen for PIH.

ALTERATION IN FAMILY PROCESS

Assessment

Assessment for alteration in family process should occur respectfully and with the family members. This is a period when bed rest for the woman results in other numbers of the family assuming care-taking roles. Open dialog should be encouraged with family members, both individually and through group process. The single parent family should also be carefully reviewed for potential support systems.

Intervention

Interventions should be centered around family members. Compliance to treatment is dependent on support systems available to the pregnant woman. Dialog should be encouraged between family members. Importance of compliance to medical management should be stressed by the home health nurse.

Outcome

Family process will function optimally so that medical treatment can be observed.

DIVERSIONAL ACTIVITY DEFICIT RELATED TO BED REST

The regimen of bed rest, while therapeutic, is likely to be stressful for the pregnant woman. Because she does not feel ill, it may be more difficult to remain in bed rather than continue with her normal daily activities. Ideally, planned diversional activities will offer mental stimulation so that the client with PIH will not view the time as wasted.

Assessment

Assessment of the client with diversional activity deficit will include educational level, hobbies, and previous experience with creative projects. Foremost, the woman's ability to comply with bed rest regimen must be assessed. The greater the number and variety of quiet activities in which the woman can

become interested, the more enjoyable the time spent in bed. Again support and assessment of this woman's emotional status is crucial. It may be helpful for her to hear that this period will end!

Interventions

Interventions should be planned to assist the woman to keep her day organized. An example would be selected television programs at certain times of the day, reading at a certain time, and crafts. Games might be reserved for the evening hours when they can be enjoyed with a spouse or a significant other. The more the woman's day has prescription and order, the less stress she may experience. In addition, encourage the client to share her schedule with friends, so they will know the best times to call or visit. Some women, particularly those women in a lower socioeconomic bracket, may not have the luxury to involve themselves in such activities. In this case, the home health visit may be the center of her day and a few extra moments with the client may be worth more than realized.

Community resources should be utilized for those clients confined to bed rest. Many volunteer programs are available through church organizations and public school systems that may bring extra support to the homes of these families. Of particular importance is the inclusion of pregnant teenagers in homebound programs when available so that their education is not interrupted by their high-risk status.

Outcome

The expected outcome for interventions planned for diversional activity deficit is that the woman will view the time spent in decreased physical activity as a period of relative enjoyment and mental stimulation and productivity. An abbreviated care plan for PIH follows.

ABBREVIATED CARE PLAN: PREGNANCY-INDUCED HYPERTENSION

Nursing Diagnosis	Assessment	Interventions	Outcomes

Alteration in Tissue Perfusion	Blood pressure
	Urine protein
	Weight
		Bed rest in left lateral recumbant position with BRP
		Diet therapy
		  Protein intake of 70–80 g/daily
		  8–10 glasses of water daily
		  Decrease fried foods
			Stable BP and optimal environment for growth of fetus.

Knowledge Deficit Related to PIH	Level of education
	Health care practices
	Social and emotional status
		Etiology of condition (PIH)
		Education
		  Etiology of disease
		  Importance of compliance
		  Potential risks for mother and baby from PIH
		  Danger signs:
		    Headache
		    Blurry vision or scotoma
		    Nausea/vomiting
		    Facial edema
		    Epigastric pain
			Client and family verbalize understanding.

Alteration in Family Process	Interaction of family-support systems Ability of women to comply with medical treatment	Develop family-centered plan with family so that all family functions and needs are addressed.	Structure and function will be optimized.
Diversional Activity Related to Bed Rest	Emotional status	Develop plan for creative activities around bed rest. Provide community resource list to client for utilization.	Increase in self-esteem so that medical treatment can be observed.

DIABETES MELLITUS IN PREGNANCY

Diabetes mellitus is considered a major medical complication in pregnancy. It is associated with increased morbidity and mortality in both mother and fetus. Approximately 1 of every 300 pregnancies is complicated by diabetes. Recent acquisition of knowledge related to management of diabetes in pregnancy has contributed to the reduction of complications and related outcomes. In most instances of strict medical management the outcomes are equal to those of nondiabetic mothers.

Pathophysiology

Pregnancy can be considered a state of metabolic stress for nondiabetics. In the normal nondiabetic woman, pregnancy is associated with profound changes in fuel metabolism. Circulating levels of glucose and amino acids are decreased and levels of free fatty acids, ketones, and triglycerides are increased. More insulin is secreted in response to glucose. Pregnancy normally has a diabetogenic effect on the mother in that women who are genetically predisposed to diabetes may develop the condition during gestation and revert to normal carbohydrate metabolism after delivery (Barrow and Ferris 1982, p 36).

Much has been written about diabetes and it has been classified as follows: Type I diabetes (formerly called *juvenile-onset*) is described as the absence of beta cell functions; insulin is necessary for carbohydrate metabolism; Type II diabetes (formerly called *maturity-onset*) refers to a condition in which insulin is produced in amounts insufficient for normal carbohydrate metabolism; this condition is frequently managed with oral hypoglycemic drugs. Gestational diabetes or Type III diabetes mellitus involves hyperglycemia that occurs during pregnancy; it generally resolves postpartum (Jovanovic, Peterson, and Fuhrmann 1986, p 9). Type IV diabetes refers

to abnormalities in glucose tolerance following pancreatic disease, endocrine disorders, or drug use.

During pregnancy, the control of diabetes may be complicated by a variety of conditions. Nausea and vomiting may lead to insulin shock in women who have Type I diabetes or, if the condition worsens to ketosis, an insulin resistance may occur. Insulin resistance may also develop if an infection is present in pregnancy. In addition, the muscular exertion of labor, particularly if little or no carbohydrates is present, may result in severe hypoglycemia (Pritchard et al 1985, p 600).

Effects of uncontrolled diabetes on the mother increase the likelihood of additional complications. These include preeclampsia, infection, increased chance of perinatal death, macrosomia, respiratory distress, and metabolic derangement of hypoglycemia and hyperglycemia. Congenital anomalies of the heart, central nervous system, the sacrum and the trachea in the infant have been associated with inherited diabetes (Pritchard et al 1985, p 601).

Assessment

Women with Type I (insulin-dependent diabetes mellitus) require the most skillful management to ensure an optimum pregnancy outcome. This management should be provided by a team approach involving the obstetrician, internist, neonatologist, nurse, and nutritionist. Ideally the woman could receive preconception counseling that would permit the selection of the appropriate time to become pregnant. Since major fetal growth occurs before the eighth gestational week, it is important that the Type I diabetic have adequate control of glycemia to avoid the major malformations that can occur during this critical period.

The Type I diabetic is at special risk during the first trimester of pregnancy for hypoglycemia, starvation, ketosis, and erratic plasma glucose values. Insulin doses frequently must be modified to meet immediate needs. This particular client should not be advised to go to the physician's office for a plasma glucose tolerance test because of the risk of hypoglycemia en route (Hollingsworth 1984 p 30). Diagnosis is made based on history of asymptomatic hyperglycemia and impairment of glucose tolerance. Some of these individuals will have been diagnosed prior to conception and may have controlled their diabetes with oral hypoglycemic drugs. These are sulfonylureas and are contraindicated during pregnancy.

Gestational diabetes varies in severity from mildly to drastically elevated postprandial and fasting blood sugar (FBS) levels. Therefore, the treatment will vary from dietary regulation alone to a regimen of dietary changes plus insulin. Treatment is important because the maternal hyperglycemia may predispose the infant to fetal abnormalities.

All pregnant women who have a history of the following risk factors should be screened with a 1 hour glucose tolerance test: previous still births; previous infants of 4,000 grams or more; previous infants with congenital anomalies; familial history of diabetes; previous obstetric complications such as pre-eclampsia or polyhydramnios; previous gestational diabetes; or age greater than 25.

NURSING DIAGNOSES

Multiple nursing diagnoses may be appropriate for the woman with diabetes in pregnancy, regardless of the type of diabetes. The most common ones will be considered here.

ALTERATION IN NUTRITION

Pregnancy is a time of accelerated carbohydrate metabolism in the body. Insulin, a hormone secreted by the pancreas, is necessary as an active transport mechanism for glucose to enter cells. Diabetes is a condition in which insulin is absent or diminished. Therefore, management of nutrition in pregnancy becomes a challenge.

Assessment

During the first half of pregnancy the major factor in carbohydrate metabolism is the need of the fetus for glucose and amino acids. As glucose and amino acids are transferred to the fetus, the tendency is toward maternal hypoglycemia. This may be symptomatic and necessitate a reduction in insulin dosage. If the woman is also experiencing nausea and vomiting, common during the first trimester, the need for insulin will be further decreased. The result of this is maternal hypoglycemia and, depending on the extent, blood glucose may approach dangerously low levels. As levels of blood glucose plummet, fat becomes fatty acids for an auxiliary fuel source. When these fatty acids cross the placenta to the fetus they are potentially damaging to neurological development or may even cause death.

In view of the factors present in the pregnant diabetic during the first half of gestation, she will probably need to increase her carbohydrate intake for this period and possibly decrease the dosage of insulin. Throughout pregnancy, it will be important to distinguish between ketoacidosis that results from inadequate insulin dosage and that occurring from starvation or insufficient carbohydrate intake.

During the second half of pregnancy there is an increasing supply of hormones that render the women diabetogenic. The woman with a predisposition to diabetes may demonstrate a glucose intolerance at this time. Pancreatic activity may be adequate to meet normal needs, but this individual does not have the reserve capacity for insulin production. The known Type I diabetic can compensate for this need by increasing her insulin dosage (Ziegel and Cranley 1984, p 303).

Interventions

Interventions for the pregnant woman with diabetes will depend on the type of diabetes present. The Type I, or insulin-dependent diabetic, will have had diabetes for a period of time prior to conception. Therefore, the nurse must obtain a thorough history of this woman with particular attention to past management of her diabetes, including any unique challenges for control.

Diabetic control will be achieved through diet and insulin, monitored by blood glucose determinations. The diet counseling should occur with a nutritionist to determine adequacy based on food preferences, life-style, and economic considerations. Caloric intake should be sufficient to permit a weight gain of 25 pounds. Usually 1800 to 2200 calories per day is sufficient. Carbohydrates and proteins should be divided to prevent wide fluctuations in blood glucose during the day. Meals should be at regular times. Often, it is easier for a diabetic woman to consume five smaller meals rather three normal-sized ones. A high protein bedtime snack may be important to avoid the risks of an overnight fast (Ziegel and Cranley 1984, p 305).

It may be helpful to the client, nurse, and nutritionist if the woman keeps a daily log of all food and liquid intake. This presents a means for ongoing assessment, diagnosis, and teaching. In addition, the log becomes evidence of the woman's active participation in the management of her pregnancy.

Insulin dosage is adjusted on the basis of blood glucose levels. (Urine testing for glucose is not a reliable method during pregnancy.) Blood glucose is a reliable method during pregnancy and provides a tremendous advantage for the pregnant diabetic. A typical home glucose monitoring schedule might be four times a day. An example would be fasting in the morning, 2 hours after breakfast, late afternoon, and evening prior to bedtime.

Insulin therapy is prescribed by the physician and normally includes a mixture of short-acting and intermediate-acting insulins. These may be administered in divided doses and the physician's prescription may provide for modification of dosage depending on the blood glucose level. Further information on insulin administration can be found in Chapter 15.

The interventions for the woman with Type II diabetes will be similar to those listed previously for the woman with Type I diabetes. They will differ in that the Type II individual may not have knowledge of home blood glucose monitoring and insulin administration. She should not take oral hypoglycemic drugs. This will be considered under the diagnosis of knowledge deficit.

The woman with gestational diabetes requires the same careful monitoring as the Type I and Type II diabetics. Evidence of placental insufficiency and possible threat to the fetus must be determined. Even with mild diabetes, the possibility of placental insufficiency increases near the end of gestation. Therefore, screening should occur between 24 and 28 weeks for all those at risk. Those who develop symptoms or have previously mentioned risk factors for gestational diabetes must be monitored more closely.

Outcome

The desired outcome for the pregnant woman with diabetes and a nursing diagnosis of alteration in nutrition is that diabetic control and fetal well-being will be maintained.

KNOWLEDGE DEFICIT RELATED TO MANAGEMENT OF DIABETES

As mentioned earlier, the woman with Type I diabetes may not require the extensive teaching as the woman with Type II or gestational diabetes. Women in the latter two categories may be much more dependent on the nurse for information, guidance, and support.

Assessment

Assessment related to knowledge deficit of diabetes includes gathering information on nutritional balance coupled with diligent data collection for risk factors indicating gestational diabetes. Unrecognized gestational diabetes results in a perinatal mortality rate much higher than that for the recognized and carefully managed woman with diabetes.

Interventions

The nurse should plan interventions for the control of gestational diabetes or Type II diabetes based on the client's fundamental knowledge of nutrition. Education must include information about proteins, fats, and carbohydrates, the function of each in the body, and alterations necessary in pregnancy. In addition to diet teaching, the nurse needs to teach the client about diabetes and the additional requirements it necessitates in pregnancy. Teaching must also include recognition of symptoms of hyperglycemia and insulin overdose. Symptoms of infection must be taught to ensure prompt reporting. The nurse will need to teach home blood glucose monitoring and insulin administration. These may require short, but frequent, teaching sessions.

The nurse may need to plan with the client regarding questions that should be asked at the weekly visit to the physician. These may include a request for an ultrasound at 20 weeks and 32 weeks to ensure adequate fetal growth and development. Nonstress testing usually begins by the 34th week. The nurse may need to instruct the pregnant woman on the importance and preparation prior to tests such as ultrasound, nonstress test, and the glucose tolerance test.

Outcome

The desired outcome of interventions related to knowledge deficit in the pregnant woman with diabetes is that she will adhere to the prescribed regimen of care to ensure a positive perinatal outcome.

PLACENTA PREVIA

Vaginal bleeding during the third trimester of pregnancy is a frightening experience for the pregnant woman. Painless bleeding resulting from placenta previa is a serious complication that occurs in approximately one of two hundred pregnancies. Other causes of vaginal bleeding in pregnancy are vaginitis, urinary tract infection, abruptio of placenta, and hemorrhoids.

Pathophysiology

Placenta previa is implantation of the placenta low in the uterus, rather than the usual fundal implantation. The placenta is placed either very near or covering the cervical os. Four classifications are used to describe placenta previa. These are a *complete placenta previa* that covers the cervical opening; a *partial placenta previa* that covers a portion of the cervical opening; a *marginal placenta previa* that occurs when an edge of the placenta lies on the margin of the os; and a *low-lying placenta previa*, a placement that lies directly next to the cervical opening (Ouimette 1986, p 101).

As the pregnancy approaches term and the lower segment of the uterus expands and the cervix begins to thin or dilate, the placenta previa in this area will become detached and bleeding occurs. Most commonly the first episode of bleeding occurs after the seventh month. The woman may experience spotting or profuse bleeding while asleep. Usually the first episode is not uncontrollable bleeding. In fact there may be several episodes of bleeding before hemorrhage occurs.

The etiology of placenta previa is unknown. It is believed that when the vasculature in the fundus of the uterus is deficient, the placenta implants at a lower level that provides a more sufficient blood supply. A large thin placenta may develop in an attempt to receive better perfusion. It is thought that the placenta implants at a different site with each pregnancy (Neeson and May 1986, p 524).

Assessment

Among the important factors associated with the incidence of placenta previa are multiparity (more than four pregnancies); age greater than 35; multiple gestation (twins, triplets, etc.); previous cesarean delivery; abnormal fetal lie; previous placenta previa; and women who have previously undergone dilation and curettage (D & C). Of women experiencing placenta previa, multiparity is the most frequent associate factor.

Since prevention of complications is the ideal approach, women who present the factors listed above should be screened by ultrasound early in pregnancy to determine placement of the placenta. Placental localization by ultrasound is approximately 95% accurate (Reeder and Martin 1987, p 751).

Physical examination of the cervix in women suspected of placenta previa or any heavy vaginal bleeding should never be performed by a nurse, either in the home or in the hospital. The potential of torrential hemorrhage exists with manual manipulation of the cervix. Every precaution must be maintained to ensure a term delivery of a healthy infant.

NURSING DIAGNOSES

Nursing diagnoses pertaining to bed rest or limited activity and anxiety related to preterm labor have been previously described. These interventions, in most instances, would apply to the woman with a pregnancy complicated by placenta previa. Therefore, the diagnosis to be described here will be related to home management of placenta previa.

KNOWLEDGE DEFICIT RELATED TO MANAGING PREGNANCY COMPLICATED BY PLACENTA PREVIA

The woman with placenta previa who is permitted to be managed on home care must be carefully selected due to the life-threatening condition that profuse bleeding can create. This woman must be reliable and have a full understanding of information necessary to management in the home (Knuppel and Drukker 1986, p 427).

Assessment

Assessment of knowledge deficit related to managing pregnancy complicated by placenta previa should be meticulously compiled. It is imperative for this woman to have transportation available at a moment's notice in the event of an emergency such as profuse bleeding.

Interventions

The nurse should plan interventions to meet informational needs of the woman with placenta previa in a factual manner. The prospect of bleeding or hemorrhage is frightening; therefore, the nurse must engage in mutual problem solving with the woman and her family as necessary details are covered.

First, the woman must plan for bed rest and the implications that presents in her home. The couple must avoid coitus as this could provoke active bleeding. She must have a round-the-clock driver and transportation available. Driving distance to the hospital should be no more than 20 minutes. The woman should have a nutritious diet and a hematocrit above 30.

She may be scheduled to visit her physician once a week for sonography and other fetal assessment (Knuppel and Drukker 1986, p 427). The woman must be taught signs of labor, infection, and implication of rupture of membranes. If any of these signs appear, she should contact her physician immediately. Cesarean section is the accepted method of delivery in most all cases of placenta previa. The woman should be prepared for this prior to hospitalization if at all possible.

Outcome

The outcome expected of the interventions directed toward knowledge deficit related to managing pregnancy complicated by placenta previa is that the woman would comply with the necessary and prescribed regimen.

ASSESSING THE HOME

Most of the high-risk conditions that have been presented in this chapter advocate bed rest and/or diet modifications resulting in a life-style change for the woman and her family unit.

Compliance with the prescribed medical regimen may depend largely on how the family unit perceives the client's condition and the emotional investment they have in the pregnancy. After a family assessment of significant support persons is conducted, the home should be evaluated (opposite).

THREATENED PRETERM (PREMATURE) DELIVERY

Preterm delivery remains the most important obstetric problem today. It accounts for ap-

---

Assessing the Home: High-Risk Pregnancy

ACCESS: Stairways and number of steps to reach dwelling. This can be a significant problem in single and multi-family dwellings. The woman may be prevented from staying in her own residence due to the number of steps to be negotiated.

BEDROOM: What room is best suited to serve as the client's bedroom? Consider:

- Location of the bedroom
- Location of stairs
- Location of kitchen
- Location of TV—TV may be the main source of entertainment

CHILDREN: Number and ages of children. What support persons are available for their care if expectant mother is on bed rest?

- Explore day care facilities, day care for after school period, foster grandparents, church and community support groups

NUTRITION: Assess the kitchen. Is there a refrigerator? What are the contents (in an attempt to establish normal eating patterns)? Is there a stove, hot plate, etc.?

- Many of the high-risk factors affect (proportionately) women from lower socio-economic background who are often limited in the areas of education and money.
- A nutritionist may be helpful in suggesting low cost meals that would meet the client's dietary needs and her family's.
- Meals on Wheels should be investigated.
- Federally sponsored program (Women, Infants, and Children) that provides

(continued)

supplemental foods for high-risk clients and children.
- Explore food banks and support groups in the community.

SAFETY MEASURES:

- Does the client have a phone? Are emergency numbers posted?
- Is there a driver that can be reached 24 hours a day.
- A driver to accompany client to doctor's appointments? Many clinics provide for taxi vouchers for clients who cannot use public transportation.
- If other children are present in the home, are electrical outlets covered? Cleaning supplies out of reach, etc? Many excellent safety pamphlets are available through poison control centers.
- As pregnancy approaches term, are baby supplies, crib, etc., available? Many "Pro life," "Right to Life" groups provide newborn supplies to needy families if enough notice is given.
- Is there an infant carseat? Many hospitals rent carseats free of charge or for a minimal fee.

proximately 75% of all cases of perinatal morbidity and mortality. In addition, a financial debt of $100,000 or more may be created for parents of infants born too soon. The term *premature* was used in the past to describe infants born before 37 weeks' gestation and with a weight of less than 2500 grams. This is confusing and the World Health Organization (WHO) recommends that infants delivered at less than 37 weeks or 259 days gestation be defined as *preterm* and that infants weighing less than 2500 grams be classified as low-birthweight (Knuppel and Drukker 1986, p 303).

Pathophysiology

The sequence of events leading to the onset of labor is better understood presently than in past decades. However, the cause of preterm labor is complicated by many factors and is poorly understood. There is considerable evidence from animal research that progesterone is important in the maintenance of pregnancy and that, when withdrawn, labor begins. It has been suggested that as the placenta produces progesterone, activity in the uterus is blocked. A decline in the production of progesterone serves to remove the block and permit the onset of labor. Currently, it is believed that this effect is accomplished primarily through production of prostaglandins by uterine decidua and fetal membranes (Queenan 1985, p 536).

The fetus may contribute to the onset of labor by its production of oxytocin. Levels of oxytocin are significantly higher in fetal blood than in maternal blood at the time of delivery. The fetus in distress may influence labor onset by passage of meconium into the amniotic fluid. Oxytocin content of meconium-stained amniotic fluid has been reported to be higher than that of clear fluid.

An additional factor in the onset of labor may be that of altered uterine blood flow. Generally, reduced blood flow is associated with increased uterine activity, while improved blood flow contributes to relaxation of the uterus. Compromise of blood flow to the uterus may be a common factor leading to preterm labor in preeclampsia/eclampsia, hypertensive disease, multiple gestation, hyponutritive conditions, and heavy smoking (Queenan 1985, p 537).

Assessment

In assessing preterm labor, the most difficult differentiation is between true and false labor. Preterm labor may be diagnosed when contractions occur at intervals of less than 10 minutes, last 30 seconds or more, and produce changes in the cervix. Once the cervix has effaced to 60% and dilated to 4 centimeters, the chances of arresting labor are small (Neeson and May 1986, p 856).

The current efforts in regard to preterm labor are in the area of identification of women at risk so that they may be taught to recognize early signs and seek interventions. However, all women should be instructed on the danger signs of preterm labor early in their second trimester. Factors that have been associated with preterm labor include the following:

Low socioeconomic status	Hypertensive disease in pregnancy
Age under 18 or over 35	Over-distended uterus (hydramnios)
Multiparity (4 or more children)	Fetal anomalies
History of premature birth	Faulty implantation of placenta
History of uterine bleeding in pregnancy	Retained intrauterine device
Urinary tract infection	Fetal death
Multiple gestation	Uterine anomalies
Smoking	Incompetent cervix

Before attempts are made to arrest preterm labor, it must be determined if further uterine stay for the fetus will be beneficial or harmful. This decision is based primarily on the maturity of the fetal lungs, because the major threat to neonatal survival is respiratory distress syndrome. This is particularly increased in infants born at less than 32 weeks. Additional threats to the preterm infant's survival are immaturity of other organs; lack of body fat; problems in thermoregulation; and increased susceptibility to intracranial trauma and hemorrhage during delivery (Neeson and May 1986, p 858).

Preterm labor is generally treated initially with hospitalization and intravenous administration of tocolytic (labor abatement) drugs. Currently, the drugs Yutopar (ritodrine), terbutaline, and magnesium sulfate are most frequently used. Once the labor is suppressed, the woman may be discharged to her home on a regimen of bed rest, oral tocolytics, and a home tocodynamometer to detect excessive contractions (Gill and Katz 1986, p 439). Home monitoring will be utilized more in the future since it is more cost-effective than hospitalization.

When preterm labor becomes too advanced to suppress, the health care workers must prepare to optimize the chances for the fetus to survive. Fetal lung maturity can be determined by a lecithin/sphingomyelin (L/S) ratio test. If this is determined to be deficient, the mother may be given Celestone (betamethasone) intramuscularly once a day for 2 days to stimulate lung maturity in the fetus.

Conditions may exist that contraindicate suppression of labor. These are ruptured membranes, maternal medical complications such as diabetes or eclampsia, intrauterine growth retardation, acute fetal distress, active bleeding or intrauterine infection.

NURSING DIAGNOSES

The most important nursing diagnoses for the care of the woman with a threatened preterm delivery will be presented.

KNOWLEDGE DEFICIT
RELATED TO PRETERM LABOR

The woman with preterm labor may be very anxious, because of the threat of delivering a small infant with decreased chances for viability. Thorough assessment of this woman with regard to teaching needs will enable the nurse to plan and meet knowledge deficits.

Assessment

The nurse must recognize those clients most prone to preterm labor. Ideally they would be taught signs and symptoms of labor and thus would seek medical attention immediately if these occurred. In addition, these individuals would also know and engage in optimum health practices to decrease their risk of preterm delivery.

Interventions

Nursing interventions for the woman with a knowledge deficit related to preterm labor should be focused on decreased activity, signs of preterm labor, prescribed medical administration, and general health practices. The interventions related to decreased activity are similar to those for the woman with pregnancy-induced hypertension. Depending on the advice from the physician, the woman should spend most of her time in bed in the left side-lying position. The woman may be permitted up for meals and to go to the bathroom. Fatigue should be avoided.

Signs and symptoms of labor on which the nurse can educate the client to report immediately are as follows:

Change of irregular contractions to a regular pattern. Medical attention should be obtained when contractions increase in intensity, duration, and frequency, and occur 10 minutes apart or closer; or greater than five contractions in 1 hour while in left lateral recumbent position.

Abdominal cramping may be associated with diarrhea.

Menstrual-like cramps

Low backache, particularly if different from any backache previously felt

Intermittent pressure in the pelvis

Change in character or amount of vaginal discharge, particularly if the discharge becomes bloody or watery (Knupple and Drukker 1986, p 313).

If the woman with preterm labor is to be managed at home on oral tocolytics such as ritodrine or terbutaline, she should be taught to take the medication at the prescribed time to maintain the therapeutic level of the drug. She should be taught the side-effects of the drug, which include headache, nausea and vomiting, jitteriness, tremulousness, and increased heart rate. Fevers, skin rashes, shortness of breath, tightness in the chest or chest pain, and a pulse greater than 140 need to be reported to the physician immediately. Fetal heart rate is usually elevated to 180 in those mothers receiving tocolytic agents. Pulmonary edema has been reported in women on both oral and intravenous ritodrine. It is a late manifestation that can occur 12 to 48 hours after the initiation of treatment. Lung sounds by auscultation should be assessed at each home visit.

General health practices that the nurse should encourage for the woman with preterm labor include omitting smoking, maintaining optimum nutrition and hydration (2500 ml/day), avoiding individuals with infections, restricting travel, and refraining from sexual intercourse and orgasm. The latter may trigger labor.

Outcome

The expected outcome of the interventions for the woman with knowledge deficit related to preterm labor is that she will be a participant in her care and adhere to the prescribed regimen to suppress labor.

ANXIETY RELATED TO POSSIBLE BIRTH OF PRETERM INFANT

The possibility of preterm labor resulting in the birth of an infant prior to the expected date is likely to engender a host of emotions in the pregnant woman. Anxiety may result from the impending threat of an interruption in meeting the mother's sociocultural needs. The mothering role, strongly socioculturally determined, is envisioned by most as caring for a robust and healthy infant. Many times, women, especially women with previous pregnancy losses, will exhibit anxious and sometimes neurotic behaviors. Again, guilt behaviors need to be recognized and redirected as they can lead to severe depression.

Assessment

The process of preparing for motherhood has been described by Reva Rubin as the *psychological tasks of pregnancy*. The first trimester is focused psychologically on the incorporation of the fetus into the woman's concept of her own baby. As she does this, thoughts become introspective and analytical while her perception of mothering and how she will mother is pondered. She begins to view herself as an individual rather than a daughter (Haber, Leach, Schudy, and Sideleau 1982, p 897).

During the second trimester, the woman is focused psychologically on the process of differentiation. This task is accomplished by the woman recognizing and acknowledging that the fetus is not actually a part of her. As she feels the baby move within her body, that baby becomes a unique individual to whom the mother begins to relate. Likewise, as movement is felt, the father of the infant becomes more emotionally involved. He may question his ability to provide for his family as he incorporates the idea of becoming a father (Haber et al 1982, p 900).

The psychological task for the third trimester has been described as *separation*. During this period the woman begins to prepare for delivery. This is accomplished through dreams, fantasies, and everyday conversations about the new baby. The couple must choose a name that will make the baby a separate and distinct individual. They begin to view the infant at a certain age in the future with a distinctive personality (Haber et al 1982, p 901).

Preterm labor, a deviation from normal expectations, creates anxiety related to a number of feelings and emotions. The mother may view the infant as a chance to fulfill unrealized dreams and therefore early birth and possible death of the infant may be viewed as cancellation of those dreams. This anxiety may be manifested as denial and the mother will delay seeking treatment because it is not time for the infant to be born according to her perception. In any event, the woman with preterm labor will be in need of a stable support system and ideally the nurse will be available to intervene as needs arise. Teaching topics should include events of hospitalization as well as childbirth education so that parents may be prepared for the birth experience.

Interventions

Preterm labor and impending birth of an immature infant may precipitate a situational crisis and nursing interventions should be directed at crisis intervention and problem solving. Inclusion of familial and extended support systems is imperative.

The nurse should direct the woman toward problem solving. This will include identification of resource and support persons. It will assist the woman to identify coping skills and begin to bring order into her life. As this begins to occur, the nurse and woman can continue to rehearse alternative approaches to problem solving. Like any alteration in daily living, this will reinforce new behavior and coping skills, provide the woman with feedback and, hopefully, enhance self-esteem. Throughout the process, the nurse acts as a role model for open, direct communication that reflects innovative thinking, flexibility, and self-awareness (Haber et al 1982, p 315).

Outcome

The expected outcome of these interventions is that the woman's anxiety will remain at a level conducive to productive problem solving.

HIGH-RISK NEWBORN

A normal newborn is born at full term gestation (38 to 40 weeks), at a weight appropriate for gestational age (2500 to 4500 grams), with no illness or congenital defects (American Academy of Pediatrics 1983). General aspects of the care of the discharged newborn will be considered in the following pages.

While stabilization usually occurs within the first 12 hours of life, many neonatal problems not apparent at birth are manifested in the first 48 to 72 hours. The American Academy of Pediatrics (1983) recommends discharge of the newborn from the hospital at 48 to 72 hours of age, providing the infant has met the following criteria:

1. The infant has successfully adapted to extrauterine life.
2. A complete physical examination has been performed, within 24 hours and preferably within 6 hours of discharge, and no abnormalities are apparent.
3. Oral feedings are tolerated with normal elimination established.
4. The infant is able to maintain a normal temperature.
5. Metabolic screening tests have been completed.
6. Methods for future medical and emergency care have been identified.

7. The home environment is appropriate and care-takers are competent and comfortable with caring for the newborn.

Currently, many facilities employ an early discharge policy, that is, discharge of mother and infant within 24 hours of delivery. Due to the element of risk involved, in that diagnostic assessment becomes intermittent rather than continuous, the American Academy of Pediatrics (AAP) Committee on Fetus and Newborn (1980) recommends that this be applied on a selective basis rather than as a general practice. Early discharge should be implemented as a component of a comprehensive plan of care including prenatal care, childbirth education and parenting education, and follow-up care for the mother and newborn. Any complication in the antepartal, intrapartal, or postpartal course, or any newborn complications should make the client ineligible for early discharge. The infant should be of term gestation and at an appropriate weight. A minimum of 6 hours' hospitalization is necessary during which time thermal homeostasis and feeding are established, and a complete physical examination is performed. Prior to discharge, maternal abilities with feeding, skin care, including cord care, use of a thermometer and temperature assessment, assessment of infant well-being, and recognition of illness should be demonstrated.

Follow-up care for the newborn is a critical component of early discharge. The infant should have a complete physical examination and assessment on the second or third day of life, with specific attention given to the evaluation of nutrition, infant behavior, urine output, stools, and assessment of jaundice. Blood for metabolic screening should be obtained. Serial examinations should be done as indicated, and the family's plans for further health care should be discussed. This should include plans for emergency treatment, as well as for periodic evaluation, immunizations, and screening (AAP 1980).

PHYSIOLOGIC JAUNDICE

Even the normal newborn faces potential complications associated with adaptation to extrauterine life. Physiologic, or developmental, jaundice occurs as a normal response to the cardiovascular changes occurring at birth. The neonate generates bilirubin at a rate of 6 to 8 mg/Kg/24 hours, or three times that of the adult, yet the newborn liver is unable to excrete the excess bilirubin. Hyperbilirubinemia is a normal occurrence in all neonates, with visible jaundice occurring in about one half. In term infants, physiologic jaundice appears after 24 hours of age, and subsides by 7 days of age. Jaundice occurring in the first 24 hours is indicative of a pathological process such as sepsis or a severe incompatibility, which will require constant diagnostic evaluation and nursing care available in the hospital (Korones 1986). While physiologic jaundice generally does not require therapy, some infants develop bilirubin levels indicating treatment with phototherapy. Bilirubin levels identified as indicative of a need for phototherapy vary widely in the literature and in practice, and depend upon such factors as the infant's age and clinical status. The AAP recommendation for home phototherapy is a level of greater than 14 but less than 18, after 48 hours of age (AAP 1985).

Traditionally this treatment has been carried out in the hospital, requiring an extended hospital stay for the infant, and separation trauma for the family. Current trends are moving toward the concept of home phototherapy programs, which avoid this parent/infant separation, as well as significantly decrease health care costs.

Entry into a home phototherapy program is by physician referral to the agency providing care. The infant should be more than 48 hours old, and at a minimum weight of 2500 grams (AAP 1985). Infants less than 2500 grams are at risk for hypothermia, hypoglycemia, feeding problems, dehydration, and complications associated with prematurity. These infants therefore require the level of care available in the hospital setting (Dortch and Spottiswoode 1986).

Phototherapy can be provided using a single quartz halogen lamp or a bank of four to eight fluorescent bulbs. The fluorescent lights may be cool-white, daybright, or special blue bulbs. The lights should be covered with a protective Plexiglas shield, and placed 12 to 30 inches from the infant. The effect of therapy depends on the amount of energy emitted in the blue spectrum, and upon the skin surface area exposed to the lights. The energy output is measured by a photometer in microwatts per square centimeter per nanometer ($uW/cm^2/nm$). A minimum level of 4 $uW/cm^2/nm$ is necessary for effective treatment (Korones 1986).

As with bilirubin levels used as a starting point for phototherapy, the levels cited at which phototherapy can be discontinued are varied; discontinuation of lights at levels below 14, with a demonstrated downward trend, is considered safe practice. Follow-up levels should be done at 12 and 24 hours to rule out rebound elevations (AAP 1985).

NURSING DIAGNOSES

Physiologic jaundice itself is considered a normal occurrence in the newborn. However, its treatment with phototherapy is not without untoward effects. This section will describe these effects as related to nursing diagnoses, and discuss assessment, planning, interventions, and outcomes.

ALTERATIONS IN ELIMINATION

Infants under phototherapy often develop loose green stools, resulting in increased stool water losses. This phenomenon is related to a transient lactose intolerance induced by the phototherapy. Insensible water losses through the skin are increased significantly as well. This effect is related to an increase in skin blood flow seen with phototherapy. Increased skin temperature may also occur, with an increase in heart rate and respiration (Korones 1985). Hyperthermia as a complication of phototherapy is most often associated with treatment in the hospital setting, where isolettes and radiant warmers are in use. In the home setting, the infant is probably at greater risk for hypothermia, as treatment requires that the infant be naked while exposed to the lights.

Assessment

Daily home visits to the infant undergoing phototherapy are necessary. On each visit, the nurse should assess the infant for signs of dehydration, such as poor skin turgor, and dry mucous membranes. A sunken fontanelle is a very late sign of dehydration. The urine may be darkened as the photodegradation products are excreted by the kidneys. Intake and output should be recorded on the flow sheet. The parents should record the number of wet diapers, and number and consistency of stools.

Interventions

The benefit of supplemental water feedings in the treatment of jaundice is not proven; however, most physicians advise its use. To prevent excess supplementation, instruct the parents to offer water only after feedings with formula, with a limit of 4 to 6 ounces per 24 hours.

The parents should be instructed to regulate the infant's room temperature to maintain the baby's temperature within a range of 97.8° – 99° F. The infant's axillary temperature should be checked at least every 8 hours, and recorded on the parents' flow sheet (Fig. 16-1) with intake and output (I&O) and feedings (Dortch & Spottiswoode, 1986).

Outcome

The infant's normal elimination pattern will be maintained.

ALTERATIONS IN NUTRITION

Phototherapy causes an increase in metabolic rate, thus increasing caloric requirements. In many cases, there is an increase in intestinal transit time as well, related to lactose intolerance. As a result, there is decreased intestinal absorption of milk and uptake of calories. The situation becomes one of diminished

---

PARENTS' RECORD

Parents, this is your record to help the nurses assess intake and output. Please record feedings (breast and bottle), urine and stool, and chart the temperature every eight hours.

TIME	FEEDINGS	URINE	STOOL	TEMPERATURE

Figure 16-1. Parents' flow sheet used to record pertinent information during phototherapy regimen. (From Dortch E, Spottiswoode P: New light on phototherapy: Home use. Neonatal Network 4: 30–34, 1986)

supply and increased demand. There is a demonstrated slowing of growth in the first week of life for infants receiving phototherapy. This is followed by a "catch-up" period in weeks 2 and 3. There are no indications that long-term growth and development are impaired (Korones 1986).

Assessment

A weight check should be done with each visit. The infant will gain weight, but in smaller amounts than expected. A weight loss may indicate inadequate calorie intake for caloric needs, or reflect excessive water losses.

Interventions

The home health nurse should also evaluate the current feeding schedule. The infant should be fed breast milk or formula at least every 4 to 6 hours, supplemented with water following the feeding. A lactose-free formula may be indicated to decrease the intestinal transit time and increase the uptake of calories. Unless the use of a lactose-free formula is necessary, there is no reason to stop or restrict breast-feeding in favor of a standard formula (Dortch and Spottiswoode 1986).

Outcome

Adequate nutrition will be maintained.

HOME PHOTOTHERAPY

Prior to setting up the home for phototherapy, the parents should be contacted and given some basic information to help them prepare for the experience. As treatment is continuous, and the infant will be kept naked under the lights, supplemental heat may be needed. The infant's room temperature must be kept at 80° to 86° F to maintain a body temperature of 98.6° to 99° F. The parents will need to purchase or borrow a heater be-fore phototherapy is started. A portable bed or crib may also be needed, if the standard crib is not suitable. Baby baskets, carriage or bassinet tops, car beds, or even a dresser drawer or cardboard box may be used.

On the first visit, the necessary supplies are taken to the home. These include the phototherapy light, photometer, eye masks, thermometer, bulb syringe, blood collection supplies, the chart, and chart forms.

The bed must be placed so that the surface of the mattress is 12 to 30 inches from the lights. Some standard cribs may be tall enough, or the mattress or entire crib may be elevated to the correct level with books or blocks. If a small bed or portable crib is used, it should be placed on a stable surface of the correct height. Safety factors to be considered include proximity to heaters, windows, and drafts, and accessibility to siblings and pets.

Temperature regulation is important as the infant will be at risk for thermal instability. If a space heater is unavailable, central heating can be used, closing all vents except those in the infant's room. Hats and booties may also be used if needed. Axillary temperatures should be monitored, and the room temperature adjusted as needed.

The chart forms should include a flow chart for the parents' use, as well as an instruction sheet and supplemental information such as displayed on page 500.

As a rule, families respond positively to home phototherapy, although many are anxious and apprehensive at the beginning. Home care involves added stress and an increased work load for the parent. In spite of this, mothers surveyed all felt positive about the experience and would repeat it. As one mother stated, "Hospitalization is much more traumatic. It was much more tiring to travel back and forth from home to the hospital than to have him home when I was doing the care." Another said, "It was worth all the work to have him home with me."

**Home Phototherapy Program
Parent Information Sheet**

Dear Parent,

Your baby's physician has contacted the Home Phototherapy Program to begin treatment of jaundice. We are pleased to provide a service that will allow your baby to receive this medical treatment in your home.

Please read the following information and instructions:

1. Your baby's physician will assume responsibility for arranging home phototherapy.

2. Prior to starting phototherapy treatment, you will be required to sign two consent forms: (a) Consent for Treatment and (b) Responsibility for Equipment.

3. You will be billed by Home Care unless arrangements can be made with your insurance carrier.

4. A registered nurse will come to your home to deliver and set up the necessary equipment.

5. The visiting nurse must see and examine your baby daily, check the equipment, instruct you in care of your baby, communicate with your baby's doctor, and obtain a bilirubin blood sample.

6. Your baby's doctor must examine your baby at least every other day. Please call his/her office to schedule these appointments, and please inform your visiting nurse of the appointment times.

7. The phototherapy treatment should be continuous except for feeding times and medical examinations.

8. Eye patches are mandatory during phototherapy. These should be removed only during feedings.

9. Your baby should be completely nude while under phototherapy.

10. Your infant's temperature (rectal) should be monitored every 8 hours. It is important to maintain the baby's temperature between 97.8° and 99.0°F through controlled room temperature.

11. You should provide breast or formula feeding at a minimum interval of 4–6 hours, encouraging the infant to drink sterile water or sugar water after each feeding.

12. It is important that you record your baby's temperature and the number of wet diapers and stools your baby has had.

13. Your visiting nurse will provide you with a pamphlet on jaundice. Please read this carefully for more information, and please ask your visiting nurse or your infant's physician any additional questions you may have.

(Dortch E, Spottiswoode P: New light on phototherapy: Home use. Neonatal Network 4:30–34, 1986)

Phototherapy can be carried out safely and effectively in the home setting, with support from the home health nurse (Dortch and Spottiswoode 1986).

POTENTIAL FOR RETINAL INJURY
Assessment

Extensive animal research has demonstrated retinal injury occurring with unprotected exposure to phototherapy lights at current therapeutic levels. While no similar effect has been noted in human infants, "it seems prudent to continue to patch the eyes of infants receiving phototherapy" (Avery 1981).

Interventions

Protective masks with eye pads should be applied whenever the infant is under the light. In applying the mask, it is important to make certain the eyes are closed. The mask should be removed during feeding, or whenever the infant is out from under the lights, and the eyes checked for signs of conjunctivitis, such as redness or discharge. Eye pads should be replaced as needed. Correct placement of eye patches is essential, as displaced masks and pads can obstruct the nares and cause respiratory distress.

Outcome

Follow-up studies of infants whose eyes were well protected during treatment with phototherapy demonstrate normal visual function (Avery 1981).

POTENTIAL IMPAIRMENT OF SKIN INTEGRITY

Assessment

The skin may become bleached during phototherapy, rendering skin color useless as a means to assess jaundice. Black infants often show a 'tanning' effect. The skin becomes more deeply pigmented with exposure to the lights. This is a separate phenomenon from the "bronze baby syndrome" observed in infants with liver disease who are treated with phototherapy. A maculopapular rash is a frequently seen side-effect, and fades quickly when treatment is stopped.

Interventions

Changes in skin coloration, whether bleaching or tanning, render visual assessment for jaundice ineffective. As changes in skin color can be quite subtle and difficult to assess, it is best to assume their occurrence and not rely on visual assessment at all. Blood samples must be drawn and serum levels checked once daily. The specimen is drawn by heelstick and .06 cc in a red-topped bullet is required. When obtaining the sample, the phototherapy lights must be turned off, and the specimen placed in an opaque container to prevent exposure to sunlight.

Parents can be assured that rashes and the changes in skin coloration are common occurrences associated with phototherapy and not harmful to the infant. The specific treatment or interventions other than normal skin care are indicated. The bleaching effect or rash will subside with discontinuation of therapy. Black infants will retain the increased pigmentation acquired under the lights (Korones 1985).

ALTERATIONS IN PARENTING

Parents involved in home phototherapy are often anxious, overwhelmed, and apprehensive as they deal with the "normal" stresses of adjusting to a new baby plus the added stress of home phototherapy. Phototherapy involves increased work, usually for the mother as primary care-taker.

Assessment

A good deal of education is needed to enable parents to administer treatment safely. Begin by assessment of the parents knowledge of the importance of hydration and recording intake and output, the use of protective eye patches, and thermoregulation. Parent education should also impart a basic understanding of jaundice and the principles of phototherapy (Dortch and Spottiswoode 1986).

Interventions

Information should be presented in as simple a format as possible with plenty of time allotted for questions and explanations. A brochure titled "I am Curious Yellow . . . What is Jaundice?" is available as a teaching reference (Woods, Hitt, and Wennberg 1983). Written guidelines should also be left with the parents, with a contact phone number, and instructions to call for assistance as needed. Parents are often concerned that they will not be able to carry out the treatment. This is a normal response, and they can be assured that the treatment will become easier. Follow-up calls, especially during the evening following setting up of the home for treatment, are helpful. Encourage parents to utilize their support system to provide them with a person who will be able to help care for the infant and lend emotional support.

The daily visit by the home health care nurse provides the parents with the opportunity to ask questions that have arisen, and gain assurance that they are providing care correctly. When surveyed at the time of treatment, parents identified the administration of the treatment and related stresses as the source of their anxiety. In post-treatment interviews, parents then identified their worry about the bilirubin levels and the possible effects on the baby as anxiety provoking, rather than the phototherapy.

Outcome

As treatment progresses, even the most apprehensive of parents gain confidence and become more comfortable (Dortch and Spottiswoode 1986). Parents will successfully cope with caring for the infant.

An assessment of the home when home phototherapy is required is outlined in the boxed material opposite.

THE HIGH-RISK INFANT

Dramatic advances in neonatal intensive care have resulted in a significant increase in the

---

Assessing the Home: Home Phototherapy

HOME PHOTOTHERAPY: Can the family afford to buy a heater or is there one available to borrow to maintain room at needed temperature?

Many heaters (kerosene, etc.) must be properly vented and maintained and should not be used in a closed area. Instructions for safe operation can be found in the operation manual or by contacting the manufacturing company.

Is there a separate room that can be maintained to provide the needed warmth for the infant?

ALL IN HOME THERAPY: Is the infant's room large enough to accommodate equipment, i.e., phototherapy, O_2 equipment, suctioning equipment?

Is the room equipped with necessary electric outlets? This information can be attained from supply company.

Notify utility companies concerning apparatus in home.

OTHER SAFETY MEASURES: If other children are in the home, are electrical outlets covered, cleaning supplies stored out of reach, etc?

Are emergency numbers posted, EMS, Dr?

Do care-givers feel comfortable administering CPR and other emergency procedures?

Dangers associated with O_2 i.e., smoking, fireplaces, heaters?

---

survival rates of progressively smaller, younger infants. Following is a description of the high-risk premature infant.

Prematurity is defined as a gestation of less than 38 weeks. Low birthweight (LBW) refers to infants born weighing less than 2500 grams; very low birthweight (VLBW) refers to infants of less than 1500 grams at birth. Extremely low birthweight (ELBW) refers to those infants weighing less than 1000 grams when they are born. Infants are further classified by relation of size to gestational age. Small for gestational age (SGA) infants weigh less than expected for their gestation, indicating intrauterine growth retardation. Appropriate for gestational age (AGA) indicates normal intrauterine growth and development. Large for gestational age (LGA) indicates excessive intrauterine growth. This multifactorial approach provides a more acute indication of the problems that may be anticipated (Ahmann 1986).

In the United States, 7% of all live births are infants of less than 2500 grams. These infants account for 66.7% of all neonatal deaths. The risk of mortality increases with decreasing gestational age, so that a premie of less than 1500 grams is 200 times more likely to die than a full-term, appropriately grown infant (McCormick 1985). However, with advances in care there has been a constant improvement in the survival of premature infants. In the 1960's infants who were less than 1000 grams were not considered viable; this lower limit is now at 500 grams. With this increased survival has come an increase in long-term morbidity, and a greater need for home health care maintenance (Ahmann 1986).

The high-risk premature infant is at risk for a wide range of physiologic disturbances. These occur because of the immaturity of all the organ systems, and as complications of invasive treatment. Table 16-1 outlines the most common disorders seen in prematurity (Ahmann 1986). An exhaustive review of all the problems is not within the scope of this text. This chapter will focus on the most frequently encountered problems, those primarily related to alterations in oxygenation.

Apnea of prematurity (AOP) is one of the most common cardiorespiratory disorders leading to a need for home care. As one of many factors associated with the occurrence of sudden infant death syndrome (SIDS), it is presented here as a model for the home care of infants at risk for SIDS.

Bronchopulmonary dysplasia (BPD) is a lung disease commonly associated with prematurity. It is presented as a model for home care of an infant with respiratory compromise.

APNEA OF PREMATURITY

Episodes of apnea, described as *the cessation of breathing for more than 20 . . . or 30 seconds*, are seen in 25% of infants who were less than 2500 grams at birth. Its incidence is inversely related to gestational age, so that it occurs in 84% of premies weighing less than 1000 grams at birth (Aranda, Trippenbach, and Turman 1983). AOP has many causes, all related to immaturity and ineffective respiratory control centers in the brain. The leading causes of recurrent apnea are hypoxia, hyaline membrane disease, and intraventricular hemorrhage (Brown 1984). AOP is a separate entity from periodic breathing, a normal finding in the premie. Periodic breathing occurs in sporadic episodes where breathing stops for up to ten seconds, and is not associated with cyanosis or bradycardia (Korones 1986).

A good deal of attention has been focused upon AOP as a possible cause of SIDS. Sudden infant death syndrome is defined as *the sudden death of any infant or young child that is unexpected by history, and in which a thorough postmortem examination fails to demonstrate an adequate cause for death* (Zebal and Friedman 1984). While AOP is certainly a contributing factor indicating high risk for SIDS, research indicates that the ac-

TABLE 16.1 Common Disorders of Prematurity

Organ System	Disorders	
	Acute	Chronic
Respiratory system	Respiratory distress syndrome Apnea of prematurity Pneumonia	Bronchopulmonary dysplasia Apnea of prematurity Tracheostomy Subglottic stenosis Croup syndromes Frequent respiratory infections
Cardiovascular system	Patent ductus arteriosus Cor pulmonale	Cor pulmonale
Central nervous system	Hypoxic brain damage Intraventricular hemorrhage Seizures	Neurodevelopmental disorders Hydrocephalus Seizures
Gastrointestinal system	Necrotizing enterocolitis Jaundice	Malabsorption syndrome Malnutrition Growth retardation
Hematologic system	Anemia	Anemia
Other	— Sepsis Meningitis Pneumonia	Hernias Retinopathy of prematurity Sepsis Recurrent respiratory and gastrointestinal infections

From Ahmann E: Home Care for the High-Risk Infant. Rockville, MD, Aspen Publishers, Inc., 1986

tual incidence of SIDS as a result of apnea is less than 10% to 20%. (Merritt and Valdes-Dapena 1984).

Other factors associated with a risk for SIDS include inadequate prenatal care; maternal cigarette smoking; infection; gender (males more frequently affected); maternal age and parity; prematurity, and a previous SIDS loss. Most SIDS deaths occur during the winter months, during sleep, and following a minor illness. Infant age is a factor, with the greatest risk at 2 to 4 months of age (American SIDS Institute 1983). "Near-miss SIDS" is a term coined to describe an apneic episode occurring in sleep where an apparently healthy baby stops breathing, becomes blue and hypotonic, and requires prolonged vigorous stimulation, or mouth-to-mouth resuscitation to recover (Kelly, Shannon, and O'Connell 1978). Any infant with a risk factor associated with SIDS, with a "near-miss" episode, or with a family history of SIDS should be managed similar to management of an infant with AOP (Ahmann 1986).

The major concerns for AOP and its management in the home are those related to alterations in oxygenation, and alterations in parenting.

ALTERATIONS IN OXYGENATION

Apnea is classified as either *central, obstructive,* or *mixed* apnea. Central apnea involves an absence of movement of the thoracic and abdominal muscles, and a lack of air flow. With obstructive apnea there is muscular activity, but no exchange of air. Mixed apnea combines the two, with central apnea followed by obstructive apnea. All can occur in a term as well as in a preterm infant (Ahmann 1986).

Assessment

During an apneic episode there is a significant decrease in blood oxygenation, leading to cyanosis and bradycardia. There may also be decreased peripheral blood flow, hypotension and hypotonia. A prolonged apnea can lead to respiratory arrest, brain damage, and death (Korones 1986).

With every home visit, the infant's heart rate, respiration, and color should be observed and documented. The apnea flow sheet should be reviewed, and the frequency and duration of any apnea or bradycardia alarms should be discussed. The parents should describe the infant's status at the time of the event, any preceding symptoms, and the amount of stimulation needed.

Short apnea events that do not set off an alarm may still cause hypoxia. Pallor, cyanosis, and hypotonia should be noted whenever observed. With these, frequent bradycardia alarms may occur. Factors other than apnea can trigger an alarm, and may indicate a need for further medical evaluation. Bradycardia alarms may occur with normal bradycardias related to stretching, hiccups, passing of stool or flatus, prolonged crying, or with feeding. A cold, fever, or immunization may cause increased alarms. Careful assessment is important and should consider factors such as the frequency and duration of the alarm, and specific signs and symptoms observed. Parents

should be encouraged to call the nurse or physician at any time, with any concerns about the monitor, alarms, or the infant's status.

Interventions

Parents' education concerning apnea (their infant's condition, monitoring, response to alarms, CPR, home record keeping, follow-up care, and criteria for discontinuing of the monitor) is a part of the hospital's discharge planning and teaching. The home health nurse should be made aware of the parents' status and further educational needs prior to the infant's discharge. In the home, the nurse should confirm that the parents are able to provide safe care. The signs and symptoms of prolonged apnea, cardiopulmonary resuscitation (CPR) procedures, and coping with false alarms should be reviewed on the first visit. Parents must be instructed in keeping a complete record of all apnea events. Figure 16-2 shows a sample form for use as an apnea record (Ahmann 1986).

CPR guidelines and emergency phone numbers should be prominently posted in the house. The local Emergency Medical Service can be notified, as many maintain a listing of high-risk individuals, including monitored infants.

The type of monitor used will be decided prior to discharge. This chapter will discuss impedance monitoring, considered to be the safest and most accurate method (Norris–Berkmeyer and Hutchins 1986). It is important to check out the monitor controls and settings in the home. If alarm limits are not set internally, they should be checked at each visit, and the parents instructed to check them frequently. The alarm should be audible throughout the house. If it is not, a remote alarm, or an intercom system is needed.

The monitor should be placed on a stable surface with 8 inches of ventilation space

CHILDREN'S HOSPITAL NATIONAL MEDICAL CENTER
PULMONARY MEDICINE
APNEA RECORD

NAME: ______________ ID #: ______________

	BABY												MACHINE									
	STATE		BREATHING			SKIN COLOR			STIMULATION				ALARM					IMPEDANCE LIGHT				
TIME AM or PM	AWAKE	ASLEEP	NORMAL	SHALLOW	NONE	NORMAL	PALE	DUSKY-BLUE	NONE	MILD	VIGOROUSLY	MOUTH-MOUTH	APNEA	CARDIAC SLOW	CARDIAC FAST	BOTH	NUMBER OF BEEPS	GREEN	YELLOW	RED	BEEPING&BREATHING (YES, NO)	COMMENTS

Source Reprinted with permission of the Pulmonary Medicine Department, Children's Hospital National Medical Center, Washington, D.C.

Figure 16-2. Apnea record. (From Ahmann E: Home Care for the High-Risk Infant. Rockville, MD, Aspen Publishers, 1986)

above and behind it. It should be placed out of reach of other children, and childproof panels used to cover the knobs. The monitor is not to be placed on any other electrical equipment, and an extension cord should not be used. The monitor should be plugged in to a grounded outlet.

Monitoring supplies needed include two sets of lead wires, disposable patches, and a monitor manual. A battery pack is optional, as is a belt apparatus with permanent electrodes. Electrodes should be placed symmetrically, and must contact the sides of the chest wall in order to pick up respiratory movements. Use of the belt is not appropriate for infants under 8 to 10 pounds. Patches should be replaced every 2 to 3 days, or as they become loose. The infant should never be bathed with the monitor on as there is a risk of electrocution. The lead wires should be threaded through the bottom of the infant's garment, to prevent the possibility of strangulation. Figure 16-3 illustrates proper placement of electrodes and belt (Bell 1984).

Rehearsals of appropriate responses to alarms are helpful in assessing the parents' ability to cope, and useful as a teaching exercise. Parents should be able to describe the necessary steps in responding to each alarm: apnea, bradycardia, and loose-lead alarms. Other care-givers should also know these procedures and be able to perform CPR. When responding to an apnea alarm the parent should:

1. Observe for respirations.
2. If none are noted, or the baby is hypotonic, stimulate the infant; appropriate methods of stimulation include
   (a) Calling to the baby
   (b) Gentle patting or stroking of the trunk or back
   (c) Gently patting, stroking, or flicking of soles of feet
   (d) Lightly slapping the soles of the feet.

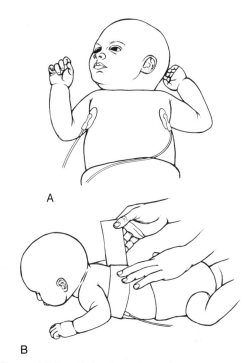

A

B

Figure 16-3. (*A*) Placement of apnea monitor electrodes. (*B*) Placement of apnea monitor belt. (Bell CW: Home Care and Rehabilitation in Respiratory Medicine. Philadelphia, JB Lippincott, 1984)

3. With no response, initiate CPR procedures.

For a bradycardia alarm, gentle stimulation is usually sufficient. For loose-lead alarms, parents will have to be able to troubleshoot. A logical approach is to start at the baby, and work toward the monitor. The cause of the alarm may be a loose or dried patch, a dirty electrode, oil or lotion on the skin, a loose belt or lead wire, broken lead wires, malfunction of the patient cable, or the monitor itself.

Each person who will be giving care must be able to demonstrate correct CPR and emergency procedures. Maintaining skills with regular review is important. Thorough practice will make coping with an actual event much easier.

With each visit, address any problems or concerns that have arisen. On-going assessment of the parents' knowledge concerning their infant's status is essential, with teaching accomplished as deficits are identified. Parental understanding of the condition and principle of monitoring is crucial for success with home monitoring (Ahmann 1986).

Outcome

Infant will establish normal breathing patterns.

ALTERATIONS IN PARENTING: HOME MONITORING

Parents facing the experience of home monitoring with the surrounding implications of an "at risk" diagnosis will be in need of continuous emotional support and on-going education. Parents of the premie with AOP will have been coping with the fear for their infant's well-being since birth. They have probably been exposed to the infant's apneic episodes in the hospital. Unlike the parents of a "near-miss" infant for whom the diagnosis of "at risk" is a sudden shock, the parents of the premie have had time to work through their feelings of grief and denial. Most have had time to learn to cope with the anxiety surrounding their high-risk situation. They will have accepted that their child is "different" and are aware of the long-term problems associated with prematurity. For many of these parents, the monitor represents a means of control over the problem, and provides a great deal of comfort (Smith 1984). In general, the diagnosis of "at risk for SIDS," regardless of cause, has a profound emotional and psychological effect upon the family. "From the outset most families in which there is an infant who is considered for monitoring are likely to have a high level of anxiety. A monitor that reduces this anxiety, whether or not it protects the infant from death, is probably a good treatment" (Southall 1983).

Assessment

The home health nurse should assess the parents for their knowledge of the interventions and their emotional response to the situation. Several visits may be needed to complete the assessment.

Interventions

The mother, as primary care-giver, usually experiences the greatest level of stress with home monitoring. Many are reluctant to trust others with the care of the infant or embarrassed to request assistance; conversely, other family members are often reluctant to assume responsibility for caring for the infant. Research data indicate that mothers were personally responsible for caring for their monitored baby for an average of 20 to 24 hours per day (Black, Hirsher, and Steinschneider 1978). The primary support person identified was the father, with the home monitoring staff ranking second. Most families felt that the home care personnel were the most experienced, and most available as a source of support for both emotional and technical concerns (Cain, Kelly, and Shannon 1980).

Home monitoring has a devastating impact upon the family's daily routine. The family will need assistance in developing new ways of coping with daily responsibilities without placing the infant at risk. While changes in life-style must be made, the family should be encouraged to maintain as normal a home life as possible, avoiding isolation, neglecting the other children, and over-protecting the affected child. They should be encouraged to make some arrangement for relief care-givers to enable them to have a break and decrease their stress and anxiety (Ahmann 1986).

With time, the level of anxiety decreases. After the first month the monitor is credited with helping the parents feel more comfortable about their infants. The monitor, rather than the infant, was often the recipient of the parents' anger and frustration, producing feelings of ambivalence. One father stated, "I felt like throwing the whole machine out the window — but, what choice did we have?" With plans to discontinue monitoring, anxiety levels peak again as parents become fearful or apprehensive (Cain et al 1980).

Planning for the discontinuing of the monitor should begin prior to coming home with a monitor. Parents should have a clear understanding of the criteria for stopping monitoring from the beginning. The general criteria for infants with apnea are:

1. The infant has been free of "life-threatening" events requiring prolonged vigorous stimulation or resuscitation for at least 3 months, or for 2 months if there have been no critical problems since the presenting episode.
2. The infant has not experienced a real monitor alarm for at least 2 months, on an apnea setting of 20 seconds, and a heart rate setting of 60 beats/minute.
3. During the asymptomatic period, the infant must have experienced the stress of an upper respiratory tract infection, DPT (diptheria – pertussis – tetanus) immunization, or another illness without recurrence of symptoms.
4. Clinical evaluation, including neurological, developmental, and physical examinations, shows that initial and any other reasons for monitoring have been resolved.
5. The infant has shown no abnormalities on cardiorespiratory recordings, if these were present at the time of the child's initial evaluation (Ariagno 1984).

Two normal sleep studies at 2 to 3 month intervals are also frequently recommended (Ariagno 1984).

The prospect of losing the monitor is an anxiety-provoking event for the parents who have come to view the monitor as a comforting, even life-saving object. As assessment indicates that monitoring is no longer needed, plans for discontinuing it should be discussed with the parents. With a gradual weaning process, the parents will have time to recognize their child's stable condition, which will facilitate their coping with elimination of the monitor procedure (Ahmann 1986).

Outcome

With support, the parents will provide optional care for the infant. A Nursing Care Plan for AOP follows.

BRONCHOPULMONARY DYSPLASIA

The premature infant's lungs lack the biochemical and mechanical properties needed for the adequate exchange of oxygen and carbon dioxide. As a result, respiratory distress develops, which requires treatment with supplemental oxygen and mechanical ventilation. While life-saving, these treatment measures can cause tissue damage that often results in a chronic respiratory insufficiency. This condition, called *bronchopulmonary dysplasia* (BPD), is characterized by airway stenosis, inefficient gas exchange, and the excessive production of bronchial secretions. The infant with severe BPD requires extended treatment with mechanical ventilation. Infants less severely affected become dependent on supplemental oxygen. Bronchopulmonary dysplasia results in decreased exercise tolerance, increased work of breathing, and a greater susceptibility to infection. This chronic respiratory compromise affects the infant as a whole, impacting on feeding, growth, and nutrition, cardiovascular function, and neuro-behavioral development.

In most cases the prognosis is good. Given time, and with meticulous care, healing eventually occurs more rapidly than tissue damage, and healthy new lung tissues develop (Ahmann 1986).

Support for home care of the chronically ill infant has increased due to escalating health care costs, a lack of pediatric rehabilitation facilities, and the adverse effects of long-term hospitalization upon infants, their families, and the health care system. Home care of the infant with BPD is less expensive than prolonged hospitalization. It provides the infant with an environment supportive of normal growth and development. The family is able to function as a family unit, including previously excluded family members, in providing care (Jackson 1986).

The major concerns related to nursing diagnoses are alterations in oxygenation, alterations in nutrition, and alterations in parenting.

ALTERATIONS IN OXYGENATION

The changes occurring in the lung of the infant with BPD can include anatomic changes, progressing to physiologic changes, and finally, alterations in pulmonary function. Infants with severe BPD often develop cor pulmonale, a form of heart disease in which the right ventricle becomes enlarged. In the recovery phase, when the lungs are growing and healthy tissue has developed, pulmonary physiology and function remain abnormal. Research data indicate that children with BPD will have abnormal chest x-ray films and pulmonary function tests until 6 to 9 years of age (Lamarre 1973; Taussig and Leman 1979). The child with BPD experiences many interrelated problems, specifically:

1. Airway stenosis
2. Hyperreactive airways
3. Hypoxemia
4. Retention of secretions
5. High risk for infection
6. Fluid retention
7. High risk for cor pulmonale

Assessment

To ensure a smooth transition from hospital to home care, coordination between the community health nurse and the hospital staff is essential. Information needed by the home health nurse includes information about the infant's hospital course, baseline vital signs, discharge medications, instructions regarding care, and plans for follow-up and emergency care. It is also important to be aware of the parents' level of understanding of the infant's condition and care, their abilities and limitations in providing care, and further teaching and support needed.

Emergency preparations are a critical component in home care of the infant with BPD. The home should have a telephone; if this is not possible an alternate plan for obtaining help in an emergency must be formulated. The electric and phone companies should be notified to place the family on a priority service list. The utility companies will then notify the family prior to any anticipated interruption of service. Emergency Medical Services should also be made aware of the family's situation to ensure a prompt response and appropriate emergency interventions. Guidelines for CPR and a list of emergency phone numbers should be posted at the phones, and at the baby's bedside. Posted information should include the home address and the nearest intersection or cross street to give as a reference point. Discharge teaching will include CPR training, which should be reviewed by the community health nurse.

Other care-givers (babysitters, other family members, etc.) also need instruction in giving CPR, and must be familiar with the plan for emergency care.

Temperature, pulse, and respirations should be assessed at each visit. Each infant will have individual baseline values, and there will be changes related to changes in position, and levels of activity. Any values above or below the infant's baseline not related to activity or emotional stress may indicate respiratory or cardiac compromise.

Lung auscultation is an essential component of the home visit. Assessment includes the quality of breath sounds as well as the presence or absence of adventitious sounds. The lengths of the inspiration and expiration phases should be compared. The infant with BPD may have a relatively long expiratory phase. Wheezing may be heard in the infant with hyperactive airways. Rhonchi are common with BPD, and may indicate increasing or thickening secretions. Rales may indicate edema, fluid overload, or pneumonia.

The infant should be observed for the signs and symptoms of respiratory distress. These include tachypnea, nasal flaring, retractions, grunting, pallor, cyanosis, diaphoresis, and edema. The infant's alertness and level of activity should be noted as general indicators of overall status. Irritability, lethargy, or loss of appetite indicate distress. Amount, consistency, color, and odor of respiratory secretions should be assessed. Increased amount or thickness of secretions, a yellow green color or a foul odor are indications of infection. Those giving care to the infant should be instructed in the assessment of vital signs, breath sounds, and respiratory secretions, and should be taught to recognize the signs and symptoms of respiratory distress. They should be given guidelines identifying situations requiring medical intervention or advice.

Interventions

Infants with BPD may be on a variety of medications in any combination including, bronchodilators, digoxin, diuretics, steroids, and electrolytes. On the first visit, and at intervals thereafter, all medications should be reviewed with the parents and care-givers. The care-givers' ability to administer each medication correctly should be demonstrated. The dose and concentration of the medications on hand should be checked against the prescription for accuracy. Medication schedules should be established that are tailored as much as possible to the family's daily activities. Helpful strategies include minimizing late night doses, grouping medication administration to several times during the day, and developing of a checklist for the care-giver's use.

Regular chest physiotherapy (CPT) is an important component in the care of the infant with BPD. The aim of CPT is to encourage the drainage of secretions from the lung. The care-giver's ability to correctly perform CPT should be established. Correct positioning is illustrated in Figure 16-4. Percussion over each lobe for one minute to loosen secretions is recommended. CPT is given as needed to clear secretions, and it will be needed more frequently for the infant with a cold or other respiratory distress causing increased or thickening of secretions.

Chest physiotherapy is always followed by suctioning. Suction is also indicated when secretions fill the oro-/nasopharynx, with increased or thickened secretions, when the presence of fluid is audible, and with signs and symptoms of respiratory distress. Most infants will require catheter suction. The catheter is inserted gently with no suction applied, and advanced until a cough reflex is elicited. Gentle suction is applied as the catheter is removed. Suction should be applied for no longer than 5 seconds. The procedure may be repeated two or three times, allowing the infant to breathe and regain color between passes. The catheter is cleansed with saline between passes and following the procedure. the care-giver's suctioning technique should be assessed for accuracy and safety, and instruction given as needed. Suction apparatus should be checked for proper functioning. A portable mouth suction device (DeLee catheter) should be available in case of electrical failure, and a bulb suction should also be at hand for emergency use.

For the infant requiring oxygen therapy, the equipment used should be checked at each visit. Oxygen and humidity settings should be checked for accuracy, and the oxygen source inspected to ensure proper function. Oxygen safety precautions should be posted in the home, and on-going assessment for compliance should be a part of each visit. An important component of oxygen safety includes choosing a reliable supplier with a 24-hour call service. A home care respiratory therapist can assist with this decision, as well as with maintaining oxygen therapy in the home.

The infant with BPD is at increased risk for infection through age 1 or 1½. Family and care-givers need to be aware of this risk, instructed in preventative strategies, and taught to recognize the signs and symptoms of infection. Strategies aimed at minimizing the risk of infection include limiting exposure to persons with upper respiratory infections, and meticulous care of respiratory care equipment.

A routine schedule for the cleaning and disinfecting of respiratory equipment is an important component in preventing respiratory infection. Cleaning should be done in a clean area, free from drafts and away from open windows or vents. Hands should be washed prior to handling the equipment. The screen-trap filter should be removed from the sink, as it can be an excellent growth area for pseudomonas. Equipment can be cleansed in warm soapy water, and a half-strength white vinegar solution used as a 20-minute soak for disinfection. Following cleaning and disinfecting, rinse thoroughly and air dry. After cleaning, equipment should be stored in a jar or plastic bag to protect from contamination between uses.

Routine assessment of the signs and symptoms is also very important. An increase in the amount of viscosity of secretions, foul odor, or yellow green color of secretions, irritability, lethargy, loss of appetite, and the signs and symptoms of respiratory distress are all early signs of infection. The physician should be notified promptly when these are noted (Ahmann 1986).

A full discussion of care of the infant with cardiac compromise is not within the scope of this chapter, and the reader is referred to other sources for in-depth information. Two important aspects of care for the infant with cor pulmonale—administration of medications and signs and symptoms of congestive heart failure (CHF)—will be discussed.

In order to ensure accurate measurement of medications, the care-giver's technique in administration should be observed. Exact measurement is critical as there is quite a small margin of difference between therapeutic and toxic levels for both digoxin and diuretics. Guidelines for digoxin therapy and the signs of toxicity are shown in the boxed material on page 515 and should be reviewed with the care-givers. The earliest signs of digoxin toxicity in the infant are nausea, vomiting, and anorexia (Whaley and Wong 1983).

Infants with cor pulmonale often develop CHF, which occurs when the heart is unable to circulate enough blood to the systemic circulation to meet the metabolic demands of

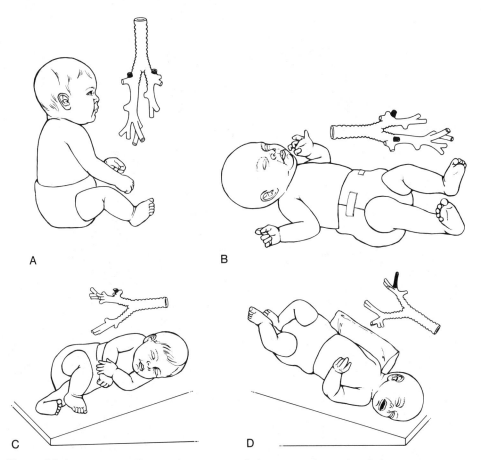

Figure 16-4. Positions for newborn postural drainage. This page: (*A*) Apical segments—upper lobes. (*B*) Anterior segments—upper lobes. (*C*) Posterior segments—upper lobes. (*D*) Right middle lobe. Other views: Page 514. (*E*) Superior segments—lower lobes. (*F*) Anterior basal segments—lower lobes. (*G*) Lateral basal segments—lower lobes. (*H*) Posterior basal segments—lower lobes. (From Schreiner RL, Kisling JA: Practical Neonatal Respiratory Care. New York City, Raven Press, 1982)

the body. The nurse should observe for signs and symptoms of CHF at each visit, and instruct the care-giver in recognition of these signs. The signs and symptoms of CHF include cardiovascular, respiratory, and other related signs. Cardiovascular signs include tachycardia, hyperdynamic precordium, gallop rhythm, peripheral cyanosis, periorbital edema, and a rapid weight gain. Distention of the neck veins is a rare manifestation of CHF in the infant. Respiratory symptoms include tachypnea, dyspnea, orthopnea, retractions, nasal flaring, grunting, and fine rales. Other related signs include hepatomegaly, feeding intolerance, anorexia, diaphoresis, oliguria, irritability, and fatigability (Ahmann 1986).

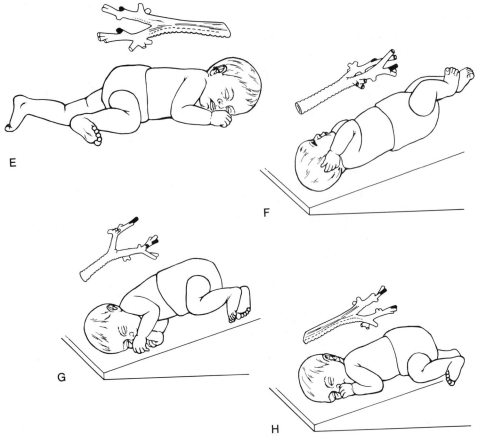

Figure 16-4. *(Continued)*

Outcome

Optimum oxygenation will be maintained.

ALTERATIONS IN NUTRITION

Assessment

The infant with BPD has problems with growth and feeding related to his high energy needs and easy fatigability. Primarily due to the increased work of breathing associated with BPD, caloric requirements are much greater than for the normal newborn. Conversely, the infant with BPD is easily exhausted and may be unable to sustain the activity of feeding. As a result there is an increase in demand complicated by a decrease in supply. This may be further complicated by the need for fluid restriction, as in the presence of cor pulmonale. At each visit the nurse should assess the infant's nutritional intake and measure growth parameters. The infant with BPD will lag behind the normal growth curve, but should show progress, albeit

Guidelines for Digoxin Administration

1. Give digoxin at regular intervals, usually every 12 hours, such as 8 AM and 8 PM.
2. Plan the times so that the drug is given *1 hour before* or *2 hours after* feedings.
3. Use a calendar to mark off each dose that is given, or post a reminder, such as a sign on the refrigerator.
4. Have the prescription refilled *before* the medication is completely used.
5. Administer the drug carefully by slowly squirting it on the side and back of the mouth.
6. Do not mix it with other foods or fluids, since refusal to consume these results in inaccurate intake of the drugs.
7. If the child has teeth, give him water after administering the drug; whenever possible, brush the teeth to prevent tooth decay from the sweetened liquid.
8. If a dose is missed and more than 6 hours have elapsed, withhold the dose and give the next dose at the regular time; if less than 6 hours has elapsed, give the missed dose.
9. If the child vomits within 15 minutes of receiving the digoxin, repeat the dose *once*; if more than 15 minutes have elapsed, do not give a second dose.
10. If more than two consecutive doses have been missed, notify the physician.
11. Do not increase or double the dose for missed doses.
12. If the child becomes ill, notify the physician immediately.
13. Keep digoxin in a safe place, preferably a locked cabinet.
14. In case of accidental overdose of digoxin, call the nearest poison control center immediately.

From Whaley LF, Wong DL: Nursing Care of Infants and Children, 3rd ed. St Louis, CV Mosby, 1987. Modified from Jackson PL: Digoxin therapy at home: Keeping the child safe. Am J Maternal Child Nurs 4(2)105–109, 1979

---

slowly. Any rapid loss or gain, or a protracted failure to gain weight are causes for concern. Parents will be concerned about their infant's growth, but can be assured the slow growth is common for the baby with BPD. A plan of care to assist in ensuring adequate nutrition should be developed with the parents.

Interventions

The simplest means of increasing caloric intake is to increase the volume of formula given. Where this is not applicable, as with fluid restriction, the caloric concentration of infant formula can be increased. A 20 cal/ounce formula can be increased to 24 cal/ounce by mixing a 13 ounce can of concentrate with just 9 ounces of water. Commercial supplements such as Polycose, Moducal, or vegetable oil can be used to provide 26 to 30 cal/ounce formula (Ahmann 1986).

Corn syrup is frequently mentioned as a calorie supplement; however research data indicate corn syrup, like honey, may contain *Clostridium botulinum* spores. Infant botulism has been associated with a failure to thrive, and sudden death. It is recommended that honey and corn syrup not be fed to infants under one year of age (Arnon 1979; California Morbidity 1984).

As the infant progresses to baby foods and table foods, high calorie food such as cheese or ice cream should be encouraged. Homemade baby food often contains less water than commercial baby food, and so delivers more calories. Caloric content can also be increased by adding butter, margarine, or oil to solid foods, and powdered milk to liquids, yogurt, puddings, and cereals (Ahmann 1986).

Outcome

Nutritional balance will be maintained.

ALTERATIONS IN PARENTING

Parents of the infant with BPD will experience many knowledge deficits related to the home management of their child. These educational needs have been discussed in earlier portions of this text. This section will focus upon alterations in parenting associated with the emotional/psychological stresses encountered in dealing with the chronically ill or handicapped infant.

Assessment

The home health nurse will assess the parents' understanding of and their response to the situation. An evaluation of their coping style and ability will provide useful information.

Interventions

Parent–infant attachment can begin as early as the preconceptual stage of planning for the pregnancy. Parental expectations of their newborn are established in the course of the pregnancy. They will often assign physical and personality characteristics to the fetus, and will develop an attachment to this imagined child. One of the developmental tasks of parenthood is the working out of the discrepancies between the imagined child and the actual infant. Before bonding can begin, the parents must grieve the imagined infant. Where the infant is sick, or malformed this normal process is severely complicated (Klaus et al 1982). Parents have been observed to experience the classic grief responses following the birth of a sick or handicapped child. Mothers often grieve as intensely for the infant requiring phototherapy who must remain in the hospital for treatment as for the infant who is severely ill, or who dies. The grief response to a chronically ill child differs from the response to death in that it is on-going, and often not resolved until the eventual death of the child. Even where eventual recovery occurs, the chronic sorrow and stresses involved may become pathologic in nature. This is manifested in various parenting disorders, ranging from overprotectiveness to physical abuse (Klaus 1982).

Chronic and recurrent sorrow are common, essentially normal responses for the parents of the chronically ill child. Parents often express feelings of failure, deprivation and disappointment. They may experience times of intense longing for the idealized, imagined child, and feel resentment toward the actual infant. Many experience guilt, or try to assign blame on self or others for this situation. These are normal responses in the process of adjusting to the chronically ill child (Ahmann 1986).

No two individuals progress through the stages of grief at the same rate, or necessarily in the same order. These individual differences in coping can cause severe family stresses, including marital difficulties and maladjustment among siblings. In order to assist the family, it is helpful to encourage individual family members to take the time to care for themselves, work through their feelings, identify and develop coping strategies, and establish supportive relationships. The family can learn to help itself by recognizing and accepting each individual's coping mechanisms and rate of progress through the grief process (Ahmann 1986).

The task of caring for the sick infant at home carries additional stress. The family, as a system, seeks to maintain order, balance, and continuity (Berdie and Selig 1981). The arrival of the chronically ill infant results in dynamic changes in the order of the family system. Dramatic emotional and role adjustments are required. As a result, previously minimal stressors may become exceptionally troublesome to family members. The community health nurse can assist the family by helping family members to identify new, appropriate patterns of interaction, to develop new problem-solving skills, and to assume altered role responsibilities.

Family role changes are a major source of stress to the family. The mother often becomes the major point of communication with the health care team, and gains the most expertise in giving care for the infant. These events change her role within the family as well as alter her self-perception, and how she is seen by others. The exclusion of others in the family from daily care of the infant can result in feelings of helplessness and failure when they are faced with giving care. It is important to train the entire family in caring for the infant and to encourage an accepting atmosphere that allows the family to feel safe in sharing feelings and seeking information regarding the infant's care.

The uncertain prognosis for the chronically ill infant is also a major stressor for the family. With repeated illnesses and hospitalization, the family experiences dramatic emotional shifts and encounters repeated crises. With uncertainty comes unpredictability in day-to-day events. This can result in feelings of loss of control, which can be very frightening to the parents. The home care nurse should respond to parents' questions with realistic, honest answers, at the parents' level of understanding. Providing information helps the family gain some level of control, and assists their participation in effective decision making regarding care.

Caring for the chronically ill infant requires a tremendous investment of physical and emotional energy by the care-givers. Parents often become so focused upon day-to-day care they become isolated from friends and other family members. The community health nurse can help alleviate exhaustion and isolation by arranging for home nursing, identifying respite care options, and helping the family identify others who can lend support. The extended family can be enlisted to assist the immediate family in many ways, such as helping with transportation, assisting with daily household chores, caring for siblings, and babysitting for the infant. Including the extended family in these ways can help them cope with their grief, feelings of denial, guilt, or blame, and their need for comfort (Ahmann 1986).

Outcome

A major role of the community health nurse in home care consists of providing practical and emotional support. This support should be based on an understanding of parents' emotional responses to their disabled child, an awareness of the family's function as a dynamic system, and recognition of factors contributing to the stresses on the family. The goal of the home health professional in this role is to help families to manage stresses effectively, resulting in optimal home health care for the chronically ill infant.

ASSESSING THE HOME

Considering that 60% of American households are composed of either one parent families or of households where both parents work, an ill infant can impose serious financial strain on the entire structure. Referrals to social workers, psychiatric consultations, exploration of community resources, including support groups, are essential for the well-being of all.

NURSING CARE PLAN: APNEA OF PREMATURITY

Nursing Diagnosis	Assessment	Interventions	Outcomes
Alterations in Oxygenation	Pallor Cyanosis Heart rate	Monitor for apneic episodes. Instruct parents in correct use of the apnea monitor. Teach parents to assess alarms and the correct responses. Teach parents and other care-givers CPR. Establish plan for emergency care. Teach parents concerning the baby's condition and the principles of treatment. Discuss infant's condition at each visit and provide information as needed. Provide contact phone numbers for parents' use. Maintain equipment and supplies. Discuss criteria for discontinuation of monitoring.	Infant will establish normal breathing pattern.
Alterations in Parenting	Knowledge Emotional response	Provide information re: baby's condition; principles of treatment.	Parents will provide optimal care for the infant.

NURSING CARE PLAN: APNEA OF PREMATURITY (*continued*)

Nursing Diagnosis	Assessment	Interventions	Outcomes
		Assess parents' ability to cope with home monitoring.	
		Provide information as indicated by assessment or request.	
		Help the family develop coping mechanisms and support network.	
		Assist in identifying respite care options.	
		Develop plan for discontinuing of monitor.	

References

High-Risk Pregnancy

Burrow GN, Ferris TF: Medical Complications During Pregnancy. Philadelphia, WB Saunders, 1982

Gill PJ, Katz M: Early detection of preterm labor: Ambulatory home monitoring of uterine activity. J Obstet Gynecol Neonatal Nurs 15: 439–442, 1986

Haber J, Leach AM, Schudy SM, Sideleau BF: Comprehensive Psychiatric Nursing, 2nd ed. New York, McGraw-Hill, 1982

Hollingsworth DR: Diabetes mellitus: Newest approaches for a successful pregnancy. Consultant 8: 29–41, 1984

Jovanovic L, Peterson CM, Fuhrmann K: Diabetes and Pregnancy: Teratology, Toxicity, and Treatment. New York, Praeger, 1986

Knupple RA, Drucker JE: High-Risk Pregnancy: A Team Approach. Philadelphia, WB Saunders, 1986

Neeson JD, May KA: Comprehensive Maternity Nursing: Nursing Process and The Childbearing Family. Philadelphia, JB Lippincott, 1986

Ouimette J: Perinatal Nursing: Care of The High-Risk Mother and Infant. Boston, Jones and Bartlett, 1986

Pritchard JA, MacDonald PC, Gant NF: Williams' Obstetrics, 17th ed. East Norwalk, CT, Appleton-Century-Crofts, 1985

Queenan JT: Management of High-Risk Pregnancy, 2nd ed. Oradell, NJ: Medical Economics Books, 1985

Reeder SJ, Martin LL: Maternity Nursing: Family, Newborn, and Women's Health Care, 16th ed. Philadelphia, JB Lippincott, 1987

Whittaker AA, Hull B, Clochesy J: Hemolysis, elevated liver enzymes, and low platelet count syndrome: Nursing care of the critically ill obstetric patient. Heart Lung 15: 402–408, 1986

Ziegel EA, Cranley MS: Obstetric Nursing, 8th ed. New York, Macmillan, 1984

High-Risk Infant

Ahmann E: Home Care for the High-Risk Infant. Rockville, MD, Aspen Publishers, Inc, 1986

American Academy of Pediatrics' Committee on Fetus and Newborn: Criteria for early infant discharge and follow-up evaluation. Pediatrics 71: 651, 1980

American Academy of Pediatrics' Committee on Fetus and Newborn: Prenatal Care. Evanston, American Academy of Pediatrics, 1983

American Academy of Pediatrics' Committee on Fetus and Newborn: Home phototherapy. Pediatrics 76: 136–137, 1985

American SIDS Institute: Sudden infant death syndrome fact sheet. Atlanta, American SIDS Institute, 1983

Aranda JV, Trippenbach T, Turman T: Apnea and control of breathing in newborn infants. In Stern L (ed): Diagnosis and Management of Respiratory Disorders in the Newborn. Reading, MA, Addison-Wesley, 1983

Ariagno RL: Evaluation and management of infantile apnea. Pediatr Ann 13: 217–221, 1984

Arnon SS: Honey and other environmental risk factors for infant botulism. J Pediatr 94: 331–336, 1979

Avery GB: Thermatology: Pathophysiology and Management of the Newborn. Philadelphia, JB Lippincott, 1981

Bell CW: Home Care and Rehabilitation in Respiratory Medicine. Philadelphia, JB Lippincott, 1984

Berdie J, Selig, AL: Family functioning in families with children who have handicapping conditions. Fam Ther 8: 189–195, 1981

Black L, Hirsher L, Steinschneider A: Impact of the apnea monitor on family life. Pediatrics 62: 681–685, 1978

Brown LW: Home monitoring of the high-risk infant. Perinatology 11: 85–100, 1984

Cain LP, Kelly DH, Shannon DC: Parents' perceptions of the psychological and social impact of home monitoring. Pediatrics 66: 37–41, 1980

California Morbidity: Honey, corn syrup, and infant botulism, 1984

Dortch E, Spottiswoode P: New light on phototherapy: Home use. Neonatal Network 4: 30–34, 1986

Jackson DF: Nursing care plan: Home management of children with BPD. Pediatr Nurs 12: 342–348, 1986

Kelly DH, Shannon DC, O'Connell K: Care of infants with near-miss sudden infant death syndrome. Pediatrics 61: 511–517, 1978

Klaus MH, Kennell JH: Parent–infant bonding. St. Louis, CV Mosby, 1982

Korones SB, Lancaster J: High-Risk Newborn Infants: The Basis for Intensive Nursing Care, 4th ed. St. Louis, CV Mosby, 1986

Lamarre A: Residual pulmonary abnormalities in survivors of idiopathic respiratory distress syndrome. Am Rev Respir Dis 108: 60–64, 1973

McCormick M: The institution of low birth weight to infant mortality. N Engl J Med 312: 82–90, 1985

Merritt TA, Valdes-Dapena M: SIDS research update. Pediatr Ann 13: 193–207, 1984

Norris-Berkmeyer S, Hutchins KH: Home apnea monitoring. Pediatr Nurs 12: 259–264, 1986

Smith JC: Psychosocial aspects of infantile apnea and home monitoring. Pediatr Ann 13: 219–224, 1984

Southall DP: Home monitoring and its role in the sudden infant death syndrome. Pediatrics 72: 133–137, 1983

Taussig LM, Lamen RJ: Chronic obstructive lung disease. Pediatrics 26: 354–392, 1979

Whaley LF, Wong DL: Nursing Care of Infants and Children. St. Louis, CV Mosby, 1983

Woods C, Hitt N, Wennberg RP: I am Curious Yellow . . . What is Jaundice?, 1983

Zebal BH, Friedman SB: Sudden infant death syndrome and infantile apnea. Pediatr Ann 13: 188–190, 1984

17

ALTERATIONS IN BODY INTEGRITY

Barbara J. Edlund
Cheryl Gardner
Karen Evans
Bonnie Wesorick
JoAnn B. Wise

There are multiple ways in which the client can experience an alteration in body integrity. In this chapter, two major alterations in body integrity will be discussed: neoplasia and acquired immunodeficiency syndrome (AIDS). The nursing diagnoses related to these conditons will be described and particular emphasis will be placed on infection control, wound care, pain, and intravenous therapy. Based upon the knowledge gained through this chapter, the home health nurse will be able to provide expert nursing care to clients who experience an alteration in body integrity. The nurse will also be able to provide teaching and support to the family as they assist the client.

NEOPLASIA

Cancer is the second leading cause of death in the United States, claiming nearly 500,000 lives per year. Although cancer can affect any portion of the body, there are certain areas more commonly affected in both men and women (Fig. 17-1).

PATHOPHYSIOLOGY

Cancer calls are derived from previously normal cell populations within the body. Malignant cells grow in inappropriate locations and do not respond to the usual restraints on

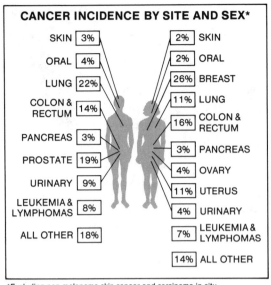

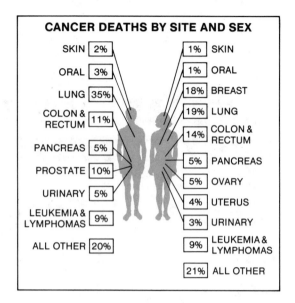

*Excluding non-melanoma skin cancer and carcinoma in situ.

Figure 17-1. Cancer incidence and deaths by site and sex (1985). (From Cancer Facts and Figures. New York, American Cancer Society, 1985)

the size of cell populations or on the rate of growth of those populations (Luckmann and Sorenson 1987).

Cancer cells are reported to have an abnormality in the membrane of the cell that results in abnormal reception of control signals; yet another explanation is that the abnormal membrane leads to abnormal responses to signals. Scientists believe that cancer develops as a result of genetic alteration caused by one or more etiologic agents, resulting in uncontrolled cellular reproduction and growth. When a defective cell divides, the new cells contain the defective molecular code within deoxyribonucleic acid (DNA).

The immune system is also involved in the development of cancer although differences of opinion exist concerning the actual involvement of the immune system. Some researchers believe that the immune system perceives cancer cells as foreign entities and

destroys them. However, certain conditions either cause a breakdown in the immune system or overwhelm it. Thus, the malignant cells reproduce more rapidly than the immune system can destroy them. One major piece of evidence for this theory is that persons with congenital or acquired immunologic deficiencies have a higher incidence of cancer than do persons with an intact immune system. For example, Kaposi's sarcoma is a type of rare cancer frequently diagnosed in clients with AIDS.

Another theory suggests that the immune system may be "blocked" in its effort to destroy tumor-associated antigens. For example, some tumors release antigens that stimulate the immune system to produce antibodies. These antibodies in turn destroy the cancerous cells. However, it appears that other malignant tumors release "blocking agents" that interfere with the action of antibodies or sensitized lymphocytes, or both, and prevent tumor destruction. Laboratory experiments demonstrate that the immune systems of experimental subjects can thwart the action of "blocking" agents by releasing "deblocking" agents, which upset the action of the blocking agents, and, in turn, allow the host's antibodies to act against the tumor cells.

Investigators are trying to determine whether the immune system controls the spontaneous regression of tumors. Spontaneous regressions of cancers occur in about one out of every 100,000 cases (Luckman and Sorenson 1987).

PROGRESSION

The spread of cancer can take many forms: direct extension, seeding of cancer cells to adjacent structures, or metastatic spread through the blood or lymphatic pathways. Growth usually occurs at the tumor periphery with direct extension to or invasion of the surrounding tissue. Malignant tumors have no sharp line of demarcation separating them from the surrounding tissue. This makes complete surgical removal of the tumor difficult. Seeding of cancer cells into body cavities occurs when a tumor erodes into these spaces and tumor cells drop onto the serosal surface.

Metastatic spread occurs when a malignant tumor invades the vascular or lymphatic channels, and parts of the tumor break loose, traveling to distant parts of the body where implantation occurs. When metastasis occurs by way of the lymphatic channels, the tumor cells lodge first in the regional lymph nodes that receive their drainage from the tumor site. The regional lymph nodes may contain the tumor cells for a time, but eventually the cells break loose and gain access to more distant nodes and to the blood stream through the thoracic duct.

STAGING

When a neoplastic growth is diagnosed, it must be further defined in terms of its extent. This diagnostic process, called *staging*, involves a systematic search for several things including

1. The characteristics of the primary tumor
2. Involvement of the lymph nodes
3. Evidence of metastasis

The "TNM" system is the most common type of system used in the defining of the staging process. "T" stands for tumor; "T1–T4" defines the increasing extent of the tumor size; "N" stands for the regional lymph nodes, with "N1–N3" indicating the advance of the nodal disease; "M0" means no metastasis, and "M1" indicates that metastasis is present. This system is summarized in Table 17-1.

The tumor grade is an evaluation of the extent to which tumor cells differ from their normal precursors. Low numeric grades are well differentiated and deviate minimally from normal, while high grades are poorly differentiated and are the most aberrant.

The histologic grade is determined by a pathologist. Tumor grading involves a histologic and anatomic description of the malignant neoplasm. The treatment protocol using the TNM staging system is summarized in Table 17-2.

NURSING DIAGNOSES

The nursing diagnoses are related to both the diagnosis of cancer and the required treatment. Aspects of chemotherapy that are now performed in the home setting will be discussed.

ALTERATION IN NUTRITION

Clients with a diagnosis of cancer may experience an alteration in nutrition due to a de-

TABLE 17.1 TNM Staging System

Tumor	
T0	No evidence of primary tumor
TIS	Carcinoma in situ
T1 T2 T3 T4	Progressive increase in tumor size and involvement
TX	Tumor cannot be assessed
Nodes	
N0	Regional lymph nodes not demonstrably abnormal
N1 N2 N3	Increasing degrees of demonstrable abnormality of regional lymph nodes. (For many primary sites, the subscript "a," *e.g.*, $N1_a$, may be used to indicate that metastasis to the node is not suspected; and the subscript "b," *e.g.*, $N1_b$, may be used to indicate that metastasis to the node is suspected or proved.)
NX	Regional lymph nodes cannot be assessed clinically
Metastasis	
M0	No evidence of distant metastasis
M1 M2 M3	Ascending degrees of distant metastasis, including metastasis to distant lymph nodes

(Reprinted with permission from the American Joint Committee for Cancer Staging and End-Results Reporting and from Clinical Staging System for Carcinoma of the Esophagus)

creased oral intake. The decreased intake may be associated with dysphagia, with anorexia caused by the disease process, or may occur as a side-effect of chemotherapy.

With chemotherapy, the client may experience persistent nausea together with vomiting. This will increase the loss of nutrients, making fewer available for needed growth. As the malignant cells proliferate, they maintain an elevated metabolic rate that necessitates continuous energy utilization.

Assessment

On the first visit to the client and on subsequent visits, the home health nurse will want to perform a total nutritional assessment. Specifically note the client's weight, triceps skinfold measurements, and complaints of weakness or fatigue. If there is concern over the client's nutritional status, it may be necessary to request laboratory studies that could add

valuable information concerning nutritional status. See Chapter 11 for a complete discussion of the appropriate techniques.

The family may be able to assist the nurse in the assessment by determining the amount of food taken by the client. The home health nurse can also assess for the presence of other problems that could interfere with the ability to digest nutrients, including nausea, anorexia, taste distortion, and stomatitis.

Interventions

Once the more direct cause of the alteration in nutrition has been identified, the home health nurse can begin to plan interventions. If the problems include nausea or stomatitis, the home health nurse will recommend interventions to decrease these problems.

One of the first interventions will be to initiate a nutritional consultation to determine what foods the individual is able to tol-

TABLE 17.2   A Treatment Protocol Using the TNM Staging System

Primary Lesions With Negative Nodes:

T1 N0:
Radiation and surgery are equally effective in controlling early primary lesions. Selection of method of treatment is based on cosmetic, functional, and expeditious considerations.

T2 N0:
Moderate exophytic lesions are effectively irradiated with excellent results. Surgery is not precluded in event of failure.

T3 N0:
Advanced lesions can be treated by irradiation, but when they invade bone or cartilage, they are better managed surgically by a composite resection. Preoperative irradiation is advisable.

T4 N0:
For very extensive lesions, combination of techniques is being considered, such as radiation therapy and chemotherapy, or preoperative radiation followed by radical surgery. Preoperative chemotherapy may be used in selected cases with concept of converting an inoperable lesion into an operable one; however, this is not a general principle.

Primary Lesions With Positive Nodes:

T1 N1:
In selected cases, irradiation and surgery can be combined, *i.e.*, primary lesion, such as tongue carcinoma or buccal carcinoma, is treated by radiation therapy followed by neck dissection.

T2–3 N2–3:
The presence of cervical node metastases is generally a surgical problem and is an indication of *en bloc* dissection of both primary and neck nodes.

T4 N3:
Massive lesions are most often inoperable. Palliative radiotherapy and/or chemotherapy are utilized.

(Reprinted with permission from Bales HW, Norante JD: Head and neck tumor. In Rubin P (ed): Clinical Oncology, p 307. New York, American Cancer Society, 1974)

erate. Consult with the physician to determine the need for addition of vitamins to the diet.

Assist the family and client to select foods that are easily chewed and swallowed. Meals should be presented in a relaxed atmosphere. If these interventions are not successful, it may be necessary to institute supplemental forms of feeding.

Chemotherapy may also produce taste distortion that will similarly interfere with the client's appetite. For clients with this problem, beef or pork may taste bitter. If this is the situation, encourage the client and family to select fish, chicken, eggs, and cheese as a source of protein. Snacks of sweetened, high-calorie, high-protein foods may be helpful in replacing needed nutrients. The physician may order zinc to be given, since it may correct the abnormalities of taste (Ulrich, Canale, and Wendell 1986).

Outcome

The client will maintain normal nutritional balance.

ALTERATION IN BOWEL ELIMINATION

Clients may experience constipation or diarrhea. Constipation is related to autonomic nerve dysfunction, decreased physical activity, and a decreased intake of the appropriate foods. Constipation may be worsened by a decreased fluid intake. Diarrhea may be aggravated by increased intestinal motility, resulting from inflammation of the gastrointestinal mucosa caused by chemotherapy.

Assessment

The client's previous bowel habits should be assessed. On each visit, assess bowel sounds, noting if they are normal, hypoactive, or hyperactive. Also assess the client for signs of either diarrhea or constipation. Question the client about the presence of pain, cramping, feeling of fullness, or pressure in the abdomen.

Interventions

Interventions to combat constipation are described in detail in Chapter 11. The most important interventions for the client with cancer include maintaining an adequate fluid intake, and increasing activity as tolerated. Periodically, it may be necessary to supplement the client's diet with medications to encourage evacuation of the bowel.

Interventions for the client with diarrhea are also described in Chapter 11. For the client with the medical diagnosis of cancer, it may be necessary to utilize opium derivative medications to limit the intensity of the episodes. Other measures can be taken to rest the bowel. These include avoiding food or fluids that act as irritants to the bowel, such as those with high-fat, high-fiber content, and spicy foods. Fluids high in caffeine, carbonated beverages, or those that are very hot or very cold may worsen the problem.

Outcome

The client will experience a normal bowel evacuation pattern.

ALTERATION IN COMFORT: NAUSEA AND VOMITING

There are several reasons why the client with cancer would experience an alteration in comfort as evidenced by the presence of nausea or vomiting. The use of chemotherapeutic agents may cause nausea and vomiting related to stimulation of the vomiting center. This occurs due to direct stimulation of the chemoreceptor trigger zone by the chemotherapeutic agents themselves. Other factors that may worsen the problem include vagal stimulation resulting from visceral irritation. Finally, cortical stimulation may also occur, increasing the likelihood of nausea or vomiting.

Assessment

Assess the client for the events that may induce nausea and vomiting. Also assess the client's weight and other indicators of nutritional status.

Interventions

The first intervention is to assist the client in identifying methods to decrease the incidence of nausea and vomiting. These include encouraging the client to eat dry foods when nauseated. Encourage the client to rest after eating, either by sitting up in a chair or lying in a high Fowler's position.

Since the cause of the nausea may be the chemotherapeutic drugs, suggest to the family and client that drugs be administered later in the day to prevent the perception of nausea. During administration of the drug, if the client experiences nausea due to its taste, the use of hard candy may be effective. The use of carbonated beverages between meals may also help to decrease nausea. Certain drugs may be ordered to reduce nausea. The home health nurse may need to instruct the family in the use of suppositories or injections.

Outcome

Client and family will be able to identify interventons that will decrease the incidence of nausea.

ALTERATION IN COMFORT: PAIN

The disease process itself can produce an alteration in comfort for any client. There can be different degrees of pain at various stages throughout the illness. Side-effects of the treatment, whether chemotherapy or radiation, may also affect comfort. To successfully implement a plan to treat this alteration in comfort, the home health nurse must develop an understanding of the physiology of and interventions to diminish pain.

Pain is a complex and elusive phenomenon. It is both sensory and perceptual in nature and, as such, is subjective (Donovan and Girton 1984). Pain has been defined as a personal and private sensation of hurt, a harmful stimulus signaling impending tissue damage, and a response to protect the organism from harm (Sternbach 1968). Probably one of the most clinically useful definitions of pain was proposed by McCaffery (1979) who stated that "pain is whatever the experiencing person says it is and exists whenever he says it does."

Theories of pain have undergone evolutionary change. New physiological evidence and psychological and clinical observations have added to our knowledge and understanding of this phenomenon (Kim 1980). Currently, the most commonly accepted and probably the most clinically useful theory of pain is the gate control theory proposed by Melzack and Wall (1965). An explanation of the nerve fibers involved in the transmission of pain is most helpful as a basis for understanding the gate control theory.

Nerve fibers are divided into three classifications: A, B, and C fibers. Classifications are based on size, action potential, and rate of conduction. The A fibers are large, myelinated, and fast-conducting. There are four subclasses of A fibers: alpha, beta, gamma, and delta. Only the role of alpha and delta fibers has been identified in the transmission of pain (Eland 1981). A-alpha fibers mediate well-localized sensations of fine touch, pressure, and kinesthetic sense. A-delta fibers mediate pain characterized by a sharp, pricking, or cutting sensation (Stephens 1980).

C fibers, on the other hand, are small, thinly myelinated or unmyelinated, and slow-conducting. These fibers mediate pain, temperature, and poorly localized touch. Both A-delta and C fibers are involved in the pain experience. The A-delta fibers are involved in the first sensation of pain experienced at the site of a trauma. This initial sharp, pricking, or cutting sensation is followed by a more generalized, dull, aching, and throbbing sensation (C fibers).

According to the gate control theory, the pain mechanism results from the interaction of three systems within the spinal cord (Fig. 17-2):

1. The cells of the substantia gelatinosa (SG) in the dorsal horn
2. The central transmission cells (T cells) in the dorsal horn
3. The afferent fibers in the dorsal column of the spinal cord

This theory postulates that the SG functions as the "gating mechanism," regulating the flow of nerve impulses; that dorsal column fibers selectively stimulate certain brain processes (central control system), influencing the regulating mechanisms of the SG, and that T cells initiate certain neural mechanisms (action system), responsible for pain perception and response (Kim 1980; Donovan and Girton, 1984; Stephens 1980).

Specifically, the large-diameter A-alpha fibers act as inhibitory fibers (Fig. 17-3) (de-

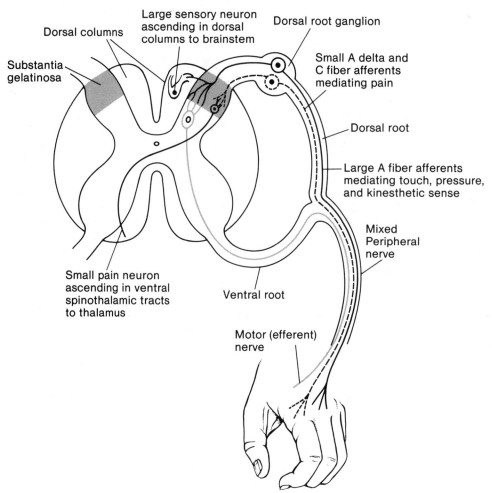

Figure 17-2.   Diagram of cross section of spinal cord, showing ventral and dorsal horns; ventral and dorsal spinal roots; and a mixed motor and sensory somatic nerve. The large A sensory fibers, conveying sensations of touch, pressure, and kinesthesia, enter the cord and synapse with: (1) large sensory fibers that travel to the brain stem in the dorsal columns on the same side; and with (2) motor fibers mediating spinal reflexes. The small A delta and C pain fibers, carrying epicritic and protopathic pain impulses, respectively, synapse in the substantia gelatinosa of the dorsal horn with sensory fibers that cross over and ascend to the thalamus in the spinothalamic tracts. A delta (epicritic) and C (protopathic) pain fibers are not differentiated in this diagram. (From Stephens G: Pathophysiology for Health Practitioners. New York, Macmillan, 1980)

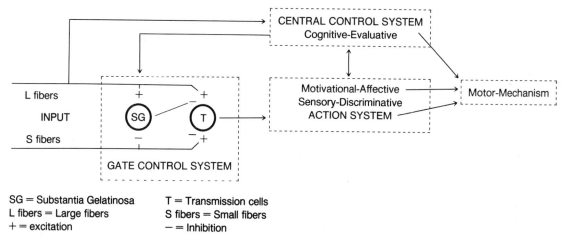

Figure 17-3. Schematic diagram of the gate control theory of pain mechanism. (From Kim S: Pain: Theory, research, and nursing practice. ANS 2(2): 43–59, 1980)

picted as −) that alter and inhibit the transmission of pain in the SG and thus "close" the gate (Erlanger and Gasser 1930). These afferent fibers can be "selectively stimulated by nonpainful impulses (electricity, touch, vibration, massage, and other stimuli) because they have a lower excitation threshold than do small diameter fibers" (Donovan and Girton 1984, p 176). A-alpha fibers enter the cord and synapse in the SG with large sensory neurons that then ascend in the dorsal column to central controls (Fig. 17-2).

The A-delta and C fibers, on the other hand, carry excitatory neurological messages (depicted as + in Fig. 17-3) to the SG (Eland 1981; Stephens 1980). Impulses from these fibers inhibit the inhibitory fibers. When the excitatory input (+) is greater than the inhibitory impulse (−), the gate opens and increases the sensory input to the T cells (Kim 1980). The T cells then activate the action system, which is directed by central controls (Fig. 17-3). The action system may be responsible for the perception of pain and for the response to pain. Arousal of the action system occurs when the individual experiences pain.

A specialized system of large-diameter fibers "directly alerts central control processes to the injury before information is processed in the substantia gelatinosa" (Eland 1981, p 166). These fibers deliver information about the nature and site of the pain and stimulate selected areas of central control that involve memory of previous experiences and response strategies (Melzack 1972). Descending signals are then transmitted to the gating mechanism in the SG. Descending central control signals contribute information about previous pain experiences, the meaning of the pain, conditioning, and emotional factors. Thus the gating mechanism is affected by the transmission of ascending afferent impulses to the brain as well as descending efferent signals from the brain (Melzack 1982; Wolf 1980).

The physiology of chronic pain is believed to be different from that of acute pain described above. It is postulated that with chronic pain, the transmission of impulses via the large fibers to the SG is decreased or even eliminated over time. This leaves the "gate" wide open for the continuous transmission of painful stimuli. It is also thought that the central control processes of clients experiencing chronic pain hold vivid and painful memories of suffering and repeated failed attempts to alleviate the pain (Eland 1981). Thus, the modifying effect of central control processes on the gate is lost in the presence of chronic pain. Melzack (1972) noted that stored painful memories, as well as the elimination of the input from the large fibers to the SG, maximize the intensity of the pain. Over time, patients with chronic pain may suffer more because of the failure of the "gating" mechanism and the mental and psychological depletions that occur (Bonica 1973; Fordyce 1976).

ACUTE VERSUS CHRONIC PAIN

The physiological effects of pain may be of either short- or long-term duration. Acute pain is the activation of what Selye described as the *general adaptation syndrome*—the fight or flight response. Acute pain is short-term in duration and is predominantly a sympathetic response (Eland 1981). In acute pain, epinephrine and norepinephrine are released, causing peripheral vasoconstriction and increases in blood pressure, perspiration, respiration, basal metabolic rate, and heart rate. Serum glucose is also elevated. Restlessness, muscular tension, apprehension, and impaired thinking may also be present.

The client in acute pain may also exhibit heightened behavioral responses. Frequent position changes, bodily rocking, walking, pacing, and holding or supporting an injured area may be increased (Donovan and Girton 1984). The client may also be motionless in an effort to avoid increasing the pain.

Acute pain, however, is time-limited, and the clinical signs and symptoms of this type of pain can only be maintained for about 24 hours. When the pain persists the body begins to adapt and the response is more parasympathetic in nature. With time, the client becomes irritable, fatigued, and apathetic. The skin becomes flushed and warm. The vital signs may be either decreased or normal. Mobility is usually limited and the client is often depressed and withdrawn (Eland 1981).

The client in acute pain presents the classic picture of an individual in pain while the client in chronic pain, over a long period of time, "presents a strikingly different picture (Donovan and Girton 1984, p 186). The longer the pain lasts, the more depleted and exhausted the client becomes. The signs and symptoms usually associated with "pain" are not exhibited. Clients in chronic pain have learned to control their expression of pain so that it is more socially acceptable (Hackett 1971). Depression, and not anxiety, becomes the predominant feature of chronic pain (Donovan and Girton 1984; Copp 1974; McCaffery 1979).

Assessment

Comprehensive assessment is the first step toward effective pain management. The nurse begins the assessment by determining what the client knows and believes about the pain. The family's knowledge and beliefs about pain should be assessed as well. The nurse determines the location and duration of the pain and its typical pattern, if any. She explores the client's past experience with pain and how the client has coped. The nurse also identifies what the pain feels like and how intense it is (use a 0 to 10 numerical scale with 0 representing no pain and 10 representing the worst possible pain). In addition, the measures that have relieved the pain and those that have made it worse are discussed. It is also important to determine the degree to which the pain is interfering with the client's life-style and the ways in which the client is currently coping.

The importance of obtaining a complete pain assessment cannot be overstressed. The assessment provides a working framework from which interventions are planned and progress measured.

Interventions

After the nurse determines what the client and family know about pain, she initiates a well-developed and thought-out teaching plan. The plan should include, as appropriate, information about the following areas:

1. Physiology of pain
2. Characteristics of chronic pain, and how it differs from acute pain
3. Analgesic intervention (discussion of drug(s), dose, interval, side-effects, tolerance, dependence, withdrawal, addiction)
4. Nonanalgesic interventions (evaluate for use of and teach as appropriate distraction cutaneous stimulation, visual imagery, relaxation, and body positioning)
5. Resources (provide information about support groups and organizations as well as sources for client and family counseling)
6. Compliance with the therapeutic regime.

Information giving is an extremely important nursing intervention. Based on the gate control theory of pain, it can alter central control's perception of the pain. Information provides the client with the opportunity to feel he can control what is happening and alter the outcome.

The goal of nursing care is to increase client comfort. This is done through a variety and combination of approaches.

1. Analgesic interventions
2. Nonanalgesic interventions (guided imagery, relaxation, distraction, cutaneous stimulation and body positioning)
3. Support and reassurance
4. Client and family teaching

5. Promotion of adequate rest and sleep (McCaffery and Hart 1976; Bulechek and McCloskey 1985; Snyder 1985).

Analgesic Intervention

Analgesic interventions are, by far, the most frequently and widely used of pain relief measures. However, in the care of clients with chronic pain, the approach to analgesic management differs from that used with acute pain. Yasko (1981) and Foley (1986) discuss the importance of administering analgesics "around the clock" and *never* as needed or required (prn). Also the route of administration must be adjusted to the patient's needs. Oral administration is the route usually used in the analgesic management of chronic pain. Equianalgesic doses should always be used when administering narcotics orally. Administration of drugs parenterally should only be used for acute pain or when chronic pain exacerbates (Yasko 1981).

Utilize narcotic and non-narcotic analgesics in combination. Narcotics (*e.g.*, morphine, codeine) act centrally, while non-narcotic analgesics (*e.g.*, aspirin, acetaminophen, nonsteroidal drugs) act peripherally to reduce pain. This combination promotes more effective pain relief (Foley 1986; Moertel and colleagues 1974). Narcotics are the drugs of choice for the relief of severe pain and non-narcotics for the relief of mild to moderate pain. The lowest possible dose of an analgesic should be used so that pain is relieved and side-effects are tolerable. The analgesics commonly used in the management of pain are listed in Tables 17-3 and 17-4. These tables provide information relative to equianalgesic dose, duration, half-life, and additional factors. They should serve as a helpful reference for the nurse who is assessing the effectiveness of a particular analgesic.

The use of potentiators (*e.g.*, Phenergan) is not encouraged because these drugs simply sedate the patient but provide no pain

TABLE 17.3   Oral Non-narcotic and Narcotic Analgesics for Mild to Moderate Pain

Analgesic	Equianalgesic Dose (mg)*	Duration (hr)	Plasma Half-life (hr)	Comments
Aspirin	650	4–6	3–5	Standard for non-narcotic comparisons; gastrointestinal and hematologic effects limit use in patients with cancer
Acetaminophen	650	4–6	1–4	Weak anti-inflammatory effects; safer than aspirin
Propoxyphene	65†	4–6	12	Biotransformed to potentially toxic metabolic norpropoxyphene; used in combination with non-narcotic analgesics
Codeine	32†	4–6	3	Biotransformed to morphine; available in combination with non-narcotic analgesics
Meperidine	50	4–6	3–4	Biotransformed to active toxic metabolite normeperidine; associated with myoclonus and seizures
Pentazocine	30	4–6	2–3	Psychotomimetic effects with escalation of dose; available only in combination with naloxone, aspirin, or acetaminophen (US)

* Relative potency of drugs, as compared with that of aspirin, for mild to moderate pain.
† Some investigators have reported that a much larger dose (propoxyphene, 130 mg; codeine, 60 mg) is effective in patients with mild to moderate pain.
(Reprinted with permission from Foley K: The treatment of pain in the patient with cancer. CA 36(4): 194–214, 1986)

relief (Yasko 1981). Continuous sedation is not the goal in chronic pain management. Rather, the goal is to keep the client as comfortable as possible while still alert and functioning.

Depression, so characteristically seen in the client with chronic pain, should be evaluated and managed. Tricyclic antidepressants (*e.g.*, Elavil, Tofranil) have been shown to be most useful in managing the depression associated with chronic pain (Donovan and Girton 1984; Foley 1986). It is important to note

that approximately 3 weeks are required before the client comes to realize the benefit of this type of medication. Also several of the antidepressants (*e.g.*, Tofranil) boost the effects of the narcotics so that the dose of the narcotic may need to be reduced (Yasko 1981).

Aspirin is an extremly useful drug in the management of mild to moderate pain. It is important to note, however, that if a client is taking more than 12 aspirin tablets (325 mg) a day, the client probably needs a stronger

TABLE 17.4   Oral and Parenteral Narcotic Analgesics for Severe Pain

Narcotic Agonists	Route*	Equianalgesic Dose (mg)†	Duration (hr)	Plasma Half-life (hr)	Comments
Morphine	IM	10	4–6	2–3–5	Standard for comparison; also available in slow-release tablets
	PO	60	4–7		
Codeine	IM	130	4–6	3	Biotransformed to morphine; useful as initial narcotic analgesic
	PO	200††	4–7		
Oxycodone	IM	15	3–5	—	Short acting; available alone or as 5 mg dose in combination with aspirin and acetaminophen
	PO	30			
Heroin	IM	5	4–5	0.5	Illegal in US; high solubility for parenteral administration
	PO	60	4–5		
Levorphanol (Levo-Dromoran)	IM	2	4–6	12–16	Good oral potency; requires careful titration in ititial dosing because of drug accumulation
	PO	4	4–7		
Hydromorphone (Dilaudid)	IM	1.5	4–5	2–3	Available in high-potency injectable form (10 mg/ml) for cachectic patients and as rectal suppositories; more soluble than morphine
	PO	7.5	4–6		
Oxymorphone (Numorphan)	IM	1	4–6	2–3	Available in parenteral and rectal suppository forms only
	PR	10	4–6		
Meperidine (Demerol)	IM	75	4–5	3–4	Contraindicated in patients with renal disease; accumulation of active toxic metabolite normeperidine produces central nervous system excitation.
	PO	300††	4–6		
Normeperidine				12–16	
Methadone (Dolphine)	IM	10		15–30	Good oral potency; requires careful titration of the initial dose to avoid drug accumulation
	PO	20			

(continued)

TABLE 17.4 Oral and Parenteral Narcotic Analgesics for Severe Pain *(continued)*

Narcotic Agonists	Route*	Equianalgesic Dose (mg)[†]	Duration (hr)	Plasma Half-life (hr)	Comments
Mixed Agonist–Antagonist Drugs					
Pentazocine (Talwin)	IM PO	60 180[††]	4–6 4–7	2–3	Limited use for cancer pain; psychotomimetic effects with dose escalation; available only in combination with naloxone, aspirin, or acetaminophen; may precipitate withdrawal in physically dependent patients
Nalbuphine (Nubain)	IM PO	10 —	4–6	5	Not available orally; less severe psychotomimetic effects than pentazocine; may precipitate withdrawal in physically dependent patients
Butorphanol (Stadol)	IM PO	2 —	4–6	2.5–3.5	Not available orally; produces psychotomimetic effects; may precipitate withdrawal in physically dependent patients
Partial Agonists					
Buprenorphine (Temgesic)	IM SL	0.4 0.8	4–6 5–6	?	Not available in US; no psychotomimetic effects; may precipitate withdrawal in tolerant patients

* IM = intramuscular; PO = oral; PR = rectal; SL = sublingual.
[†]Based on single-dose studies in which an intramuscular dose of each drug listed was compared with morphine to establish the relative potency. Oral doses are those recommended when changing from a parenteral to an oral route. For patients without prior narcotic exposure, the recommended oral starting dose is 30 mg for morphine; 5 mg for methadone; 2 mg for levorphanol, and 4 mg for hydromorphone.
[††]The recommended starting doses for these drugs listed in Table 17.3.
(Reprinted with permission from Foley K: The treatment of pain in the patient with cancer. CA 36(4): 194–214, 1986)

medication (Yasko 1981). In large amounts, aspirin can affect platelet aggregation and lead to thrombus formation, adding further complications. With regard to the management of mild to moderate pain, research (Moertel and colleagues 1972) has shown that two aspirin or acetaminophen tablets (650 mg) offer as much pain relief as the following orally prescribed medications: codeine (32 mg); Demerol (50 mg); Talwin (30 mg); Darvon (65 mg); 5 Darvon-N (100 mg); and Dilaudid (125 mg).

The side-effects of the analgesics, particularly the narcotics, need to be monitored. The drowsiness that accompanies narcotic analgesics should lift in about 48 to 72 hours. If the drowsiness continues beyond this time, the dose needs to be readjusted. A standing protocol approved by the physician for respiratory depression due to over-treatment with a narcotic should also be readily available.

Constipation is probably one of the most troublesome side-effects for the client on long-term narcotic analgesics. It can, however, be effectively managed by using a routine bowel preparation. This needs to be started the day the client begins using a narcotic analgesic. The client may require more than the normal recommended adult dose and schedule usually prescribed for occasional constipation. The nurse needs to assist the client in arriving at a dosage that effectively manages the problem. One to two tablespoons of Chronulac (lactulose), one to two times a day, have been shown to be very effective in preventing constipation in patients on long-term narcotic analgesics.

Nausea and vomiting may occur as an expected side-effect and not as an allergic reaction to narcotic analgesics (Yasko 1981). The problem can be managed by keeping the client on an antiemetic for 48 to 72 hours until the nausea and vomiting subside. If the vomiting persists, discuss the situation with the client's physician.

With chronic pain management, there is often confusion related to drug tolerance, physical dependency, and drug addiction (Catalano 1985). An understanding of the concepts is important in client care. Drug tolerance can occur with repeated administration of analgesics. The drug loses its effectiveness first in its duration of action and then in its analgesic effect. It is important to teach the client that drug tolerance can occur and is usually resolved by increasing the dosage of the medication under the physician's direction (Yasko 1981). "Physical dependence is an altered physiological state characterized by the appearance of a withdrawal or abstinence syndrome when the drug is suddenly withheld" (Donovan and Girton 1984, p 230). Physical dependence can occur after 24 hours on a narcotic. Therefore, it is important that drugs not be abruptly discontinued but rather that the dosage be gradually reduced in conjunction with the physician's knowledge/direction.

Drug addiction is a different entity from drug tolerance and physical dependence. It is an "overwhelming involvement with obtaining and using a drug for its psychic effect rather than for medically or socially approved reasons" (McCaffery 1980, p 37). The risk is low, McCaffery (1980) noted, when narcotics are given for the purpose of pain relief. Health care providers should consider that major factors leading to addiction include noneffective treatment of chronic pain; a decrease in the dosage; and an increase in the interval between administration of the drug. When pain is not relieved, clients can become desperate in their behavior to prove that they have pain. This situation should not occur if the goal of pain management is effective pain relief. Analgesic intervention should be used on a consistent and regular basis, increasing or decreasing the dosage as needed in order to make the patient as comfortable as possible.

Noninvasive Interventions

Chronic pain is more effectively managed by a multiple modality approach than it is by a single intervention (Yasko 1981). The noninvasive interventions, as a category of pain relief measures, provide therapeutically useful techniques that assist in alleviating pain. These techniques include distraction, cutaneous stimulation (massage, heat or cold, vibration, pressure and electrical stimulation — transcutaneous stimulation [TNS, TENS]), relaxation, guided imagery, hypnosis, and body positioning (McCaffery 1979).

The basis for the effectiveness of these techniques lies in the gate control theory. Distraction, relaxation, guided imagery, and hypnosis decrease the motivational–affective processing, that is the unpleasant affective quality of pain (Eland 1981). Heat or cold and positioning of the body reduce small-diameter fiber irritation, thus altering sensory message transmission to the T cells. Massage, rubbing, pressure, vibration and electrical stimulation increase large-diameter fiber transmission. The reduction of small-diameter fiber irritation and the increase of large-diameter fiber transmission work to "close the gate" and prevent the further transmission of painful stimuli (Eland 1981).

A detailed discussion of each of the noninvasive pain relief methods is beyond the scope of this chapter. However, there are many excellent sources of information on the subject, among them the writings of McCaffery (1979), Bulechek and McCloskey (1985), Snyder (1985), Donovan and Girton (1984). To assist the nurse in identifying which techniques would be more beneficial in certain clinical situations, Donovan (1985) has compiled a set of observations on pain relief methods (Table 17-5). During the assessment process, the nurse must be alert to the cues clients are giving about how they perceive and cope with pain. These cues can then be utilized in planning which techniques will work best to deal effectively with the pain.

Clients who experience chronic pain often have difficulty obtaining adequate sleep and rest. A number of factors contribute to this problem. Lack of sensory stimulation, as often occurs with immobility, can contribute to frequent dozing and catnaps during the day. This is because the wakefulness center (in the reticular activating system in the brain stem) must be bombarded continually by stimuli in order for the client to remain alert. When the stimuli are diminished or absent, the client continually dozes. The later in the day this continues, the more likely the client is to approximate the pattern of nightly sleep. Thus, when it is time for sleep, the client is not sleepy. More than likely, the client is also taking "round the clock" analgesics, which may affect his level of alertness, further contributing to frequent dozing during the day. Fitful nights of sleep, coupled with early morning awakenings as is seen with depression, contribute to the overwhelming fatigue experienced by clients in chronic pain.

Management of this problem must address a number of factors. First of all, sleep and rest must be separate. Early morning naps are encouraged, while late afternoon or early evening naps are discouraged. Mobility and activity, as appropriate for the client, should be encouraged. Physical activity during the day increases restful, physically restoring sleep (NREM sleep) (Kleitman 1969). Activity, mobility, and positioning increase large-diameter fiber transmission, thus "closing the gate" to the further transmission of painful stimuli. Activity can also influence positively the client's self-concept and feelings of self-worth.

In addition, a client should adhere, when feasible, to a regular schedule identifying bedtime and awakening time (Kales and Kales 1970). The use of the bed for activities other than sleep or sex should be discour-

TABLE 17.5 Use of Observations of Patient, Family, and Care-givers

Observation		Pain Relief Methods to Consider Based on Observations
Attitude toward noninvaasive methods	Accepting Skeptical	Noninvasive methods Start with medications, then sell noninvasive methods.
Attitude toward medications	"The Answer" Resistant	Start with medications. Noninvasive methods; sell medications
Level of trust in health care system	High Lacking	Any intervention may be suggested. Start with what the patient thinks will work best.
Perceptions	Detailed Global	Specify intervention in detail. Capitalize on trust and previous success.
Interactions	Provide relief No relief	Distraction Do not use distraction.
Use of medications	Regular and effective Regular/not effective	Continue and evaluate for use of noninvasive methods. Titrate dose and add local/regional methods or refer for pain clinic evaluation if pain is severe and not responding to any type of intervention.
Depression		Evaluate for use of tricyclic antidepressants.
Anxiety	Pain controlled Pain not controlled	Listen, psychotherapy, tranquilizers Control pain.
Expectations	Positive Negative	Meet as much as possible, or if not realistic, assist patient to modify. Assist patient to modify.

(Reprinted with permission from Donovan M: Nursing assessment of cancer pain. Semin Oncol Nurs 1(2): 109–115, 1985)

aged. Sleep needs to be associated with the bed. Getting a client out of be during the day, then, becomes most important. Adhering to a nightly routine can facilitate night sleep. Such measures as a shower, tub bath, glass of warm milk, repositioning, straightening sheets, as well as analgesics and sedatives, can assist in promoting a good night's rest (Eland 1981).

Outcome

The client will experience comfort and control of pain.

ALTERATION IN ORAL MUCOUS MEMBRANE

With the advent of chemotherapeutic drugs, stomatitis is a common problem for the clients with cancer. The drugs interfere with the normal development of the rapidly dividing mucosal epithelial cells. In addition, dehydration, decreased salivary flow, and poor oral hygiene may worsen the problem.

Assessment

The family can assist in monitoring the client for mouth ulcerations. On each visit, the home health nurse must also assess the client's mouth for signs of dry, reddened mucosa with areas of skin breakdown. The client may also complain of oral pain, dysphagia, and thickened saliva.

Interventions

Instruct the client and family in the importance of oral hygiene. This hygiene should include frequent rinsing with either hydrogen peroxide or baking soda with water. The teeth should be cleaned, using a soft toothbrush. Recommend that the client avoid use of substances that can dry the mouth, including mouthwashes with alcohol bases or lemon–glycerine swabs. Increasing the amount of fluid will assist in prevention of stomatitis (Ulrich, Canale, and Wendell 1986).

If problems continue, the home health nurse may need to approach the physician for antifungal or antibacterial agents. Once prescribed, these must be given carefully, according to the directions of the manufacturer. Failure to utilize these preparations appropriately will result in their inability to treat the problem.

Outcome

The client will maintain a healthy oral cavity.

SENSORY–PERCEPTUAL ALTERATION

The use of chemotherapeutic agents may cause damage to the eighth cranial nerve. This causes tinnitus and/or hearing loss.

Assessment

On each visit, the home health nurse will evaluate the client's hearing. Instruct the family to report any problems in hearing. Encourage them to monitor the client for some of the more subtle indications of a hearing loss, including inappropriate responses to questions, and moving closer to others when they speak.

Interventions

Encourage the client and family to evaluate continually for the problem. Monitor for additional problems when other ototoxic drugs are used, such as furosemide or gentamicin.

If a decrease in hearing is evident, utilize techniques to assist the client in overcoming the deficit. These include reducing environmental noise, asking the family to speak louder and to face the client when speaking.

Outcome

The client will experience minimal alterations in hearing.

ANXIETY

There are numerous reasons for the client to experience anxiety. The recognition of the diagnosis will increase the possibility of anxiety. The effects of some of the chemotherapy or radiation treatments may also encourage anxiety. The realization of the future related to the cancer may also cause the client to experience anxiety.

Assessment

Assess the client for signs of anxiety including tenseness, irritability, restlessness, tachycardia. If the client is noncompliant, consider the possibility of anxiety. The presence of persistent pain or side-effects from the therapy may also heighten anxiety.

Interventions

The family can be extremely helpful in assisting the client to cope with anxiety. Encourage them to provide the client with a peaceful environment. On each visit, assure that the client has been provided with adequate information concerning treatment and care. Encourage both the client and family to talk with you, expressing their fears and anxiety. Instruct the client in relaxation techniques that can be employed to decrease anxiety at specific times (Ulrich, Canale, and Wendell 1986).

If these interventions are ineffective, the physician can be contacted to prescribe minor tranquilizers or sedatives. Although these provide for short-term assistance only, they may be needed to assist the client over particularly difficult times.

Outcome

The client will be able to utilize methods to decrease anxiety. The client will also report a decrease in anxiety and tension.

ALTERATION IN SKIN INTEGRITY

Clients with cancer may develop an alteration in skin integrity. Wound care of pressure sores in the home is provided under very different circumstances than in the traditional hospital setting. The home health nurse and the family members, or possibly even friends, are the primary deliverers of wound care and assessors of the progress of wound healing. Physician involvement is minimal when compared to the hospital setting. Those providing care must be depended on for accurate observatons and assessments.

Friction, shearing, debilitating secondary conditions, and poor nutritional status are factors that may contribute to skin breakdown. In general, immobilization and the resulting increased pressure against the skin are the most common origins.

If pressure is unrelieved, nutrients and oxygen cannot reach the skin and underlying tissues and waste products cannot be removed. Such failure of exchange in the capillary bed results in cell destruction and, if uncorrected, tissue necrosis occurs. High pressure exerted for a short time and minimum to moderate pressure applied for an extended period are equally injurious. If this pressure is not decreased to below capillary closure pressure, irreverisble damage may occur. Such damage may occur in only 1 to 6 hours, depending on the general physical condition of the patient, preexisting condition of the skin, and the amount of pressure being applied.

When cellular necrosis occurs, an inflammatory process is initiated. Vasodilatation is the initial event, followed by a hyperemic response. Deep cellular tissue damage can occur at this stage if the situation remains unremedied. Although the bulk of the injury is well below the skin, while this process is occurring the skin surrounding the necrotic tissue becomes erythematous and continues to increase in size. As the deterioration of the tissue accelerates, bleeding may occur at the wound edges. Bacterial invasion into the wound bed may also occur, producing a purulent exudate that may result in an increased depth of the wound.

WOUND HEALING

Inflammation is the initial response to all tissue injuries. The intensity and duration of this acute inflammatory response is determined by external localized factors and internal systemic factors.

Leukocytes are the dominant cells that invade the injured tissue. Plasma proteins and red blood cells also migrate to the area. This period of leukocytosis lasts for approximately the first 72 hours postinjury. During this time, phagocytes invade the area and destroy debris. If the wound is relatively superficial and free from infection, the inflammatory stage is brief. However, if the wound becomes infected the phase becomes chronic and wound healing is delayed. If there are no complicating internal factors such as anemia or malnutrition, the length of the acute inflammatory stage is determined by the external localized factors. Poor or inappropriate wound care may result in chronic inflammation and delays the granulation process.

If there are no hindrances, in about 72 hours new fibroblasts develop and mobilize from the wound edges across the wound bed. Reepithelialization can be seen as new tissue develops at the periphery of the wound. Collagen also forms and the new tissue gains tensile strength. The new granulation tissue is fragile and needs protection from injury until collagen synthesis is complete. This may take 4 to 6 weeks, depending on the size and depth of the wound.

Assessment

Staging of the wound provides a consistent, universal identification of the wound involvement when used by health care professionals. The taxonomy for wound staging is displayed in the boxed material opposite.

Another way of describing ulcers is as *split-* and *full-thickness ulcers.* Split-thickness ulcers incorporate stages I and II and full-thickness includes stages III and IV. This system may offer increased clarity since it is sometimes difficult to differentiate between a

---

Taxonomy for Staging of Wounds

STAGE I

A reddened inflamed area with superficial excoriation may be present.

STAGE II

Injury extends through the dermis but not to underlying tissue.

STAGE III

Injury extends through subcutaneous fat and fascia. Muscle may be involved.

STAGE IV

Injury extends through the muscle and possibly to the bone.

---

stage II and stage III ulcer or between a stage III and stage IV ulcer.

On each visit, assess the appearance of the wound. In particular, note if it is clean or draining purulent material. Based on this observation, the necessary wound care or type of dressing should be prescribed. Since wound healing is greatly affected by degree and duration of immobilization, continence, nutritional status, and presence of chronic debilitating secondary conditions, an accurate assessment of these aspects is very important. If these factors are not well-balanced, healing will be impaired, even with good wound care.

The client's appetite, availability of someone to prepare food, and to feed the client either orally or via tube must be assessed and monitored. Assess for the presence of continence. The cause, type, frequency, and duration may be a factor in determining the type of wound care needed. Identification of secondary conditions such as diabetes mellitus, peripheral vascular disease, and other chronic disease processes is necessary because such processes will influence the degree of pressure relief needed, as well as the nutritional and medication requirements.

An accurate assessment of the family members (or friends) involved in the daily wound care is critical. Their availability, educational capabilities, motivation, and compliance with prescribed wound care and treatment plus financial resources will impact greatly on the external and internal factors involved in wound healing. Frequency and complexity of dressing changes, adequate turning, good hygiene, providing adequate nutrition, and administration of medications will depend on a family member being available on a 24-hour basis.

Interventions

Modalities for Stage I and Stage II (Split-Thickness) Ulcers

The presence of clean, nondraining wounds makes possible the greatest and most flexible variety of wound care. Damp to dry dressings remain the most commonly used. Saline should be the solution of choice since hydrogen peroxide, Dakin's solution, and povidone iodine (Betadine) interfere with re-epithelialization of a granulating wound.

The needed supplies (saline, gauze sponges, and tape) are readily available and relatively inexpensive. However, the degree of family involvement required is greater than is involved in the use of any other type of dressing. Someone should be available to change these dressings three times a day, preferably on an 8-hour schedule. The client and family should be taught the correct dressing procedure, including fluffing the gauze, wringing it as completely dry as possible, and placing it on the wound so that it does not overlap and potentially macerate surrounding tissue. This compliance is needed for optimum wound care.

If the wound is on the sacrum and the patient is incontinent, the dressing and wound are easily contaminated by stool and/or urine. Another type of dressing should be considered to prevent deterioration of the wound.

Sprays and other topical products such as Granulex may be utilized. Again someone must be available to apply the spray every 6 to 8 hours or the product is ineffective. Fecal incontinence provides the same potential for wound contamination as damp to dry dressings. The use of Granulex is not difficult and is easily taught. Use of other topical products such as bourbon and bismuth, Mercurochrome, alum, and a host of others have the same pro's and con's in use as Granulex.

All of these dressings employ the principles of dry wound healing. Keeping wounds clean and dry is a principle accepted by many physicians and consequently may be more frequently prescribed.

Synthetic semipermeable wound films have increased in popularity in the past 5 years. Such dressings include Op-Site, Tegaderm, Bio-clusive, Uniflex, and Operaflex. These wound films utilize the principles of moist wound healing.

Use of wound films is indicated for stages I and II clean ulcers. Presence of purulent exudate or debris is an *absolute* contraindication either for initiating or for continuing use as a dressing. When in doubt, a culture should be obtained. There are several advantages to the use of wound films with a clean, split-thickness ulcer. Fewer dressing changes are required. As long as good adhesion exists and there is little accumulation of fluid under the dressing, it can be left in place up to 7 days; however, a more realistic time is generally 3 to 5 days.

Wound films provide a bacterial barrier and yet allow for vapor exchange. The wound bed is not disturbed when dressings are changed since the film does not adhere to moist tissue. Therefore new granulation tissue is not damaged. Although more expensive per package than gauze, they may be actually more cost-effective than damp to dry dressings because of the decreased dressing changes required.

There are some limitations in use. Teaching the family how to apply the product is not generally difficult; however, the preparation of the wound and surrounding skin is extremely important. No wound film will adhere to moist or oily skin. There must be a minimum of one inch overlap of the film onto contact, dry, fat-free skin. Ideally, the overlap should be 1½ to 2 inches.

The wound bed should be gently cleaned with saline, and patted dry before applying the film. If applied to the buttocks, sacrococcygeal area, or to the heels, it is desirable to tape all the edges with a paper or silk-type tape, using a picture frame technique. If any sign of infection occurs, the wound film should be discontinued immediately. The family consequently must be able to recognize signs and symptoms of infection and be relied upon to notify the home health nurse. With these factors of such importance, the family capability and compliance are essential.

Another limitation exists when fecal incontinence is present and the wound is on the sacrum. The edges of the wound film sometimes lose adhesion and "roll-up" due to position changes or turning. Then there is the potential for stool to become trapped under the dressing and contaminate the wound.

Wound films may also be used after granulation is complete. The film acts as a second skin and protects the new granulation tissue until collagen is synthesized and tensile strength has returned.

Wafer dressings are another example of those utilizing moist healing principles. Duoderm and Ulcer Dressing are examples of the wafer concept. Such dressings are occlusive rather than semipermeable and have been reported to increase significantly the process of wound reepithelialization when compared to dry dressings.

There are components in the wafer dressing that, once in contact with the wound, contribute to formation of a moist gel. It is this gel that prevents the wound bed from drying out and maintains the moist environment. The advantages and disadvantages offered are essentially the same as for wound films. These dressings do well on sacral wounds if there is fecal incontinence, since they protect the wound totally. Additionally, when the edges are properly taped in a picture-frame fashion, there is less potential for curling edges than with a wound film. Since wafers are significantly more expensive than wound films, their use may be determined by whether or not the wound film adheres and whether fecal incontinence is a factor.

Granulation of wounds sometimes appears to reach a plateau and little progress is seen. It then becomes necessary to reevaluate the current wound care and dressings. Since wound films are less expensive, they are frequently selected over wafers; however, if the reepithelialization does not occur at a reasonable rate, a wafer may be indicated.

Stage I and Stage II Ulcers, Draining, Infected

Fortunately, most split-thickness (stage I and stage II) ulcers do not drain purulent material or become necrotic unless there is a complete lack of wound care. With good wound care and control of indirect factors such as pressure, these wounds will heal quickly. However, if the inflammatory stage becomes chronic due to infection, the dressings and type of wound care are limited. Wound films and wafer dressings are absolutely contraindicated in such cases since maintenance of a moist wound would stimulate the growth of infectious material. Damp to dry dressings are the primary means of "cleaning up" such wounds.

If drainage is present, povidone iodine damp to dry dressings, changed every 8 hours, are the primary therapy. Once the drainage stops and the wound is clean, the other dressings described for stage I and stage II ulcers may be implemented. If damp to dry dressings are continued, a saline solution should be used.

If there is necrotic tissue present, the wound must be debrided.

Wound films and wafers may be used to soften or break down eschar. Meticulous observation and a dressing change regimen are required. Dressings used for this purpose should be changed every 48 hours. If left in place longer, eschar and debris may liquify and cover the wound bed, causing undesirable results.

Enzymatic debriding can occur through the use of such agents as Elase and Travase. However, for treatment to be effective, the wound bed must be cleansed thoroughly and these agents applied precisely according to manufacturer's directions. Selection of the appropriate enzyme for the type of wound is also critical. Elase is specific for fibrin removal. Travase is proteolytic in nature and will debride the soft, gelatinous spongy sticky material found on some wounds. It is ineffective against fibrin and collagen.

Modalities for Stage III and Stage IV (Full-Thickness) Ulcers

There have been no recent significant developments in dressings or innovative wound care for full-thickness ulcers. Damp to dry dressings should be changed every 8 hours. Clinitron therapy is of value; however, it is generally unavailable in the home unless the family has excellent insurance coverage or unlimited financial resources. Wound care of these ulcers is the most demanding on the family.

Saline damp to dry dressings usually are indicated. If the wound becomes infected or necrotic tissue is present the physician must decide whether or not to admit the patient to an acute care hospital. The home health nurse will likely be required to increase the number of home health visits to provide needed observation and to better assess the state of the wound. Povidone iodine damp to dry dressing may be used if the wounds drain purulent material.

Wound exudate absorbers such as Debrisan, Hydragran, and other absorption dressings may be used to wick away such drainage from the wound bed. These dressings do not debride; they absorb and trap undesirable exudate.

There are stage III ulcers that will granulate over a prolonged period of time and under ideal circumstances if optimum wound care, maximum pressure relief, and good nutrition are provided. These efforts are controlled by the family and its resources, the home health nurse, and the physician. The general procedures for decubitus and pressure area care are outlined in the boxed material on page 544.

Dry and Moist Wound Healing Wounds heal in either a dry or moist environment. In this context, *moist* implies that the wound is bathed or covered in its own physiologic solution, not infectious or purulent drainage. Utilization of moist wound healing is applicable only to clean wounds.

In dry wound healing, a layer of desiccated exudate forms over the wound bed and creates a scab. (Exudate in this context is fluid resulting from a tissue injury and does not imply an infectious process). The underlying tissue also dehydrates. The new epithelial cells move through the dried tissue to the moist interface below. From there the cells move across the wound to form granulation tissue.

General Procedure for Decubitus and Pressure Area Care

Equipment:

Cleansing solution

Normal saline solution

Heat lamp

Medicated ointment (if prescribed)

Disinfectant solution

Dressing (if necessary)

Irrigation kit (if needed)
  Sterile irrigation syringe (50 ml)
  Sterile irrigation solution
  Sterile basin
  Padding for linen

Procedure:

1. Wash hands carefully before and after caring for the immobilized client.

2. Assist the family to turn the immobilized client at least every 2 hours. Each time the client is turned, inspect the skin for signs of pressure areas, which include discoloration (redness or whiteness), lack of sensation, and breaks in the skin. Gently massage bony prominences with lotion.

3. Place the client in a variety of positions, including prone. If a recliner is available, place the client in various positions of reclining to vary the pressure on the skin. The client may be placed in the prone position for variation. Be sure that breathing is not inhibited. Rolled pads may be used to keep body parts in proper alignment; however, be sure that the pads themselves do not cause pressure.

4. Cleanse the pressure sore. Agents used in cleansing include hydrogen peroxide and povidone iodine. These solutions should be rinsed off with saline solution.

5. Irrigate the decubitus ulcer if there is a good deal of drainage. Place padding under the ulcer area to catch the irrigation fluid.

6. Open the sterile basin and pour sterile irrigation fluid (usually normal saline) into the basin.

7. Don sterile gloves and draw up the solution into the syringe. Gently irrigate the ulcer, allowing the solution to flow away from the ulcer onto the padding.

8. The dry method of treatment includes using heat, such as a heat lamp, to dry the tissue for a period of 20 minutes, with the lamp kept at a distance of 18 to 20 inches (45 cm to 50 cm). The skin must be checked every 5 minutes during treatment. The area may then be covered with a bandage or left open to room air. **Never use a sun lamp or infrared lamp for decubitus care.**

9. The wet method includes dressings that create a moist environment. After the area is cleansed, a transparent material such as Op-Site is placed on the area to seal in the body's normal defensive secretions, such as the leukocytes, plasma, and fibrin.

10. The dressing is left in place until it becomes dislodged; then it is replaced. This type of dressing is transparent so the wound is visible for continuing assessment.

11. Do not place rubber or plastic next to the client's skin. The more desirable

bed coverings are sheepskin, egg crate mattress, and other coverings designed to decrease pressure and enhance circulation.

(Adapted from Walsh J, Persons CB, Wieck L: Manual of Home Health Care Nursing. Philadelphia, JB Lippincott, 1987)

The concept of moist wound healing has gained popularity since the mid-1970s. Winter in England (1971) did much research to substantiate the validity of this process. By covering a clean, noninfected wound with a semipermeable or occlusive dressing, the physiologic fluid in the wound is maintained and not lost on the traditional gauze dressing. Consequently, the exposed dermal layer is kept moist and viable and this in turn, results in unhindered leukocytosis. Also, the new epithelial cells can migrate easily across the moist wound bed ultimately to cover the entire wound surfaces. Since such dressings do not adhere to the wound bed, new granulation tissue is not disturbed when dressings are changed. Such dressings also create a barrier against bacteria that may prevent chronic inflammation from occurring.

Expenditures for egg crate mattresses, alternating pressure pads, water mattresses, and decubitus pads are generally reimbursed by Medicare and Medicaid. Such items available to the general public are usually of lesser quality than those available to hospitals so frequent turning is even more essential. If the patient has private insurance coverage, Clinitron or KinAir therapy may be available and provided with justification from the physician. The home health nurse will make the assessment and provide the documentation for such justification.

Outcome

The skin should remain intact. If skin integrity is altered, the nursing interventions begin to restore the integrity.

POTENTIAL FOR INJURY: INFECTION

Nosocomial, or hospital acquired, infections account for substantial morbidity and mortality each year. In 1984, the National Nosocomial Infection Surveillance System collected and analyzed data from a large sample of U.S. hospitals. This data indicated an average rate of 33.5 nosocomial infections per 1,000 discharges. The study further indicated that, in a significant number of cases, the infection either contributed to or caused death. Due to shortened hospital stays, patients may leave the institution while in the incubated state of an infection and therefore shortly after discharge may manifest symptoms of a nosocomial infection.

COMMON SITES FOR INFECTION

The home-bound client who was previously hospitalized and experienced such common medical interventions as indwelling catheters (Foley, nasogastric, chest tubes, peripheral or central intravenous lines), antibiotics, and surgery will be susceptible at the common nosocomial sites. The sites of infection in order of frequency are the urinary tract, surgical wounds, respiratory tract, and the skin. The common causative agents and their sites are documented in the boxed lists on page 546.

Most of the organisms listed are normal resident flora. They are harmless in their usual sites and prevent colonization, invasion, and infection by pathogenic organisms. They can, however, produce disease when relocated. Man's own flora (endogenous) becomes a threat when the balance has been interfered with by antibiotics, chemotherapy, or alteration of the immune system. A detailed description of these commonly found organisms can be found in Table 17-6.

Several factors have an important effect on an individual client's ability to resist infection (Fig. 17-4). Nutritional deficiencies due to

---

Common Invading Organisms

Escherichia coli (E. coli)

Pseudomonas

Staphylococcus aureus

Enterococcus

Klebsiella

Staphylococcus epidermidis

Enterobacter

Proteus

Serratia

Streptococcus (B)

Pneumococcus

Haemophilus influenzae

Virus (herpes)

Other

Sites and Common Invading Organisms

RESPIRATORY	URINARY
Pseudomonas aeruginosa	*Escherichia coli*
Staphylococcus aureus	*Enterococcus*
Klebsiella	*Pseudomonas aeruginosa*
Pneumococcus	*Klebsiella*
Streptococcus (B)	**WOUND (SURGICAL)**
Haemophilus influenzae	*Staphylococcus aureus*
BACTEREMIA	*Enterococcus*
Coagulase negative *Staphylococcus*	*Escherichia coli*
Staphylococcus aureus	**WOUND (CUTANEOUS)**
Escherichia coli	*Staphylococcus aureus*
Candida	Coagulase negative *Staphylococcus*
	Escherichia coli
	Pseudomonas aeruginosa

---

inadequate intake of protein calories, vitamins, and minerals will weaken the immune system. Any invasive or irritating devices such as central peripheral IV, Foley catheters and nasogastric tubes, ill fitting dentures, or oxygen devices challenge the immune system by disturbing the first line of defense—the skin barrier.

Diseases such as diabetes, liver disease, malignancies, diseases of the spleen, massive trauma, and addiction to drugs, alcohol or tobacco can contribute to reduced host defenses to infection. Age is also an important factor, with the young and the elderly having a more fragile immune system.

Drugs used as part of client therapy, including steroids, antibiotics, anesthesia, cyclosporins, or chemotherapy, will affect the function of the immune system. All of these drugs decrease its effectiveness.

Treatment modalities such as radiation may also weaken the patient's normal abilities to cope with exposure to invading organisms by decreasing the effectiveness of the immune system.

The stress of illness or surgery, loss of sleep, bereavement, or loss of control may also alter the patient's normal defenses against infection.

TABLE 17.6 Commonly Found Organisms

Organism	Site of Infection	Reservoir
Escherichia coli	Urinary tract or perianal abscess	Endogenous or hands of health care provider
Pseudomonas	Respiratory tract Other moist areas	Equipment and supplies Environment
Staphylococcus aureus	Surgical and cutaneous wounds	Endogenous Hands and nasal droplets of provider of care
		A recent strain has been found to be methicillin resistant.
Gram-negative organisms	Normal flora	Endogenous and hands of provider of care
Enterococcus		
Enterobacter	Tube feedings	
Proteus		
Klebsiella	Intravenous solutions	
Serratia	Moisture Respiratory equipment and Foley bags	
Fungus	Total parenteral nutrition	Endogenous; overgrowth is seen in use of antibiotics and chemotherapy
Staphylococcus epidermidis	Prosthetic devices Central catheter lines	Endogenous and hands of provider of care Has affinity for plastic

Assessment

Assess the client for the presence of any etiologic or contributing factor for the development of infection. Personal factors that relate to a high risk for infection include stress, inadequate coping patterns, substance abuse, and poor hygiene. Other personal contributing factors include inadequate knowledge and immunization.

Assess the client's skin and mucous membranes for any disruption. Assess for the presence of invasive devices (IV's, Foley catheters) that may increase the risk for infection. Evaluate the client's nutritional status.

An external assessment must also be completed. The home health nurse should assess for equipment, moisture, stagnant solutions, airborne contamination, and vehicles for contamination. Note also the presence of possible vectors in the environment including mosquitoes, flies and rats. Even family pets must be considered as possible vectors for infection.

Assess the client for the presence of objective signs of infection. These include fever, diaphoresis, blood pressure changes, fatigue, and headache. The signs related to specific areas of the body are shown in Table 17-7.

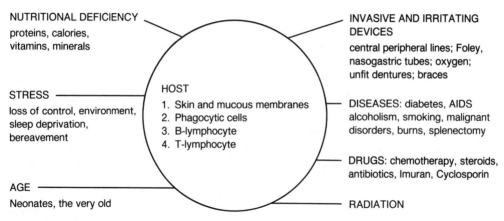

Figure 17-4. Factors that alter immune system and enhance risk for infection. (From Wesorick B. Practice challenge: Potential for infection. In Creating the Future, p 129. American Association of Critical Care Nurses, 1985)

TABLE 17.7 Symptoms of Infection for Specific Body Areas

Body Area	Symptoms
Genitourinary Tract	Dysuria, pyuria, itching, cloudy, bloody urine, frequency, urgency, specific gravity; complaints of pressure; odor. Flank pain, suprapubic and CVA tenderness
Skin	Wound (poor approximation); erythema, warmth, pain, flushing, vascularity, lesions, weeping, blisters, maculo/papular rashes, itching, discharge (color, amount, odor)
Mucous Membranes	eyes, oral, nasal, vaginal, perineal; sinusitis, itching, erythema, pain, lesions, discharge, weeping, blisters.
Respiratory	*Lower:* cough, cyanosis, sputum, infiltration, chest x-ray, dyspnea, chest/pleuritic pain, congestion, fever
	Upper: ear, nose, and throat pain; rhinorrhea
Bacteremia	Restlessness, confusion, all general symptoms
Gastrointestinal Tract	Diarrhea, distention, flatulence, alteration in bowel sounds, abdominal asymmetry, pain, melena, nausea, vomiting
Central Nervous System	Headache, nuchal rigidity, confusion, change in personality, level of consciousness, nausea, vomiting

Interventions

Instruct the family in techniques to assist in monitoring for the signs and symptoms of infection. If infections continue, it may be necessary to suggest to the physician that cultures be obtained.

Measures that can be used to reduce the risk of infection may be beneficial. In certain circumstances, it may be necessary to protect the client from other persons with infection. Instruct the family in the importance of allowing the client to use his own eating utensils and not sharing them with other members of the family. Impress upon the family and client the importance of maintaining good nutritional status. Encourage the client to consume a minimum of 2500 cc of fluid daily.

If the client is treated with antibiotics, it is important for the home health nurse to assess the client for therapeutic and nontherapeutic effects of the drugs.

At times, it will be necessary for the home health nurse to suggest the institution of isolation precautions within the home. There are many reasons for isolation and these dictate the type of precautions to be taken (Table 17-8).

Outcome

The client with cancer will remain free from infection.

IMPAIRED PHYSICAL MOBILITY

Clients with cancer may experience impairment in physical mobility for several reasons. The normal disease process may be the most likely reason for problems. The consequences of the disease process, including side-effects from the drugs, sensory deficits, and motor deficits may also interfere with mobility. As the disease progresses, physical mobility may worsen.

Assessment

Assess the client for the range of his abilities for mobility. These will include muscle strength and weakness, foot or wrist drop, and complaints of fatigue. Talk with the family to determine the client's normal habits and if the current situation is unusual.

Interventions

The home health nurse in consultation with the client and family will be able to identify measures that will work to improve activity tolerance. These measures include adequate rest periods and optimal nutritional status. The client can also be instructed in techniques that may limit energy expenditure during routine activities. Examples include sitting while brushing the hair or teeth.

Assist the family in developing the skills needed to assess the client's tolerance for activity. Pertinent signs include chest pain, shortness of breath, or complaints of extreme fatigue after exercise or activity. Encourage the client progressively to engage in as many activities as possible.

Outcome

The client will demonstrate an increased tolerance for activity and optimal level of physical mobility.

SEXUAL DYSFUNCTION

Many sexual changes can occur after the diagnosis of cancer is confirmed. Both men and women may experience a decreased libido due to a number of reasons, including disturbance in self-concept, fear, pain, and fatigue. Therapy with alkylating agents may also lead to ovarian and/or testicular failure. Impotence may also occur due to hormonal imbalance and psychological changes.

(Text continues on p 553)

TABLE 17.8 Isolation Precautions

Category: Strict
Requirements

Room	Ventilation	Apparel	Articles	Diseases
Private; should not share with other family members.	Some conditions require special ventilation.	Masks, gowns, gloves are indicated for direct care or contact.	Contaminated articles must be left in the room or placed in paper bags and boiled or soaked in bleach to clean and disinfect.	Diphtheria, pneumonic plague, smallpox, varicella (chickenpox), zoster.

Category: Contact
Requirements

Room	Ventilation	Apparel	Articles	Diseases
Private; may share room with siblings or others with the same disease or condition.	Normal room air.	Masks for those who come in close contact; gowns or aprons if soiling is likely; gloves for touching infective materials.	Contaminated articles must be left in the room or placed in paper bags and the contents boiled or soaked in bleach to clean and disinfect.	Respiratory infection in infants and children; diphtheria (cutaneous), group A streptococcus, endometritis, herpes, impetigo, influenza in infants and young children; certain multiple-resistant bacterial infections; pediculosis, viral pneumonia, rubella, scabies, draining infected wounds.

Category: Respiratory
Requirements

Room	Ventilation	Apparel	Articles	Diseases
Private; may share room with others with similar condition.	Normal room air.	Masks for those who come in close contact; no gowns or gloves.	Articles that come in contact with respiratory secretions should be bagged and disinfected by boiling or soaking in bleach.	Measles, meningitis, meningococcal pneumonia, meningococcemia, mumps, whooping cough, pneumonia (*Haemophilus influenzae*) in children.

Category: Tuberculosis (AFB Isolation)
Requirements

Room	Ventilation	Apparel	Articles	Diseases
Private; door kept closed; may share with others with same condition.	Special ventilation required.	Masks only if client is coughing and cannot be relied on to cover mouth.	Articles are rarely involved in the transmission of tuberculosis; articles should be cleaned and disinfected or discarded.	Tuberculosis

Category: Enteric Precautions
Requirements

Room	Ventilation	Apparel	Articles	Diseases
Private room is needed only if the client has poor hygiene habits; may share the room with others who have the same condition.	Normal room air.	Masks are not indicated; gowns or aprons only if soiling is likely; gloves only when touching infective materials.	Articles that have come in contact with infective materials should be bagged and cleaned by boiling or by soaking in bleach or other	Amebic dysentery, cholera, acute diarrhea, enterocolitis, enteroviral infection, gastroenteritis, type A viral hepatitis, viral

(continued)

TABLE 17.8 Isolation Precautions (*continued*)

Category: Enteric Precautions
Requirements

Room	Ventilation	Apparel	Articles	Diseases
			disinfectant.	meningitis, poliomyelitis, typhoid fever, viral pericarditis, myocarditis, or meningitis.

Category: Drainage/Secretion Precautions
Requirements

Room	Ventilation	Apparel	Articles	Diseases
Private room is not indicated.	Normal air.	Masks are not needed; gowns or aprons only if soiling is likely; gloves only when touching infective materials.	Articles contaminated with infective material should be discarded or bagged and decontaminated by boiling or soaking in bleach or a disinfectant.	Abscess, burn infection, conjunctivitis, infected decubitus ulcer, skin infections, wound infections.

Category: Body/Fluid Precautions
Requirements

Room	Ventilation	Apparel	Articles	Diseases
Private room if hygiene is poor (*i.e.*, if person does not wash hands after handling infective material).	Room air.	No masks; gown or apron if soiling of clothing with blood or body fluids is likely; gloves if touching blood or body fluids.	Articles contaminated with blood or body fluid should be bagged and decontaminated by boiling or soaking in bleach or disinfectant.	Acquired immune deficiency syndrome, arthropod-borne viral fevers (yellow fever, Colorado tick fever), hepatitis B, hepatitis non-A, non-B, leptospirosis, malaria, relapsing fever, syphilis.

Assessment

Assess the client for verbalization of sexual concerns. Work with the client to determine the influence of chemotherapy on the normal sexual process. Investigate the degree of the client's knowledge about the problems and potential explanations for the problems.

Interventions

As a major intervention, the home health nurse must establish a relationship with the client that will facilitate the ability to discuss sensitive issues. Encourage the client to express concerns and feelings. Other specific interventions for sexual dysfunction can be found in Chapter 11.

Outcome

The client will be able to verbalize feelings about sexuality.

ALTERATION IN SELF-CONCEPT

The client with an alteration in body integrity due to cancer may experience a disturbance in self-concept related to several variables. While undergoing therapy, the client may experience changes in appearance including alopecia and weight loss. Skin pigments may also be altered due to the effects of chemotherapeutic agents. The end result of all of these changes is that the client may also develop an increased dependence on others and an ultimate change in life-style.

Assessment

On initial assessment, the home health nurse will want to assess the client for any changes in appearance that may be related to the drugs and their side-effects. The nurse should also evaluate the client's role within the home and family and identify if the diagnosis and treatment of cancer has changed the family system. Note any disruptions in communication between the client and family. Comprehensive assessment of self-concept is crucial to developing an appropriate and individualized plan of care.

Interventions

Positive changes in self-concept occur as clients assume greater control of their physical condition. The home health nurse can assist the client to verbalize his feelings about the illness and treatment. Help the client to identify the factors most likely to interfere with maintenance of a positive self-concept.

Encourage the family to assist the client in maintaining independence, insofar as is possible. Identify positive behaviors and promote a positive image. Offer the client and family information concerning psychological counseling and community support groups. Encourage the client to develop an interest in hobbies and social activities.

The home health nurse can offer specific strategies for some of the conditions leading to the disturbance in self-concept. For alopecia, inform the client that hair loss can be expected following initiation of chemotherapy. Loss of hair can be minimized by brushing hair with a soft brush and avoiding the use of harsh shampoos. Use of an ice cap during administration of the drugs may help to prevent hair loss.

For changes in skin pigment, inform the client that these changes are generally transient. The client should be encouraged to avoid exposure to direct sunlight, since exposure may increase pigmentation.

Outcome

The client will begin to experience adaptation to the changes in self-concept.

GRIEVING

All of the changes imposed by the diagnosis of cancer, together with the threat of an impending death, may cause the client increased feelings of grief.

Assessment

The home health nurse will assess the client's perception of the diagnosis of cancer. The family may be able to offer important information concerning the client's response to changing patterns of health. Monitor the client for physical signs of grieving, such as anorexia, insomnia, and noncompliance.

Interventions

The home health nurse can be instrumental in assisting the client to recognize his coping skills. On each visit, encourage the client to express his feelings. Alert the client to the possibilities of participating in counseling services or community support groups.

Outcome

The client will begin to establish mechanisms to work through the grieving process.

KNOWLEDGE DEFICIT

The client with cancer will undergo multiple therapies. A major role for the home health nurse is to assure that the client possesses adequate knowledge to participate actively in his care, as is feasible. In addition, the client should be provided with adequate information so he can participate in necessary decision making.

Assessment

The client's knowledge concerning several areas of treatment must be evaluated. Many clients may be undergoing therapy through a central venous catheter, Ommaya reservoir, or infusion pumps. The home health nurse plays an important role in assuring that the client and family is presented with the information needed in order to work with this equipment.

Interventions

The Broviac/Hickman catheter is a silicone rubber, radiopaque right atrial catheter that can be used for any client receiving intermittent or continuous IV therapy. The distal end of the catheter lies in a position similar to that of a subclavian IV catheter, and the proximal portion is located in a tunnel of subcutaneous tissue along the anterior chest wall.

The client should be taught the appropriate technique for changing the dressing, instilling medication, and flushing of the catheter. The client and family should also be taught specifics concerning the routine care of the Hickman catheter and potential complications. All of these techniques are outlined below and on pages 555 and 556.

(Text continues on p 557)

Home Care of the Hickman Catheter
(Instructions Given to the Client)

DRESSING CHANGE

Dressings over the Hickman catheter exit site should be changed on Mondays, Wednesdays, and Fridays. Make certain to change the dressing three times a week and choose a time convenient for you.

Procedure:

1. Wash hands.

2. Carefully remove the old dressing.

3. Open a sterile gauze packet.

4. Open the alcohol and Betadine solutions.

(continued)

5. Pour alcohol and Betadine on the center of separate gauze sponges and grasp them by the edges.

6. Start at the point where the catheter exits the skin; cleanse the skin with alcohol, using a circular motion. Once you have cleaned the area, do not go back over the same spot again. Use as many alcohol gauze pads as necessary until they appear snow white.

7. Starting at the point where the catheter exits the skin, cleanse the skin with Betadine, using a circular motion. Once you have cleaned the area, do not go back over the same spot again.

8. Allow the Betadine to dry (this usually takes 30 seconds).

9. Apply a small amount of Betadine ointment to the catheter area.

10. Using a dressing, and handling only the edges, cover the catheter site.

IRRIGATING THE HICKMAN CATHETER WITH HEPARINIZED SALINE

This procedure is necessary to prevent blood clots from forming inside the catheter. Heparin is a medication that prevents the formation of blood clots. Therefore, it is mixed with a liquid called *saline*; it comes prepared in a small vacuum bottle called a *vial*. Using a syringe, you will be taught how to withdraw this solution from the vial and how to inject the solution into the rubber cap of the Hickman catheter. Routine heparinization of the catheter will prevent blood clots from forming inside the catheter when it is not in use.

Procedure:

1. Wash your hands.

2. Cleanse the top of the vial of heparinized saline with alcohol.

3. Inject 3 cc of air into the vial.

4. Invert the vial and withdraw 5 cc of heparinized saline. Check the syringe very carefully for air. If air is present, it must be removed.

5. Replace the protective needle cover and lay down the filled syringe.

6. Cleanse the top of the irrigation cap with alcohol.

7. Remove the protective needle cover and insert the needle into the center of the irrigation cap. Be careful not to pierce the catheter with the needle.

8. Remove the bulldog clamp (if in use).

9. Before you completely empty the syringe (having approximately ½ cc left in the syringe), replace the bulldog while still pushing the heparinized saline. This prevents a backflow of blood into the catheter.

10. Discard the syringe and needle in a puncture-proof container.

SPECIAL CONSIDERATIONS DURING IRRIGATION:

1. On Mondays, Wednesdays, and Fridays, change the special piece of tape on the catheter where the bulldog clamp is attached. This helps to prevent kinking of the catheter. Always place the bulldog clamp near the injection cap.

2. Change the irrigation cap once a week. Make certain to fill the irrigation cap

(continued)

with heparinized saline prior to attaching it to the Hickman catheter. This will prevent air from getting into the catheter. Make sure that the bulldog clamp is clamped when changing the irrigation cap.

3. *Never have both the bulldog clamp and the irrigation cap off at the same time.* If this happens, air could get into the line and cause problems.

4. Never force the irrigation solution into the catheter. If you are unable to irrigate the catheter easily, check for kinks in the catheter or check to see if the bulldog clamp has been removed completely.

5. Your physician may want you to heparinize the catheter once or twice a day.

(Reprinted with permission of Spartanburg General Hospital, Spartanburg, SC)

Principles for Teaching the Client with a Hickman Catheter

RECOGNIZING COMPLICATIONS

It is extremely important that all procedures be done with the chance of bacterial contamination in mind. Bacteria are everywhere—on spotless counters, newly laundered clothes, and freshly washed hands. Outside the body, these bacteria are relatively harmless. If these same bacteria should enter the blood stream, infection can result. This complication can be minimized by use of sterile techniques.

Do not be afraid to use alcohol sponges. They are inexpensive and constitute the primary defense against contamination. If you think you may have contaminated a solution, do not compound the error by ignoring it. Discard it. An entire month's supply costs less than a few days in the hospital.

Do not experiment. If you think you have discovered a better way to do one of the procedures, discuss it with your IV nurse *before*, not after, trying it. The procedures you will learn have been developed to protect you. They may not be as simple or as quick as you would like, but they are safe if you follow instructions.

AIR EMBOLISM: This danger, the entrance of air into the blood stream, is very unlikely to happen. If the catheter cap is removed without having the catheter clamped, air may be sucked into the line by negative pressure generated in the chest during breathing. If the catheter is filled with air, it will be best to insert the catheter cap while you are lying on your left side and to remain in the position for at least 30 minutes. This will keep the air in the heart and allow it to dissolve in the blood or escape slowly into the lungs.

BLOOD BACK-UP: If a small amount of blood begins to leak around the capped end of the catheter, most likely the cap has been attached improperly. Clamp the catheter, prepare supplies necessary to reheparinize the catheter, including a fresh cap. Reheparinizing will flush the blood out of the catheter to avoid clot formation. After reheparinizing, replace the cap carefully and snugly so as to avoid another accidental leak.

Never use scissors around your catheter. Use only the special clamp that has been attached to your catheter.

CATHETER INJURY: If your catheter becomes injured in any way, clamp the catheter just below the injured portion, using your bulldog clamp, and come to the emergency room. Your catheter will need to be repaired.

The client may also be undergoing intravenous therapy. The techniques for care of this equipment are outlined in the displayed material below.

Finally, clients and family members should be taught the specifics of the individual chemotherapeutic agents used in the treatment plan.

Outcome

The client and family will possess the knowledge needed for participation in client care.

Guidelines for Home Intravenous Therapy

PART I: STARTING THE IV

Equipment:

IV solution/medications

IV tubing

Tourniquet

Razor or depilatory cream (if required)

Alcohol sponges

Sterile 4×4 gauze pads

Iodophor ointment (optional)

Padded arm board

Freshly laundered bath towel to protect linen

IV drip controller

If using an intermittent infusion device (heparin lock):
  Commercially prepared heparin flush or 10 ml of heparin flush solution in a syringe (1 unit heparin to 10 ml normal saline)

Procedure:

1. Wash your hands. Spike the IV fluid with the tubing. Prime the tubing and clamp it. Suspend the IV on an IV pole or substitute.

2. Thread the tubing through the IV drip controller.

3. Apply the tourniquet above the proposed puncture site.

4. Remove excess hair from the site if necessary, using a razor or depilatory cream.

5. Wash your hands thoroughly.

6. Prepare the insertion site with iodophor solution and allow it to dry. Reapply the tourniquet.

7. Holding the needle bevel up and at a 45° angle, puncture the skin lateral to the vein.

8. Reduce the angle of the needle to the skin, and gently insert the needle ½ cm (¼ in) into the vein. Observe the flashback chamber or syringe for retrograde blood flow.

9. Advance the device using the appropriate technique.
   For the catheter-through-the-needle device
   • Stabilize the needle with one hand. Advance the catheter through the needle with the opposite hand, until the full length has been inserted.
   • Engage the needle and catheter hub.
   • Withdraw the needle and catheter from the vein until about 4 cm (1½ in) of the catheter is exposed. Remove the plastic sleeve. Withdraw the stylet.
   • Attach the primed IV tubing to the catheter hub and begin the infusion.

(continued)

- Apply the needle guard over the needle bevel.

For the catheter-over-the-needle device

- Stabilize the needle hub with one hand. Advance the catheter over the needle and into the vein with the other hand. Withdraw the needle from the catheter and connect the primed IV tubing. Begin the infusion.

For the butterfly or heparin lock

- Gently advance the needle into the vein until the total length has been inserted.
- For a butterfly device, remove the protective cap and connect the primed IV tubing. Begin the infusion.
- For a heparin lock, flush the tubing with a heparin flush by piercing the resealable cap.

10. Secure the infusion device with tape.

11. Apply iodophor ointment to the infusion site. (Optional: Dress with a sterile 4 × 4 gauze pad and an occlusive dressing.)

12. Write the date, time, type of device, and the person starting the IV on the tape. Adjust the infusion rate.

PART 2: MAINTENANCE OF THE INTRAVENOUS ROUTE

1. Apply an arm board to immobilize the IV site, if applicable.

2. Change the IV tubing every 48 hours and the container every 24 hours. Palpate the site through the dressing for tenderness, and observe for signs of phlebitis every 8 hours. Attempt to rotate the site every 72 hours, if possible.

3. Change the dressing if necessary, following the same procedure as when the IV was inserted.

4. Keep the drip chamber at least half full of fluid to prevent air embolus.

5. Discontinue the IV when therapy is completed:
   Clamp the tubing. Remove the dressing. Remove the cannula with one smooth movement. Hold pressure on the site with a 4 × 4 gauze pad until bleeding stops. Cover with an adhesive bandage. Dispose of equipment and cannula in the trash.

The client and/or family should:

1. Change the IV dressing if it is wet, soiled, or loose.

2. Check the IV site for signs of infection. Monitor vital signs for elevated temperature or pulse rate indicating a possible infection.

3. Check IV fluids for the presence of particulate matter, cloudiness, or cracks. (Do not infuse these solutions. Bring them to the attention of the home health nurse or vendor.)

4. Maintain the integrity of the IV line. Remove air bubbles if they appear in the tubing. Keep the drip chamber at least half full to prevent air embolus.

5. Check the drip rate.

6. Add new containers of IV fluid to the line when necessary.

7. Monitor intake and output using household measuring devices and a flow sheet.

8. Cover the IV site with a resealable plastic bag or plastic wrap during bathing or showering. If showering is attempted, the extremity with the IV will have to be kept outside the shower.

This is only feasible if a shower curtain is used. A wet dressing allows bacteria to penetrate and infect the IV site.

9. Wear clothing with a large sleeve opening so that the top can be removed while the infusion is in progress, if necessary. A robe is usually suitable, because the arm openings are larger. An oversized shirt is also appropriate.

(Adapted from Walsh J, Persons CB Wieck L: Manual of Home Health Care Nursing. Philadelphia, JB Lippincott, 1987)

ABBREVIATED CARE PLAN: ALTERATION IN BODY INTEGRITY: CANCER

Diagnosis	Assessment	Interventions	Outcomes
Alteration in Nutrition	Weight Weakness Fatigue Nutrition history	Initiate a nutritional consultation. Assist family and client in selection of foods.	Client will maintain normal nutritional balance.
Alteration in Bowel Elimination	Bowel habits Diarrhea Constipation Pain Cramping Fullness	Maintain adequate fluid intake. Increase activity as tolerated. Administer medications as needed.	Client will experience a normal bowel evacuation.
Alteration in Comfort: Nausea and Vomiting	Weight Complaints of nausea	Encourage client to eat dry foods when nauseated. Administer drugs as needed.	Client and family will identify methods needed to decrease incidence of nausea.
Alteration in Comfort: Chronic Pain (etiology to be individualized)	Knowledge and beliefs Past experience Coping ability Past therapies	Provide narcotic and narcotic analgesics in combination as needed. Monitor the effectiveness of the analgesics used. Utilize noninvasive pain relief measures concurrently with analgesic measures.	Client will indicate that pain is better. Client actively participates in the planning and implementing of self-care, suggesting modifications as necessary. Client reports he is able to rest and sleep

(continued)

ABBREVIATED CARE PLAN: ALTERATION IN BODY INTEGRITY: CANCER (*continued*)

Diagnosis	Assessment	Interventions	Outcomes
		Monitor the effectiveness of the noninvasive measures used.	more comfortably than previously.
		Be flexible and make adjustments as needed.	Client reports mobility and activity (needs to be individualized).
		Encourage client participation in planning care.	
		Encourage client to monitor own pain management plan and suggest modifications as appropriate.	
		Provide continual support and reassurance.	
		Provide adequate rest by	
		• Encouraging mobility and activity	
		• Adhering to a regular schedule	
		• Discouraging late afternoon naps	
		• Adhering to a nightly routine	
		• Utilizing analgesics and sedatives as needed	
Alteration in Oral Mucous Membrane	Mouth ulcers Oral pain	Encourage frequent oral hygiene. Evaluate need for antifungal or antibacterial agents.	Client will maintain healthy oral cavity.

ABBREVIATED CARE PLAN: ALTERATION IN BODY INTEGRITY: CANCER (*continued*)

Diagnosis	Assessment	Interventions	Outcomes
Sensory–Perceptual Alteration	Hearing ability	Monitor for decreased hearing.	Client will maintain adequate hearing.
Anxiety	Tenseness Restlessness	Provide peaceful environment. Encourage client and family to express feelings. Instruct in relaxation exercises.	Client will report a decrease in anxiety and tension.
Alteration in Skin Integrity	Appearance of wound Continence Nutritional status Family's ability	Wet to dry dressing. Change as necessary.	Skin remains intact.
Potential for Injury: Infection	Contributing factors Skin and mucous membranes Fever Malaise	Institute measures to decrease risk of infection. Administer antibiotics as needed.	Client will remain free from infection.
Impaired Physical Mobility	Muscle strength Fatigue Foot/wrist	Identify measures to improve activity tolerance. Assist family to support client's mobility.	Client will demonstrate an increased tolerance for activity.
Sexual Dysfunction	Verbalization of concerns	Establish therapeutic relationship. Encourage expression of feelings.	Client will verbalize feelings about sexuality.
Alteration in Self-Concept (etiology to be individualized)	Appearance Communication	Stress client's assets versus liabilities. Confine the effect of the disability only to those areas affected. Encourage mobility and activity.	Client will report an improved sense of self.

(*continued*)

ABBREVIATED CARE PLAN: ALTERATION IN BODY INTEGRITY: CANCER (*continued*)

Diagnosis	Assessment	Interventions	Outcomes
		Encourage participation of client in planning care.	
		Encourage development and utilization of support systems.	
		Communicate interest and support of client.	
		Encourage expression of feelings of discouragement, anger, frustration, etc.	
		Encourage positive self-talk.	
		Initiate referral for counseling if necessary.	
		Set obtainable goals for client.	
Grieving	Client's perception	Assist client to recognize coping skills.	Client will begin to establish mechanisms to work through the grieving process.
	Client's response	Refer to counseling or support services.	
Knowledge Deficit	Treatment	Teach client/family care of the invasive lines.	Client and family will possess the knowledge needed to participate in care.
	Hickman catheter		
	Intravenous catheters		

ACQUIRED IMMUNE DEFICIENCY SYNDROME

Acquired immune deficiency syndrome (AIDS), first recognized only 5 years ago, has become a medical and social phenomenon of staggering proportions. To date, over 20,000 cases of AIDS have been reported in the world, with nearly 14,000 occurring in the United States (Jackson 1986). Two to five times that number of persons have been reported to have AIDS-related conditions. AIDS is increasing at an alarming rate, and many researchers and clinicians feel that the cases seen today represent only a small fraction of individuals actually infected. At present, there is no cure for AIDS; however, some of the complications of the disease *can* be treated. Vast amounts of research, literature, and information have been published and disseminated to nurses and other health care personnel, but little has been directed specifically to the nurse providing care in the home. With the realities of diagnosis related groups (DRGs) and reimbursement issues, home health care for AIDS patients has become a viable alternative to hospitalization. By utilizing and incorporating a basic understanding of AIDS, the home health nurse can be prepared to meet both the specialized physical and emotional needs of her client with caring sensitivity.

PATHOPHYSIOLOGY

AIDS is caused by a retrovirus, first isolated in France in 1983, where it was known as the *lymphadenopathy-associated virus (LAV)*. It was then isolated independently in the United States in 1984, and called the *human T-cell lymphotropic virus III (HTLV-III)*. A retrovirus is a ribonucleic acid (RNA) virus able to manufacture deoxyribonucleic acid (DNA), which may then be inserted into the host cell's genetic code. This virus specifically attacks the T_4 lymphocytes, a type of white blood cell (WBC). To be specific, the virus enters the T cell and incorporates itself into the DNA in the cell's nucleus. When the T cells are stimulated by an antigen, as they would be in the presence of an infection, the virus replicates itself, kills the T cell, and consequently spreads to invade and kill other T cells (Daniels 1985). Without the protection afforded by the body's T cells, an individual may fall victim to a variety of opportunistic infections that rarely cause disease in those with an intact immunological system.

The incubation period of AIDS is unknown; however, it has been hypothesized that it may be up to 5 years, and possibly 10 years. Seroconversion usually occurs 2 to 6 months after exposure to the virus, and patients may have a transient febrile illness 1 to 2 months after becoming infected. This period is usually followed by an asymptomatic phase, which may last from several months to a few years. If symptoms do occur, they may range from simple malaise and fever to AIDS-related complex to end-stage AIDS. AIDS-related complex (ARC) is a syndrome marked by nonspecific symptoms (extreme malaise, fever, night sweats, weight loss, diarrhea, and generalized lymphadenopathy) suggesting AIDS and an altered immune status, but without opportunistic infections. ARC may last for 1 to 2 years after infection (Minkoff 1986).

AIDS itself is defined by the Centers for Disease Control as *the occupance of a disease at least moderately predictive of a defect in cell-mediated immunity, occurring in a person with no known cause for decreased resistance* (Gostin 1986). These diseases include Kaposi's sarcoma, primary esophagitis due to *Candida*, herpes simplex or cytomegalovirus, lymphoma of the central nervous system, *Pneumocystis Carinii* pneumonia, and unusually extensive mucocutaneous herpes simplex of greater than 5 weeks' duration.

Most AIDS patients die, not from the disease itself but from the multiple infectious processes they develop. Therefore, the patient's quality and duration of life is ultimately dependent on the prevention and treatment of these infections.

NURSING DIAGNOSES

Many nursing diagnoses can be recognized in this patient population, and are dependent on the patient's individual response to his disease. Several diagnoses with particular relevance to the AIDS client will be examined, together with appropriate assessment, planning, and intervention strategies.

ACTIVITY INTOLERANCE

Profound fatigue and malaise, persisting for several weeks with no obvious cause, is one of the most common clinical features of AIDS. It is usually accompanied by fever and weight loss. These symptoms may occur both before and after an opportunistic infection develops and after the actual diagnosis of AIDS has been established. It must be kept in mind that activity intolerance may also be a result of the drug therapy necessary to treat the infections, or from the pain associated with lymphoma or Kaposi's sarcoma lesions.

The fever may be either low-grade and persistent, or episodic and spiking to 39°C and higher. It is often a debilitating problem, and while some are able to tolerate it without great difficulty, others cannot work or actively care for themselves. The cause of the fever is often difficult to identify, and may be due to one, or several, of the myriad of infections that can affect AIDS patients (DeVita, Hellman, and Rosenberg 1985).

Another cause of the fatigue and weight loss usually present in AIDS clients is the copious watery diarrhea with which many of these clients are afflicted. Homosexuals with AIDS may have a wide range of bowel complaints, caused by a multitude of organisms that cause symptomatic disease in the gay population. For some clients, the problem is more aggravating than medically significant. For others, however, the diarrhea can be so profuse and associated with so much nausea and vomiting that it accounts for a body weight loss of up to 30%. Symptomatic therapy using antimotility drugs and dietary alteration is successful in some clients but total parenteral nutrition may be needed in others.

Assessment

Initial assessment of the activity level of these clients should include the identification of causative and/or precipitating factors. These may then be dealt with specifically and individually. How the client perceives himself as able to perform his activities of daily living is important to consider. Vital signs, especially pulse and respiration, are significant indicators of how much activity can be tolerated. Dyspnea, shortness of breath, tachycardia, pallor, and vertigo all direct attention to a client's inability to maintain his former activity level.

Interventions

A major goal in caring for the AIDS client with activity intolerance is to assist him in dealing with the factors that are contributing to his fatigue, and help him manage them within the individual limits of his ability. Care may be planned around rest periods, or when pain medication is maximally effective. The AIDS client should be encouraged to participate in planning his activities, and given information that provides evidence of his progress, if appropriate. Another goal is to protect the client from injury that may be caused by his inability to tolerate activity. It may be necessary to assist the client in learning safety measures, and to provide him with devices such as a wheelchair or walker in order to protect him from harm. Family and/or significant others need to be included in assisting with these activities (Lederer and colleagues 1986).

Outcome

The expected outcome for the AIDS client with activity intolerance would be that he learns to develop less strenuous ways of performing the affected activity in a safe and comfortable manner.

IMPAIRED SKIN INTEGRITY

Kaposi's sarcoma is a complication of AIDS that occurs in about 35% of all cases, and is the most frequently diagnosed malignancy in AIDS. It is a cancer of the skin and connective tissues that can cause an impairment of skin integrity, compromising it as an effective barrier against infections.

Most AIDS clients who present with Kaposi's sarcoma first do so with isolated skin lesions that start on the feet or ankles, and progress proximally. The lesions range from pink, slightly raised nodules to the more distinctive dark blue or purple brown plaques. These lesions are usually painless, and are not often open or ulcerated. Extracutaneous lesions are most frequently found in the gastrointestinal tract, with the second most common incidence in the respiratory tract. For some AIDS patients it is a rapidly progressing disease with involvement of virtually every body organ. In spite of its aggressive nature, Kaposi's sarcoma is rarely fatal (Daniels 1985).

Assessment

The first step in assessing for impairment of the skin surface includes inspection for intactness, noting not only the presence of open and closed lesions, but also the general color, elasticity, and turgor of the client's unaffected skin. The presence and/or absence of sensation, redness, tenderness, excoriation, and pain must be assessed over the entire body surface, as well as over those areas affected by the lesions. Maintaining the protective function of the skin is of particular importance in AIDS clients, who may be fatally compromised by any break in the skin's defense.

Interventions

Interventions useful in maintaining the skin's integrity include bathing, massage, the application of moisturizing lotions, and frequent turning and repositioning of the bedfast client. Stringent handwashing before and after direct contact with the patient, and after contact with articles used for care is the surest way of protecting both client and nurse from the transmission of disease. Gloves, gowns, and masks are not routinely needed unless the care-giver is handling body fluids or has a contagious disease. Particular attention should be paid to the thorough cleansing of the perianal area in order to avoid skin breakdown. Protective measures, such as an egg crate mattress or foam protectors, may need to be utilized. If the client is able to tolerate them, foods high in proteins, minerals, and vitamins can be provided in order to facilitate skin healing. If the lesions are open or ulcerated, they should be gently cleansed with warm, soapy water and rinsed twice a day. Wet to dry dressings or Neosporin ointment may then be applied, and the lesion covered with a Telfa pad (Lillard 1984).

Outcome

The primary measurement of successful intervention is that the client's skin is free from excoriation and erythema. If open lesions exist, the client should be free of further skin breakdowns, with a decrease in the size of the involved areas.

ALTERATIONS IN ORAL MUCOUS MEMBRANES

The oral mucous membranes of an AIDS client may be altered due to the development of oral candidiasis (thrush). It is caused by an overgrowth of the normal mouth flora, and may occur as the initial manifestation of the disease, or after the documentation of Kaposi's sarcoma or another opportunistic infection. Oral candidiasis is characterized by grey or white "cottage cheeselike" patches in the mouth and throat. In some clients the patches may develop into ulcers that are extremely painful and interfere with nutritional intake. *Candida* esophagitis is also common in AIDS, causing symptoms such as dysphagia and retrosternal pain.

Assessment

In assessing the client with oral *Candida*, an examination of the lips, buccal membranes, gums, teeth, and hard and soft palate is necessary. These structures should be inspected not only for signs of thrush, but for color, signs of inflammation, the presence of any lesions, cracks, and evidence of bleeding as well. Assessment of the client's understanding of the need for good oral care and his ability to perform that care merit equal consideration. His identification of substances that irritate the oral mucus, such as tobacco, alcohol, and food seasonings, should be documented (Lederer 1986).

Interventions

Interventions helpful in dealing with this problem include brushing the teeth with a soft child's toothbrush or toothettes after meals, followed with use of a one half-strength H_2O_2 mouthwash. A suspension of Mycostatin (5 cc) or ketoconazole (200 mg) every morning or Mycelex troches five times a day are often readily effective in resolving *Candida* infections. However, most AIDS clients relapse within days or weeks of termination of the therapy, and so must be maintained on whatever agent has been found to be effective for the rest of their lives (Lillard 1984).

Outcome

Effective interventions should result in the client's ability to maintain an intact oral mucosa, free of irritation and inflammation.

IMPAIRED GAS EXCHANGE

The client with AIDS can suffer from impaired gas exchange secondary to diffuse pneumonia. By far the most common complication of AIDS is *Pneumocystis Carinii* pneumonia (PCP), which has been diagnosed in 58% of AIDS victims and is the major cause of death in this group. This type of pneumonia can cause intermittent symptoms, such as dyspnea, shortness of breath, and copious sputum production that may either develop rapidly over several days or insidiously over many weeks or months (Daniels 1985).

Assessment

Assessment for impaired gas exchange includes inspection, auscultation, and palpation for the presence or absence of breath sounds (noting rales, rhonchi, and wheezing), respiratory rate, and production of sputum, as well as the more objective measurements of arterial blood gases and blood chemistry levels. Of particular importance to note are the behavioral changes that occur with decreased oxygen levels, such as anxiety, irritability, and restlessness (Schietinger 1986).

Interventions

There are several interventions that can be implemented to assist the AIDS client with impaired gas exchange at home. The temporary administration of oxygen and assistive breathing devices may be useful. The home health care nurse should stay with and reassure the client during periods of acute respiratory distress. Many clients benefit from instruction in relaxation techniques to improve their breathing pattern. High Fowler's position will prevent aspiration, and an oral morphine solution may be administered to reduce the respiratory rate by decreasing anxiety and dyspnea. If the client is coughing or producing sputum, disposable tissues should be kept within reach, together with a receptacle for soiled tissues. There is no need for the care-giver to wear a mask, unless there is direct and sustained contact with an actively coughing client, or when the client needs to be suctioned. Of course, the home health nurse should wear a mask if she has a cold or cough, in order to protect the client (Garvey 1985).

Outcome

The expected outcome for the AIDS client with impaired gas exchange would be that he is free from respiratory distress. The ideal measurement of this would be arterial blood gases that are within normal limits for the individual client and subjectively free from respiratory distess.

POWERLESSNESS

Virtually every aspect of an AIDS client's life is affected by his disease. Not only must he deal with the constant media reminders of the threat AIDS poses to his own mortality, but also with its debilitating and disfiguring effects on his everyday life. Most AIDS victims are 25 to 49 years old—an age group in which the most crucial developmental tasks include establishing an identity, becoming self-reliant, and refining an adult life pattern. Suddenly faced with ill health, many of these young adults experience feelings of overwhelming powerlessness (Bryant 1986). The loss of control experienced by the AIDS client is, by necessity, often due to his new reliance on others to help meet his physical needs. Though not acutely ill, he may be forced to depend on friends, volunteers, and/or paid workers for such basic activities of daily living as grocery shopping and laundering. Because of his physical status, or in some cases, public prejudice and ignorance,

the AIDS client may lose his employment and income, with resulting loss of economic status. Loss of positive body image, closely associated with self-esteem in this age group, also contributes to feelings of helplessness and despair (Baumgartner 1985).

Assessment and Interventions

Assessment, through both verbal expressions and nonverbal indicators such as anger, apathy, listlessness, and depression, help the home health care nurse determine those situations in which the client feels powerless. A major contributing factor may be the care-giver's (sometimes unconscious) control of the information given to the client. Health care professionals often use terminology unfamiliar to the lay person, and respond to the adult as though he were a child. Clarifying terms that are unfamiliar, supplying health information, and helping the client understand possible options in care can reduce significantly any feelings of helplessness (Kelly 1985).

Allowing the client choices by giving him a major role in planning his own daily care and providing for flexibility in care as indicated by the client can reinforce his feelings of self-control. Setting obtainable goals and making sure to include the client in decision making about his care routine will bolster his sense of independence. In many cases, simply encouraging the client to express his feelings of powerlessness and to identify contributory factors is helpful.

Outcome

Successful interventions will result in the client's verbalization of a feeling of control over his environment and plan of care, and participation in that care.

SOCIAL ISOLATION

The client with an established diagnosis of AIDS risks the loss not only of friends, work colleagues, and casual acquaintances, but also that of family and lovers. Due to both ignorance and fear of contagion, many persons with AIDS suffer rejection and abandonment. For some, the diagnosis forces them to reveal homosexuality or drug use to family and colleagues, who may react with anger or revulsion. Many young gay men have relocated to large cities such as New York, and are thousands of miles from their families of origin. Even if the family is able to be reengaged and actively involved in the client's care, long-standing feelings of alienation by the client may not be surmountable (Jackson and Goldman 1986).

Ashamed of physical or psychological deterioration, an AIDS client may isolate himself both socially and sexually. For the person to whom sexual intimacy is a major form of communication and contact, it is especially wrenching. Some cope with these feelings of isolation by turning to drugs, alcohol, or suicide.

Assessment

Assessment can be accomplished by observing the pattern of interaction between the client and his family and friends. The client may also verbalize feelings of loneliness, fear or inadequacy, or react to perceived isolation with indecisiveness, restlessness, and withdrawal.

Interventions

By remaining at home, the AIDS client is often more comfortable and better able to deal with his feelings of isolation. A supportive relationship with his health care provider and the familiar environment of home will encourage him to verbalize his feelings of isolation. In many communities, private-, locally- and state-funded AIDS service organizations are available to provide buddies, support groups, and counseling to the client and his significant others (Stoller 1985).

Outcome

With successful interventions, the client should demonstrate acceptance of those factors that are perceived to contribute to his social isolation, and identify persons and resources available to him.

Media sensationalism, fear, and prejudice have been the hallmarks of the AIDS epidemic. It is up to the professional health care worker to provide accurate information to both the lay public and her client. A client's sexual orientation or life-style may be considered unacceptable to the general community. It is important for the care-giver to examine thoroughly her own feelings and fears in order to determine whether they will influence her ability to provide compassionate, nonjudgmental care. Our obligation to supply sensitive, supportive, and practical care to our clients is in no way diminished by the spectrum of AIDS.

POTENTIAL FOR INFECTION

The client with AIDS experiences a depression in the functioning of the immune system that increases the potential for infection. Other variables that increase the likelihood of infection include poor nutritional status and the presence of multiple microorganisms. The use of antimicrobial agents directly alters the normal flora, which will increase the likelihood of development of an infection.

Assessment

Encourage the family and client to monitor the client's temperature frequently. Evaluate the client for symptoms of infection, including respiratory distress, production of sputum, headache, and alterations in mentation. On each visit, evaluate the skin for presence of signs of inflammation or infection.

Interventions

The client, family, and friends should be encouraged to wash their hands frequently to decrease the spread of infection. The client should be in a clean, well-ventilated environment. Gloves should be worn during direct contact with secretions/excretions or when there is a break in the skin of the care-giver's hands. If infection is suspected, laboratory studies such as a complete blood count or culture and sensitivity studies may be required. Once the location of infection and causative agents have been identified, antibiotic therapy may be ordered.

Outcome

The client will be free from infection.

DECREASED FLUID VOLUME

Hydration can be a problem in the client with AIDS. Specifically, copious diarrhea, poor nutritional status, profuse sweating, and vomiting may cause depletion of fluid and electrolytes.

Assessment

Monitor the client for decreased skin turgor and dry mucous membranes. The client may also experience postural hypotension, tachycardia, decreased urine output, and thirst. Periodic determination of body weight will be helpful in identifying excessive fluid loss.

Interventions

Work with the family to encourage the client to increase fluid intake. Fluids such as Gatorade may be best since they also allow the replacement of needed electrolytes. Other interventions are directed towards interfering with the diarrhea or vomiting causing the fluid volume deficit.

Outcome

The client will maintain normal fluid balance.

POTENTIAL FOR INJURY: ALTERED CLOTTING FACTORS

AIDS initiates several changes that will affect clotting. There is an alteration in hepatic function leading to a decreased absorption of vitamin K. Other factors include the presence of autoimmune antiplatelet antibodies, malignancies, and circulation endotoxins that alter coagulation. Eventually, the alteration in clotting will lead to bleeding.

Assessment

Assess the client for any evidence of bleeding. Monitor all body fluids for the presence of blood. Note any oozing of blood from portions of the body. Monitor for any changes in vital signs consistent with bleeding.

Interventions

Continual assessment of the potential for bleeding is required. Encourage the family to participate in making the client's environment safe from hazards that could worsen the problems of bleeding. Procedures that may increase bleeding should be avoided or monitored. These include injections and rectal temperatures. Instruct the client to avoid the use of aspirin, since it may increase bleeding.

Outcome

The client will be free from bleeding episodes or the effects of the bleeding will be minimized.

ALTERATION IN NUTRITION

Multiple factors limit the client's ability and interest in eating. Nausea and vomiting and the presence of lesions in the mouth may interfere with the ability to eat. Intestinal changes in mobility may also serve to decrease appetite. Diarrhea may lead to excessive gastrointestinal loss and malabsorption. The metabolic need for nutritional substrates may be increased by the presence of a fever.

Assessment

On the initial visit and periodically after that time, a complete nutritional assessment should be completed (see Chapter 11). Other parameters to assess include bowel sounds and weight. The client's ability to chew, taste, and swallow should be monitored.

Interventions

The family can assist in monitoring the client's dietary intake. It may be necessary for the home health nurse to recommend a dietary consultation to assure adequate intake of nutrients and calories. The dietary regimen should be flexible enough to allow for the individual tastes of the client. The caloric intake should be recorded and carefully monitored.

Frequent mouth care may be helpful in decreasing mouth pain and thus encouraging the client to eat. Care should be exercised to provide a clean, quiet environment during mealtimes. If these interventions are not effective, home parenteral or enteral nutrition may be needed.

Outcome

The client will maintain normal nutritional status.

ALTERATION IN COMFORT

Discomfort and pain are common problems for the client with AIDS. These sensations are usually related to the presence of malignancies or infections that may lead to lesions and tissue necrosis. Other symptoms such as headaches, chest pain, and night sweats may also occur. Abdominal cramping and rectal pain associated with diarrhea may also be present.

Assessment

Note the location, intensity, frequency, and time of onset of pain. Assess the client for other indications of pain including restlessness, tachycardia, and nonverbal signs.

Interventions

A complete discussion of interventions for pain can be found earlier in this chapter. Other interventions that may be beneficial include repositioning and massage. Analgesics may be necessary, particularly in later stages of the disease. Activities for the client should be planned for times when the client is most rested.

Outcome

The client will utilize techniques that will increase comfort.

KNOWLEDGE DEFICIT

Although the media discusses AIDS and its treatment frequently, many people do not understand the reality of the disease. Once diagnosed with AIDS, the client and family require additional information and continual updates.

Assessment

Assess the client and family for their knowledge of the disease process, treatment, and complications. Be careful to assess for inaccurate information since there is a great deal of misinformation currently available.

Interventions

Teach the client and family the symptoms of the disease, including the presence of infections and neoplasms. Assure that they have an accurate understanding of the transmission of the disease. Safety concerns should be paramount; client and family should be aware of ways to decrease the possibility of transmission. The home health nurse can play a valuable role in assisting the client and family to utilize this information in their daily lives. Encourage them to consult with the home health nurse when specific questions arise. An important aspect of teaching is to allow the family and client to express their feelings as they learn about the disease and its consequences.

Outcome

The client and family will verbalize understanding of the disease, its treatment, and its complications.

ABBREVIATED CARE PLAN: AIDS

Nursing Diagnosis	Assessment	Interventions	Outcomes
Activity Intolerance	Causative/precipitating factors Client perception	Monitor for signs and symptoms of activity intolerance. Plan care around rest periods or when pain medication is maximally effective. Protect from injury. Encourage client's participation in planning activities.	Client will develop less strenuous ways of performing affected activity.
Impairment of Skin Integrity	Inspection Color, elasticity, redness, pain	Keep skin clean and dry. Reposition, apply lotions, and massage skin as needed. Provide well-balanced diet high in protein and vitamins. Keep open lesions clean and apply wet	Client will maintain skin integrity.

(continued)

ABBREVIATED CARE PLAN: AIDS (*continued*)

Nursing Diagnosis	Assessment	Interventions	Outcomes
		to dry dressings or Neosporin ointment, then cover with Telfa pad.	
Alterations in Oral Mucous Membranes	Thrush Color Inflammation Lesions Cracks	Brush teeth with soft child's brush or toothettes. Utilize medication that has been effective for client. Limit substances that are irritating to mucosa.	Client will maintain an intact oral mucosa.
Impaired Gas Exchange	Breath sounds Respiratory rate Sputum	Provide administration of O_2. Reassure client and instruct in relaxation techniques. Position in high Fowler's. Provide pain medication as needed.	Client is free of respiratory distress.
Powerlessness	Anger Apathy Information	Use terminology familiar to client. Encourage participation of client in planning care. Set obtainable goals for client. Encourage expression of feelings of powerlessness.	Client will demonstrate feelings of control.
Social Isolation	Interaction between client and others Feelings of loneliness, fear	Communicate interest and support for client. Encourage development and	Client will experience a decrease in feelings of isolation.

(continued)

ABBREVIATED CARE PLAN: AIDS (*continued*)

Nursing Diagnosis	Assessment	Interventions	Outcomes
		utilization of support systems.	
		Initiate referral for counseling if necessary.	
Potential for Infection	Temperature Respiratory distress Sputum	Wash hands frequently. Utilize appropriate isolation procedures. Administer antibiotics as needed.	Client will be free from infection.
Decreased Fluid Volume	Skin fungus Mucous membranes Weight	Increase fluid intake. Decrease diarrhea or vomiting.	Client will maintain normal fluid balance.
Potential for Injury: Altered Clotting	Evidence of bleeding Oozing	Continually assess for bleeding. Provide a safe environment. Avoid procedures that may increase bleeding.	Client will be free from bleeding episodes.
Alteration in Nutrition	Nutritional assessment Bowel sounds Ability to chew, taste, swallow	Recommend dietary consultation. Record dietary intake.	Client will maintain normal nutritional status.
Alteration in Comfort	Location Intensity Frequency	Reposition and massage. Administer analgesics. Plan activities around rest periods.	Client will utilize techniques to increase comfort.
Knowledge Deficit	Knowledge of disease, treatment, complications Feelings	Teach symptoms. Stress safety concerns. Consult with home health nurse for questions.	Client and family will verbalize understanding of disease, treatment, and complications.

References

Neoplasia

Bonica J: Fundamental considerations of chronic pain therapy. Postgrad Med 53(6): 81–90, 1973

Bulechek G, McCloskey J: Nursing Intervention: Treatments for Nursing Diagnoses. Philadelphia, WB Saunders, 1985

Catalano R: Pharmacology of analgesic agents used to treat cancer pain. Semin Oncol Nurs 1(2): 126–140, 1985

Copp LA: The spectrum of suffering. Am J Nurs 74(3): 491–495, 1974

Donovan M: Nursing assessment of cancer pain. Semin Oncol Nurs 1(2): 109–115, 1985

Donovan MI, Girton SE: Cancer Nursing Care. East Norwalk, CT, Appleton-Century-Crofts, 1984

Eland J: Pain. In Hart L, Reese J, Fearing M (eds): Concepts Common to Acute Illness, pp 164–196. St. Louis, CV Mosby, 1981

Erlanger J, Gasser HS: The action potential in fibers of slow conduction in spinal roots and somatic nerves. Am J Physiol 92(1): 43–82, 1930

Foley K: The treatment of pain in the patient with cancer. CA, 36(4): 194–214, 1986

Fordyce A: Behavioral Methods for Chronic Pain and Illness. St. Louis, CV Mosby, 1976

Hackett T: Pain and prejudice: Why do we doubt that the patient is in pain? Med Times 99(2): 130–141, 1971

Kales A, Kales J: Evaluation, diagnosis and treatment of clinical conditions related to sleep. JAMA 213: 2229–2235, 1970

Kim S: Pain: Theory, research and nursing practice. ANS 2(2): 43–59, 1980

Kleitman N: Basic rest–activity cycle in relation to sleep and wakefulness. In Kales H (ed): Sleep Physiology and Pathology. Philadelphia, JB Lippincott, 1969

Luckmann J, Sorensen KC: Medical–Surgical Nursing: A Psychophysiologic Approach. Philadelphia, WB Saunders, 1987

McCaffery M, Hart L: Undertreatment of acute pain with narcotics. Am J Nurs 76(10): 1586–1591, 1976

McCaffery M: Nursing Management of the Patient With Pain, 2nd ed. Philadelphia, JB Lippincott, 1979

McCaffery M: Patients shouldn't have to suffer: How to relieve with injectable narcotics. Nursing 80, 10(10): 34–39, 1980

Melzack R, Wall PD: Pain mechanisms: A new theory. Science 150(3699): 971–979, 1965

Melzack R: The Puzzle of Pain. New York, Basic Books, 1972

Melzack R: The Challenge of Pain. New York, Basic Books, 1982

Moertel C, Ohmann D, Taylor W et al: Relief of pain by oral medication. JAMA 229: 55–59, 1974

Moertel C, Ohmann D, Taylor W et al: A comparative evaluation of marketed analgesic drugs. New Engl J Med 286: 813–815, 1972

Stephens G: Pathophysiology for Health Practitioners. New York, Macmillan, 1980

Sternbach PA: A Psychophysiological Analysis. New York, Academic Press, 1968

Snyder M: Independent Nursing Interventions. New York, John Wiley & Sons, 1985

Ulrich SP, Canale SW, Wendell SA: Nursing Care Planning Guides: A Nursing Diagnosis Approach. Philadelphia, WB Saunders, 1986

Winter GD: Healing of skin wounds and the influence of dressings in the repair process. In Harkiss KJ (ed): Surgical Dressing and Wound Healing, pp 44, 60. Bradford England, Bradford University Press, 1971

Wolf, L: Pain theories: An overview. Top Clin Nurs 2(1): 9–18, 1980

Yasko J: Guidelines for Pharmacological Intervention for the Control of Chronic Pain (copyrighted handout), 1981

Yasko J: Guidelines for Chronic Pain Control (copyrighted handout), 1981

AIDS

Baumgartner G: AIDS. Psychosocial Factors in the Acquired Immune Deficiency Syndrome. Springfield, Il, Charles C. Thomas, 1985

Bryant J: Home care of the client with AIDS. J Community Health Nurs 3(2): 69–74, 1986

Daniels V: AIDS, the Acquired Immune Deficiency Syndrome. Hingham, MA, MTP Press, 1985

DeVita V, Hellman S, Rosenberg S (eds): AIDS: Etiology, Diagnosis, Treatment, and Prevention. Philadelphia, JB Lippincott, 1985

Garvey E: Guidelines for caring for the AIDS patient in the home setting. NITA 8(6): 481–483, 1985

Gostin L: Acquired immune deficiency syndrome: A review of science, health policy, and law. In Pharm M (ed): AIDS and Patient Management: Legal, Ethical, and Social Issues. Owings Mills, MD, Rynd Communications, 1986

Jackson P, Goldman C: AIDS. J Pract Nurs 35(4): 26–31, 1986

Kelly M: Nursing Diagnosis Sourcebook. East Norwalk, CT, Appleton–Century–Crofts, 1985

Lederer J, Marculescu G, Gallagher J, Mills P: Care Planning Pocket Guide: A Nursing Diagnosis Approach. Reading, MA, Addison–Wesley, 1986

Lillard J, Lotspeich P, Gurich J: AIDS in home care: Maximizing helpfulness and minimizing hysteria. Home Healthcare Nurse 2(6): 11–14, 16, 1984

Minkoff H: Acquired immunodeficiency syndrome. J Nurse–Midwifery 31(4): 189–193, 1986

Schietinger H: A home care plan for AIDS. Am J Nurs 86: 1021–1028, 1986

Stoller B: AIDS. J Pract Nurs 35(4): 26–31, 1985

INSULIN ASSISTS*

I. INSULIN DEVICES TO HELP THE LOW-VISION DIABETIC CLIENT ACCURATELY AND INDEPENDENTLY GIVE INSULIN

1. B–D Magniguide
2. Insulgage with Holdease
3. Dos-Aid
4. Inject-Aid

II. SELECTING THE APPROPRIATE DEVICE

Questions to Ask	Suggestions
1. Does the client need syringe magnification or an insulin measuring device?	When assessing if magnification is sufficient, make sure the client can see the line calibrations, not just the larger numbers.
2. Does the client need to measure a mixed dose?	*Insulgage* is the safest for mixed dose measuring.
3. Does the client's dose change frequently?	With *Dos-Aid* and *Inject-Aid,* dose setting can be changed easily by changing the screw setting.
4. Does the client have adequate hand dexterity to use a device?	*Dos-Aid* seems easiest for limited hand dexterity.
5. Is the client able and motivated to learn the device?	*Insulgage, Dos-Aid* and *Inject-Aid* all need a motivated and able learner.
6. Can the visually impaired diabetic reset the device for a new dosage or must a sighted person do this?	*Insulgage* is the only device with which the client can be truly independent (it comes in raised numbers and braille numbers). New dose setting for

*(Used with permission of the Visiting Nurse Association of Allegheny County (PA), 1985)

Questions to Ask	Suggestions
	Inject-Aid and *Dos-Aid* must be made by a sighted person.
7. Is cost a factor?	*Inject-Aid* is the cheapest ($4.95). Some insurances will reimburse cost with a physician's prescription.

NOTE: Even though there are some very reliable and accurate devices using glass syringes, it has been found repeatedly that sterilizing and reassembling the glass syringe is frustrating and difficult for the older client and almost impossible for the blind person.

INDEX

Page numbers in *italics* indicate figures; those followed by *t* indicate tables.

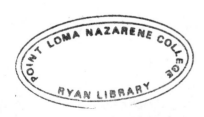